AF412791

EVALUATION AND TREATMENT OF MYOPATHIES

CONTEMPORARY NEUROLOGY SERIES AVAILABLE:

EVALUATION AND TREATMENT OF MYOPATHIES

Robert C. Griggs, M.D.
Professor and Chairman of Neurology
Professor of Medicine, Pathology, and Pediatrics
University of Rochester School of Medicine and Dentistry
Rochester, New York

Jerry R. Mendell, M.D.
Professor and Chairman of Neurology
Professor of Pathology
Director of The Neuromuscular Disease Center
The Ohio State University College of Medicine
Columbus, Ohio

Robert G. Miller, M.D.
Clinical Professor of Neurology
University of California, San Francisco
Chairman of Neurology
Director of Neuromuscular Research
California Pacific Medical Center
San Francisco, California

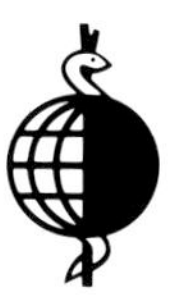 F. A. DAVIS COMPANY • Philadelphia

F. A. Davis Company
1915 Arch Street
Philadelphia, PA 19103

Printed in the United States of America

Last digit indicates print number: 10 9 8 7 6 5 4 3 2 1

Medical Editor: Robert W. Reinhardt
Medical Developmental Editor: Bernice M. Wissler
Production Editor: Crystal S. McNichol

As new scientific information becomes available through basic and clinical research, recommended treatments and drug therapies undergo changes. The authors and publisher have done everything possible to make this book accurate, up to date, and in accord with accepted standards at the time of publication. The authors, editors, and publisher are not responsible for errors or omissions or for consequences from application of the book, and make no warranty, expressed or implied, in regard to the contents of the book. Any practice described in this book should be applied by the reader in accordance with professional standards of care used in regard to the unique circumstances that may apply in each situation. The reader is advised always to check product information (package inserts) for changes and new information regarding dose and contraindications before administering any drug. Caution is especially urged when using new or infrequently ordered drugs.

Library of Congress Cataloging-in-Publication Data

Griggs, Robert C., 1939–
    Evaluation and treatment of myopathies / Robert C. Griggs, Jerry
R. Mendell, Robert G. Miller.
        p.   cm. — (Contemporary neurology series ; 44)
    Includes bibliographical references and index.
    ISBN 0-8036-4410-8 (hardback : alk. paper)
    1. Neuromuscular diseases.   2. Muscles—Diseases.
3. Neuromuscular manifestations of general diseases.   I. Mendell,
Jerry R. (Jerry Roy), 1942–   . II. Miller, Robert G. (Robert
Gordon), 1942–   . III. Title. IV. Series.
    [DNLM: 1. Neuromuscular Diseases—diagnosis.   2. Neuromuscular
Diseases—therapy.   W1 C0769N v. 43 1995 / WE 550 G857e 1995]
    RC925.G75   1995
    616.7′44—dc20
    DNLM/DLC
    for Library of Congress   94-10338
                                                                            CIP

We dedicate this book to our wives, Rosalyne, Joyce, and Chris, whose support and encouragement made possible this book and the careers that led up to it.

FOREWORD

Why does any book need a foreword? And why am I the one to write this one? The two answers converge. I have been working in the field of neuromuscular disease for 45 years, which gives me a perspective that is not available to the authors themselves. More important, perhaps, are the constraints of modesty. I can make statements about the book (and the authors, too) that might be unseemly if they came from the authors. In doing so, I hope I can generate enthusiasm about the book for readers from all the numerous fields involved in the care of patients with neuromuscular diseases that are often difficult or impossible to reverse. The authors themselves are the ones who have really made the text interesting, comprehensive, and accessible.

But that leads to another question: There is already a plethora of books on neuromuscular diseases. Why yet one more?

There is a ready answer for that one, too. And it has to do with the authors. Robert C. Griggs, Jerry R. Mendell, and Robert G. Miller are such an unusual combination of neurologists that they can provide a unique volume, one that differs from all others in several important ways.

First, each of the authors is an experienced clinician as well as an experienced and productive clinical investigator. This combination gives all of them, individually and together, an extraordinary point of view.

Second, their individual research perspectives are sufficiently different to be complementary. Miller is the clinical physiologist, a leader in electromyography and nerve conduction studies. Mendell started as a muscle morphologist; his work has incorporated immunologic and genetic approaches. Griggs worked first in metabolic studies and, in the last 3 years, he was among the investigators who mapped the genes for disease of sodium channels. All three authors have been leaders in developing double-blind controlled therapeutic trials, an achievement that was too long delayed in neuromuscular disease—and a contribution that has not been sufficiently recognized. There is now no going back; trials can only improve in the future. In carrying out those trials, each author gained intimate knowledge about the practical needs of patients and their caregivers.

Third, these three are not merely the editors of this book; they have actually written it. Their personal attention to the writing provides a coherence that often seems to be missing in the multiauthored and edited volumes that now seem mandatory as knowledge has proliferated. This book thereby differs from other major publications of the 1990s: the *Handbook of Clinical Neurology* volumes on myopathies and motor system diseases; the sixth edition of Walton's perennial favorite, *Diseases of Voluntary Muscle*; and the second edition of the monumental two-volume *Myology*, edited by Andrew Engel and Clara Franzini-Armstrong. Each of these has earned a special niche. Each provides not only examples of the value of gathering the expertise of multiple authors but also the inconsistencies of chapters written by multiple authors. In this book, all three authors have participated in the writing of each chapter, providing seamless and clear descriptions throughout.

Fourth, the amazing research advances of the past decade are described in ample detail. The excitement of molecular genetics is described in chapters on Duchenne and Becker muscular dystrophies, the gene amplification disease (myotonic dystrophy), facioscapulohumeral muscular dystrophy, mitochondrial diseases, hyperkalemic periodic paralysis and the myotonias, and metabolic myopathies. The immunocytochemical advances that have led to the better understanding of dermatomyositis and polymyositis and increasing diagnostic importance of inclusion-body disease are described. Immunology has also gone molecular, and there may yet be specific immunotherapy for these inflammatory myopathies.

Fifth, each of the trio is an outstanding teacher. That comes through in the selection of illustrations and tables as well as in the organization and presentation of the text.

Finally, the book is intensely practical in orientation. Although the latest research advances have been described clearly and thoroughly, it has been done with a clinical emphasis. The authors tell the reader how to take a history, how to examine the patient, how to evaluate the family background, how to decide which diagnostic tests should be done for which patients, and how to think about the limitations of each diagnostic test. Therapy is considered in detail, not only drug therapy but also physical treatments and ways to enhance the quality of life for people with disabling and sometimes fatal diseases. The authors have aimed this book for the practicing physician, whether experienced or novice; the clinician, the house officer, or the medical student; and the specialist in neuromuscular disease, the general neurologist, or the pediatrician. Other health-care workers — nurses, physical therapists, and occupational therapists — can also benefit.

The advantages of this volume promise that it, too, will become a favorite.

Lewis P. Rowland, M.D.
Neurological Institute
Columbia-Presbyterian Medical Center
New York, New York

PREFACE

This book is written by clinicians for clinicians. Each of the authors is active in the management of patients with neuromuscular diseases. We also attend general neurologic and medical patients and appreciate the need to decide which patient needs extensive evaluation for neuromuscular disease and which does not. Thus we set out to write a practical book on managing muscle disease in an era of rapid change. In addition to writing about specific diseases, we have addressed common problems, such as fatigue and myalgias, and have outlined our approach to the patient. We chose to work together on this text because our backgrounds bring together the perspectives of neurology, internal medicine, physiology, pathology, molecular biology, and experimental therapeutics.

Neurology was once a specialty noted for therapeutic nihilism, and most myopathies had no treatment. Such is no longer the case. Rehabilitative and symptomatic therapy is now available for all patients with neuromuscular disease. Moreover, specific treatments that arrest or reverse the symptoms of myopathy are available for many disorders: the periodic paralyses, the myotonias, many inflammatory myopathies, selected metabolic myopathies, and most myopathies associated with systemic disease. Even the weakness of Duchenne muscular dystrophy, the most dreaded of muscle diseases, can be improved by medication. And this is just the beginning. Knowledge of the genetic defect and missing or defective gene product has already led to clinical experiments with myoblast transfer aimed at correcting the gene lesion. These developments are truly revolutionary and herald the beginning of a new era for the management of neuromuscular diseases.

In this text, we emphasize both the clinical evaluation of the patient and the practical use of important diagnostic studies. We briefly present pertinent information on normal morphology and physiology to aid in the discussion of pathogenesis. In diseases for which the cellular and molecular pathobiology have been partially explained, we indicate current thinking. Specific or supportive treatment is now available for most myopathies; the individual disease discussions present the current approach to therapy. Illustrative cases from our own experiences have been chosen to highlight the clinical features of major diseases and serve to emphasize the characteristic features — or at times the puzzling features — encountered in evaluating the patient.

In Part I of this book, Chapter 1 provides the evolving, working definition of myopathies, a concise overview of the organization of the motor unit, and sufficient information on the structure and function of muscle to define terms and concepts used throughout the volume. Chapter 2 describes and illustrates the important features of the history, the physical examination, and the diagnostic studies used in the evaluation of the patient. Chapter 3 sets forth an approach to the family history and genetic evaluation of the patient, as well as information useful for the clinician who employs molecular biologic techniques in everyday practice.

Part II (Chapters 4 through 10) examines individual diseases, describing clinical evaluation, laboratory studies, pathophysiology, genetics, and treatment of each disorder. Chapter 10 reviews the myopathies that occur as a manifestation of systemic disease.

In Part III, we consider the evaluation and management of common patient complaints of pain and fatigue, and we outline the supportive care of the patient with chronic muscle disease, as well as the management and prevention of the complications of myopathies.

In the past 25 years, our understanding of muscle disease has changed from mere clinical phenomenology to the identification of a precise biochemical or genetic defect in many patients with myopathies. The pace of change is such that still-obscure causes of disorders soon will be fathomed and elucidated.

Robert C. Griggs, M.D.
Jerry R. Mendell, M.D.
Robert G. Miller, M.D.

ACKNOWLEDGMENTS

The authors thank Ms. Lisa Oppelt for her careful and highly competent secretarial and administrative work on this book. We thank the Muscular Dystrophy Association for many years of generous support of our clinical and research programs. We also thank the nurses and other staff of the Clinical Research Centers of our institutions, who have assisted with the many studies of our patients. Finally, we thank our patients, many of whom participated in research with their major motivation being the good of others.

CONTENTS

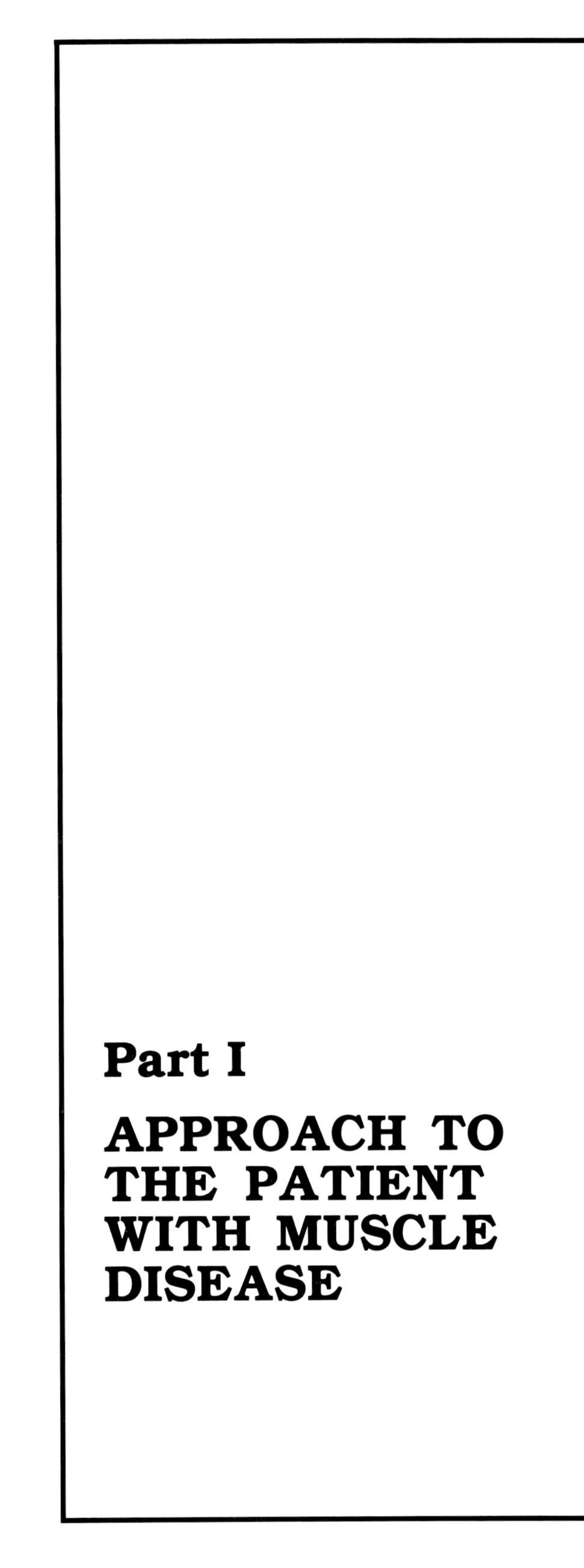

Part I

APPROACH TO
THE PATIENT
WITH MUSCLE
DISEASE

Chapter 1

STRUCTURE AND FUNCTION OF NORMAL MUSCLE

THE MOTOR UNIT

A knowledge of the normal motor unit is essential to understanding the pathophysiology of many neuromuscular diseases and interpreting muscle pathology and electromyography.

The motor unit is the final common pathway for motor activity in the nervous system, and muscle is the final effector of the motor unit. The motor unit (Fig. 1–1) is composed of the anterior horn cell, its peripheral axon, the axon's terminal branches, the associated neuromuscular junctions, and the muscle fibers they innervate. Muscle fibers from a single motor unit are spatially dispersed throughout as much as 30% of the muscle,[7] and only a few fibers innervated by the same anterior horn cell are contiguous.

The number of motor units varies greatly between muscles, from 100 in the intrinsic muscles of the hands to approximately 1000 in certain leg muscles.[4] The number of muscle fibers per motor unit varies from as few as 10 in the extraocular muscles, to nearly 2000 in leg muscles such as the gastrocnemius[14]; the total number of muscle fibers per muscle varies more than 1000-fold, from 1000 fibers in the extraocular muscles, to more than 1 million in large thigh muscles.

MUSCLE FIBER TYPES

Motor units differ not only in size but also in the biochemical and physiologic properties of their muscle fibers. A number of biochemical, histochemical, and physiologic classifications have been proposed.[3,4,8,32] Figure 1–2 gives a classification useful in the interpretation of muscle pathology. On the basis of histochemistry, muscle fibers can be divided into three major types, which correlate with physiologic properties: type 1 fibers (slow-twitch oxidative), type 2A (fast-twitch oxidative glycolytic), and type 2B (fast-twitch glycolytic). A motor unit is composed of a uniform muscle fiber type, corresponding to type 1, 2A, or 2B motor units. The histochemical profile of normal human muscle is illustrated in Figures 1–2 and 1–3. The adenosine triphosphatase (ATPase) stain is most reliable in differentiating fiber types, and the three fiber types can be best demonstrated with preincubation at pH 4.6. Under these conditions type 1 fibers appear dark, type 2A are light, and type 2B are intermediate. With preincubation at pH 4.3, another fiber type appears, the 2C fibers, which are thought to be undifferentiated. In development they precede the appearance of types 2A and 2B and are believed

3

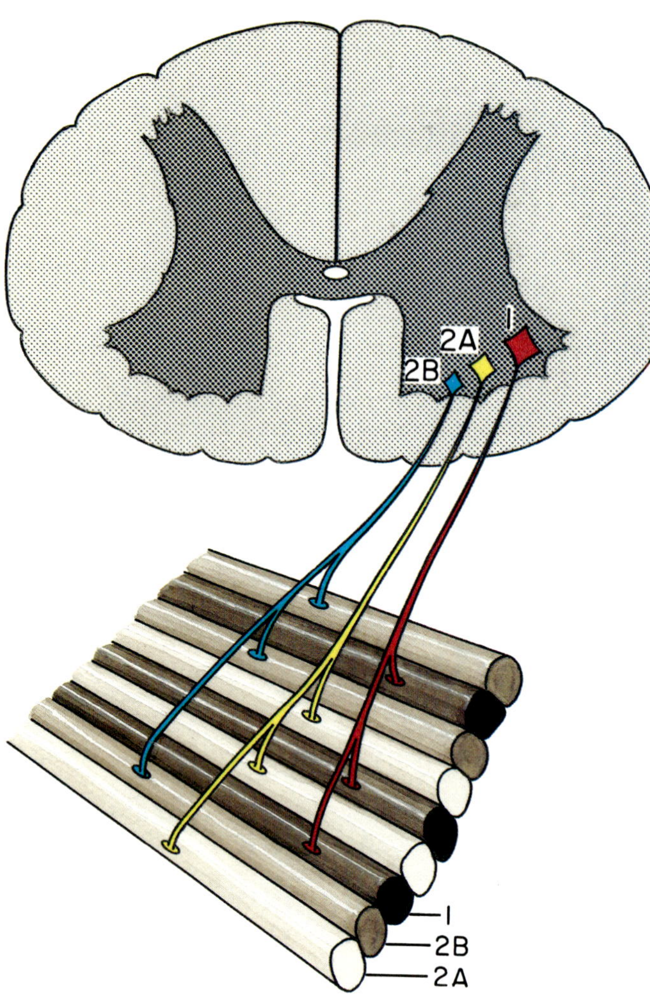

Figure 1–1. Diagram of a cross-section of the spinal cord showing three motor neurons and their motor units. Type 1 motor units are slow-twitch oxidative and are innervated by the largest motor neurons; type 2A motor units are fast-twitch oxidative glycolytic and have intermediate size motor neurons; type 2B motor units are fast-twitch glycolytic and have the smallest motor neurons. Each motor unit is composed of the same muscle fiber types (1, 2A, 2B). The muscle fibers appear as they would in ATPase stain pH 4.6.

to differentiate into one of these types. Motor units are never composed of only type 2C fibers.

Oxidative enzymes and lipid content correspond to the physiologic properties. Type 1 fibers are richest in lipid and oxidative enzymes, type 2A are intermediate, and type 2B have the least (see Fig. 1–2).

Analysis of histochemical fiber type is useful in the interpretation of muscle pathology. Preferential abnormalities of a single fiber type occur in certain muscle disorders: for example, type 2B fibers atrophy in cachexia and disuse atrophy. In myotonia congenita, type 2B fibers may be absent,[9] and in myotonic dystrophy, type 1 fibers may be preferentially atrophied.[12]

Neural Control of Muscle Fiber Type

Experimental studies in animals and clinical observations in humans indicate that the anterior horn cell determines the characteristics of the muscle fibers it supplies.[35] All muscle fibers within the same motor unit are identical in histochemical and physiologic type. This determination of muscle characteristics by motor nerve can be demonstrated using cross-innervation experi-

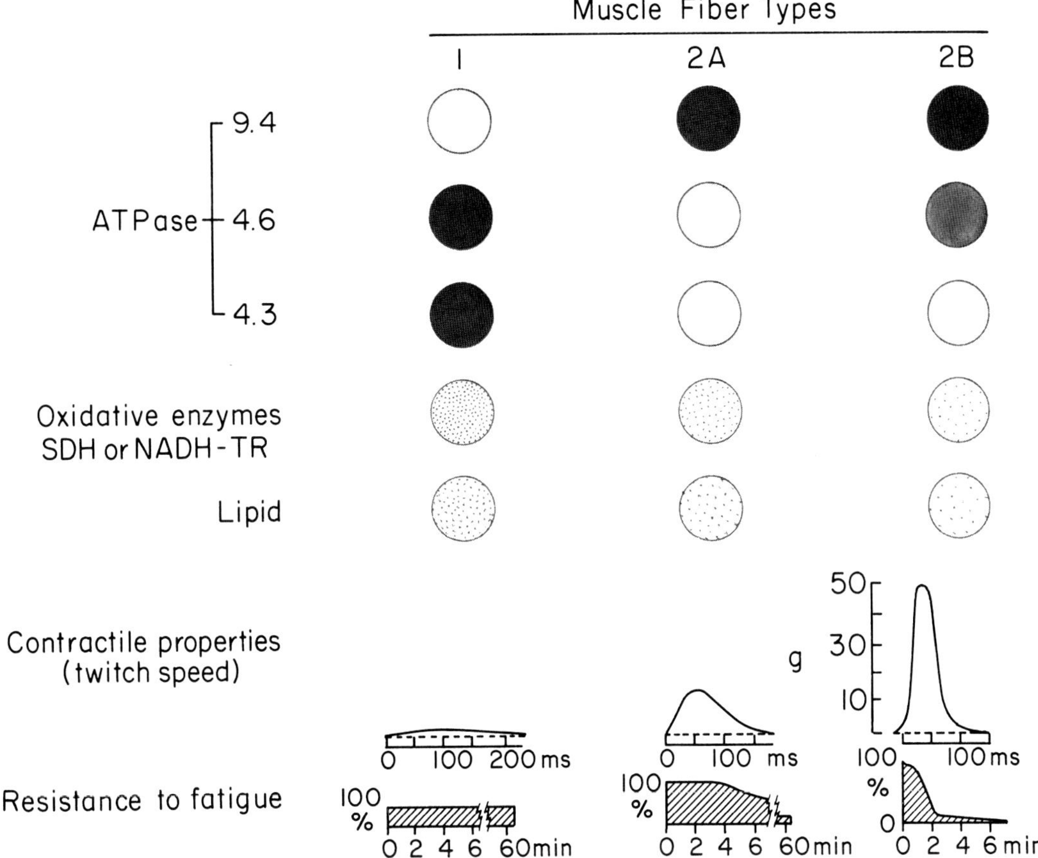

Figure 1–2. Histochemical and physiologic properties of muscle fibers: type 1 (slow-twitch oxidative); type 2A (fast-twitch oxidative glycolytic); and type 2B (fast-twitch glycolytic). The upper portion shows the staining properties in ATPase at pH 9.4, 4.6, and 4.3. Type 1 fibers show more oxidative enzymes and lipid, type 2A fibers show intermediate amounts, and type 2B fibers demonstrate the least amounts. The lower portion demonstrates greater force generation but also greater fatigability in type 2B fibers and low force but excellent fatigue resistance in type 1 fibers. Type 2A fibers are intermediate in these properties.

ments in animals. For example, if the nerve to the pure type 1 soleus muscle of a guinea pig is exchanged with a nerve innervating a muscle of mixed fiber type (cross-innervation), subsequent examination of the soleus muscle demonstrates a mixture of muscle fiber types.[35] Although no human muscles are composed of only one fiber type, these experiments are relevant to the interpretation of human muscle biopsies, because reinnervation of muscle often follows denervation, leading to *type grouping* (large areas of muscle composed of fibers of the same type).

The exact means by which individual nerve fibers determine muscle fiber type is not clear, but the pattern of firing of the neuron is probably a major factor. Experiments in animals have demonstrated that different patterns of electrical stimulation can change the biochemical and physiologic properties of muscle fibers.[5,33]

Activation of Motor Units According to Muscle Fiber Type

With each body movement, the central nervous system selectively activates motor units having muscle fiber characteristics best suited to perform

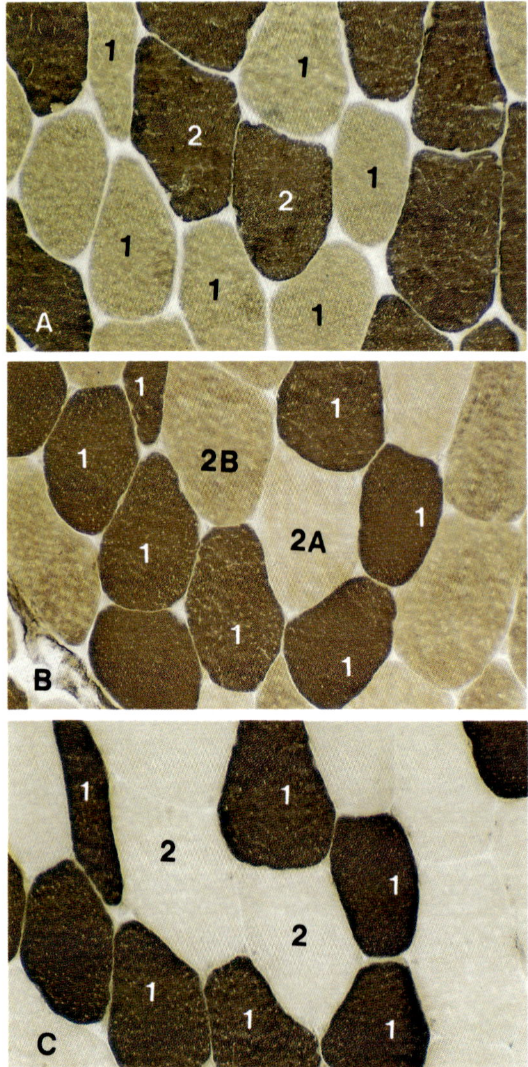

Figure 1–3. Serial sections of normal skeletal muscle showing the same muscle fibers in ATPase stains at different pH. (*A*) At pH 9.4, two fiber types are seen: type 1 (light) and type 2 (dark). (*B*) At pH 4.6, three fiber types are seen: type 1 (dark); type 2A (light); and type 2B (intermediate). (*C*) At pH 4.3, the reversal of fiber types is complete, demonstrating only two types: type 1 (dark) and type 2 (light).

the required task. Motor units with type 1, slow-twitch, slowly fatiguing muscle fibers are designed for continuous and prolonged activity. Their energy supply for ATP generation is derived from substrate metabolism through the oxidative pathways of mitochondria.[40] Motor neurons innervating type 1 muscle fibers are small in diameter; recruitment occurs with low-intensity exertion or contraction (Fig. 1–4).[19] To perform higher-intensity effort, such as lifting a heavy weight, larger, higher-threshold, more rapidly conducting motor neurons are recruited. These large neurons innervate type 2A fast-twitch, oxidative-glycolytic muscle fibers.[19] With very high intensity exercise or maximal exertion of the muscle, the neurons innervating the type 2B, fast-twitch, rapidly fatiguing, glycolytic fibers are recruited.[32]

SEQUENTIAL RECRUITMENT OF MOTOR UNITS

The physiologic properties of motor units and their response to voluntary contraction are such that each muscle possesses a stereotyped pattern of recruiting and an orderly sequence for the activating of its motor units.[29] Low-intensity or endurance activity depends primarily on type 1 fibers. Type 2 motor units are activated only with rapid or forceful contraction.[19] This fact underlies, in part, the ability of muscles to gain size and strength with repeated heavy exertion. An increase in the myofibril content of muscle fibers, and possibly a small increase in the number of muscle fibers, occur with repeated heavy exertion.[10,18] By contrast, endurance training increases capillary density and the size and numbers of mitochondria.[23]

EFFECT OF TRAINING ON HUMAN MOTOR UNITS

Several attempts have been made to change contractile properties of motor units in humans, but most studies have not demonstrated significant conversion of fiber type.[11] On the other hand, a comparison of sedentary individuals

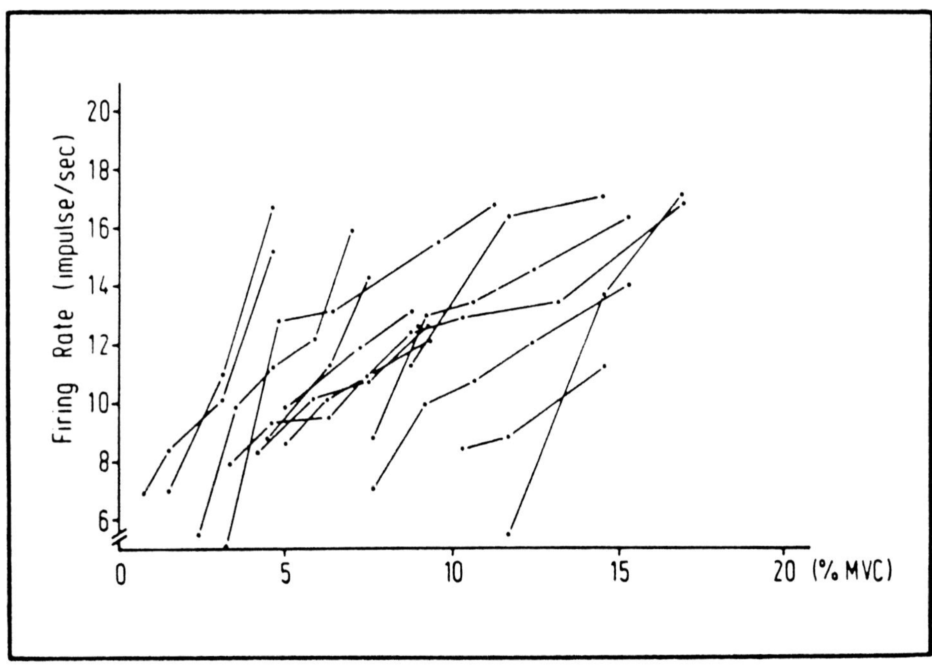

Figure 1–4. Representative curves from normal first dorsal interosseous muscle of single motor unit firing rates at different levels of voluntary contraction. MVC = maximum voluntary contraction strength.

with athletes of various types has yielded differences in motor unit pools.[34] A predominance of slow-twitch fibers is found in athletes trained for endurance events, and the number of fast-twitch fibers is greater in weight lifters than in untrained people.[34] The distribution of fiber type in sedentary individuals did not change after a period of exercise training, however.[34] It appears that the motor unit pool may vary considerably from individual to individual but that this variation is largely determined by genetic differences. It remains possible that exercise training during growth and development may significantly influence the motor unit pool of an adult. A lack of activation of some motor units may underlie the weakness common in many sedentary persons and in disabled or hospitalized patients.[17]

VOLUNTARY CONTROL OF MOTOR UNIT ACTIVITY

Relationship of Size to the Recruitment of Single Motor Units

According to the so-called size principle, the larger the cell body of the motor neuron, the higher the conduction velocity of its axon and the stronger the muscular contraction produced when it is stimulated.[38] Larger motor neurons are also *recruited* into activity at higher thresholds during reflex action, and with intracellular, electrical stimulation.[6] Both indirect and direct evidence demonstrates that small (type 1) motor units are recruited before larger (type 2) units and that the sequence of motor unit recruitment is the same with each voluntary contraction.[28]

Firing Rates of Single Motor Units

Two mechanisms increase the force of voluntary contractions in human muscle: either inactive motor units may

be recruited, or the firing rate of already active units may be increased[27] (see Fig. 1–4). The electrical behavior of single muscle fibers during moderate contraction of human muscles is the same as that of the corresponding nerve fiber, and the gradual increase in the strength of contraction is associated with an increase in firing frequency of the active motor units.[6] Frequency modulation, an increase or decrease in motor unit firing, has been suggested as the most important factor in fine control of muscle contraction.[28] The order of recruitment and relative roles of the two types of motor units are adapted both to the speed and to the strength of contraction.[1]

Impaired Voluntary Control of Motor Units

A patient who is malingering or cannot exert full effort because of pain will have a ratchetlike and "give way" quality on muscle testing. This "give way" weakness results from the normal, rapid derecruitment of motor units that occurs with sudden relaxation; the patient then reinitiates voluntary effort, giving a ratchetlike quality to the contraction as the examiner tests strength.

Patients with central nervous system disorders are often weak and characteristically fatigue easily. Such patients may demonstrate marked slowing of rapid movements, as well as spasticity and hyperreflexia. Patients with upper motor neuron disease have great difficulty in both initiating and maintaining motor unit recruitment, so that they exhibit symptoms that result from disordered motor control and impairment of fine movements.[36] Muscle power often increases with encouragement during examination, as the patient slowly recruits additional motor units.

MECHANISMS OF MUSCULAR CONTRACTION

Striated muscle is made up of myofilaments arranged in an interdigitating

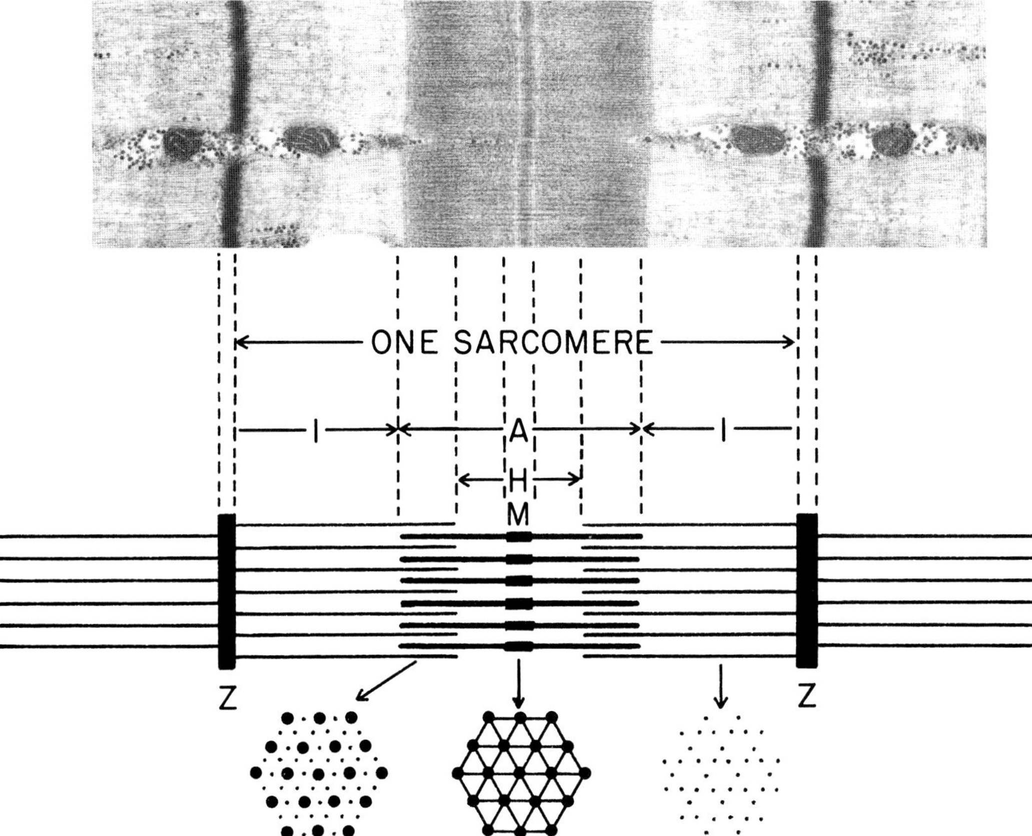

Figure 1–5. Electron micrograph of a sarcomere of skeletal muscle with each band labeled. Transverse sections through the sarcomere at various levels demonstrate different arrays of filaments, as illustrated at the bottom.

array of thick and thin filaments. These filaments form a repeating pattern of cross striation along the entire length of the muscle fiber. A single unit of the pattern is called a sarcomere. Figure 1–5 shows the characteristic division of the sarcomere into A and I bands, the H zone, and the Z line. Thick filaments, confined to the A band, are composed of the protein, myosin. The thin filaments extend from each side of the Z line through the I band and penetrate into the thick filaments in the A band. These filaments are composed of another protein, actin. The absence of thin filaments in the center of the A band gives rise to the H zone in the sarcomere. The M line is a thickening in the center of the myosin, or thick, filaments.

Transverse sections through the sarcomere at various levels demonstrate different arrays of filaments. Each thick filament is surrounded by six thin filaments, and each thin filament is surrounded by only three thick filaments (see Fig. 1–5). Thus, there are twice as many actin as myosin filaments. Cross sections through the H zone show only myosin, and cross sections through the I band show only actin. The myofibrils of the muscle fiber are surrounded by an intracellular matrix, the sarcoplasm.

Biochemistry of Contraction

Myosin (the thick filament) is a complex protein with a molecular weight of approximately 500,000 daltons. It is an ATPase: that is, it hydrolyzes ATP to form ADP and inorganic phosphate. This reaction is activated by calcium ions and inhibited by magnesium ions. The proteolytic enzyme trypsin splits the myosin into two fragments, light meromyosin and heavy meromyosin. Only heavy meromyosin acts as an ATPase.

Isolated actin (the thin filaments) exists in two forms: G-actin (globlular actin), with a molecular weight of 60,000 daltons, and F-actin (fibrous actin), which is a polymer of G-actin. Neither form of actin has ATPase activity. Actin filaments have three different components: actins, troponins, and tropomyosin. The bases of the actin filaments insert into the Z discs. The Z disc is composed of filamentous proteins that run across both the actin and myosin myofibrils, attaching them to each other. The portion of the myofibril between successive Z discs is the sarcomere (see Fig. 1–5).

The initiation of contraction depends on the two proteins troponin and tropomyosin. Troponin is a globular protein (molecular weight 50,000 daltons), which can reversibly combine with calcium ions. Tropomyosin is a fibrous protein (molecular weight 70,000 daltons). Troponin and tropomyosin sensitize the actomyosin ATPase to the presence of calcium ions. Calcium ions combine with troponin to prevent the inhibition of the actomyosin ATPase by the troponin-tropomyosin system. Thus, the combination of calcium ions with troponin allows contraction to proceed.

The Sliding Filament Theory

Before 1954, most theories concerning the mechanism of muscular contraction involved the coiling of long protein molecules, like the shortening of a helical spring. In that year two groups independently formulated the sliding filament theory, according to which the A band does not change length when the muscle is stretched or shortened.[20-22] In this view, contraction is brought about by movement of the thin (actin) filaments between the thick (myosin) filaments. The sliding is thought to be caused by a series of cyclic reactions between the projections (cross bridges) on the myosin filaments and active sites on the actin filaments.

According to the sliding filament theory, the isometric tension is directly proportional to the number of cross bridges that can be formed between the thick and thin filaments.[16] Thus, at long lengths, the tension is proportional to the degree of overlap of the filaments. Tension develops as qualitative changes occur in the relations between elements of the sarcomere (Fig. 1–6). Above 3.65 μm (fully stretched muscle) there is no cross-bridge interaction, and therefore no tension development. Between 3.65 and 2.25 μm, the number of cross bridges increases linearly with the decrease in length, and the increase in isometric tension is also linear. From 2.25 to 1.95 μm, the number of cross bridges remains constant and, therefore, tension is constant.[16] Below 1.95 μm, the thin filaments overlap, and tension is reduced. At 1.65 μM, the A filaments abut the Z lines and tension falls off sharply. Thus the force generated by a muscle is critically dependent on its length.

Excitation-Contraction Coupling

The stimulus for contraction of a muscle fiber is initiated by an impulse from its motor nerve, setting off a sequence of events:
1. The nerve impulse
2. Transmitter release
3. The end plate potential
4. The action potential
5. Calcium release
6. Contraction

The details of contraction have been reviewed earlier. A description of the excitation-contraction coupling process (steps 4 and 5) follows.[15]

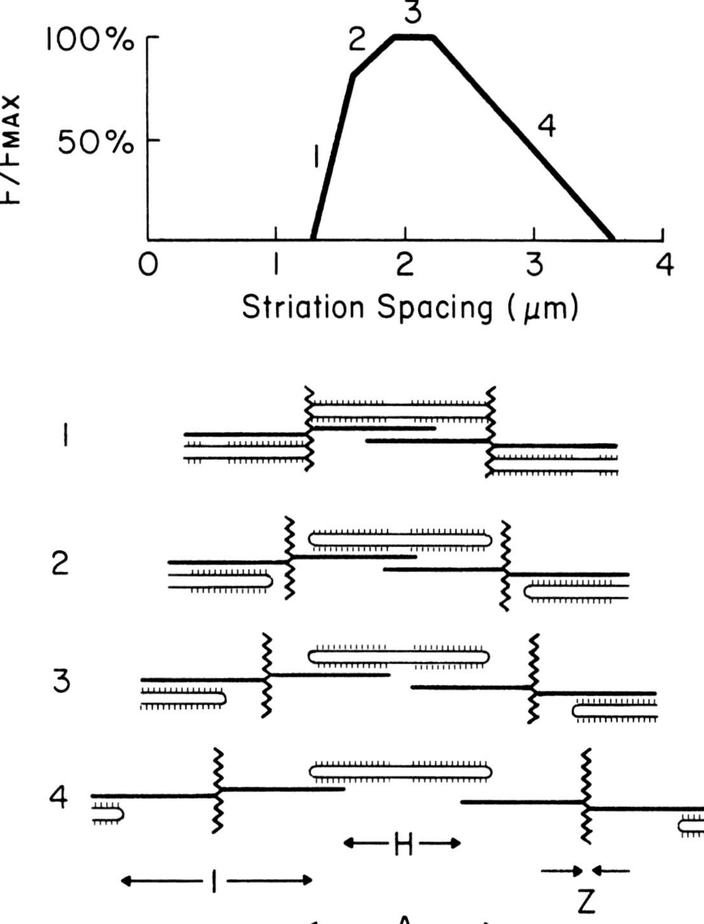

Figure 1-6. The length-tension diagram shown here for a single sarcomere illustrates the important clinical point that muscular force generation is reduced in muscles at very short length (because of compression of thick filaments) and also when stretched to long length (because some cross bridges cannot engage the thin filaments).

THE IMPORTANCE OF CALCIUM IONS

Depolarization of the membrane cannot itself be the ultimate trigger for the contraction process, because glycerinated fibers have no physiologically active membrane and yet are still able to contract and relax.

A rise in calcium ion concentration in the sarcoplasm immediately after stimulation was first demonstrated by injecting the protein aequorin (which comes from jellyfish and emits light in the presence of calcium ions) into a muscle with very large individual muscle fibers.[37] When the muscle fiber was stimulated, the aequorin produced a faint glow of light, indicating the presence of calcium ions inside. Increased stimulus strength, accompanied by depolarization, caused greater light intensity, reflecting increased release of calcium ions and increased muscle tension.

INTERNAL MEMBRANE SYSTEMS

How does excitation at the cell surface cause release of calcium ions inside the fiber? A specific inward-conducting tubule called the transverse (T) tubule is continuous with the sarcolemma and extends into the muscle in close proximity to the sarcoplasmic reticulum (Figs. 1-7 and 1-8). Action potentials spread

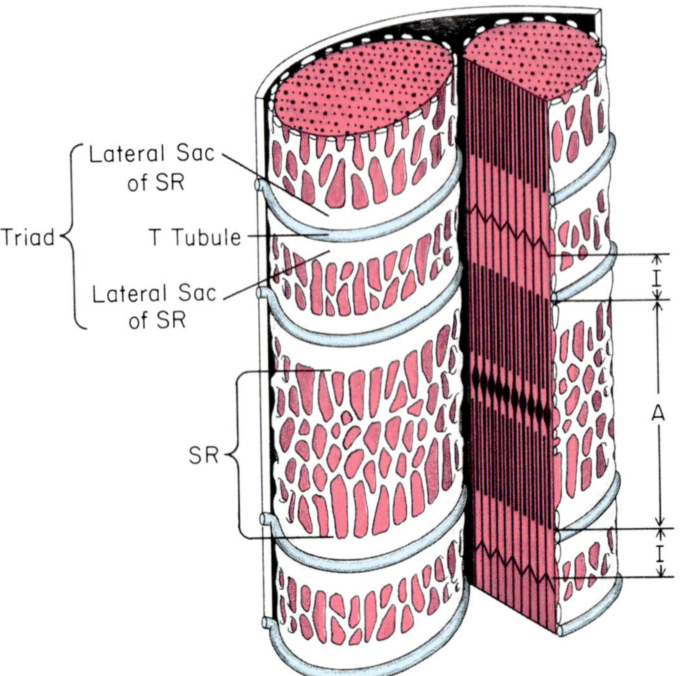

Figure 1–7. Sarcoplasmic reticulum (SR) and transverse tubules (T tubules) of skeletal muscle. The T tubules represent invagination of the sarcolemma that communicate with the extracellular space. The SR is an intracellular membranous system. Lateral sacs represent expansions of the SR. The lateral sacs and T tubule form the triad, which can be found at the A band-I band junction in mammalian skeletal muscle. A sarcomere is labeled showing A and I bands.

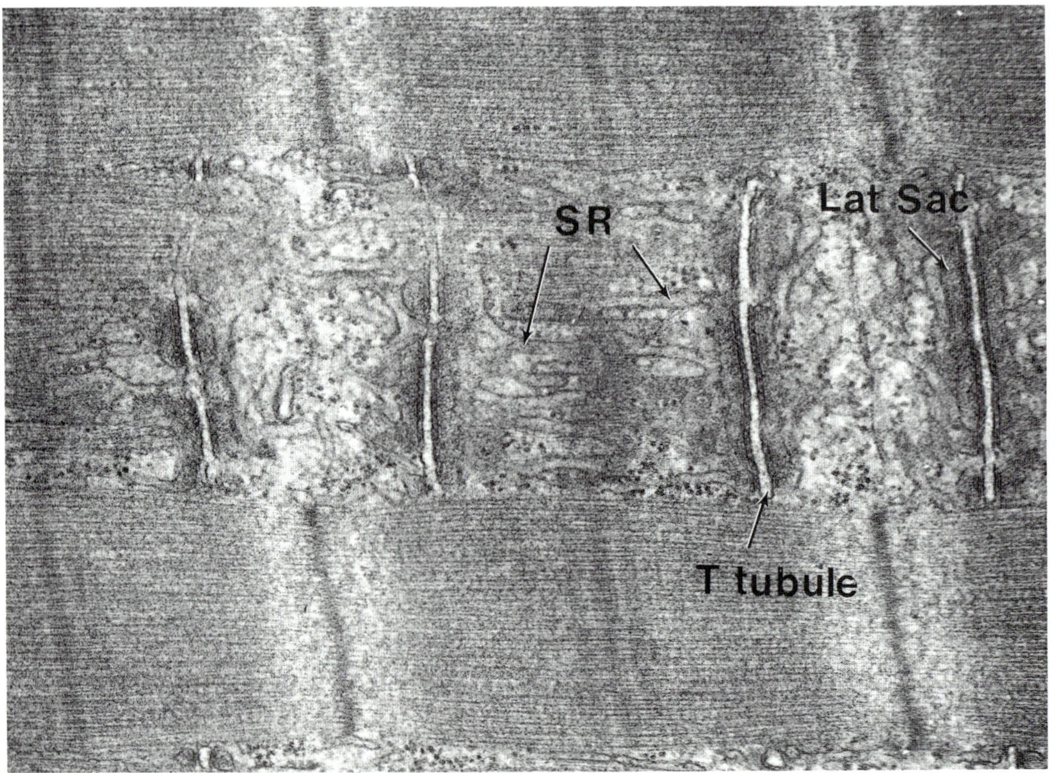

Figure 1–8. Electron micrograph of normal human muscle showing transverse tubule (T tubule), sarcoplasmic reticulum (SR), and lateral sac of SR.

from the surface membrane via transmission along T tubules that penetrate the muscle fiber. The action potentials of the T tubules cause release of calcium from the sarcoplasmic reticulum. The T tubules of mammalian muscle are paired networks located at the junction of the A band and I band.[31] The chemical messenger, inositol triphosphate, has been proposed as a mediator of intracellular signal transduction between depolarization of the T tubule and release of calcium from the sarcoplasmic reticulum.[37]

THE COUPLING PROCESS

The interaction between the actin and myosin filaments, which constitutes contraction, depends on the presence of ATP, magnesium ions, and calcium ions. In resting muscle, ATP and magnesium ions are present in concentrations required for contraction (3 and 10 mM, respectively), but calcium concentration is held at a low value (10^{-7} to 10^{-8} M) by the calcium pump in the sarcoplasmic reticulum.[15] When the calcium concentration in the region of the myofilaments rises above 10^{-7} to 10^{-6} M, the action of the troponin-tropomyosin system on the actomyosin ATPase system is inhibited, and contraction occurs. Maximum contractile activity occurs when calcium concentrations are in the region of 10^{-5} to 10^{-4} M. At the end of the excitation period, the T tubules are no longer depolarized.

Calcium ions are removed from the sarcoplasmic fluid by a calcium pump and stored in the sarcoplasmic reticulum. The protein calsequestrin binds calcium effectively and facilitates its storage. Relaxation of contraction occurs when calcium concentration falls to 10^{-7} to 10^{-8} M.

CYTOSKELETON

Muscle cells, like all eukaryotic cells, have a cytoskeleton that consists of fibrillar structures composed principally of proteins.[24] These cytoskeletal pro-

Table 1 – 1 CYTOSKELETAL ELEMENTS AND PROTEINS

MICROFILAMENTS
  Profilin
  Alpha-actinin
  Gelsolin
  Fragmin
  Severin
INTERMEDIATE FILAMENTS
  Desmin (skeletin)
  Vimentin
  Filamin
MICROTUBULES
  Tubulin
ELASTIC FILAMENTS
  Nebulin
  Titin (connectin)
MICROTRABECULAE (GROUND SUBSTANCE OR LATTICE)
ANCHORING OR ATTACHMENT SITES (COSTAMERES)
  Vinculin
  Spectrin
  Ankyrin
  Dystrophin

teins are important for cellular shape and cell movement, for maintaining the position of elements within the cell, and for cell division. The fibrillar structures of the cytoskeleton include microfilaments, intermediate filaments, and microtubules, as well as elastic filaments and microtrabeculae[39] (Table 1 – 1). In muscle cells, the cytoskeleton includes additional proteins that anchor fibrillar structures to the sarcolemma (at so-called costameres) and to contractile proteins. Skeletal muscle function demands that the muscle cell have elastic properties so that the cell can adapt to the deformation produced by muscle contraction.

Characterization of the function of proteins in the cytoskeleton remains incomplete,[25] but roles of several proteins have been determined. Titin (also called connectin) is a long, flexible, filamentous protein that links Z discs to thick myosin filaments in the sarcomere; it constitutes nearly 10% of myofibrillar protein. The high molecular weight of titin (approximately 1 million daltons) has made it difficult to isolate and study. Titin probably represents a major elastic component of muscle. Along with another large protein called nebulin (molecular weight approximately 500,000 daltons), titin runs in longitudinal filaments that give muscle cells their resting tension.[25,39] Alpha-actinin is an actin-binding protein found in both muscle and nonmuscle cells. Alpha-actinin plays an important role in anchoring actin to intracellular structures.[2] Other cytoskeletal proteins whose distribution and function have been partially characterized include desmin, which is found in intermediate filaments localized to the neuromuscular junction; vinculin, which binds actin myofilaments and may attach actin to the sarcolemma in the Z-disc region; and ankyrin, which, along with vinculin, spectrin, and dystrophin, is localized to the plasma membrane at sites of Z-disc attachment.

The genetic control of the proteins of the cytoskeleton and the function of each protein have assumed major clinical importance with the discovery that two allelic forms of muscular dystrophy (Duchenne dystrophy and Becker dystrophy) are caused by a genetic defect in a single cytoskeletal protein, dystrophin.[30] Dystrophin's function appears to be to link the actin cytoskeleton of muscle to the extracellular matrix of muscle via a glycoprotein complex that spans the sarcolemma.[13]

SUMMARY OF MUSCLE FUNCTION: RELATIONSHIP TO MYOPATHIES

Coordinated firing of the motor neuron produces depolarization of all muscle fibers within a motor unit. This depolarization spreads throughout the entire muscle fiber, results in calcium release, and culminates in contraction of the myofibrils. Myofibrils are composed of actin and myosin myofilaments that are attached to the muscle cell membrane (sarcolemma) by cytoskeletal proteins. The cytoskeletal proteins give muscle fibers their shape and their resting tone and transmit the force of muscle contraction to the sarcolemma, to produce overall shortening of the muscle fibers. Relaxation of the muscle fiber occurs when calcium is taken up by the sarcoplasmic reticulum.

The force of muscular contraction is increased through only two mechanisms: (1) recruitment of additional individual motor units or (2) increasing firing rates in already active motor units — or through a combination of these two. The discharge of each motor neuron produces depolarization of all muscle fibers within that motor unit. Depolarization spreads through the entire muscle fiber, producing calcium release and contraction of the myofibrils. The actin and myosin myofilaments within each myofibril are anchored to the cytoskeleton and to the muscle cell membrane by a variety of proteins including alpha-actinin, vinculin, and dystrophin. These cytoskeletal proteins give muscle fibers their structural integrity and transmit the force of muscle contraction to the muscle membrane, producing muscle fiber shortening. Muscle fiber relaxation occurs when calcium is taken up by the sarcoplasmic reticulum.

Certain myopathies result from specific gene defects that produce discrete abnormalities in one of the processes of muscle contraction and relaxation. For example, myotonic disorders and periodic paralysis are the result of abnormalities within the muscle cell membrane. On the other hand, structural defects in Duchenne and Becker muscular dystrophies are produced by abnormalities in a cytoskeletal protein. Finally, a genetic error in metabolism usually produces dynamic symptoms (e.g., McArdle's disease, mitochondrial myopathy, or carnitine palmitoyltransferase deficiency). In some metabolic defects, however, such as carnitine deficiency or acid maltase deficiency, progressive degeneration of individual muscle cells may occur and produce progressive proximal weakness.

A good understanding of the normal mechanisms of muscle contraction, muscle structure, and muscle energetics will provide a firm basis for understanding individual myopathies.

REFERENCES

1. Belanger AY and McComas AJ: Extent of motor unit activation during effort. J Appl Physiol 51:1131, 1981.
2. Blanchard A, Ohanian V, and Critchley D: The structure and function of α-actinin. J Muscle Res Cell Motil 10:280, 1989.
3. Brooke MH and Engel WK: The histographic analysis of human muscle biopsies with regard to fiber types, I. Adult male and female. Neurology 19:221, 1969.
4. Brooke MH and Kaiser KK: Muscle fiber types: how many and what kind? Arch Neurol 23:369, 1970.
5. Buller AJ, Eccles JC, and Eccles RM: Interactions between motoneurones and muscles in respect of the characteristic speeds of their responses. J Physiol (Lond) 150:417, 1960.
6. Burke RE: Motor units in mammalian muscle. In Sumner AJ (ed): The Physiology of Peripheral Nerve Disease. WB Saunders, Philadelphia, 1980, p 133.
7. Burke RE, Levine DN, Tsairis P, and Zajac FE III: Physiological types and histochemical profiles in motor units of the cat gastrocnemius. J Physiol (Lond) 234:723, 1973.
8. Burke RE, Levine DN, Zajac FE III, Tsairis P, and Engel WK: Mammalian motor units: Physiological-histochemical correlation in three types in cat gastrocnemius. Science 174:709, 1971.
9. Crews J, Kaiser KK, and Brooke MH: Muscle pathology of myotonia congenita. J Neurol Sci 28:449, 1976.
10. Edström L and Ekblom B: Differences in sizes of red and white muscle fibres in vastus lateralis of musculus quadriceps femoris of normal individuals and athletes. Relation to physical performance. Scand J Clin Lab Invest 30:175, 1972.
11. Edström L and Grimby L: Effect of exercise on the motor unit. Muscle Nerve 9:104, 1986.
12. Engel WK: Selective and nonselective susceptibility of muscle fiber types. A new approach to human neuromuscular diseases. Arch Neurol 22:97, 1970.
13. Ervasti JM and Campbell KP: Membrane organization of the dystrophin-glycoprotein complex. Cell 66:1121, 1991.
14. Feinstein B, Lindegård B, Nyman E, and Wohlfart G: Morphologic studies of motor units in normal human muscles. Acta Anatomica 23:127, 1955.
15. Fleischer S and Inui M: Biochemistry and biophysics of excitation-contraction coupling. Annu Rev Biophys Biophys Chem 18:333, 1989.
16. Gordon AM, Huxley AF, and Julian FJ: The variation in isometric tension with sarcomere length in vertebrate muscle fibres. J Physiol 184:170, 1966.
17. Hainaut K and Duchateau J: Muscle fatigue, effects of training and disuse. Muscle Nerve 12:660, 1989.
18. Hall-Craggs ECB: The longitudinal division of fibres in overloaded rat skeletal muscle. J Anat 107:459, 1970.
19. Henneman E, Somjen G, and Carpenter DO: Functional significance of cell size in spinal motoneurons. J Neurophysiol 28:560, 1965.
20. Huxley AF and Niedergerke R: Structural changes in muscle during contraction. Interference microscopy of living muscle fibres. Nature 173:971, 1954.
21. Huxley H and Hanson J: Changes in the cross-striations of muscle during contraction and stretch and their structural interpretation. Nature 173:973, 1954.
22. Huxley HE: The mechanism of muscular contraction. Sci Am 213:1026, 1965.
23. Jones DA, Rutherford OM, and Parker DF: Physiological changes in skeletal muscle as a result of strength training. Quarterly Journal of Experimental Physiology 74:233, 1989.
24. Lazarides E: Intermediate filaments: A chemically heterogeneous, developmentally regulated class of proteins. Annu Rev Biochem 51:219, 1982.
25. Maruyama K: Connectin, an elastic filamentous protein of striated muscle. Int Rev Cytol 104:81, 1986.
26. McComas AJ, Fawcett PRW, Campbell MJ, and Sica REP: Electrophysiological estimation of the number of motor units within a human muscle. J Neurol Neurosurg Psychiatry 34:121, 1971.
27. Miller RG and Sherratt M: Firing rates of human motor units in partially dener-

vated muscle. Neurology 28:1241, 1978.

28. Milner-Brown HS, Stein RB, and Yemm R: Changes in firing rate of human motor units during linearly changing voluntary contractions. J Physiol (Lond) 230:371, 1973.

29. Milner-Brown HS, Stein RB, and Yemm R: The orderly recruitment of human motor units during voluntary isometric contractions. J Physiol (Lond) 230:359, 1973.

30. Monaco AP, Neve RL, Colletti-Feener C, Bertelson CJ, Kurnit DM, and Kunkel LM: Isolation of candidate cDNAs for portions of the Duchenne muscular dystrophy gene. Nature 323:646, 1986.

31. Peachey LD and Franzini-Armstrong C: Structure and function of membrane systems of skeletal muscle cells. In Peachey LD, Adrian RH, and Geiger SR (eds): Handbook of Physiology. American Physiological Society, Bethesda, MD, 1983, p 23.

32. Peter JB, Barnard RJ, Edgerton VR, Gillespie CA, and Stempel KE: Metabolic profiles of three fiber types of skeletal muscle in guinea pigs and rabbits. Biochemistry 11:2627, 1972.

33. Salmons S and Vrbová G: The influence of activity on some contractile characteristics of mammalian fast and slow muscles. J Physiol (Lond) 201:535, 1969.

34. Saltin B and Gollnick PD: Skeletal muscle adaptability: Significance for metabolism and performance. In Peachey LD, Adrian RH, and Geiger SR (eds): Handbook of Physiology. American Physiological Society, Bethesda, MD, 1983, p 555.

35. Samaha FJ, Guth L, and Albers RW: The neural regulation of gene expression in the muscle cell. Exp Neurol 27:276, 1970.

36. Shahani BT (ed): Electromyography in CNS Disorders: Central EMG. Butterworth, Boston, 1984.

37. Somlyo AP, Walker JW, Goldman YE, Trentham DR, Kobayashi S, Kitazawa T, and Somlyo AV: Inositol trisphosphate, calcium and muscle contraction. Philos Trans R Soc Lond Biol 320:399, 1988.

38. Stuart DG and Enoka RM: Motoneurons, motor units, and the size principle. In Rosenberg RN (ed): The Clinical Neurosciences, Vol 5. Churchill Livingstone, New York, 1983, p 471.

39. Wang K: Cytoskeletal matrix in striated muscle: The role of titin, nebulin and intermediate filaments. Adv Exp Med Biol 170:285, 1984.

40. Warmolts JR and Engel WK: Open-biopsy electromyography. I. Correlation of motor unit behavior with histochemical muscle fiber type in human limb muscle. Arch Neurol 27:512, 1972.

Chapter 2

EVALUATION OF THE PATIENT WITH MYOPATHY

DEFINITION OF MYOPATHY
CLINICAL EVALUATION
DIFFERENTIAL DIAGNOSIS
LABORATORY EVALUATION
ELECTRODIAGNOSIS
MUSCLE BIOPSY
NERVE BIOPSY

The majority of patients with muscle symptoms do not have a definable disease of muscle. Paradoxically, patients who complain of weakness and tiredness usually have normal strength. On the other hand, many patients with objective weakness, particularly when it develops slowly, do not report weakness as a symptom. Patients who have symptoms but no known disease are hard to discuss. Chapter 11 reviews the current state of knowledge about normal fatigue and muscle pain and suggests diagnostic and management strategies useful for these patients.

Although breakthroughs in molecular genetics have defined the genetic lesion in many myopathies, for most muscle diseases we still do not know the reason for many symptoms and signs. In two or three decades, today's understanding of a disease such as Duchenne dystrophy will appear much as the work of Duchenne and Erb in the late 1800s appears to us now. When Erb first performed biopsies on muscle, clinical scientists believed that they knew the cause of progressive muscular dystrophy: replacement of muscle by connective tissue and fat. What more could be learned? We now know that a protein (dystrophin) is missing in all muscles of patients with Duchenne dystrophy. However, many muscles are normal early in life and some (such as extraocular muscles) never become weak. Why? What is the function of dystrophin? Dystrophin is present in all mammalian species muscle, but in some mammals (e.g., mice) it can be genetically absent, and the animals will still have normal strength.

DEFINITION OF MYOPATHY

Because the cause of many muscle diseases is unknown, we often must use a flexible definition of *myopathy*. In the context of a neuromuscular disease, myopathy implies that the disorder to be discussed reflects, in fact, a disease of muscle, rather than of the central nervous system, anterior horn cell, peripheral nerve, or neuromuscular junction. Moreover, major questions confront students at all levels of sophistication as to the site of the primary defect in the various neuromuscular diseases.

By convention, the neuromuscular diseases are classified into four categories, subdividing the two cells of the motor unit—the neuron and the muscle cell—into disorders of (1) anterior horn cell, (2) peripheral nerve, (3) neuromuscular junction, and (4) muscle. Certain clinical and laboratory criteria have been used to defend this subdivision (Tables 2–1 and 2–2). Unfortunately, because the pathogenesis of most myopathies is unknown, disease

17

Table 2–1 DEFINITION OF MYOPATHY: CLINICAL CRITERIA

CLINICAL FEATURES SUGGESTIVE OF
  MYOPATHY
  Distribution of weakness—proximal,
    symmetric
  Muscle bulk—preserved or enlarged
  Muscle palpation (unreliable)—indurated,
    tender
  Muscle percussion—diminished muscle
    contraction
  Reflexes—parallel muscle strength
CLINICAL FEATURES CONTRAVENING
  MYOPATHY
  Distal weakness
  Fasciculations—suggest anterior horn cell
    disease
  Tremor—suggests peripheral neuropathy or
    anterior horn cell disease
  Sensory signs (or symptoms)–suggest
    peripheral neuropathy
  Pathologic fatigue—suggests neuromuscular
    junction defect
  Early absence of reflexes

currently believed to be exclusively in muscle may eventually prove to result, in part, from an abnormality of the neuron. For example, corticosteroid "myopathy" merits the name chiefly because weakness predominates in proximal muscles. Many other criteria, however, belie the term: serum levels of creatine kinase, the muscle enzyme, are usually normal, and muscle morphol-

Table 2–2 LABORATORY FINDINGS SUGGESTIVE OF MYOPATHY

Serum enzymes
  Elevations of creatine kinase (>four-fold)
Electromyography
  Potentials—brief, low-voltage, polyphasic
  Recruitment—increased
  Interference pattern—full in weak muscles
  Fasciculations—absent
Nerve conduction
  Normal; normal impulse transmission with
    repetitive nerve stimulation
Muscle biopsy
  Muscle fiber necrosis and regeneration;
    central nuclei
  Hypertrophy, abnormally round muscle fibers
  Increase in endomysial connective tissue

ogy shows only atrophy, rather than traditional indications of a myopathy, such as muscle necrosis.[84] Although electromyography (EMG) may show a myopathic pattern with small, numerous action potentials,[69] such abnormalities are not specific for myopathy and can be found in other disorders in which a primary defect in muscle is not implicated, such as neuromuscular junction diseases (for example, myasthenia gravis and the Lambert-Eaton syndrome).[92] The pathogenesis of corticosteroid-induced weakness ultimately is related to elevated steroid levels and is probably mediated by direct effects on muscle. Whether corticosteroids also alter neuronal firing pattern, the neuromuscular junction, muscle hormone receptors, or still other factors, is unclear. Thus, the term *corticosteroid myopathy* is widely accepted even though the pathophysiology of the disorder remains uncertain.

Similarly, in acid maltase deficiency, biochemical analysis can identify a specific deficiency of enzyme activity in muscle, and the morphologic and biochemical alterations can be reproduced in cultured muscle.[5] Nevertheless, co-existing disease is present in anterior horn cells and peripheral nerve, and various features of the muscle biopsy and of electromyography have led some authors to propose that denervation contributes to the clinical picture.[42] As in many disorders in which the pathogenesis of weakness is not yet known, clinical and laboratory findings in these patients do not adequately define the site of pathology; but the weight of evidence favors myopathy.

The Hereditary Myopathies

Lacking a satisfactory scientific definition of myopathy, this text includes the gamut of hereditary disorders implicating muscle dysfunction, including:

1. The muscular dystrophies, with caveats concerning their pathogenesis

2. Disorders whose biochemical abnormalities are expressed in muscle

Table 2-3 SOME INHERITED DISORDERS WITH FREQUENT SUBCLINICAL OR SLIGHT MUSCLE INVOLVEMENT

Ataxia telangiectasia (Louis-Bar syndrome)
Spinocerebellar degeneration
  Friedreich's ataxia
  Refsum's disease
Lipoprotein disorders
  An-alphalipoproteinemia (Tangier disease)
  A-betalipoproteinemia (Bassen-Kornzweig
    syndrome)
Hematologic disorders
  Hemoglobinopathies
  Acanthocytosis
  McLeod syndrome
Connective tissue disease
  Marfan's syndrome
  Ehlers-Danlos syndrome
Mucopolysaccharidoses
Sphingolipidoses
Dysmorphic syndromes
  Noonan's syndrome
  Cornelia de Lange syndrome
  Prader-Willi syndrome

3. Disorders with distinctive morphologic alterations in muscle
4. Disorders characterized by abnormalities of the muscle membrane

Gene-mapping studies have confirmed that the genetic defects of muscular dystrophy are present in somatic cells other than muscle. Many of these inherited disorders fulfill our definition of myopathy if muscle weakness is a major feature of the illness. In some disorders, however, although muscle is clearly involved, myopathy is overshadowed by more evident disease in other tissues (Table 2-3). If myopathy can dominate the picture, failing to classify the disease first and foremost as a myopathy may simply be the result of another specialty claiming it first. Thus, carnitine deficiency is usually classified with the myopathies, but it also can present as an encephalopathy[37] or as a primary cardiomyopathy.[87]

The Inflammatory Myopathies

This text includes both primary and secondary inflammatory myopathies.

The categorization of one disease as an inflammatory myopathy (such as dermatomyositis) can be arbitrary, because inflammation is often lacking, whereas inflammation can be present in a hereditary disease such as fascioscapulohumeral muscular dystrophy. Historical classifications will persist until the pathogenesis of each myopathy is understood.

Myopathies Due to Systemic Diseases

Chapter 10 summarizes these conditions. Impressive muscle pathology can occur in many disorders in which clinical evidence for muscle dysfunction is often minimal or absent. Sarcoidosis, polyarteritis, amyloidosis, parasitic infections, and neoplasms may be recognized in the muscle of patients without muscle weakness. A substantial number of metabolic defects such as the leukodystrophies, lipoprotein disorders, and hereditary ataxias (see Table 2-3) also may produce muscle pathology, but they rarely present with myopathy.

CLINICAL EVALUATION

To diagnose and treat the patient with weakness due to neuromuscular disease, the lesion must be localized to the appropriate portion of the motor unit. Systematic clinical evaluation is needed to localize disease to the anterior horn cell, peripheral nerve, neuromuscular junction, or muscle. Some neuromuscular disorders have distinctive symptoms and physical findings that suggest the diagnosis. Table 2-1 lists abnormalities on examination that occur singly or in various combinations in different myopathies.

In most patients with myopathies, the major problem is weakness; less commonly, muscle pain or cramping appear first. Patients with prominent complaints of pain often have diseases of joint, bone, or nerve rather than of muscle. Patients with depression, anemia, or systemic illness may also complain of weakness, although they usually mean a generalized sense of *asthenia*. Through a careful examination and history, the true nature of the patient's problem usually can be determined.

History

WEAKNESS

In most cases, motor signs precede motor symptoms. Athletes or very strong individuals may notice a loss of strength before it is apparent to the examiner. In taking the history, the clinician must ask the patient about his or her ability to perform a specific activity, because patients often are able to ignore slowly progressive weakness by unconsciously compensating for loss of strength. Often only an acute or abrupt change will prompt a complaint of muscle weakness; patients may avoid medical attention until they encounter difficulty carrying out specific tasks. In addition, historical features can help to define the regional distribution of weakness (Table 2–4), and the loss of a specific ability such as climbing stairs, getting up from the floor, or opening jars can document the evolution and course of a disease.

FATIGUE

The "fatigue" that occurs in healthy persons *must be distinguished from pathologic fatigability* resulting from a defect in neuromuscular transmission, from a defect in muscle metabolism, or from upper motor neuron dysfunction.[10,20] The symptom of fatigue must also be separated into *pathologic fatigability* characterized by loss of *function*, and *asthenia* characterized by loss of *"energy."* Examples of pathologic fatigability include dysconjugate eye movements, ptosis, dysphagia, and dysarthria, which occur particularly in myasthenia gravis and related conditions. In contrast, patients with asthenia may require bed rest, need frequent naps, and complain that they have no energy, but they rarely report fatigue of specific muscle groups.

Fatigability due to a failure of neuromuscular junction transmission can often be demonstrated electrophysiologically by repetitive nerve stimulation of selected muscles (see p. 52). Fatigue resulting from impaired muscle metabolism often requires provocative exercise testing (see p. 258). Fatigue of other components of motor function such as suprasegmental control (the upper motor neuron) or the muscle contractile

Table 2–4 SIGNS AND SYMPTOMS OF MUSCLE WEAKNESS

Location	Signs and Symptoms
Ocular	Ptosis, double vision, dysconjugate or limited eye movements
Facial	Sclera visible while sleeping or during eyelid closure, inability to "bury the eyelashes," smile, whistle
Palatal	Nasal escape of liquids, nasal speech
Pharyngeal	Weight loss, difficulty swallowing, recurrent pneumonias secondary to aspiration of liquid or food, cough or dyspnea during meals
Trunk	Accentuated lumbar lordosis, scoliosis, protuberant abdomen, difficulty sitting up from supine
Shoulder and arms	Winging of scapulae, difficulty lifting objects above the head, inability to do push-ups
Forearm and hand	Finger or wrist drop, inability to make a tight fist and blanch the knuckles, inability to prevent escape from hand grip
Pelvic	Waddling gait, difficulty stepping up onto a chair, rising from a squat (with one or both legs), rising from a chair (with or without using hand support)
Leg and foot	Inability to hop or walk on toes, walk on heels, or spread or curl toes

apparatus is difficult to evaluate clinically and is particularly troublesome to distinguish from volitional and motivational factors; some techniques (interpolated twitch, intermittent tetanic stimulation) recently have been developed to help with these issues.[48] In upper motor neuron dysfunction, fatigability occurs very rapidly when the patient attempts to maintain a maximum muscular contraction. EMG recordings have demonstrated a concomitant decrease in the total number and the firing rate of recruited motor unit potentials.[78] Thus electrophysiologic studies may help to reveal whether fatigability results from an abnormality in neuromuscular transmission or in suprasegmental control of the firing of the anterior horn cell.

MUSCLE PAIN, CRAMPS, AND STIFFNESS

Myalgias in association with acute viral illness and postexertional muscle pain are part of everyday experience. Muscle discomfort in these instances is usually self-limited and differs from the complaints of muscle pain that result from a hereditary or acquired abnormality of muscle metabolism, from an inflammatory myopathy, or from a toxic myopathy (Table 2–5). Components other than muscle fibers, including connective tissue, blood vessels, nerves, and tendons, often are responsible for muscle pain. Still more commonly, joint pain may be referred to adjacent muscles. Joint diseases such as polymyalgia rheumatica, rheumatoid arthritis, or lupus erythematosus often present with muscle pain and stiffness.

Patients use subjective terms to describe muscle pain; words such as "cramp," "charley horse," "spasm," "seizing up," "lameness," "rheumatism," or "leaders" often tell more about a patient's cultural heritage than about his or her muscle function. Many patients with muscle pain turn out to have a definable disease of muscle,[57] but many do not. In fact, most patients with myopathies have little or no muscle pain.

Fibrositis or *fibromyalgia* is a common but poorly understood disorder.[14,98] Patients complain bitterly of muscle pain and tenderness and often can identify specific areas of tender muscle or skin (trigger points), but muscle biopsy fails to demonstrate specific abnormalities.[36] As discussed further in Chapter 11, sleep disturbances are frequent in such patients.[15]

Table 2–5 MAJOR CAUSES OF MUSCLE PAIN, CRAMPS, AND STIFFNESS

The most common cause of muscular pain are other than primary muscle disease:
  Circulatory insufficiency
  Joint disease
  Bone disease
  Neuropathy
  Anterior horn cell disease
  Fasciitis
Muscle disorders are often painless. Those with pain include:
  Inflammatory myopathies—dermatomyositis; polymyositis; myositis with collagen vascular disease; viral, bacterial, and parasitic myositis
  Substrate-utilization defects—glycogenolysis, glycolysis, fatty-acid oxidation, purine nucleotide cycle
  Toxic myopathies—alcohol, narcotics, clofibrate, zidovudine
  Endocrinopathies—hypothyroidism, hyperthyroidism, hypoparathyroidism, hyperparathyroidism
  Metabolic disorders—lowered sodium, potassium, calcium, magnesium, phosphate; elevated sodium, calcium
  Myotonia (occasionally painful)

A *muscle cramp* is associated with involuntary, high-frequency discharge of many motor units and is promptly relieved by stretching the affected muscle.[95] Muscle cramp must be differentiated from a muscle *contracture*, which is related to defects in carbohydrate metabolism. Although associated with painful shortening of the muscle belly and sustained contraction of the muscle, contractures are electrically silent when studied by electromyography.[67]

Muscle cramps are frequent in diseases of the anterior horn cell, such as amyotrophic lateral sclerosis, and in disorders of the peripheral nerve, if the axon is affected. Less common diseases that can result in muscle cramps include the *stiff-man syndrome*, where cramps originate in the anterior horn cells, and *Isaac's syndrome*, a disorder in which continuous firing of muscle fibers is associated with muscle stiffness and hyperhidrosis, and in which cramps originate in the distal peripheral nerves. Cramps of neurogenic origin can be blocked by pharmacologic agents. Quinine, which stabilizes the muscle membrane, is often helpful, but agents that prevent repetitive nerve discharges, such as carbamazepine or phenytoin, are more frequently effective.

Two well-characterized metabolic glycolytic defects of skeletal muscle that are associated with painful contractures are muscle phosphorylase deficiency (McArdle's disease) and phosphofructokinase deficiency. In both of these disorders, failure of energy production results from an enzyme deficiency that blocks glycogen or glucose metabolism. These patients develop a hard, contracted muscle during vigorous exercise (see Chapter 6). In carnitine palmitoyltransferase (CPT) deficiency, oxidation of long-chain fatty acids is impaired, and many of these patients experience muscle pain and discomfort, usually described as a "tightness" rather than a muscle cramp (see Chapter 9).

In normal individuals, muscle cramps are commonly encountered during swimming and at night. Swimmers are particularly prone to develop cramping of the calf muscles, which appears to be related to a passive shortening of the gastrocnemius muscle during swimming with the ankle plantar flexed. Neural input superimposed on this passively shortened muscle without concomitant resistance or tension to limit the contractile response produces a painful muscle cramp. A similar mechanism is thought to produce nocturnal leg cramps, in which the muscle once again is passively shortened because of ankle plantar flexion. During normal muscle activity, an inhibitory feedback input to the spinal cord from the Golgi tendon organ protects against a muscle cramp.[95]

Most of us have been advised that using salt tablets prevents the muscle cramps associated with exercise. Overwhelming evidence suggests, however, that normal physiologic mechanisms avoid significant ion shifts even in intense exercise. Dehydration with decreased plasma volume appears to be a more likely cause of cramps, although the exact mechanism of their origin is unknown.[16]

PARESTHESIAS AND DYSESTHESIAS

Paresthesias and dysesthesias are characteristic of peripheral nerve or central nervous system disease; their occurrence in a weak patient points away from a diagnosis of myopathy.

Examination

DEMONSTRATION AND QUANTITATION OF WEAKNESS

Muscle strength can be tested by manual testing and from observation of functional activity (see Table 2–4). Functional assessment is particularly useful in children unable to cooperate with muscle testing. On the other hand, manual muscle testing can be used to quantify muscle strength by applying a

Table 2-6 MEDICAL RESEARCH COUNCIL (MRC) MANUAL MUSCLE TESTING SCALE[50]

MRC Grade	Degree of Strength
5	Normal
4	Able to oppose resistance
3	Able to oppose gravity
2	Able to move with gravity eliminated
1	Trace movement
0	No movement

grading system. The most widely used system is the 0 to 5 scale developed by the Medical Research Council (MRC) of Great Britain (Table 2-6).[50] One major problem inherent in this scale is that grade 4, "opposing some resistance," together with grade 5 (normal strength), often encompass 80% to 90% of the range of muscle strength.[12] The scale has been modified to address this problem by adding pluses and minuses (Table 2-7); this useful change subdivides the large range of grade 4 strength.[28]

Devices for Quantitation of Strength. The need to quantify strength or document a change with therapy has led to the use of a variety of myometers.[21,47] Most clinicians do not use these devices, as most require the physician to undergo several days of training before precise, reproducible measurements can be obtained, and patient motivation has a marked and variable effect on testing. One exception is the hand dynamometer, which requires little training for accurate use. For example, the JAMAR hand dynamometer (Asimow Engineering Company, Santa Monica, CA) was found reliable in measuring hand grip strength when tests were compared between different observers.[31]

Strength Testing in Young Children. Children less than 5 years of age often are unable to cooperate with testing. Moreover, strength testing in childhood may be difficult because of the lack of criteria for what constitutes normal strength. In young children, function testing can provide a reproducible means of assessing muscle function (Table 2-8). Careful analysis of gait on either running or walking, watching a child getting up from the floor (Gowers' sign) (Fig. 2-1), flexing the neck on the chest in a supine position (Fig. 2-2), and elevating the arms to see if winging occurs (Fig. 2-3) are all helpful approaches. Lifting the child with the examiner's hands in the axillae detects shoulder girdle weakness if the patient's shoulder girdle rises upward. Whereas the normal child involuntarily exerts downward pressure against the examiner's hands, the weak child will "fall through on suspension." Abnor-

Table 2-7 EXPANDED MRC SCALE FOR MANUAL MUSCLE TESTING

Modified MRC Grade	Degree of Strength
5	Normal strength
5-	Equivocal, barely detectable weakness
4+	Definite but slight weakness
4	Able to move the joint against combination of gravity and some resistance*
4-	Capable of minimal resistance
3+	Capable of transient resistance but collapses abruptly
3	Able to move through full range against gravity without resistance to the movement
3-	Able to move against gravity but not through full range
2	Able to move with gravity eliminated
1	Flicker of movement
0	No movement

*The subdivisions 4S (a strong 4), 4 (a moderate 4), and 4W (a weaker 4) are often useful.

Table 2–8 TESTING OF MUSCLE FUNCTION IN YOUNG CHILDREN

Muscle Group	Sign or Symptom
Ocular	Limitation in eye movements, ptosis
Bulbar function	Cry, speech, suck, tongue
Neck flexion	Head control (Fig. 2–2)
Shoulder girdle	Suspension
Hip and trunk	Gait and running ability
Trunk and proximal leg	Gowers' sign (Fig. 2–1)
Respiratory	Use of accessory muscles; paradoxical diaphragm movement

mal findings on these tests are not specific for myopathy, however; patients with other causes of proximal weakness show identical signs.

MUSCLE BULK

Muscle Atrophy. Atrophy and hypertrophy of muscle are difficult to quantitate because of the marked variation among normals. Atrophy is particularly difficult to estimate in children because of overlying adipose tissue. A visual judgment of muscle bulk is more reliable than measurements, because the circumference of the limbs, chest, and abdomen do not accurately assess the adiposity of the patient. Atrophy is easier to appreciate when it is asymmetric. Small muscles are not necessarily abnormal unless the patient is weak; this is especially true in elderly patients. Such an appearance occurs frequently in normal children or in adults who have "down weighted" to achieve greater speed in long-distance running and other endurance sports.

Myopathies characteristically produce less atrophy than neuropathies when degrees of weakness are comparable. This preservation of muscle bulk in myopathies may reflect damaged muscle fibers that generate little or no force, as well as replacement of muscle fibers by connective tissue and fat.[34a]

Muscle Enlargement. An isolated or symmetric increase in the size of an individual muscle or a group of muscles may occur with exercise. Abnormal enlargement may result from increased spontaneous activity such as occurs with myotonia (Table 2–9). This results in true hypertrophy of muscle fibers.[29] Enlargement reflecting an increase in fat and connective tissue may produce pseudohypertrophy, although the pseudohypertrophy in Duchenne dystrophy is not exclusively the result of fat and connective tissue replacement, because some muscle fibers are truly hypertrophied in this condition.[29] Muscle enlargement is usually recognized as abnormal only when selected individual muscles are enlarged in comparison with other normal or atrophied muscles; for example, the calves in Duchenne dystrophy, or the extensor digitorum brevis muscle in limb-girdle and other muscular dystrophies (Figs. 2–4A and B). Muscles also can enlarge from infiltration by amyloid or parasites.[29]

Several disorders other than primary myopathies can produce focal enlargement and masses in muscle. Such swelling can accompany generalized muscle disease due to inflammatory infiltrates or calcium deposits. Single or multiple muscle masses in the absence of weakness can reflect neoplastic involvement, focal myositis, infection, ec-

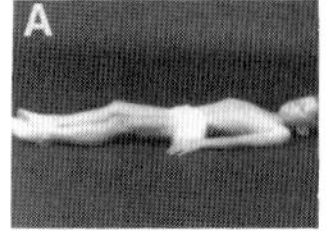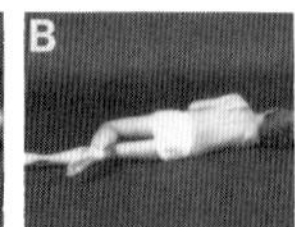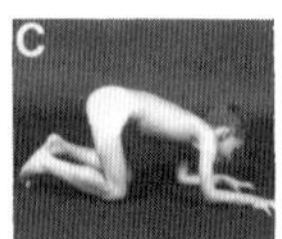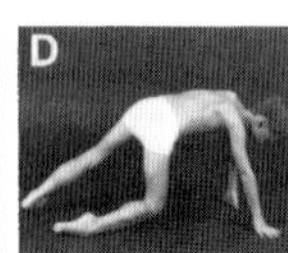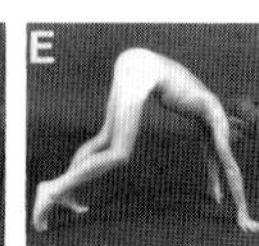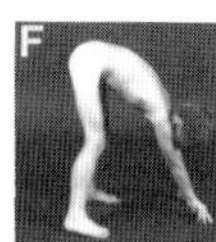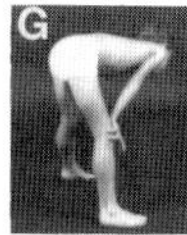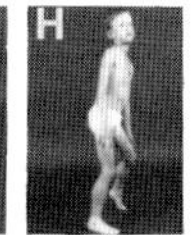

Figure 2–1. Gowers' sign. A patient with Duchenne dystrophy is shown rising from the floor. The most common cause of weakness in young boys is Duchenne dystrophy, but Gowers' sign is present in any disorder characterized by proximal weakness. To stand, the patient must roll from supine to prone (*A* and *B*), push off the floor (*C–E*), lock his knees (*F*), and then "climb up his legs" (*G* and *H*).

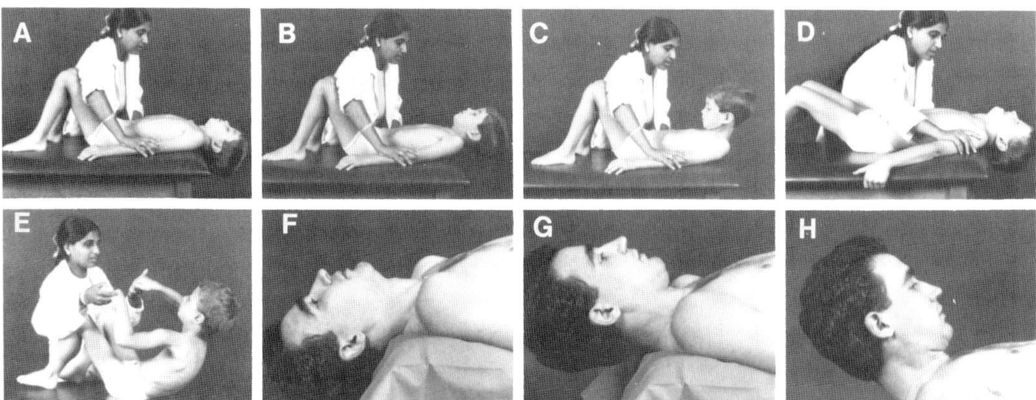

Figure 2–2. Testing neck flexion. (*A–C*) Normal child. (*D*) Neck flexor weakness in Duchenne dystrophy. The patient is unable to lift his head against gravity. It is important to fix the shoulders on the examining table. (*E*) Severe neck flexor weakness (grade 2 MRC) is present even from infancy in patients with Duchenne dystrophy. (*F–H*) Whereas the patient with Duchenne dystrophy is able to hold the head up only if gravity is partially eliminated, this patient with Becker dystrophy can lift his head against gravity.

topic ossification, or tendon rupture (Fig. 2–4C).

MUSCLE PALPATION

Palpation of weak, stiff, painful, or enlarged (or symptomatic) muscles may provide diagnostic clues. Calcium deposits are usually discrete and may be separable from surrounding tissues. Neoplasms and inflammatory lesions may also be defined. On the other hand, the texture of muscle, often described as "fibrotic," "doughy," or "flabby," is usually not diagnostic. Muscle tenderness is not a specific sign, and it rarely accompanies inflammation confined to the muscle unless there is extension into the overlying fascia. Pitting edema

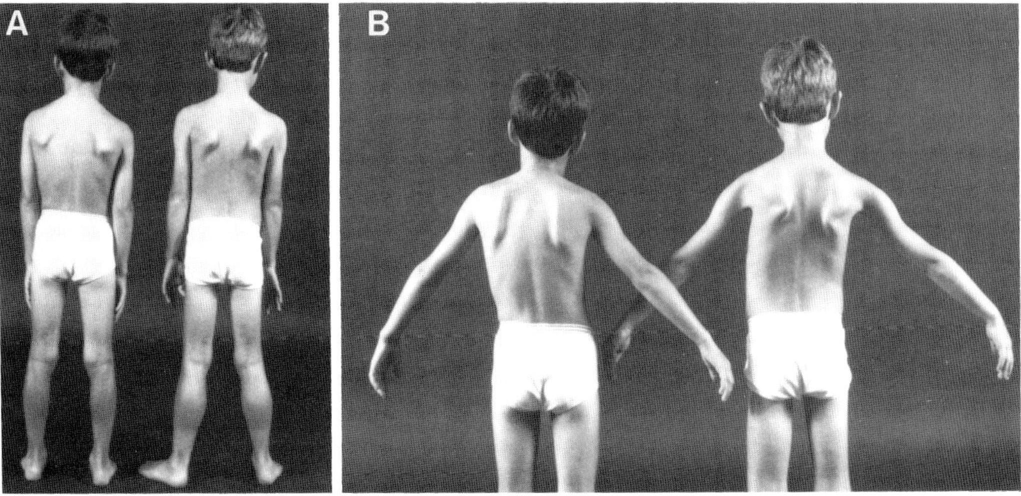

Figure 2–3. Scapular winging. Brothers with Duchenne dystrophy are elevating their arms. Protrusion of the scapulae is present bilaterally.

Table 2–9 CAUSES OF GENERALIZED OR FOCAL MUSCLE ENLARGEMENT

MUSCLE FIBERS HISTOLOGICALLY NORMAL
Exercise
Spasticity (especially with high cervical spinal cord disease)
Myotonic disorders — myotonia congenita, paramyotonia congenita, hyperkalemic periodic paralysis
Flier's syndrome (acanthosis nigricans, insulin resistance)

MUSCLE FIBERS HISTOLOGICALLY ABNORMAL
Muscular dystrophy — Duchenne, Becker, limb-girdle
Spinal muscular atrophy — Kugelberg-Welander disease
Radiculopathies
Glycogen storage disease — adult acid maltase
Endocrinopathies — hypothyroidism, acromegaly

INFILTRATION WITH PATHOLOGIC MATERIAL
Connective tissue and fat — muscular dystrophy
Parasitic infestations — e.g., cysticercosis, schistosomiasis
Amyloidosis
Sarcoidosis

FOCAL ENLARGEMENT OR MASSES
Myositis
Granulomas (esp. sarcoidosis)
Ectopic ossification
Calcinosis
Ruptured tendons
Neoplasms

confined to the muscle is uncommon, but in dermatomyositis (particularly the childhood form) edema of the subcutaneous tissue involving the arms is a valuable sign.

FATIGUE

Pathologic fatigue is the hallmark of neuromuscular junction disease, but as noted earlier (p. 20), some degree of fatigue is normal. Fatigue may also be the result of limited effort. Useful, objective clinical signs that are not likely to result from poor motivation include worsening of ptosis (Fig. 2–5), the development of dysconjugate eye movements, the peek sign (lid opening after initial closure during a Bell's phenomenon),[63] and the development of rhinolalia (nasal speech). Patients cannot mimic these abnormalities by decreased effort, and voluntary efforts cannot simulate ptosis (compare the two parts of Fig. 2–5).

MYOTONIA

In some myopathies, myotonia may be the only clinical sign that indicates an underlying muscle disease. Myotonia is the sustained contraction of muscle caused by spontaneous repetitive depolarization of the muscle membrane. The phenomenon arises directly from the muscle membrane and persists in the absence of nerve supply.[9] Myotonia is clinically and electrophysiologically distinct from a true muscle cramp or from the unusual neuromyotonia, which requires an intact innervation by the peripheral nerve.[6] True muscle cramps, which result from spontaneous discharge of motor nerves, occur either when the muscle is at rest or after muscular contraction and can

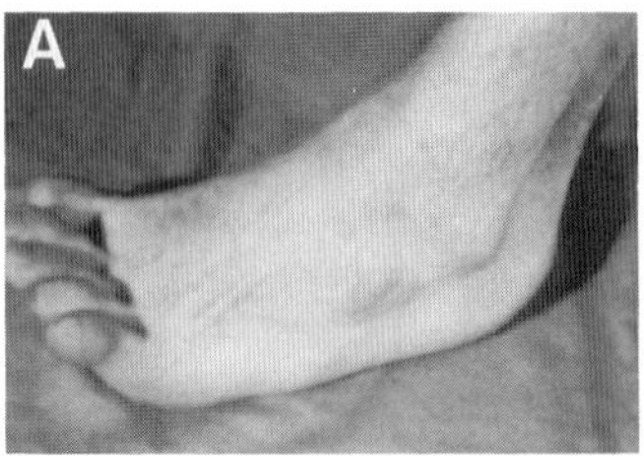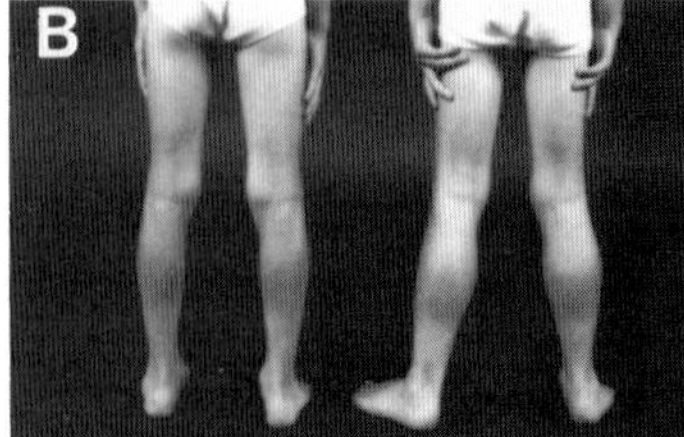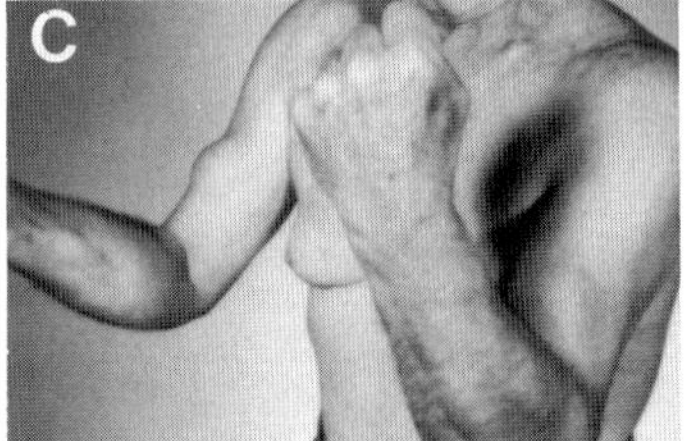

Figure 2–4. The extensor digitorum brevis muscle (*A*) is enlarged in many patients with muscular dystrophy. The patient shown has limb-girdle dystrophy. (*B*) Other muscles may show similar hypertrophy, particularly the calves in Duchenne dystrophy (compare the normal on the left with his affected brother), Becker dystrophy, and limb-girdle dystrophy. The tongue may enlarge also (see Figure 2–18C). (*C*) Bilateral rupture of biceps muscle tendons produced focal enlargement of muscle.

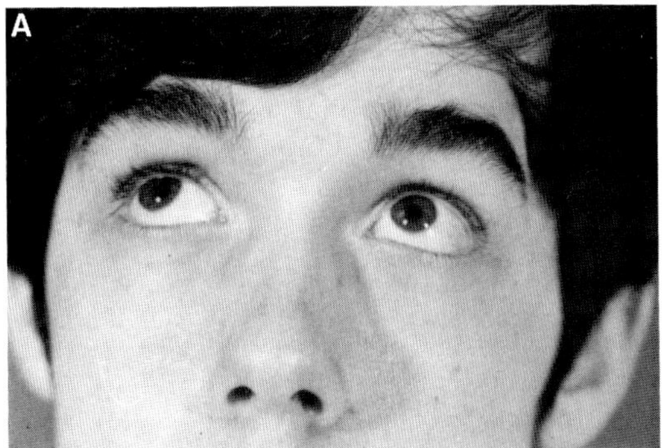
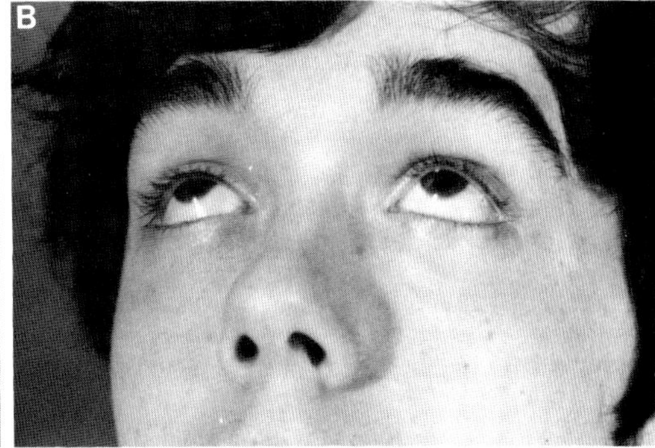

Figure 2–5. A reliable sign of fatigue in neuromuscular junction diseases is the "curtain sign" of progressive ptosis. While looking upward (*A*), the patient gradually develops ptosis (*B*).

occasionally be provoked by strong muscular contraction in strength testing. They produce a firm mounding-up of the muscle, which is promptly eliminated by stretching it. Such cramps are usually intensely painful, whereas myotonia is usually painless. (For exceptions see Chapter 9). Neuromyotonia (previously known as neurotonia and Isaac's syndrome) manifests as continuous muscle rippling and stiffness at rest. It results from bursts of very high frequency discharges of peripheral nerve.

Myotonia can be elicited either by having the patient forcefully contract a muscle (e.g., eye closure or clenched fist) (*action myotonia*, Fig. 2–6) or by tap-

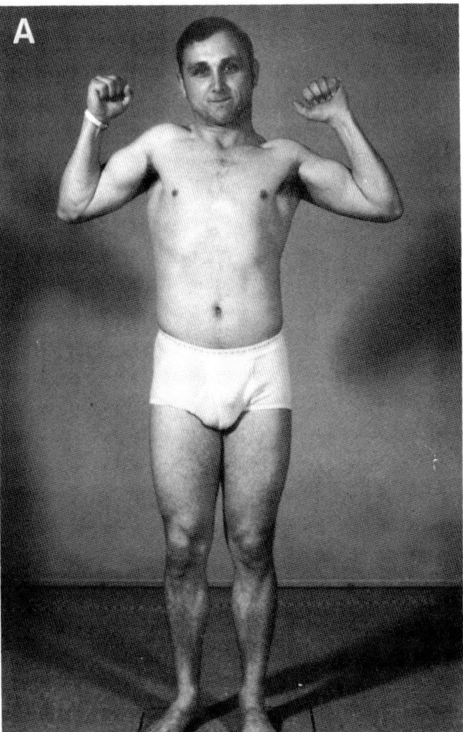
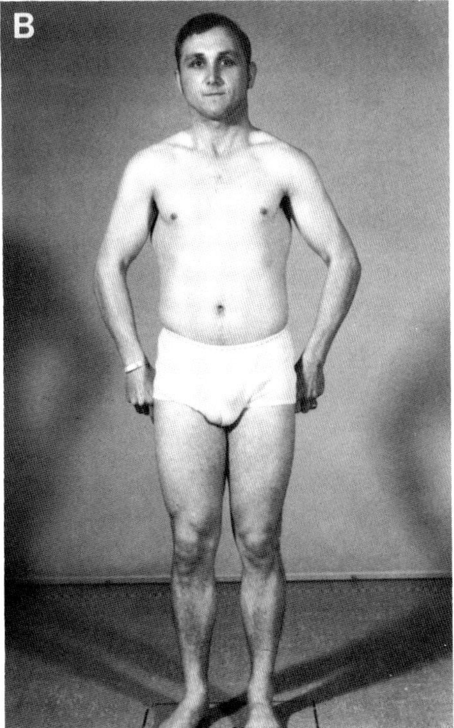

Figure 2–6. Severe action myotonia. A patient with myotonia congenita contracts his arm muscles (*A*) and is then unable to relax (*B*).

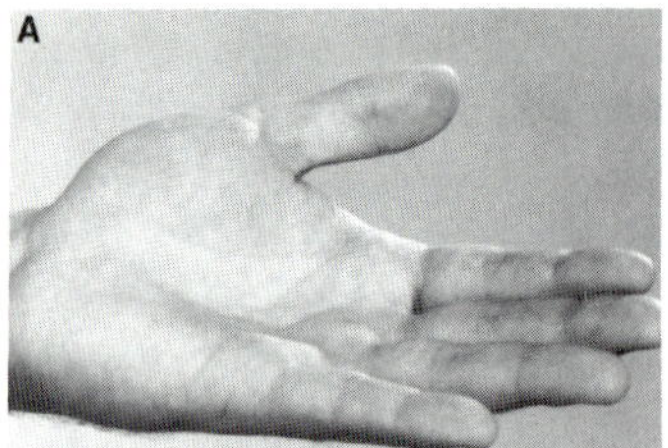
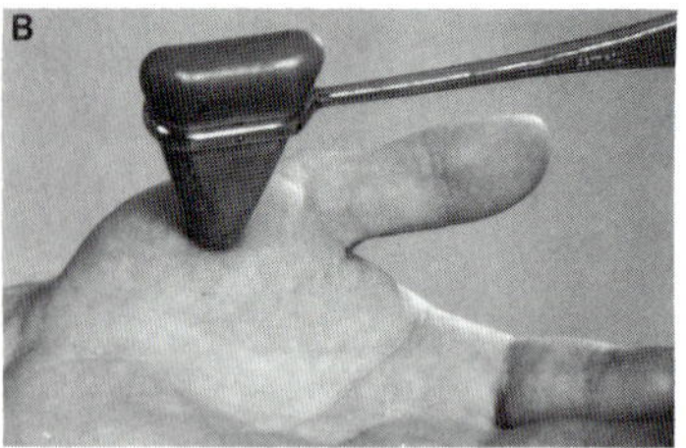
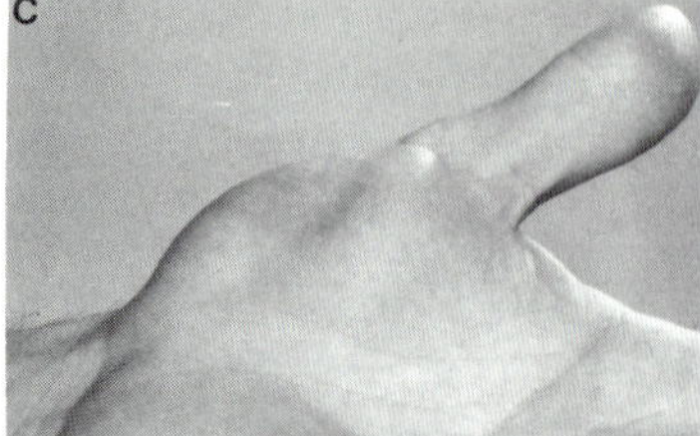

Figure 2–7. Percussion myotonia. (*A*) The relaxed thenar eminence is (*B*) struck with a reflex hammer. A persistent contraction ("dimple") is visible for 10 seconds or longer in this patient with paramyotonia congenita.

ping a muscle (*percussion myotonia*, Fig. 2–7). To elicit percussion myotonia, the muscle belly is struck sharply with a soft device such as a reflex hammer. In the normal patient, percussion of the finger extensors produces extension that lasts less than half a second. In the patient with myotonia, the fingers remain partially extended and then gradually fall. Similarly, percussion of the tongue (by tapping a tongue blade [see Fig. 2–8]) or thenar eminence can produce a sustained contraction that results in a local depression. This depression in the tongue is termed the "napkin-ring sign" and elsewhere is termed "dimpling."

Myotonia is usually more prominent in the cold or after prolonged rest with the body in a fixed posture. Myotonia typically diminishes with repeated exercise. If myotonia worsens with repeated activity, it is termed *paradoxical myotonia* (Fig. 2–9). The myotonic phenomenon can arise from a number of genetically distinct disorders of muscle membrane (see Chapter 9).

Percussion myotonia must be distinguished from the normal *muscle percussion response* and *myoedema*, respectively (Fig. 2–10). When percussed with a reflex hammer, the muscle is briefly depolarized and contracts, resembling a muscle stretch reflex. This contraction may be confusing in patients with neuropathies, who usually have hypoactive reflexes, because the muscle percussion response remains

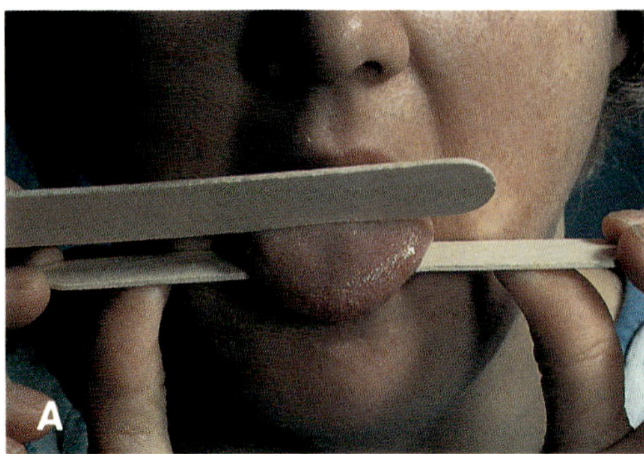
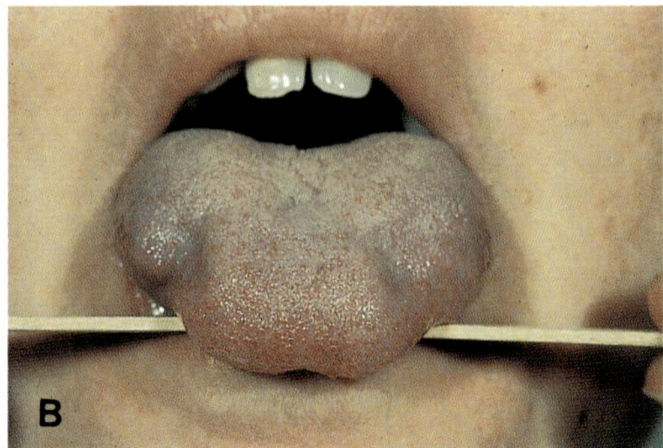

Figure 2–8. Percussion myotonia: the napkin-ring sign. The tongue is tapped lightly between two tongue blades (*A*). A persistent contraction (resembling a ring) remains for 5 to 10 seconds (*B*).

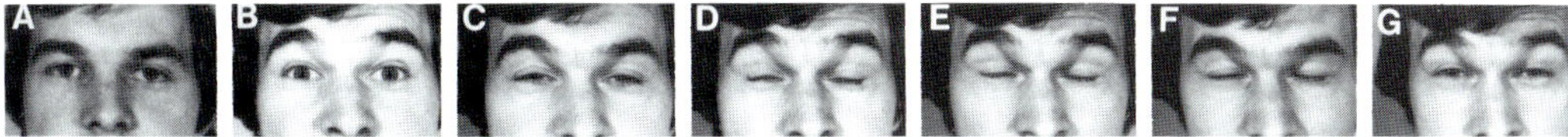

Figure 2–9. Paradoxical myotonia. The patient (*A*) is instructed to close and open his eyes forcefully five times in a row (*B–F*) and develops progressively greater difficulty in opening his eyes, which persists for 1 full minute after cessation of activity (*G*). This myotonia is termed "paradoxical" because in most conditions myotonia decreases ("warms up") with repeated activity. (Modified from Riggs JE, Griggs RC, and Moxley RT: Acetazolamide-induced weakness in paramyotonia congenita. Ann Intern Med 86:169–173, 1977, with permission.)

brisk,[66] presumably because denervated muscle fibers continue to be subject to mechanical depolarization.

MYOEDEMA AFTER PERCUSSION

Myoedema (see Fig. 2–10) is a localized, persistent, electrically silent swelling after percussion that reflects a local contraction induced by the release of calcium ions from the sarcoplasmic reticulum.[58] It is not pathologically significant but must be distinguished from myotonia: myoedema produces swelling whereas myotonia produces dimpling.

SPONTANEOUS MOVEMENTS OF MUSCLE

Muscle twitches or *fasciculations* may be an important sign of neuromuscular disease and may also be a presenting symptom. They result from the spontaneous contraction of muscle fibers within a motor unit and arise from ectopic electrical activity, usually in the distal axon.[72] Fasciculations most frequently accompany motor neuron disease and, less commonly, peripheral nerve disorders. They are diagnostically significant when they accompany weakness, but they may occur in normal individuals, particularly in tense individuals or following exercise (so-called benign or contraction fasciculations).[26] They also can accompany certain metabolic disorders such as hyperparathyroidism, hyperthyroidism, and hypomagnesemia and may reflect the toxic effects of drugs, including theophylline, caffeine, terbutaline, lithium, and anticholinesterase agents. Fasciculations may be obscured by overlying adipose tissue, but they are readily seen in the tongue (unprotruded) and the interosseous muscles. Fasciculations are rarely an early complaint in most neuromuscular diseases; in fact, many patients with severe weakness

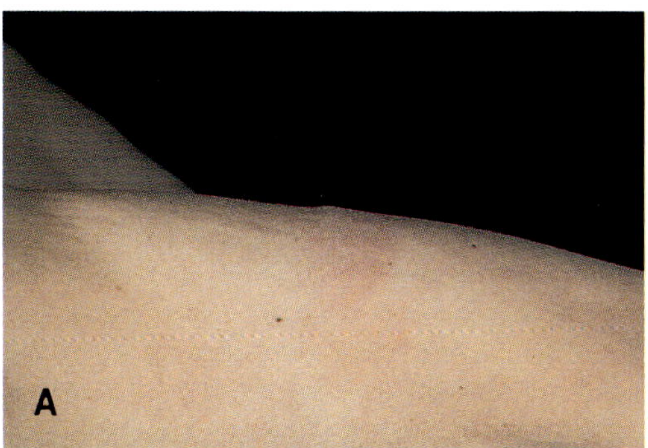
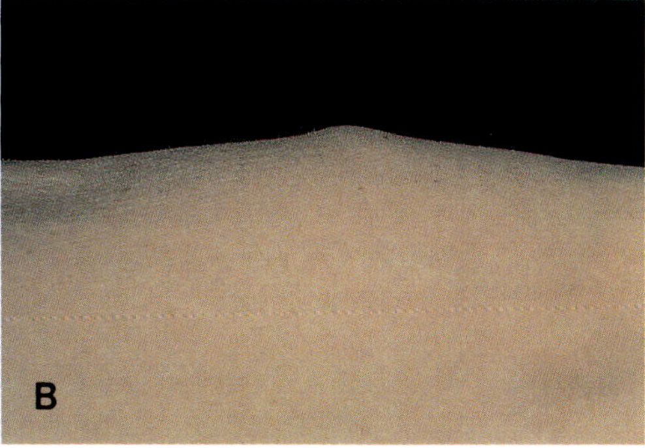

Figure 2–10. Normal muscle percussion response. A pinch of the biceps (*A*) produced a mounding (myoedema). A brisk tap of the wrist extensors produced a mound of myoedema (*B*) that persists for 1 to 3 seconds. The muscle contraction is electrically silent after a brief, mechanically-induced depolarization. Such a normal response is most easily seen in individuals lacking subcutaneous fat.

are surprisingly unaware of their presence. It is the exceptional patient with motor neuron disease who presents with florid fasciculations preceding the onset of weakness.

Myokymia, a pattern of muscle contraction that produces a "writhing" or rippling appearance in the involved area, is the result of spontaneous discharge of large motor units. Myokymia indicates neuronal disease[2]; denervation is followed by sprouting from adjacent neurons, with enlargement of the motor unit territory.

Minipolymyoclonus results from the spontaneous contraction of enlarged motor units (see below) in patients with motor neuron disease and produces small-amplitude movements of fingers and toes when an extremity is at rest.[82] Similar but accentuated movements occur when patients hold their hands in the outstretched position. *Tremor*, attributed to weakness,[74] is almost invariably present in patients with symptomatic weakness due to nerve disease. This tremor is probably an exaggeration of the normal physiologic tremor that results from the synchronized discharge of enlarged motor units in patients who have a reduced number of surviving motor neurons.[1]

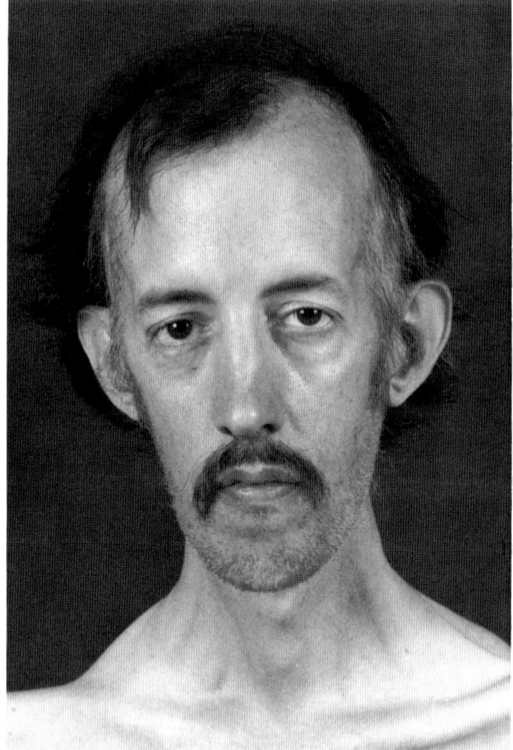

Figure 2–11. Facial features of adult-onset myotonic dystrophy: narrow, hatchet facies, frontal balding, and temporalis muscle wasting.

GENERAL EXAMINATION

Neuromuscular diseases may be suspected in individuals with various skeletal abnormalities including narrow facies, high-arched palate, pectus deformities of the chest, scoliosis, pes cavus or pes planus, and hammer toes. Associated cardiac and pulmonary abnormalities are discussed in Chapter 12. Primary muscular diseases, except for myotonic dystrophy, are associated with remarkably few nonmuscular problems.

Facial Appearance. Certain facies are diagnostically distinctive. For example, the facial appearance of adult-onset (Fig. 2–11) or congenital (Fig. 2–12) myotonic dystrophy is typical and important to recognize. The narrow,

atrophic or "hatchet" face may be present when other manifestations of the disease are minimal or absent. A somewhat similar facial appearance, however, can occur in centronuclear (myotubular) myopathy (Fig. 2–13) and nemaline (rod) myopathy (Fig. 2–14). In contrast, in myotonia congenita (Fig. 2–15) or paramyotonia congenita, muscle contraction and possibly masseter muscle hypertrophy produce an abnormal appearance that is particularly apparent during cold exposure. Facial weakness in facioscapulohumeral muscular dystrophy produces a glum appearance (Fig. 2–16), in which the sclera is frequently visible during gentle lid closure, although the sclera may also be exposed in other disorders with facial weakness.

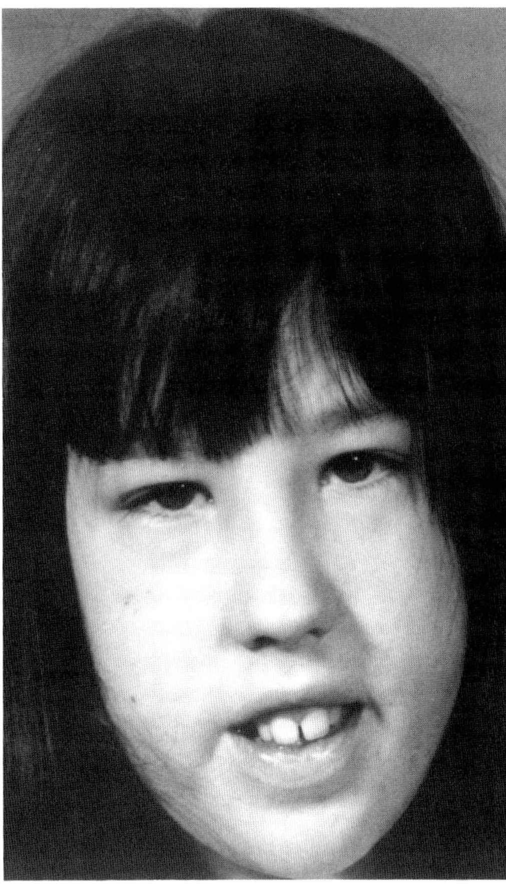

Figure 2–12. Congenital myotonic dystrophy. Dysmorphic features: a tented upper lip and facial diplegia.

Ptosis produces a characteristic facial appearance, especially if accompanied by frontalis muscle contracture and redundancy of the upper eyelids. Ptosis is usually present in oculopharyngeal muscular dystrophy (Fig. 2–17), Kearns-Sayre syndrome, and familial progressive ophthalmoplegia. Patients with myasthenia gravis may present a similar appearance, but typically they also display lower facial weakness that produces a "snarling" appearance. Efforts to smile accentuate the effect, because the initial normal upturn of the corners of the mouth is followed rapidly by a downturn as facial muscles fatigue.

The Tongue. Inspecting lingual muscles for atrophy and fasciculations is important. Normal variations that may be confusing include the scrotal or geographic tongue, as well as prominent rugations or deep clefts that can be confused with atrophy. Also, tremblings in a normal, incompletely relaxed tongue often resemble fasciculations. Nevertheless, tongue atrophy is easily detected in patients with amyotrophic lateral sclerosis and other motor neuron diseases (Fig. 2–18). A distinctive, triple-furrowed tongue can also be a useful sign of tongue muscle atrophy and is

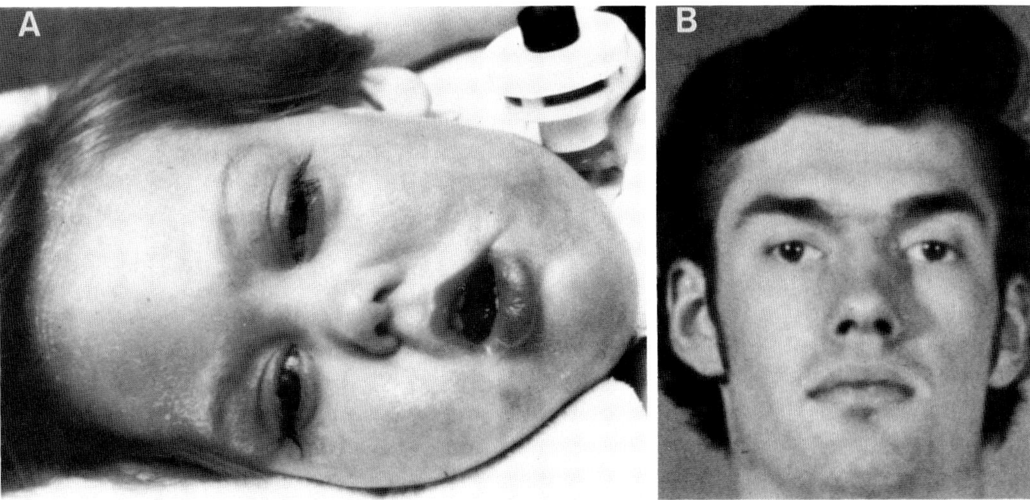

Figure 2–13. Centronuclear myopathy. (*A*) Infantile onset with ophthalmoparesis, facial diplegia, and respiratory failure. (*B*) Juvenile onset with elongated face, bilateral ptosis, and slight facial weakness.

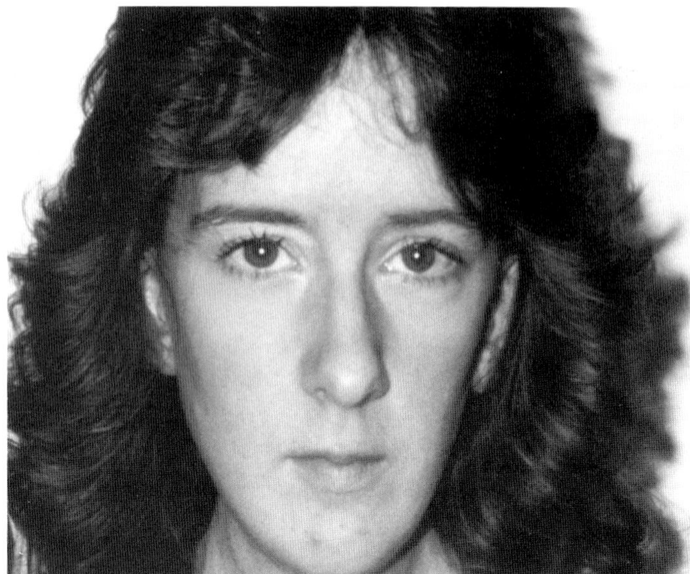

Figure 2–14. Nemaline myopathy. Elongated face with bifacial weakness.

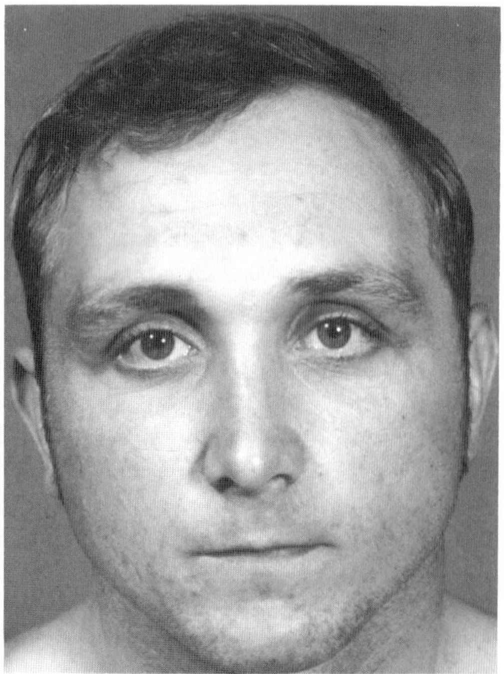

Figure 2–15. Myotonia congenita. Hypertrophy of masseter muscles produces a distinctive facial appearance.

found in severe myasthenia gravis and in myotonic dystrophy.

Enlargement of the tongue is frequent in late stages of Duchenne dystrophy and occasionally occurs in acid maltase deficiency. It is also noted occasionally in myopathies of systemic illness such as amyloidosis, hypothyroidism, and acromegaly.

GAIT

Walking reveals weakness of hip-stabilizing and trunk musculature. Compensation for truncal weakness results in a lordotic posture. A waddling gait is caused by an inability to prevent hip drop or hip dip as the leg swings through. When quadriceps weakness is severe, the patient keeps the leg fully extended to prevent the knee from buckling. This maneuver becomes obvious when the patient demonstrates "back kneeing" or a genu recurvatum. Quadriceps weakness is also associated with "toe walking," which permits the

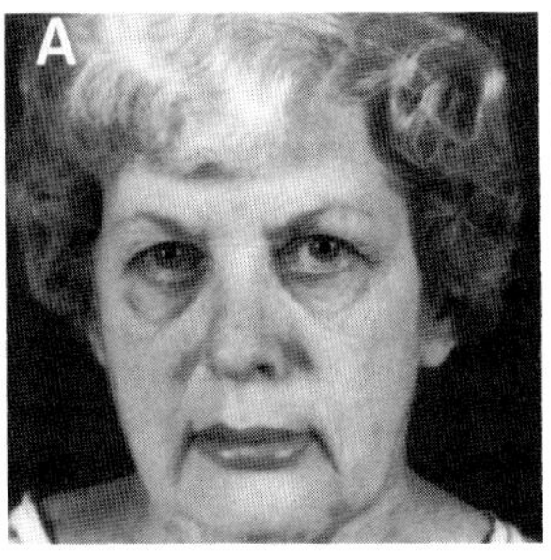

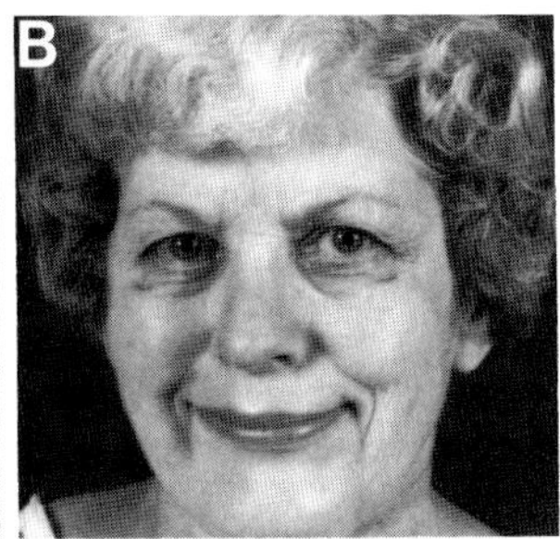

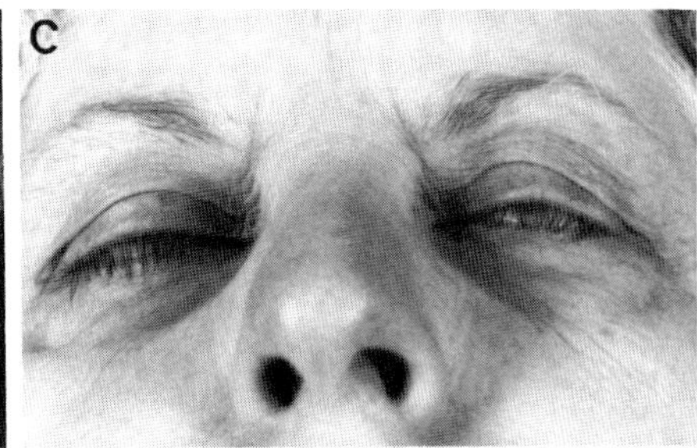

Figure 2–16. Facioscapulohumeral dystrophy. (*A*) Characteristic facial appearance. Weakness of the lower portion of the face produces a pouting expression that is often worsened by an effort to smile (*B*). (*C*) With lid closure, sclera are exposed. Patients often appear to "sleep with their eyes open."

stabilizing action of the gastrocnemius muscle. This muscle can act to extend the knee while producing plantar flexion. This "toe walking" is accompanied by shortening of the Achilles tendon. Some muscle conditions, such as myotonic dystrophy, distal myopathy, or facioscapulohumeral dystrophy, all of which can cause early foot drop, result in a steppage gait identical to that observed in peripheral neuropathies. If severe proximal and distal weakness coexist, the patient takes short, circumducting steps with the knee held in an extended (locked) position to prevent catching the toes on the floor.

REFLEXES

Muscle stretch reflexes may be preserved in myopathies until there is profound loss of strength (see Table 2–1). Myotonic dystrophy is an exception. These patients are hyporeflexic or areflexic when muscles are still relatively strong, raising the possibility of an associated neural component.[64,70] Patients with congenital myotonic dystrophy may have a spastic diplegia due to central nervous system disease.[93]

DIFFERENTIAL DIAGNOSIS

The myopathies have a relatively small number of distinct clinical presentations, each of which has a defined list of likely diagnoses. The following sections describe these presentations and indicate clinical features useful in establishing that a patient has, in fact, a primary muscle disease.

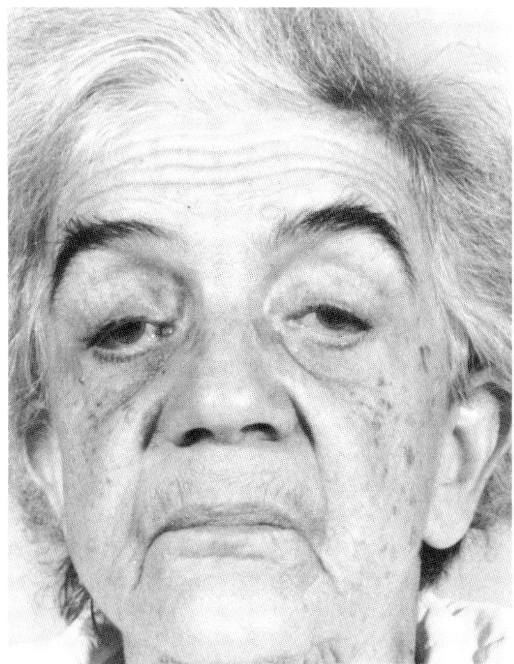

Figure 2–17. Oculopharyngeal dystrophy in a French-Canadian woman. Ptosis and a compensatory frontalis muscle contraction are present.

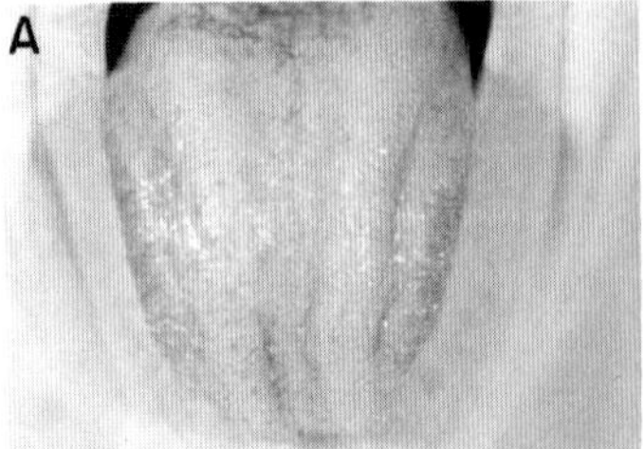
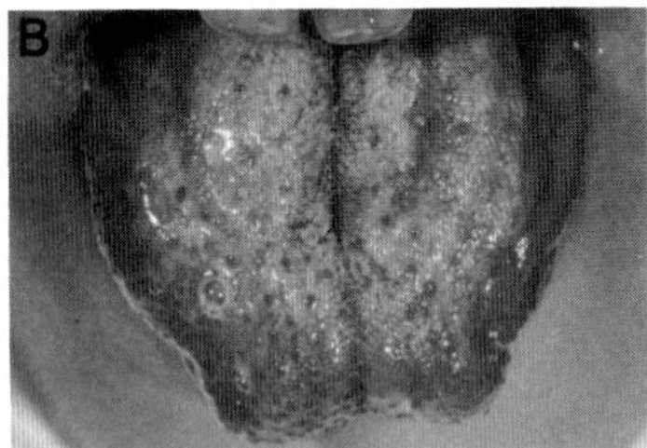
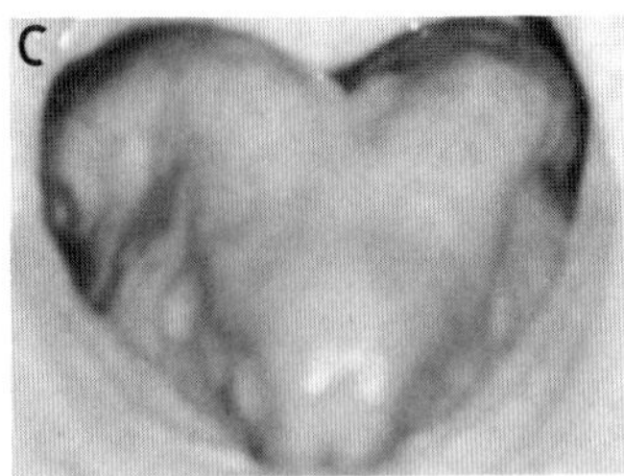

Figure 2–18. Tongue atrophy and hypertrophy. (*A*) Myasthenia gravis—the triple-furrowed tongue. (*B*) Myotonic dystrophy—a less-frequent cause of triple-furrowed tongue. (*C*) Duchenne dystrophy—hypertrophy of the tongue.

Disorders Presenting at Birth with Hypotonia

Although all neuromuscular causes combined account for far fewer floppy infants than do central nervous system causes,[60] spinal muscular atrophy, congenital myopathies, congenital muscular dystrophy, congenital myasthenia gravis, and rare forms of peripheral neuropathies must all be considered (Table 2–10). As a rule, myopathy and other neuromuscular diseases are sug-

gested if the patient appears alert but has hypoactive or absent tendon reflexes. Skeletal abnormalities such as pes cavus, high-arched palate, pectus excavatum, and joint contractures also suggest a neuromuscular basis for hypotonia. Rarely, superimposed anoxic brain damage in a patient with a myopathy that produces respiratory failure may cause hyperreflexia.

Disorders Presenting in Infancy

Spinal muscular atrophy (Werdnig-Hoffman disease) is the most common neuromuscular disease presenting in infancy. It varies in severity and may start prior to birth or at any time in the first months of life. The cases with earliest onset are often the most severe and may culminate in respiratory failure. Fasciculations of the tongue and limb muscles help establish the diagnosis, although limb fasciculations may be obscured by overlying adipose tissue. Spinal muscular atrophy is not treatable and does not improve.

Some conditions presenting in infancy that either remit spontaneously or improve with treatment include infantile botulism,[91] congenital myotonic dystrophy,[93] cytochrome oxidase deficiency (see Chapter 6), congenital myasthenias,[24] or infantile myasthenia gravis.[25] Rare forms of acquired, treatable, inflammatory demyelinating neuropathies in infancy have also been reported.[81]

Table 2–10 DISORDERS PRESENTING AT BIRTH WITH HYPOTONIA (THE FLOPPY INFANT)

CENTRAL HYPOTONIA* †(most common cause of hypotonia at birth)
MYOPATHIES
  Congenital myotonic dystrophy*
  Centronuclear (myotubular) myopathy*
  Muscular dystrophies—congenital
  Congenital fiber-type disproportion*
  Central core disease
  Nemaline (rod) myopathy
  Glycogen storage diseases (acid maltase and phosphorylase deficiencies)
  Lipid storage diseases (carnitine deficiency)

OTHER NEUROMUSCULAR DISEASES
  Spinal muscular atrophy (Werdnig-Hoffman disease)
  Congenital and infantile myasthenia gravis
  Congenital amyelinating and hypomyelinating neuropathies
  Hereditary motor and sensory neuropathies, type I and type II

ARTHROPATHIES

*Frequently present with respiratory difficulties.
†Central nervous system disorders of many types.

Table 2–11 NEUROMUSCULAR DISEASES PRESENTING AS PROGRESSIVE WEAKNESS IN CHILDHOOD

MYOPATHIES
Muscular dystrophy—Duchenne, Becker, Emery-Dreifuss, facioscapulohumeral,* limb-girdle, congenital
Inflammatory myopathies—dermatomyositis, polymyositis,* inclusion body myositis*
Lipid storage myopathy—carnitine deficiency
Glycogen-storage disease
Acid maltase deficiency
Endocrine-metabolic disorders—hypokalemia, hypocalcemia, hypercalcemia
Central core disease
Nemaline myopathy
Centronuclear myopathy
Mitochondial myopathies
Rigid-spine syndrome

SPINAL MUSCULAR ATROPHY
Kugelberg-Welander disease

NEUROMUSCULAR JUNCTION DISORDER
Myasthenia gravis
Lambert-Eaton syndrome

NEUROPATHY
Chronic inflammatory demyelinating polyneuropathy
Hereditary motor and sensory neuropathies

*Rarely presents in childhood.

Disorders Presenting in Childhood with Progressive Proximal Weakness

Duchenne dystrophy is the commonest cause of progressive weakness in boys. In girls, spinal muscular atrophy, limb-girdle dystrophy, and dermatomyositis are the most commonly encountered (Table 2–11). Spinal muscular atrophy is distinguishable from a myopathy by the presence of tremor, minipolymyoclonus, or fasciculations.

Disorders Presenting in Adulthood

PROGRESSIVE PROXIMAL WEAKNESS

Acute weakness that evolves over a matter of hours is rarely a myopathy; much more frequently, it results from neuromuscular junction or peripheral nerve disease (Table 2–12). The major exception is the muscle dysfunction produced by electrolyte or metabolic derangements. Myopathy produced by infectious and inflammatory diseases often causes acute muscle pain, resulting in apparent weakness.

Slowly progressive proximal weakness in adults is usually due to myopathy (Table 2–13). This fact leads to the erroneous, circular argument that all proximal weakness results from myopathy, as opposed to other forms of neuromuscular disease. This, of course, is not true, and it is misleading to describe

Table 2–12 NEUROMUSCULAR DISEASES CAUSING RAPIDLY PROGRESSIVE WEAKNESS

MYOPATHIES
Inflammatory
Idiopathic—polymyositis, dermatomyositis; paroxysmal rhabdomyolysis
Viral—influenza, Coxsackie B
Parasitic—trichinosis
Protozoal—toxoplasmosis
Metabolic—glycogen and lipid disorders, especially carnitine palmitoyl transferase deficiency
Endocrinopathies—hyperthyroidism, corticosteroid-related
Electrolyte imbalance—hypokalemia and hyperkalemia, hypocalcemia and hypercalcemia, hypophosphatemia, hypermagnesemia
Periodic paralysis

NEUROMUSCULAR JUNCTION
Myasthenia gravis
Lambert-Eaton syndrome
Botulism
Hypermagnesemia
Others

NEUROPATHY
Guillain-Barré syndrome
Porphyria
Diphtheria
Proximal diabetic neuropathy

ANTERIOR HORN CELL
Poliomyelitis
Amyotrophic lateral sclerosis (rarely progresses rapidly)

RADICULOPATHY
Cytomegalovirus polyradiculopathy

Table 2–13 CAUSES OF SLOWLY PROGRESSIVE PROXIMAL WEAKNESS IN ADULTHOOD

MYOPATHIES
  Muscular dystrophies—limb-girdle, facioscapulohumeral, Becker, Emery-Dreifuss
  Inflammatory—polymyositis, dermatomyositis, inclusion body myositis, viral (HIV)
  Metabolic—acid-maltase deficiency, lipid-storage, mitochondrial
  Endocrine—thyroid, parathyroid, adrenal, pituitary disorders
  Toxic—alcohol, corticosteroids, local injections of narcotics; colchicine, chloroquine

NEUROMUSCULAR JUNCTION
  Myasthenia gravis
  Lambert-Eaton syndrome

NEUROPATHY
  Chronic inflammatory demyelinating polyradiculoneuropathy
  Proximal diabetic neuropathy

ANTERIOR HORN CELL
  Spinal muscular atrophy
  Amyotrophic lateral sclerosis

proximal weakness using the term "proximal myopathy." Neurogenic disease can cause proximal weakness; of the slowly progressive neuropathies, chronic inflammatory demyelinating polyneuropathy is the best example. Hyporeflexia and sensory involvement usually distinguish this disorder from myopathies. Patients with generalized myasthenia gravis also have proximal weakness, but fatigue is conspicuous, and most also have involvement of ocular and bulbar muscles. The less common myasthenic syndrome (Lambert-Eaton), frequently characterized by fatigue and autonomic symptoms as well as proximal weakness, is often mistakenly diagnosed as a myopathy. The anterior horn cell disorders, amyotrophic lateral sclerosis and spinal muscular atrophy, may present with proximal weakness, although the weakness is often asymmetric (see Chapter 9). The presence of fasciculations and, for amyotrophic lateral sclerosis, hyperreflexia (as well as other signs of upper motor neuron involvement) help to distinguish these conditions from myopathy.

PROGRESSIVE DISTAL WEAKNESS

Distal weakness (Table 2–14) is usually caused by peripheral neuropathy or anterior horn cell disease. The most common myopathy presenting with distal weakness is myotonic dystrophy. More rare causes of distal muscle weakness due to primary muscle disease include inclusion body myositis, distal myopathy, scapuloperoneal and facioscapulohumeral dystrophies, centronuclear (myotubular) myopathy, and nemaline myopathy. Selective bilateral weakness of the gastrocnemius and soleus muscles strongly suggests the autosomal recessive, distal myopathy of Miyoshi.[7] In this condition, and in some other causes of distal myopathic weakness (such as scapuloperoneal dystrophy), the extensor digitorum brevis muscle is hypertrophied, a sign seldom seen in neurogenic disease. Virtually none of the myopathies associated with systemic disease present primarily with distal weakness.

Table 2–14 CAUSES OF PROGRESSIVE DISTAL WEAKNESS IN ADULTHOOD

MYOPATHIES
  Myotonic dystrophy
  Distal myopathy (four major forms)
  Scapuloperoneal syndrome
  Facioscapulohumeral dystrophy
  Inclusion body myositis
  Nemaline myopathy
  Centronuclear myopathy

METABOLIC DISORDERS
  Debrancher deficiency
  Phosphorylase *b* kinase deficiency
  Lipid storage myopathy (usually proximal)

PERIPHERAL NEUROPATHY (MOST TYPES)

ANTERIOR HORN CELL
  Spinal muscular atrophy
  Amyotrophic lateral sclerosis

PROGRESSIVE OCULAR MUSCLE OR BULBAR WEAKNESS

The reasons for the remarkable sparing of ocular muscles in most myopathies remain a mystery. On the other hand, certain muscle disorders primarily affect the ocular muscles (Table 2–15). Ptosis alone is seen in myotonic dystrophy, whereas ptosis plus extraocular muscle involvement occurs in mitochondrial myopathies, oculopharyngeal muscular dystrophy, and centronuclear myopathy. Because their dysconjugate gaze is long-standing, these patients rarely complain of double vision, which is a frequent complaint of those with recent-onset myasthenia gravis and other neuromuscular junction disorders.

The extraocular muscles show no significant weakness in most peripheral neuropathies or in amyotrophic lateral sclerosis. The reason they are spared is unknown, although it may be partially explained in peripheral neuropathy by the relatively short length of the axons that innervate them. The sparing of the eye muscles in motor neuron disease is accounted for less easily; weakness of extraocular muscles may develop in patients with motor neuron disease who live for many years with chronic ventilatory support.

Table 2–15 NEUROMUSCULAR DISEASES CAUSING PROGRESSIVE OCULAR MUSCLE WEAKNESS

MYOPATHIES
Kearns-Sayre syndrome, other mitochondrial myopathies
Ocular muscular dystrophy
Oculopharyngeal muscular dystrophy
Myotonic dystrophy (uncommonly)
Centronuclear (myotubular) myopathy
Hyperthyroidism

NEUROMUSCULAR JUNCTION
Myasthenia gravis
Lambert-Eaton syndrome (uncommon presentation)
Congenital myasthenia
Infantile botulism

Table 2–16 NEUROMUSCULAR DISEASES CAUSING PROGRESSIVE BULBAR WEAKNESS

MYOPATHIES
Oculopharyngeal muscular dystrophy
Myotonic dystrophy
Inflammatory myopathy
　Polymyositis
　Dermatomyositis
　Inclusion body myositis
Scapuloperoneal syndrome
Hyperthyroidism (rare)

NEUROMUSCULAR JUNCTION
Myasthenia gravis
Lambert-Eaton syndrome

PERIPHERAL NEUROPATHIES
Chronic inflammatory demyelinating polyneuropathy (rare)
Diphtheritic polyneuropathy

ANTERIOR HORN CELL
Amyotrophic lateral sclerosis
Progressive bulbar or pseudobulbar palsy
X-linked bulbospinal muscular atrophy (Kennedy syndrome)

Bulbar weakness, including difficulty swallowing, coughing, and speaking, is unusual in most myopathies but does occur in inclusion body myositis, polymyositis, and dermatomyositis and is prominent in oculopharyngeal dystrophy and myotonic dystrophy. Bulbar weakness may be seen in certain other myopathies but is more characteristic of neuromuscular junction and motor neuron disorders (Table 2–16).

OTHER PRESENTATIONS OF MYOPATHIES

Myopathies may also present with episodic weakness, myoglobinuria, muscle pain, or myotonia. Unexplained respiratory failure occasionally is the first sign of several myopathies (see Chapter 12).

LABORATORY EVALUATION

Blood Studies

CREATINE KINASE

The serum creatine kinase (CK), previously termed creatine phosphokinase, is the single most useful blood study for the evaluation of patients with neuromuscular disease. CK catalyzes the reversible reaction of adenosine triphosphate (ATP) and creatine to form adenosine diphosphate (ADP) and phosphocreatine. It is elevated in the majority of patients with myopathies but may be normal in slowly progressive muscle disorders. Even in the more progressive disorders such as Duchenne dystrophy, however, the CK falls toward normal late in the course, as muscle mass diminishes.[74] The CK level may be helpful in distinguishing different forms of muscular dystrophy. For example, the ambulatory patient with Duchenne muscular dystrophy invariably has a CK value at least 10 times (and often up to 100 times) normal, whereas in most other myopathies, such as limb-girdle muscular dystrophy, there are lesser elevations.[12,59]

Many times the CK will rise modestly (usually to less than 10 times normal) in neuromuscular diseases of neuropathic cause. Examples include the spinal muscular atrophies and amyotrophic lateral sclerosis.[96] The elevation probably reflects damage to muscle fibers that are struggling to cope with increased demands placed on weak muscles.

Elevations in CK can occur with minor muscle trauma, viral illnesses, or strenuous exercise and on a hereditary basis.[35,45,61] The CK is higher in black individuals (Table 2–17).[11] *In a patient without muscle weakness or pain, it is unusual for a slightly (threefold or less) elevated CK to be caused by an unsuspected or developing myopathy.* The most common cause of abnormally high CK blood levels (hyperCKemia) in asymptomatic persons is recent exercise or injury. We repeat the CK determination after 5 days of rest without vigorous exercise, and pursue further evaluation only if the CK elevation persists. If the CK elevation is less than two to three times normal, evaluation is frequently unrewarding, but if the level is increased more than fivefold, subjects often prove to have an underlying myopathy that has not yet emerged clinically.

Table 2–17 CAUSES OF SUSTAINED ELEVATIONS OF CREATINE KINASE WITHOUT CLINICAL NEUROMUSCULAR DISEASE

Exercise (acute or chronic)
Black race
Enlarged muscles
Muscle trauma—frequent falls, injections, EMG needles
Active psychosis or delirium
Drug use—alcohol, narcotics, and others
Endocrine disorders—hypothyroidism, hypoparathyroidism
Presymptomatic myopathies—muscular dystrophy (all forms), polymyositis, McArdle's disease
Carrier state—Duchenne and Becker dystrophies
Hereditary hyper-CK-emia
Malignant hyperthermia

CK occurs as three isozymes: MM, the principal form in cardiac and skeletal muscle; MB, occurring in a higher proportion than normal in regenerating cardiac and skeletal muscle; and BB, occurring predominantly in brain.[89] The relatively higher amount of CK-MB in diseased heart muscle once led to the hope that one might recognize coexisting cardiac disease within the myopathies by an elevation of CK-MB, but elevated CK-MB is found within the skeletal muscle—and consequently in the serum—of patients with active myopathy or even with chronic strenuous exercise,[79,80] so that it is an unreliable indicator.

The CK level may not be elevated in some myopathies or may even be *lowered* by a number of factors, as indicated in Table 2–18.[45,94] Occasionally,

Table 2–18 CAUSES OF NORMAL CREATINE KINASE LEVEL IN THE PRESENCE OF ACTIVE MYOPATHY

Muscle wasting (must be profound)
Corticosteroid administration*
Hereditary factors*
Collagen diseases*
Alcoholism*
Hyperthyroidism*

*It is likely that muscle wasting is the cause of lowered CK in each of the conditions listed.

benign elevations of CK appear on a genetic basis.[51,85]

Serum tests for other muscle enzymes are considerably less valuable than determining the level of CK. The aspartate aminotransferase and lactate dehydrogenase levels, although less markedly elevated than CK, are often obtained more routinely, and if found to be elevated, may provide an early clue to possible myopathy. Similarly, alanine aminotransferase and aldolase levels may be slightly elevated. All four of these other enzymes, however, are present in liver and other tissues at levels equal to or greater than those in muscle and consequently have little or no value in the evaluation and follow-up of patients with neuromuscular disease. Gamma-glutamyl transferase (GGT), which is found at low levels or is absent in normal muscle, is usually normal in patients with neuromuscular disease. Because GGT is elevated in patients with hepatocellular disease, its determination can be helpful in evaluating the patient with an elevated CK for the presence of coincidental liver disease, although GGT is elevated in patients with myotonic dystrophy who show no clinical or other laboratory evidence of liver disease.[3]

SERUM CREATININE

Patients with severe muscle wasting from any cause, including myopathy, have serum creatinine values below normal. Levels of 0.1 to 0.4 mg/100 mL (normal 0.8–1.2 mg/100 mL) are frequent[32] and can lead to an underestimation of the severity of coincidental renal disease. Occasionally, depressed serum creatinine values provide a clue that muscle wasting is more profound and long-standing than the clinical findings suggest.

OTHER BLOOD STUDIES

Abnormal serum potassium or calcium levels should prompt consideration of a related endocrinopathy or malignancy or of an acquired metabolic disorder (see Chapter 10). Complications of myopathies may occasionally cause alterations in the results of routine blood studies. For instance, respiratory insufficiency may lead to hypoxia and hypercapnia, which in turn cause an elevated hematocrit and serum bicarbonate level.

Urine Studies

Serum and urine may contain myoglobin as an accompaniment to muscle breakdown, particularly in metabolic disorders of muscle (Chapter 6). When large quantities are excreted, urine tests for blood are positive. Smaller increases in serum or urine myoglobin may be detected in slowly progressive muscle diseases and even in the carrier state for disorders such as Duchenne dystrophy.[27]

Measurement of the 24-hour urinary creatinine excretion provides a convenient estimate of skeletal muscle mass.[30] Precise and accurate measurements of creatinine excretion depend on consuming a diet free of animal flesh prior to and during the period of urine collection and on a careful 24-hour urine collection.[30] Creatine, the precursor of creatinine, is made by the kidney and other organs and then taken up by muscle, where it is used to synthesize creatine phosphate. Creatine phosphate and creatine are in turn broken down to creatinine, which is then excreted in the urine. Creatine excretion depends even more than does creatinine on dietary intake of meats and is of little value in the clinical setting.[30,33] Only when a patient receives a meat-free diet for several days prior to and during an inpatient evaluation can one make reliable measurements of creatinine and creatine excretion.

Muscle Imaging Procedures

Plain roentgenography of muscle is only helpful in the evaluation of mass lesions for calcium, fat, or tumor. On the

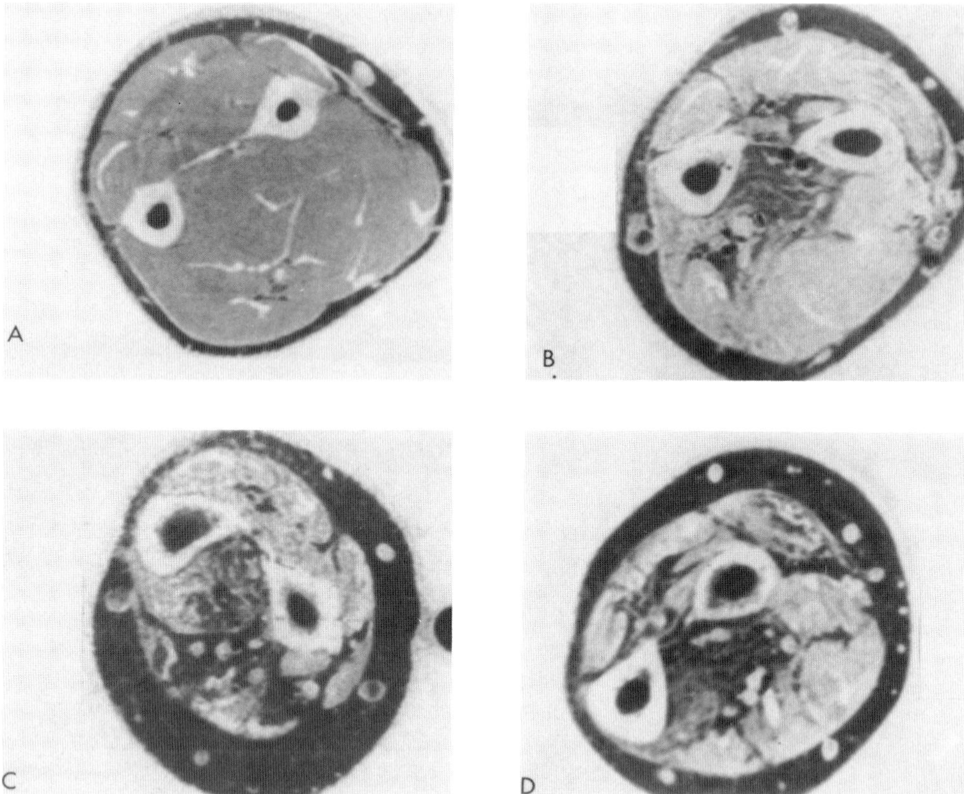

Figure 2–19. Computed tomographic scans of the thigh. (*A*) Normal. (*B*) Focal replacement of muscle by fat. (*C* and *D*) Focal and diffuse replacement of muscle by fat. (Scans courtesy of William Torch.)

other hand, computed tomography and magnetic resonance imaging of muscle show distinctive and diagnostically helpful abnormalities in many muscle diseases. In particular, a distinction between fat and muscle can be made (Fig. 2–19), helping to differentiate true hypertrophy from pseudohypertrophy of muscle. In addition, it has been suggested that inflammatory myopathies can be distinguished from muscular dystrophy.

to disordered neuromuscular transmission, or is the result of an upper motor neuron lesion should be clarified by needle electromyography and nerve stimulation studies. The findings are generally not specific, however, and must be taken in context with other clinical findings to arrive at a particular diagnosis.

This book mainly focuses on electrodiagnostic findings that characterize myopathies.

ELECTRODIAGNOSIS

In general, the major value of electromyography is to shed further light on the pathophysiology of weakness and fatigability. Whether the weakness is of a neurogenic or myogenic origin is due

The Technique of Electromyography

A concentric or monopolar needle electrode is used to record electromyographic activity. Disposable concentric needle electrodes are reliable, well tolerated by patients because they are very sharp, and have no risk of transmitting infection to the patient. The electrical activity of the muscle is amplified and displayed for visual analysis on an oscilloscope. An auditory signal accompanies the visual record. The patient lies relaxed and is periodically asked to contract the muscle under study. The needle electrode is moved into numerous sites in each muscle. At each site the electrical activity is evaluated in three steps:

1. With the muscle totally relaxed.

2. While the patient voluntarily contracts the muscle slightly, the characteristics of individual *motor unit potentials* (amplitude, duration, and phases) are observed.

3. The patient is asked to contract the muscle maximally, and the *recruitment pattern* is analyzed.

Abnormal Spontaneous Activity

Spontaneous activity arising from the endplate is associated with some discomfort for the patient. The shape and discharge frequency help to differentiate spontaneous activity from fibrillations and positive waves. Normal spontaneous endplate activity (Fig. 2–20) is initially negative (upgoing), often dis-

charges profusely at high frequencies, and rapidly attenuates upon needle movement away from the endplate.

Fibrillations (Fig. 2–21A) are spontaneous electrical discharges that are initially positive, very brief in duration (1–3 ms), and low in amplitude (less than 600 μV). Although fibrillations can occasionally be rhythmic and rapid, they can be identified with certainty only when slow and irregular.

Positive sharp waves (Fig. 2–21B) exhibit a different shape, with a marked initial positive deflection, and gradual repolarization and slow hyperpolarization phases. Positive sharp waves have the same pathophysiologic significance as fibrillations and represent the spontaneous discharge of an injured muscle fiber. Discharge patterns are similar to those of fibrillations.

Fibrillations and positive waves, although common in neurogenic disorders, are also present in virtually any muscle disease and indeed even in neuromuscular junction disorders (such as botulism). Their presence, even in a muscle disorder, implies that the muscle fiber has been disconnected from its nerve supply. This can follow segmental necrosis, when a part of the fiber downstream from the necrotic area becomes isolated from the endplate region of the fiber. In general, fibrillations and positive sharp waves are numerous in active

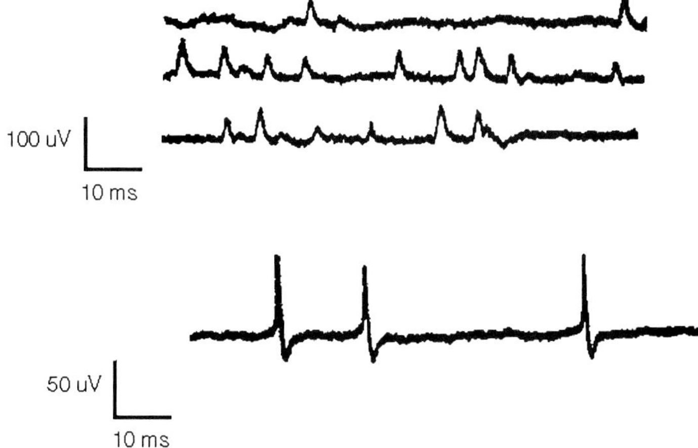

Figure 2–20. Two types of normal endplate activity, recorded with a concentric needle electrode: initially negative diphasic potentials (*bottom*) and negative spikes (*top*).

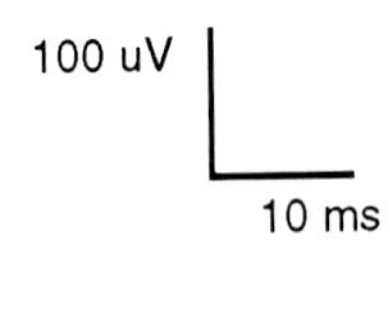
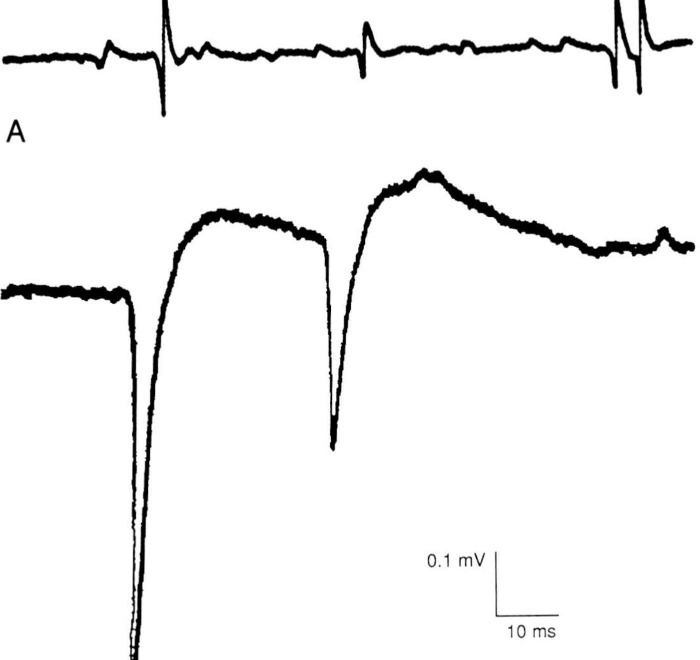
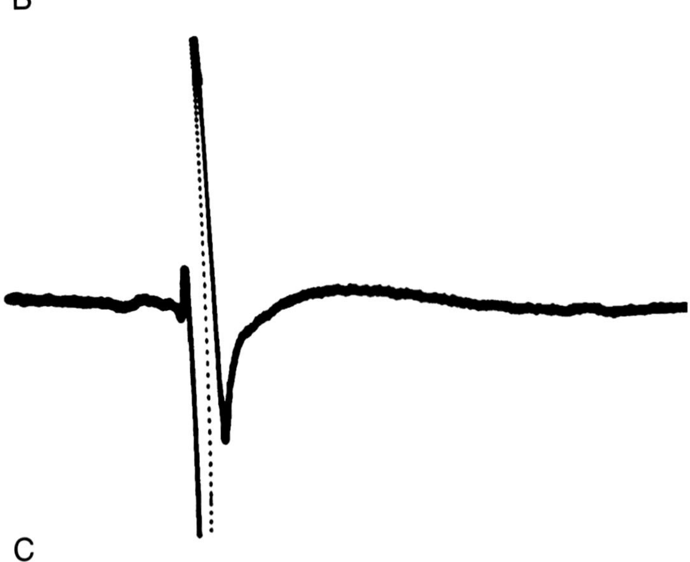
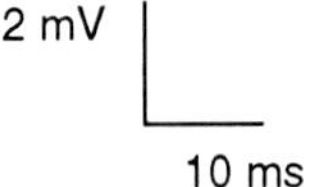

Figure 2–21. (*A*) Needle EMG recording of fibrillations. (*B*) Positive sharp waves. (*C*) Fasciculation.

disease and inconspicuous in disorders that are very slowly progressive or indolent. This point may be particularly useful in evaluating, for example, a patient with inflammatory myopathy, in whom the presence of profuse fibrillations and positive waves suggests active disease.[49]

Fasciculation potentials (Fig. 2–21C) represent the spontaneous discharge of one or more motor units and are most common in chronic neurogenic disorders. Fasciculations typically discharge singly, or slowly at a rate between 1 and 5 per second,[88] and they are larger in amplitude and longer in duration than fibrillations. Fasciculations are the result of irritability of the neuronal cell body or axon.[73,97] They may be benign, as in tense or incompletely relaxed muscle, or a sign of serious underlying neuronal disease, particularly motor neuron disease.

Complex repetitive discharges (previously called high-frequency discharges or pseudomyotonia) are particularly common in patients with inflammatory myopathy but may be found in many other disorders.[62] Both the onset and cessation are abrupt and the shape is usually complex and polyphasic, consisting of action potentials from groups of muscle fibers firing at high frequencies and in near synchrony (Fig. 2–22A). The presence of large numbers of complex repetitive discharges indicates active disease.

Cramp is the high-frequency discharge of many muscle fibers and is usually associated with intense muscular pain. The electromyogram of a cramp shows a full recruitment pattern on the oscilloscope screen (Fig. 2–22B). The cramp is usually abolished by muscle stretch, with abrupt cessation of motor unit discharges.

Myotonia (see p. 342) occurs both with insertion or movement of the needle electrode and when muscle is percussed or voluntarily contracted. Myotonic discharges are high-frequency discharges of single muscle fibers, which wax and wane in both amplitude and frequency (Fig. 2–22C). The discharges appear as either positive waves or brief (<5 ms) spikes and vary in frequency from 40 to 80 Hz. Myotonia is almost always a sign of primary muscle disease and appears in the hereditary myotonic disorders, periodic paralysis, myositis, acid maltase deficiency, and hypothyroidism. Myotonic discharges may be found in any of these conditions, even without clinical evidence of myotonia.

Neuromyotonia appears in the clinical disorder of continuous muscle fiber activity (Isaac's syndrome) (see p. 22), where there is continuous muscle rippling and stiffness;[62] neuromyotonia also occurs in tetany. Neuromyotonic discharges are single muscle fiber potentials that fire at rates of 150 to 300 Hz (Fig. 2–22D); because of the very high rate of firing, the potentials often decrease in amplitude during the long, continuous runs of activity.[44] The discharges are not affected by voluntary activity of the muscle.

Voluntary Activity

THE NORMAL MOTOR UNIT

The *motor unit potential* is the sum of the action potentials of the individual muscle fibers in the activated motor unit that lie within the field of the recording electrode. Normally, no more than 10 to 30 fibers contribute to the shape of the motor unit potential, and it is likely that only 3 to 8 fibers contribute to the high-amplitude, negative phase seen during a typical clinical EMG study (Fig. 2–23, top).[17] The configuration of a motor unit potential may be monophasic, diphasic, triphasic, or polyphasic (more than four phases). The shape of the motor unit potential in normal individuals is influenced by the person's age, the muscle being studied, and the type of electrode used.[34]

Activation of motor units during weak voluntary muscle contraction permits the analysis of motor unit configuration. Duration, amplitude, and polyphasic wave activity are initially measured by visual inspection of the screen. In

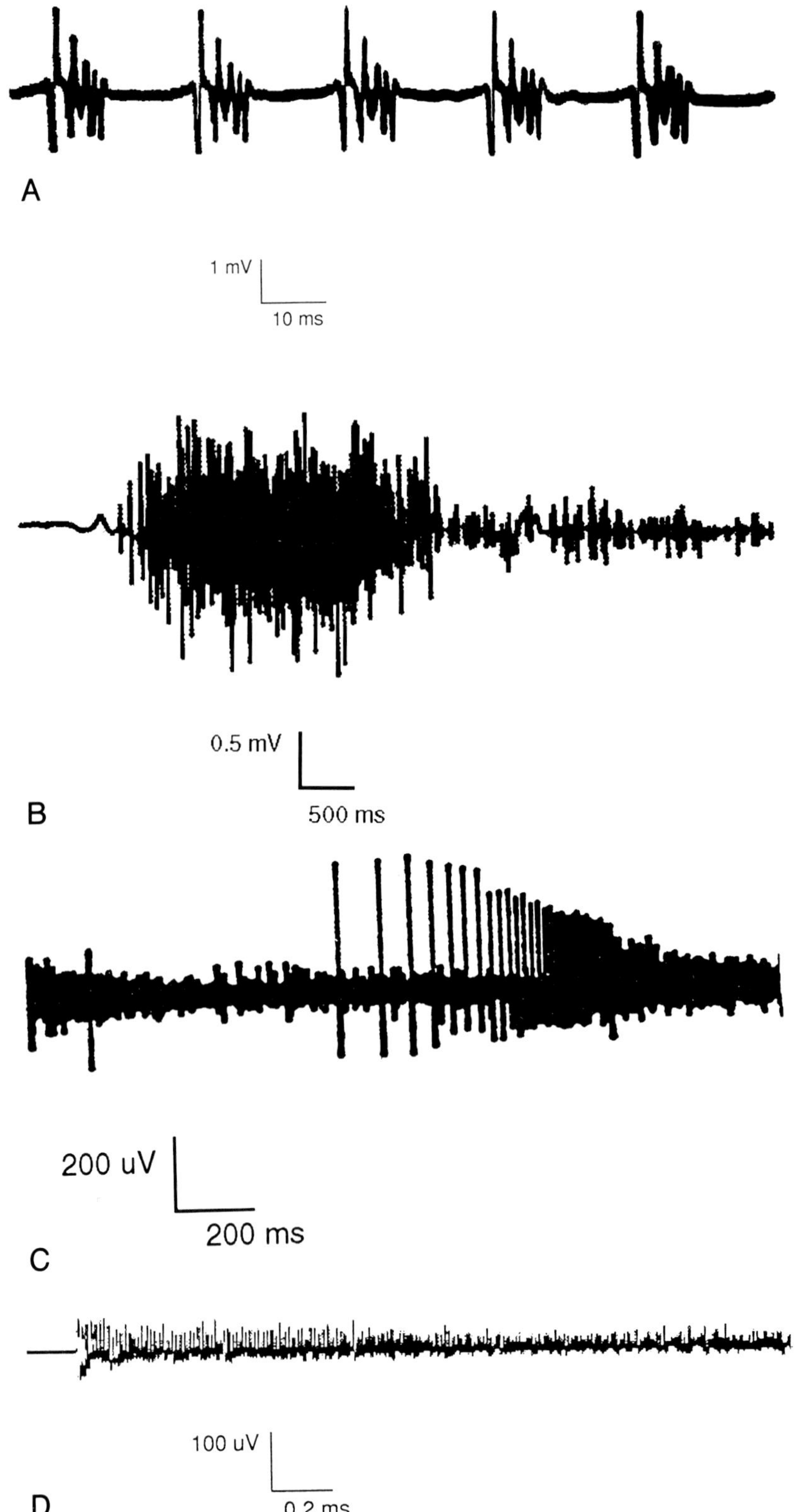

Figure 2–22. (*A*) Complex repetitive discharge. (*B*) Muscle cramp. (*C*) Myotonic discharges. (*D*) Neuromyotonia.

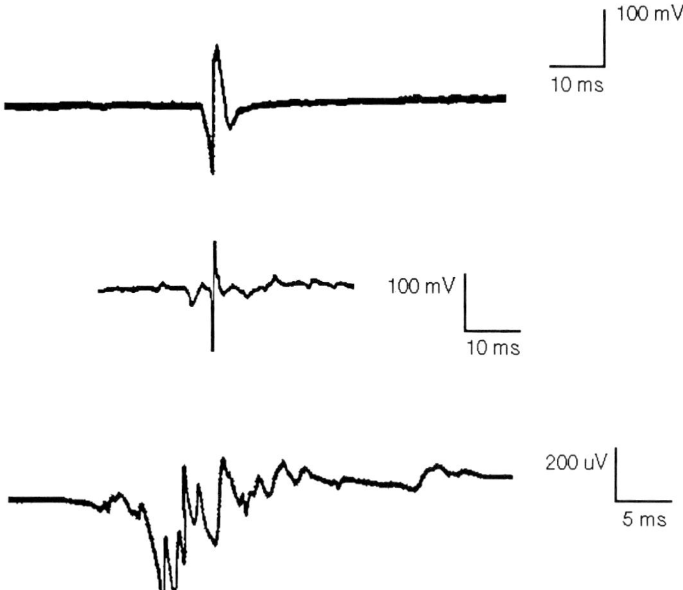

Figure 2–23. (*Top*) Normal motor unit potential. (*Middle*) Myopathic motor unit potential. (*Bottom*) Neurogenic motor unit potential.

neurogenic weakness, motor unit potentials are enlarged in amplitude, duration, and polyphasic wave activity (Fig. 2–23, bottom); they can be identified by a louder sound on the auditory output (thunk). Short-duration motor unit potentials are found in diseases with either anatomic or physiologic loss of muscle fibers from the motor unit territory or atrophy of individual muscle fibers (Fig. 2–23, middle). The amplitude and duration of motor unit potentials may be artifactually reduced by incorrect filter settings during EMG testing. An electrical short circuit in a recording electrode or connecting cables, or a reduction in surface area on the recording electrodes after improper sharpening, may produce similar artifactual disturbances of motor unit configuration.

SHORT-DURATION MOTOR UNITS

In primary muscle disease, motor unit potentials are brief in duration and reduced in amplitude. (These are termed "myopathic" potentials, with the caveat that follows.) All forms of muscular dystrophy, inflammatory myopathy, and congenital myopathy usually feature "myopathic" motor unit potentials, but short-duration and low-amplitude motor unit potentials also may occur in neuromuscular junction disorders (for example, botulinin intoxication, the myasthenic [Lambert-Eaton] syndrome, and myasthenia gravis) and during early reinnervation after nerve injury. On the other hand, not all disorders of muscle have abnormal motor unit configuration; for example, the motor unit potentials may be normal in both amplitude and duration in patients with disuse atrophy of muscle or thyrotoxic myopathy.[13]

Polyphasic motor unit potentials (Fig. 2–24A) have, by definition, five or more phases. Thus, at least five areas or phases of the potential can be found on different sides of the baseline. It is useful to consider the incidence of polyphasic potentials within the muscle when performing quantitative needle EMG. Normal muscle contains up to 12% polyphasic potentials, but the percentage may rise as high as 25% or more in neuropathy and myopathy. Small differences may be difficult to determine

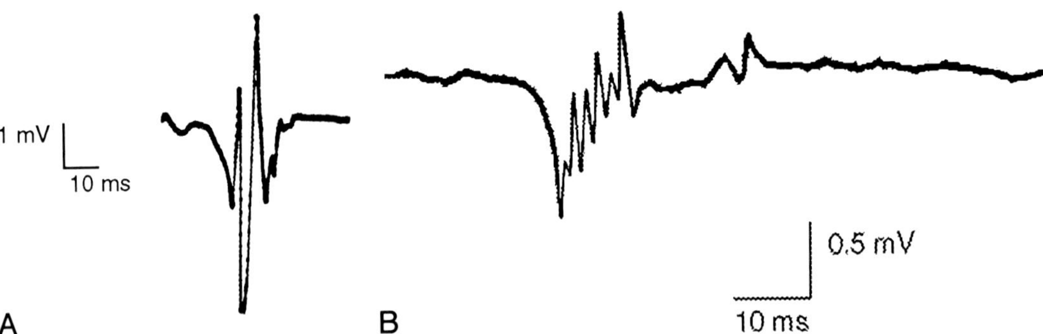

Figure 2–24. (*A*) Polyphasic motor unit potential. (*B*) Long-duration motor unit potential.

without quantitative techniques.[13] An accurate analysis of excessive polyphasic wave activity requires a systematic investigation of at least 20 motor unit potentials rather than simple visual inspection (see Quantitative Electromyography, below).

LONG-DURATION MOTOR UNITS

Long-duration motor units (Fig. 2–24B) are frequently seen in patients with chronic myopathy as well as neuropathy. Fiber splitting and reinnervation presumably lead to the increased duration of motor units in long-standing myopathy. Satellite potentials, small and delayed components of the motor unit that are frequently time-locked to its main component, may be very long in duration.[49] These long-duration motor units occur in conditions such as chronic polymyositis, recurrent myoglobinuria,[68] Emery-Dreifuss muscular dystrophy,[56] and inclusion body myositis.[23] Thus, electrodiagnostic findings of long-duration motor units make differentiation between a chronic, severe primary muscle disease and neuropathy very difficult. This confusion is particularly characteristic of inclusion body myositis, where long-duration motor units are accompanied by marked fibrillation wave activity, a reduced recruitment pattern in weak muscles, increased fiber density, and increased jitter.[23] This issue has been addressed by Partanen and Lang[65] in a study correlating amplitude and duration of individual motor units with duration of disease in polymyositis. Early in the course, the duration and amplitude of motor unit potentials were clearly reduced, but in patients with long-standing or relapsing polymyositis, the duration and amplitude of many motor unit potentials increased. In this setting, two populations of motor units often coexist: simple potentials (less than five phases) of abnormally brief duration, and complex polyphasic potentials (five or more phases) of prolonged duration. Using quantitative EMG to identify a population of simple potentials with reduced duration usually is of great help in recognizing the myopathic nature of the disorder.[13,90]

Quantitative Electromyography

Quantitative EMG measures the configurations of the motor unit potential and the recruitment pattern.[13] The duration and peak-to-peak amplitude (Fig. 2–25) of at least 20 different motor unit potentials are usually obtained in seven to nine insertions and are measured at a gain of 0.1 mV/cm. Measurements are usually made with a concentric needle electrode while the patient gives a weak contraction. The mean duration is de-

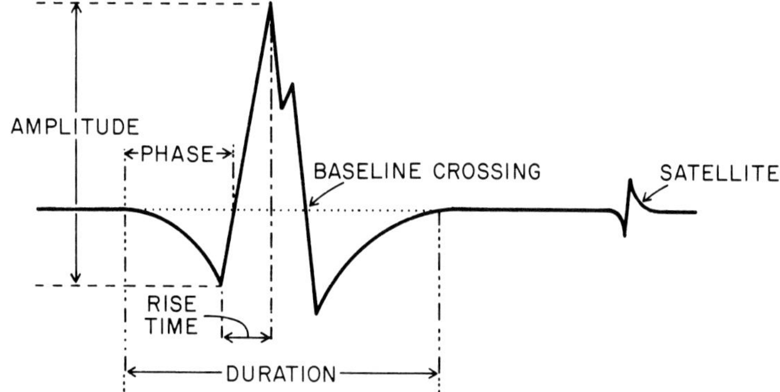

Figure 2–25. Schematic representation of motor unit potential parameters.

termined both for potentials of simple shape and for those exhibiting polyphasia. The incidence of polyphasic potentials is determined and compared with the 95% confidence limits for age-matched normal subjects. Abnormality is defined by a duration of motor unit potentials differing from the normal mean by more than 20% or by an amplitude differing by more than 40%.[13] More than 12% polyphasia is abnormal. In addition, the pattern of recruitment is recorded at full effort using a continuous, direct-writing strip chart (Fig. 2–26, top); the amplitude of the total electrical activity, termed "the envelope" (disregarding solitary high peaks), is measured. In subjects more than 15

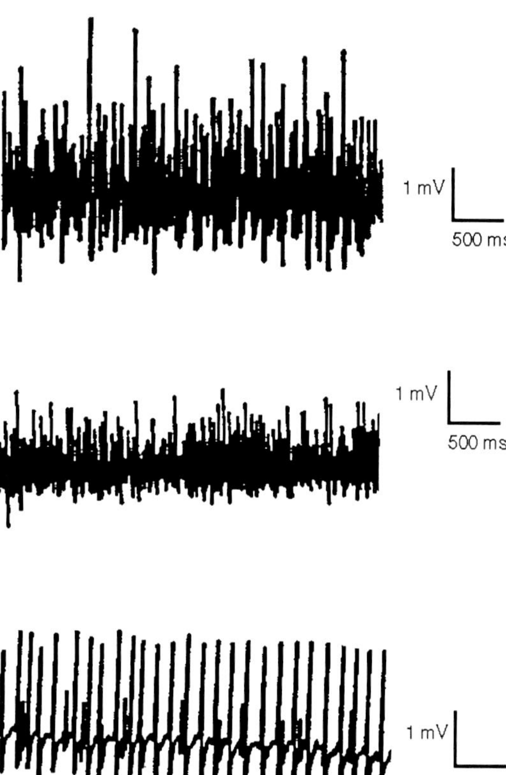

Figure 2–26. Maximum voluntary contraction of normal tibialis anterior (*top*), early recruitment in myopathy (*middle*), and reduced recruitment with high discharge frequencies in neuropathy (*bottom*).

years old, values less than 2 mV suggests myopathy.

In patients with myopathy (Fig. 2–26, middle), the average duration of the motor unit potential is shortened by 20% to 60%, reflecting loss of fibers. In more advanced weakness, the shortening of the duration results from the loss of the slow initial component and the terminal component of the motor unit potential because of the reduced fiber density in the periphery of the motor unit. Alterations in motor unit amplitude have less diagnostic significance because this measurement depends on the distance between the generator and the needle electrode. A reduced amplitude may be seen as often in neuropathy as in myopathy.

The amplitude of the recruitment pattern developed at full effort parallels the changes in duration and amplitude of individual motor units and is reduced in muscular dystrophy and other myopathies. *In general, however, a full pattern of recruitment (motor unit potentials filling the oscilloscope screen) in a weak muscle indicates early recruitment and strongly suggests myopathy* (see Fig. 2–26, middle). In long-standing neurogenic weakness seen with a chronic neuropathy, the recruitment pattern is that of individual motor units even at maximum effort (Fig. 2–26, bottom).

The electrodiagnostic evaluation of a patient with rapidly evolving muscle weakness is often difficult. When weakness is acute and severe and motor unit potentials are obviously reduced in duration and amplitude with early recruitment, the diagnosis of myopathy is highly likely. In patients with less marked weakness, where the changes in motor unit potential are more subtle, or in those with a more protracted illness and some long-duration motor units, the use of quantitative techniques is especially applicable. Although these techniques take more time, computer-assisted measurement of motor unit potentials can now be used to facilitate their application.

Electrical Stimulation Tests: Nerve Conduction Studies

Because neurogenic disorders may produce weakness that mimics the clinical features of a muscle disease, ruling them out by evaluating motor and sensory nerve conduction is important. In particular, acquired demyelinating neuropathies such as the Guillain-Barré syndrome and chronic inflammatory demyelinating polyneuropathy may be mistaken for myopathies clinically but will usually show slowing of nerve conduction (Fig. 2–27). In myopathies, on the other hand, nerve conduction studies generally are normal.

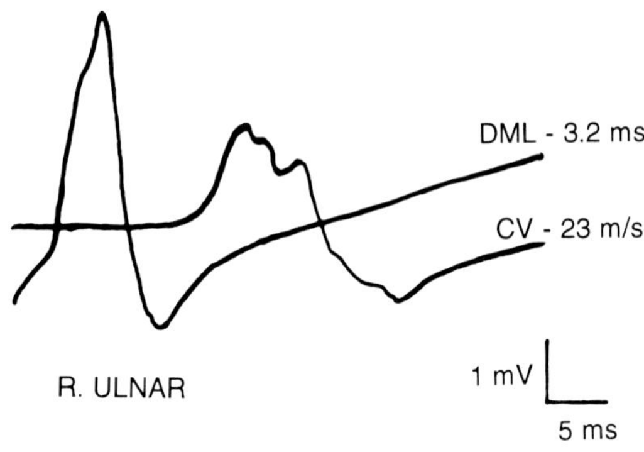

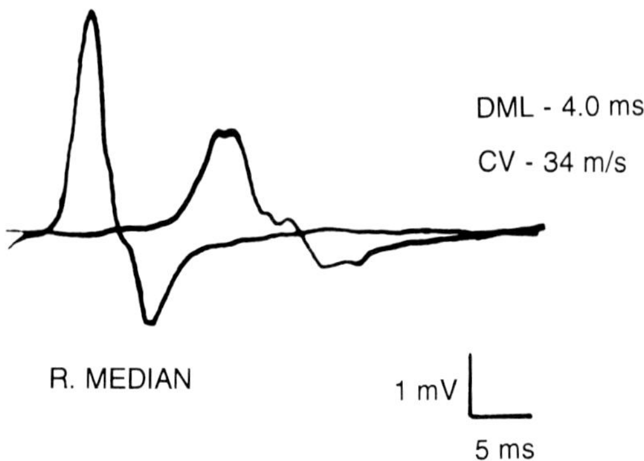

Figure 2–27. Motor nerve conduction studies in a patient with chronic inflammatory polyradiculoneuropathy, illustrating dispersion and slowing secondary to demyelination. DML = distal motor latency; CV = conduction velocity.

These studies are also important in differentiating demyelinating from axonal neuropathies.

In evaluating the weak patient, an important advantage of nerve conduction studies is that results do not depend on patient cooperation. If the muscle response to nerve stimulation is greater than one would expect from the voluntary activity, the cause for the weakness is proximal to the point of stimulation.[48] Such weakness may result from upper motor neuron dysfunction or from incomplete effort.

Factors that contribute to nerve conduction slowing in normal subjects include reduced limb temperature, age over 65 years or age less than 5 years, and submaximal stimulation.[55] Temperature is an extremely important factor that is commonly ignored. Reduced temperature of an extremity decreases nerve conduction velocity in normal nerves. In patients with cool limbs, especially those with arterial insufficiency or muscle wasting and loss of normal insulating tissue, velocity decreases 2.5 m/s for each degree that skin temperature falls below 34°C.[55] Age-related changes must be considered in infants and elderly patients.

MOTOR NERVE CONDUCTION

Technique of Testing. Stimulating electrodes are either hand-held or securely taped on clean skin over the nerve at the point of stimulation. An electrical stimulus is applied to the nerve at an intensity approximately 25% greater than that required to produce a maximum response of the muscle. The compound muscle action potential (CMAP) is recorded, amplified, and displayed on a cathode ray oscilloscope (Fig. 2–28). A stimulus artifact

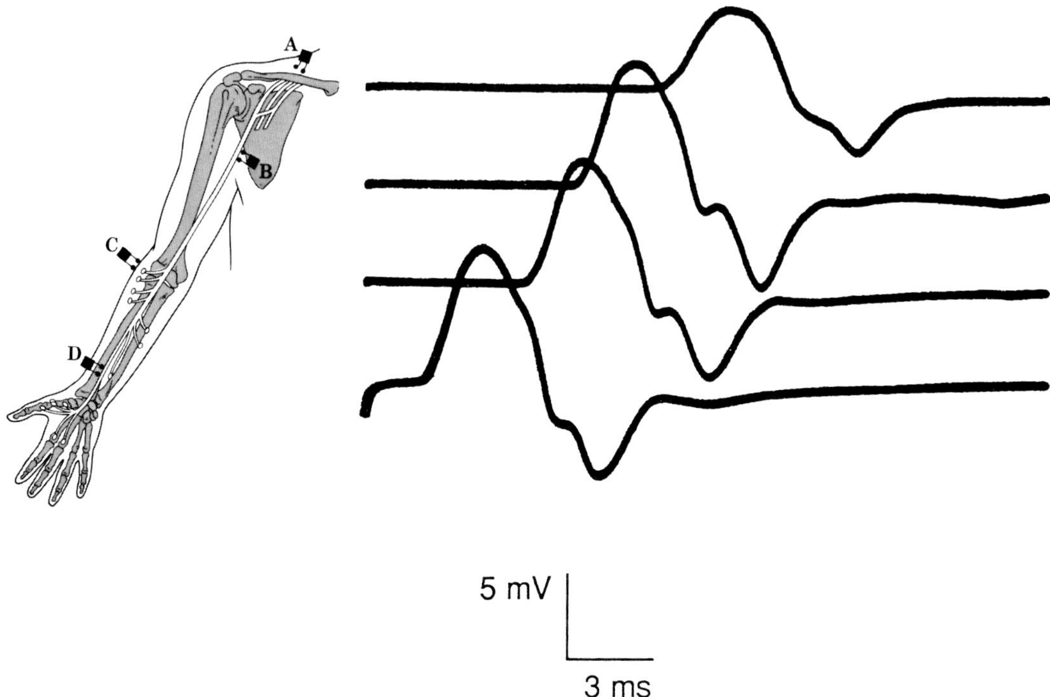

Figure 2–28. Evoked compound muscle action potentials (CMAPs) recorded over the abductor pollicis brevis muscle. (*Left*) The median nerve was stimulated at four different sites (*A–D*), producing similar CMAPs (*right*) after different latencies.

appears on the record at the moment of stimulation of the nerve; after several milliseconds, the action potential of the muscle begins. The delay between the stimulus and the muscle action potential is the time for impulse conduction from the point of stimulation of the nerve, including time across the neuromuscular junction. The CMAP of the muscle is the summation of the potentials of all the muscle fibers that respond to nerve stimulation. The response is normally a biphasic potential with an initial negative (upgoing) phase. The latency of the muscle potential is measured from the onset of the stimulus artifact to the onset of the negative phase. A stimulus is then given at a second point along the course of the nerve. The difference in latency between the two points of nerve stimulation permits calculation of the conduction velocity of the most rapidly conducting nerve fibers in that segment (see Fig. 2–28A–D). The amplitude of the CMAP, usually measured from baseline to negative peak, is expressed in millivolts. The size of the evoked muscle action potential is proportional to the number and size of responsive muscle fibers.

Changes in the amplitude of the CMAP can be followed over time to estimate the amount of functioning muscle tissue. Table 2–19 gives normal data for the most commonly studied peripheral nerves.[38]

Abnormalities of Motor Nerve Conduction. There are two major categories of motor nerve conduction abnormalities:

1. Normal or slightly slowed conduction velocity with reduced CMAP amplitude, a pattern typical of axonal neuropathies but also seen in some severe myopathies.

2. Marked slowing of nerve conduction velocity (less than 70% of the lower limit of normal), often with a relatively normal CMAP amplitude in response to distal simulation but a smaller or desynchronized response to proximal

Table 2–19 NORMAL VALUES— NERVE CONDUCTION STUDIES

MOTOR NERVES

	Amplitude*	Distal Latency†	Conduction Velocity‡
Median	4	4.5	50
Ulnar	4	3.4	50
Peroneal	2	6.5	40
Tibial	4	7.0	40

SENSORY NERVES

	Amplitude*	Distal Latency§
Median	9	3.7
Ulnar	8	3.4
Sural	7	4.3

*Lower limit of normal amplitude of the evoked action potential, measured from baseline to negative peak (motor, median nerve; sensory, ulnar nerve).
†Upper limits of normal latency to onset of the evoked response (ms) from stimulation at the second wrist crease or the ankle.
‡Lower limit of normal conduction velocity between elbow and wrist, or knee and ankle (ms).
§Upper limits of normal (ms) latency to peak stimulation of digital nerves, recording at second wrist crease for median and ulnar sensory nerves. Stimulation at calf, 14 cm proximal to recording site at lateral malleolus for sural nerve.

stimulation. This finding suggests a primary demyelinating neuropathy.[43]

Reduced CMAP amplitude with normal conduction velocity may also reflect abnormal neuromuscular transmission (especially Lambert-Eaton syndrome or botulism) or abnormal muscle membrane function, such as myotonic disorders or periodic paralysis. *These abnormalities are useful diagnostically but will be missed without careful attention to CMAP amplitude.* The technique and clinical relevance of this form of testing are discussed below in the section on repetitive nerve stimulation and in Chapter 9.

SENSORY NERVE CONDUCTION

Technique of Testing. The compound sensory nerve action potential

(SNAP) is recorded with surface electrodes placed over the cutaneous sensory nerve or with needle electrodes placed subcutaneously near the nerve. A maximal stimulus is applied, which in normal individuals produces a low-amplitude (usually less than 50–60 μV), triphasic response; an initial small positive phase is followed by a much larger negative phase and another small positive phase. The shape of this potential results from the summation of the nerve action potentials of the large myelinated sensory nerve fibers. The sural nerve and cutaneous nerves such as the digital branches of the median and ulnar nerves are routinely studied (see Table 2–19). Sensory potentials can be recorded from the digital nerves using ring electrodes around the fingers. The potential is recorded over more proximal portions of the nerve (antidromic conduction), or they can be recorded over the mixed nerve with stimulation of the sensory fibers of the digital nerves (orthodromic conduction). The latency of the sensory response is measured from the stimulus artifact to either the onset of the response (from which a conduction velocity of the fastest fibers may be estimated) or, more frequently, to the peak of the negative phase.

Abnormalities of Sensory Nerve Conduction. Abnormalities include (1) a reduction in the amplitude of the sensory action potential, (2) a prolongation of duration, (3) a slowing of conduction velocity or prolonged distal latency, or (4) the absence of, or inability to record, the SNAP. An abnormality of the nerve action potential indicates neuropathy. The sensory action potential is normal in myopathies, diseases of the neuromuscular junction, abnormalities of the muscle membrane, diseases of the anterior horn cell, and in sensory nerve lesions proximal to the dorsal root ganglion. Virtually all of the conditions discussed in this book are associated with normal sensory nerve conduction studies.

REPETITIVE NERVE STIMULATION

Repetitive nerve stimulation is valuable in the diagnosis of disorders of neuromuscular transmission, either presynaptic or postsynaptic. It is also helpful in evaluating disorders of the muscle membrane. In neuromuscular transmission disorders, muscle weakness is the result of failure of endplate potentials to reach the threshold necessary to trigger muscle action potentials.[43] Muscle fibers then fail to contract, and patients experience both weakness and fatigue. For the endplate potential to exceed the threshold and for depolarization to produce a muscle action potential, it is necessary to have (1) a sufficient release of acetylcholine from nerve terminals and (2) a normal number and sensitivity of postsynaptic acetylcholine receptors. Patients with insufficiencies of either type will experience pathologic fatigue and weakness. Repetitive nerve stimulation at low rates in such patients usually produces a decrement in the amplitude of the CMAP during the first few stimuli. The progressive decline in amplitude of the CMAP reflects the loss of individual muscle fiber action potentials that contribute to the larger potential at the start of repetitive stimulation. Different patterns of response are obtained in presynaptic and postsynaptic disorders, as well as in defects of muscle membrane excitation, as discussed below.

Technique of Testing. The examiner selects one or more muscles for recording the CMAP and applies a series of supramaximal stimuli (usually 5–10) to the motor nerve supplying that muscle, at a rate of 2 Hz. The muscles selected usually include the intrinsic hand muscles, trapezius, deltoid, biceps brachii, tibialis anterior, and facial muscles.[76,83] Several technical factors must be considered to avoid false-positive and false-negative results. False-negatives may result from cold temperature (warming to skin temperature of 37°C greatly increases test sensitivity) or ingestion of anticholinesterase medication, which should be avoided for 12 hours if it is safe to do so. False positives result from movement of electrodes, submaximal stimulation, or failure to immobilize the limb. A true decremental response is quite reproducible. High-frequency stimulation also may result in false-positive results. This type of stimulation, which is painful and produces artifactual movement, should rarely be necessary.

Abnormalities of Repetitive Nerve Stimulation. *Myasthenia Gravis.* Myasthenia gravis results from a reduced number of available acetylcho-line receptors in the postsynaptic muscle membrane. Muscle fibers may fail to fire after either low or high rates of nerve discharge or electrical stimulation.[83] In many patients, the first noted CMAP is almost always normal, followed by a decrement ($>10\%$) with either 2-Hz or 3-Hz stimulation (compare Figs. 2–29A and B). The decrement is usually maximal between the first and second responses, without much further decline by the fourth or fifth potential. Normal subjects show a transient slight ($<20\%$) increase in the amplitude of the CMAP (facilitation) immediately following brief exercise (either voluntary or by involuntary tetanic contraction). This is thought to be related to

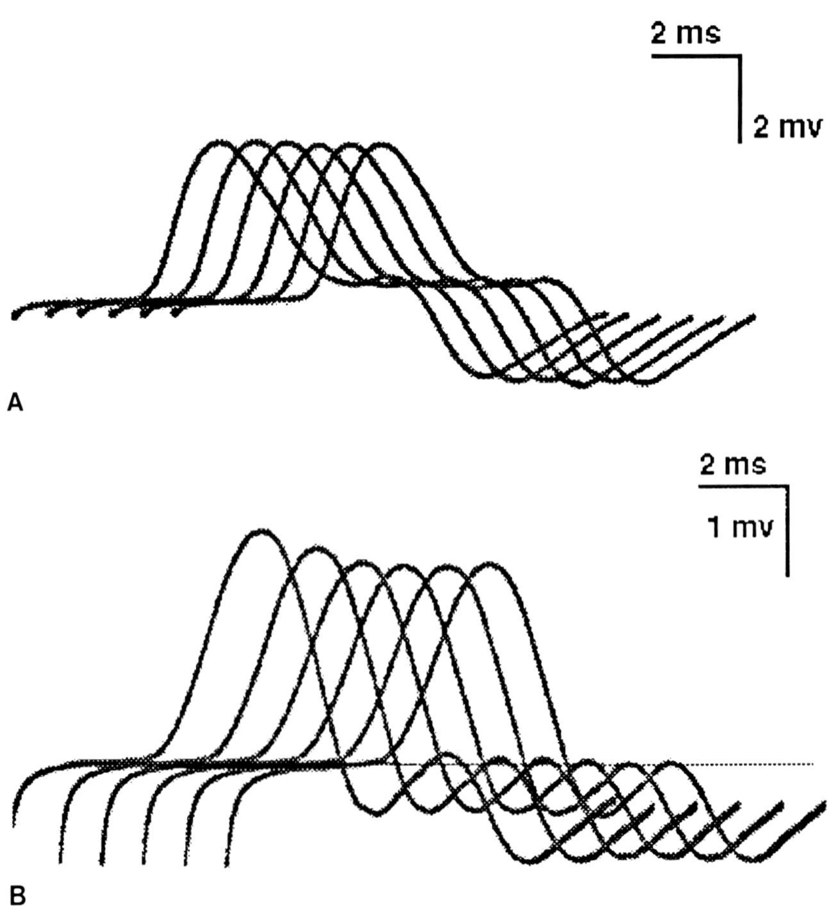

Figure 2–29. (*A*) Normal response to repetitive stimuli (3 Hz). (*B*) Decremental response to repetitive stimuli (3 Hz) in myasthenia gravis.

mobilization of acetylcholine vesicles. In myasthenia gravis, facilitation immediately following exercise often results in an increase of as much as 40% in the amplitude of the first response compared with that obtained from unexercised muscle. This increase is accompanied by a lessening of the decrement observed prior to exercise. A few minutes after exercise, the amplitude of the first potential declines, and the decremental response compared with the pre-exercise response increases. This postactivation exhaustion reflects a reduced output of acetylcholine from the nerve terminal after a period of tetanic muscle contraction.[43] In normal individuals the reduced acetylcholine output will have little effect because of the abundance of acetylcholine receptors on each muscle fiber. In myasthenia gravis, however, the reduction in the number of acetylcholine receptors diminishes the margin of safety.

In recent years, single-fiber electromyography, a highly sensitive means of detecting neuromuscular transmission dysfunction, has been used to evaluate patients with excessive fatigue.[76,77,83] If repetitive nerve stimulation studies are negative (which occurs in 20%–30% of patients with myasthenia gravis, especially those with mainly ocular involvement) single-fiber EMG may be employed. The variability of discharge between two muscle fibers in the same motor unit (jitter) (Fig. 2–30) provides a quantitative measure of abnormal neuromuscular transmission. The main disadvantage of the technique is that it may be abnormal in many neuromuscular diseases; however, a normal finding in a patient with limb fatigue casts strong doubt on the diagnosis of myasthenia.

Lambert-Eaton Myasthenic Syndrome and Other Presynaptic Abnormalities. In contrast to myasthenia gravis, the CMAP in the Lambert-Eaton myasthenic syndrome is markedly reduced in amplitude. Immediately following brief exercise (or tetanic nerve stimulation), however, the amplitude of the

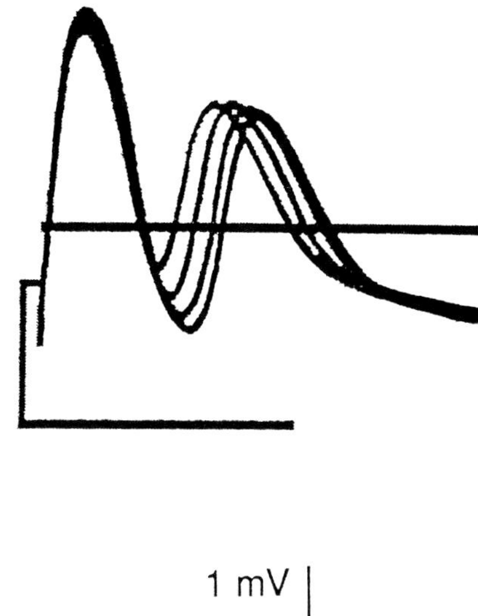

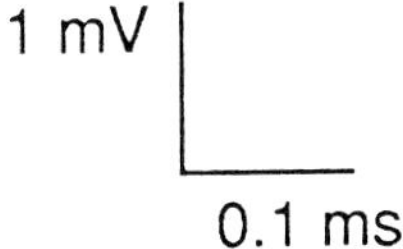

Figure 2–30. Single-fiber EMG recording of two muscle fiber action potentials. The variability of the second fiber with respect to the first is the basis for calculating jitter.

muscle response increases 2- to 20-fold because of pronounced enhancement of postactivation facilitation (compare Figs. 2–31A and 2–31B).

The Lambert-Eaton myasthenic syndrome results from destruction of the active zones on the nerve terminal, causing inadequate release of acetylcholine. Other disorders that impair function of the nerve terminal are listed in Table 2–20.[86] Pronounced facilitation of the CMAP and improved strength are produced in all of these conditions in response to high rates of repetitive nerve stimulation or a strong voluntary contraction. The high firing frequencies lead to an increased concentration of calcium in the region of the nerve terminal, and this in turn stimulates a greater release of quanta of acetylcholine. In most of these conditions, there is also a decremental response to 2- or 3-Hz stimulation, which may be more

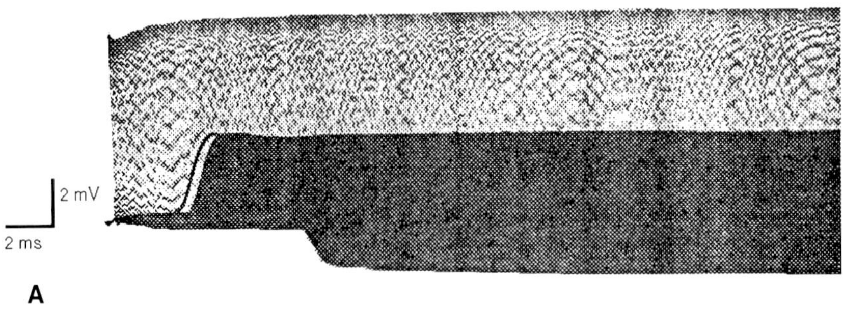

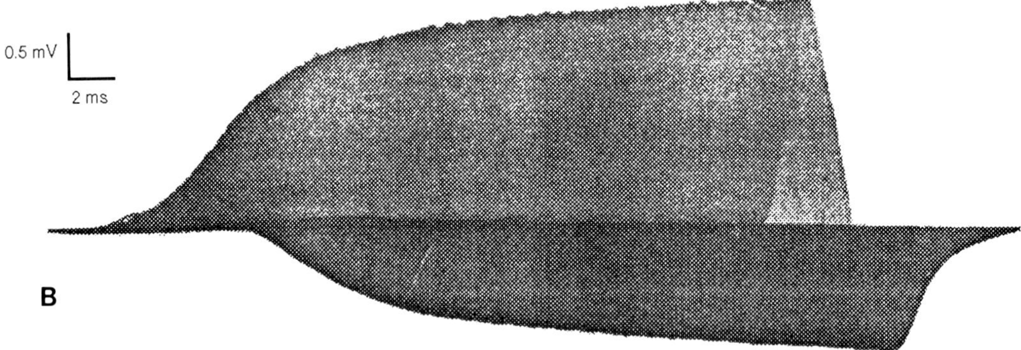

Figure 2–31. Repetitive nerve stimulation (50 Hz) of the abductor digiti minimi in a normal subject (*A*) and in a patient with Lambert-Eaton syndrome (*B*).

Table 2–20 PRESYNAPTIC NEUROMUSCULAR JUNCTION DISORDERS

Botulism
Black widow spider bite
Metabolic disturbances
  Hypermagnesemia
  Hypocalcemia
Medication
  Aminoglycoside antibiotics
    Streptomycin
    Neomycin
    Kanamycin
    Gentamicin
    Tobramycin
    Amikacin
    Polymyxins
  Anticonvulsants
    Phenytoin
    Trimethadione
  Antiarrhythmics
    Quinidine
    Procainamide
    Lithium

conspicuous after exercise-induced postactivation facilitation.

MUSCLE BIOPSY

Indications for Biopsy

If the clinical features and the laboratory and EMG results suggest muscle disease, a muscle biopsy is definitely appropriate. On the other hand, if clinical and laboratory features indicate a neurogenic cause for weakness, the muscle biopsy is rarely diagnostic. A muscle biopsy cannot differentiate anterior horn cell from peripheral nerve disease or a demyelinating from an axonal neuropathy. These distinctions are usually made by electrophysiologic testing or possibly nerve biopsy.

Selection of Biopsy Sites

The choice of muscle on which to perform the biopsy must be carefully determined by the clinical features of each patient. For practical purposes, in the upper extremities the muscles of choice are either the deltoid or biceps muscles; in the lower extremities, the quadriceps (usually vastus lateralis) is preferable. Moderately affected muscles (MRC grade 4) are chosen over those severely involved (MRC grade 0–2) because of the possibility of obtaining samples too late in the course of the illness to demonstrate the distinguishing features of a specific disorder. It is important to avoid muscles that may be damaged by unrelated conditions. This is particularly true for sites of recent muscle trauma (including EMG needle studies), previous poliomyelitis, local injections, or known circulatory disturbances. A biopsy of certain muscle groups in which the tendon insertion extends throughout the muscle (so-called pennate muscles, including the gastrocnemius) may give rise to confusion, because inadvertent sampling of a myotendinous junction causes difficulty in interpretation (see below).

Tissue Removal and Preparation

NEEDLE BIOPSY

The indications for needle biopsy versus open muscle biopsy are not universally agreed on. Both have advocates, and to a great extent the experience of the clinician and the expertise of the laboratory processing the tissue will favor one technique over the other. Advantages of needle biopsy include the lack of a scar and the possibility of sampling from more than one muscle, as well as from multiple sites in a muscle, and performing serial biopsies if necessary. The disadvantages include a smaller and difficult-to-orient sample and a specimen less satisfactory for electron microscopy. A larger incision is needed for the open biopsy, but the overall discomfort is probably similar with both procedures. The size of a needle biopsy (100–300 mg of muscle) is suitable for many histologic and biochemical studies.[19,22]

OPEN BIOPSY

Open biopsies permit the taking of larger specimens, which may be necessary for the biochemical study of muscles; a larger specimen also increases the likelihood of demonstrating focal disease such as vasculitis and decreases sampling errors.[18] Open biopsies allow a sample of muscle to be fixed at the in situ length, either in a clamp or fastened to a stick, prior to plunging into fixative (buffered glutaraldehyde) for ultrastructural examination. Open biopsies generally yield samples about 8 to 10 mm in length and about 4 to 5 mm in cross-sectional diameter (cylindrical in shape).

The fresh tissue sample is mounted on a chuck, usually held in place by gum tragacanth and plunged for at least 10 to 15 seconds into isopentane cooled to $-160°C$. For best tissue sampling, the frozen muscle should extend out of the gum tragacanth so that sections will not be surrounded by embedding media. Sections measuring 8 to 10 μm in thickness are used for a battery of histologic and histochemical stains, which permit most of the subcellular organelles and several of the enzyme systems to be systematically analyzed for specific abnormalities (Table 2–21).

Histologic Techniques[18]

For general histology, hematoxylin and eosin (H&E) and a modified Gomori trichrome are most useful. The latter particularly allows visualization of mitochondria and the tubular system of muscle, which is highlighted by red staining. The ATPase stain done with preincubation at pH 9.4, 4.6, or 4.2 allows a thorough evaluation of histochemistry fiber types (see Fig. 1–3). The

Table 2–21 BATTERY OF STAINS AND HISTOCHEMICAL REACTIONS

Stains and Histochemical Reactions	Usefulness
H&E, modified trichrome	General histology and cellular detail
ATPase (pH 9.4, 4.6, 4.3)	Muscle fiber types
Oxidative enzymes (NADH, SDH, cytochrome oxidase)*	Mitochondrial disorders (ragged red fibers); tubular aggregates†, target fibers, central cores
Oil red O	Lipid storage disease
PAS	Glycogen storage disease
Acid phosphatase	Lysosomes
Congo red, crystal violet	Amyloidosis
Myophosphorylase	McArdle's disease
Phosphofructokinase (PFK)	PFK deficiency
Myoadenylate deaminase (MADD)	MADD deficiency

*NADH = nicotinamide adenine dehydrogenase; SDH = succinic dehydrogenase.
†Tubular aggregates are stained by NADH but not SDH.

NADH tetrazolium reductase (NADH-TR) highlights sarcoplasmic reticulum, T tubules, and mitochondria. The mitochondria can be selectively stained with a succinic dehydrogenase (SDH) reaction or with cytochrome oxidase, a respiratory chain enzyme. Oil red O demonstrates neutral fat and is especially useful in lipid-storage myopathies. Glycogen content can be assessed by the periodic acid–Schiff (PAS) reaction. In patients with muscle fatigue and rhabdomyolysis syndromes, specific enzymes that can be assessed by histochemistry include myophosphorylase, phosphofructokinase, and myoadenylate deaminase.

ELECTRON MICROSCOPY

Electron microscopy is only necessary under very specific conditions. One form of inflammatory myopathy, inclusion body myositis, can be confirmed by ultrastructural examination (see Chapter 5). Mitochondrial myopathies (Chapter 8) and certain congenital myopathies such as nemaline (rod) myopathy can be better characterized by electron microscopy. Usually the presence of tubular aggregates, which may be strongly suspected on the basis of the histochemical profile of NADH-TR–positive and SDH-negative material in type 2 fibers, requires ultrastructural confirmation (see Fig. 6–16). Ultra-

structural examination is not necessary in biopsy analysis for muscular dystrophy.

IMMUNE STAINING

The demonstration of immune deposits is particularly relevant in dermatomyositis, where immunoglobulin (especially IgM and IgG) and complement (C3, C9, and membrane attack complex) are distinctive[39,40] (see Fig. 5–6). Localization of dystrophin antibody to the sarcolemmal membrane is now available for assessment of Duchenne dystrophy (see Fig. 4–12). Lymphocyte subclasses can be identified using mononuclear antibody staining[4] (see Fig. 5–8).

Differentiating Neuropathy from Myopathy

HISTOLOGIC FEATURES OF NEUROPATHY

When muscle weakness is neurogenic, histologic changes are usually easy to recognize (Table 2–22). The most characteristic change is atrophy, resulting in the appearance of small *angular* fibers not selective for fiber types. Early in the disease, scattered atrophic fibers are present, which stain darkly with oxidative enzymes (Fig. 2–32). Later, groups of angular fibers can be seen (Fig. 2–33A). In H&E and tri-

Table 2–22 MUSCLE BIOPSY FEATURES DIFFERENTIATING MYOPATHY FROM NEUROPATHY

Features	Myopathy	Neuropathy
Muscle fiber size/shape	Variability in size (small to hypertrophied), or grouped round fibers	Small angular fibers; groups of small fibers
Nuclei	Increased internal nuclei	Atrophied fibers with nuclear clumps (pyknotic)
Necrosis/phagocytosis	Common	Rare
Inflammation	Variable	None
Connective tissue	Increased	Normal (unless end stage)
Fiber-type changes	Type predominance or preferential involvement in some diseases	Type grouping

chrome stains, the loss of myofibrils leaves behind clumps of pyknotic nuclei (Fig. 2–33B). In some denervating disorders, *target fibers*, which may be a sign of reinnervation, are present. Target fibers generally have a clear central or eccentric zone surrounded by a dense intermediate zone and a relatively normal periphery, giving the appearance of three zones (Fig. 2–34). Not all target fibers exhibit the densely stained intermediate region, however. Targets preferentially affect type 1 fibers. *Type grouping*, unequivocal evidence of reinnervation, is recognized by a loss of the usual mosaic pattern of fiber types, which is replaced by large groups (greater than 40 in number) of homogeneous fiber types (Fig. 2–35). Type grouping occurs because reinnervation converts the muscle-fiber types of a denervated motor unit to that of the adopting motor neuron.

In spinal muscular atrophy, where denervation occurs very early in life, the muscle biopsy appearance is quite distinctive. Large groups of hypertrophied type 1 fibers are intermixed with fascicles of small type 1 and type 2 fibers. In these atrophic fascicles, the type 1 fibers are usually smaller than the type 2 fibers (Fig. 2–36).

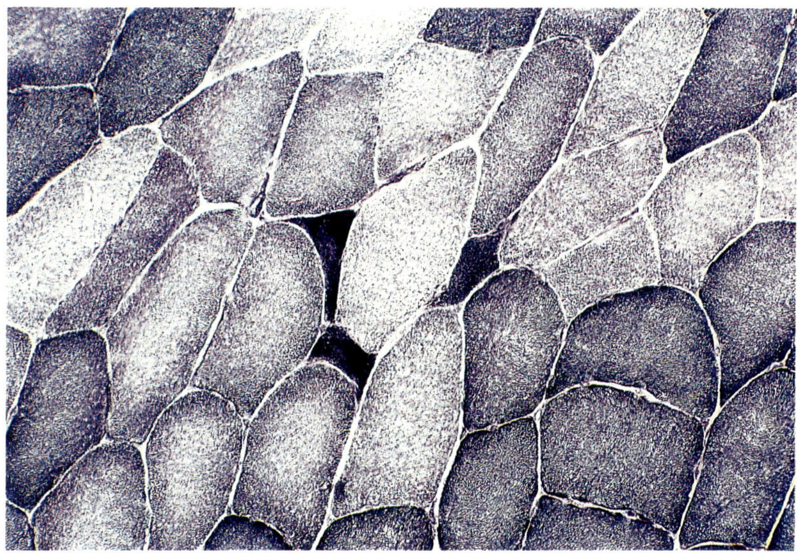

Figure 2–32. Early neurogenic atrophy. The three small, dark, angular fibers are characteristic of denervation atrophy (NADH-TR).

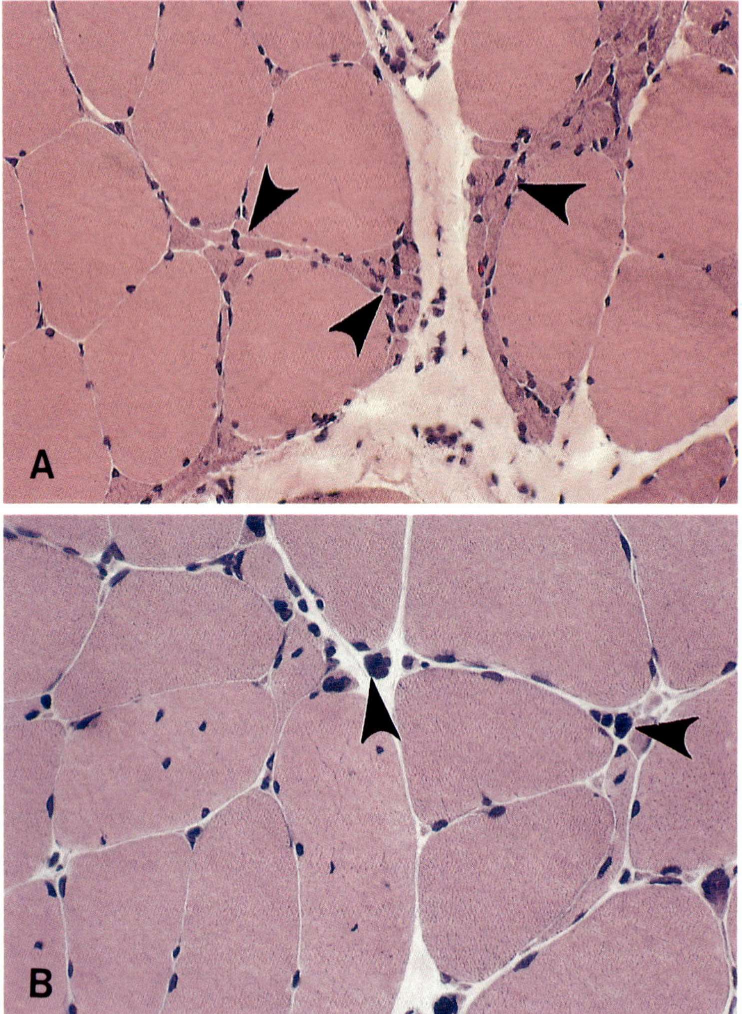

Figure 2–33. Neurogenic atrophy. (*A*) Groups of angular fibers (*arrowheads*) are clustered between and around normal muscle fibers. (*B*) Pyknotic nuclear clumps (*arrowheads*) represent the end result of muscle atrophy (H&E).

Type grouping must be distinguished from fiber *type predominance*. In most muscle biopsies, fiber types 1, 2A, and 2B are equally represented, each comprising about one third of the total.[18] In type predominance, one type of fiber makes up more than 55%[18] (Fig. 2–37). Although type predominance can be caused by reinnervation, some myopathies alter the ratio of fiber types; type 1 fiber predominance appears in Duchenne and Becker muscular dystro-phies and in congenital myopathies, including central core disease and nemaline (rod) myopathy.

HISTOLOGIC FEATURES OF MYOPATHY

The features that indicate a primary muscle disease (see Table 2–22) include muscle fiber *necrosis* (degeneration) and *phagocytosis* (Fig. 2–38).

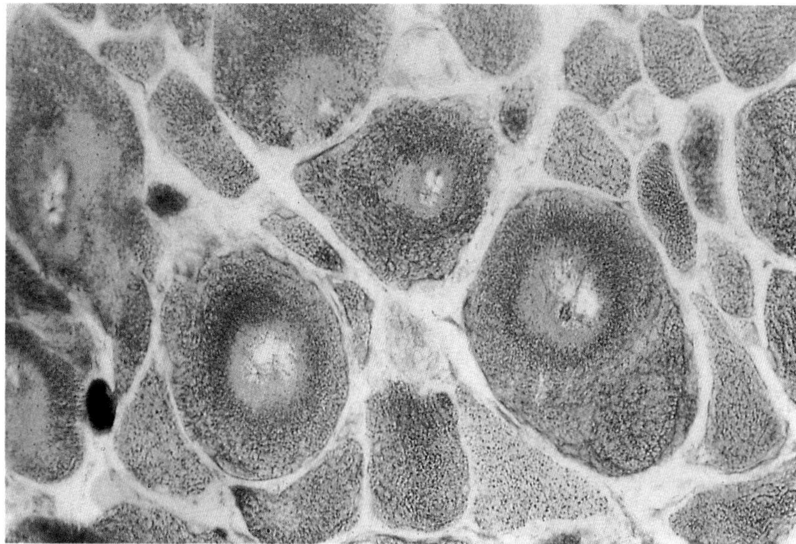

Figure 2–34. Target fibers. Muscle fibers show central light zone surrounded by a densely stained region (NADH-TR).

Muscle has substantial regenerative capabilities. When the muscle fiber is injured, resting mononucleated muscle precursor cells, called satellite cells, are stimulated to proliferate and either fuse with the injured muscle fiber or fuse with one another to form *regenerating fibers*. These are typically basophilic in the H&E stain because of rich RNA content (Fig. 2–39). During regeneration, muscle fiber nuclei often assume a central or paracentral location. An increase to more than 3% internal nuclei is considered abnormal.

Fiber splitting (Fig. 2–40) is prominent in chronic myopathies such as limb-girdle dystrophy. It is a normal occurrence at a myotendinous junction, since the muscle fiber splits as it inserts into the tendon; a section through this area must be interpreted with caution. Fiber splitting usually occurs in a previously injured area of the muscle fiber.

Connective tissue frequently proliferates when muscle fibers are lost. This *endomysial connective tissue proliferation* is especially prominent in certain disorders, like Duchenne muscular dystrophy (Fig. 2–41). In chronic myop-

athies, irrespective of their cause, excess endomysial connective tissue typically is accompanied by increased variability in fiber size, internal nuclei, and fiber splitting.

Cell infiltration or inflammation may occur in many conditions. When muscle fibers undergo necrosis from any cause, macrophages are recruited to the site of injury (see Fig. 2–38). In addition, mononuclear inflammatory cells participate in muscle fiber breakdown and can be seen invading muscle fibers prior to necrosis, especially in polymyositis (Fig. 2–42). Using mononuclear antibodies, invading cells can be further subtyped. In the inflammatory myopathies, T cells, both helper (CD4) and cytotoxic/suppressor (CD8) participate in the process.[4] Even in conditions that are not primarily immune-mediated, such as Duchenne muscular dystrophy, CD8-positive cells invade muscle fibers (see Fig. 4–9). Cellular and perivascular infiltration are the hallmark of the three major types of inflammatory myopathies: dermatomyositis, polymyositis, and inclusion body myositis. The muscle biopsy also can serve as a diagnostic

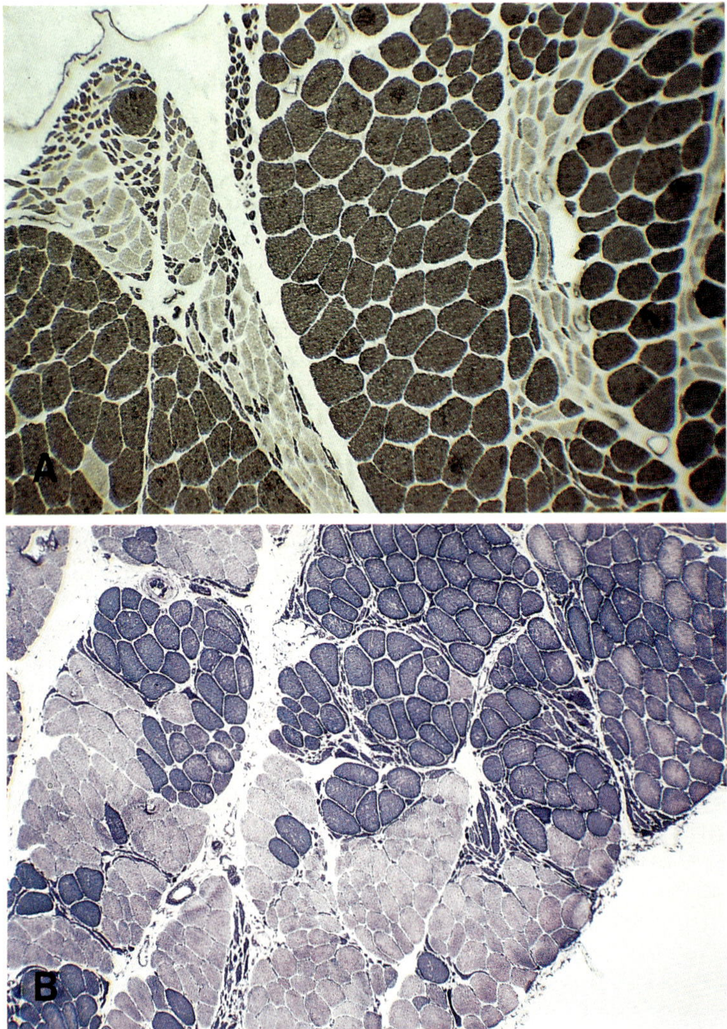

Figure 2–35. Type grouping. (*A*) Fascicles show loss of mosaic pattern, replaced by large groups of type 2 fibers. ATPase pH 9.4. (*B*) Muscle fascicles composed almost exclusively of either light, type 2 fibers or dark, type 1 fibers (NADH).

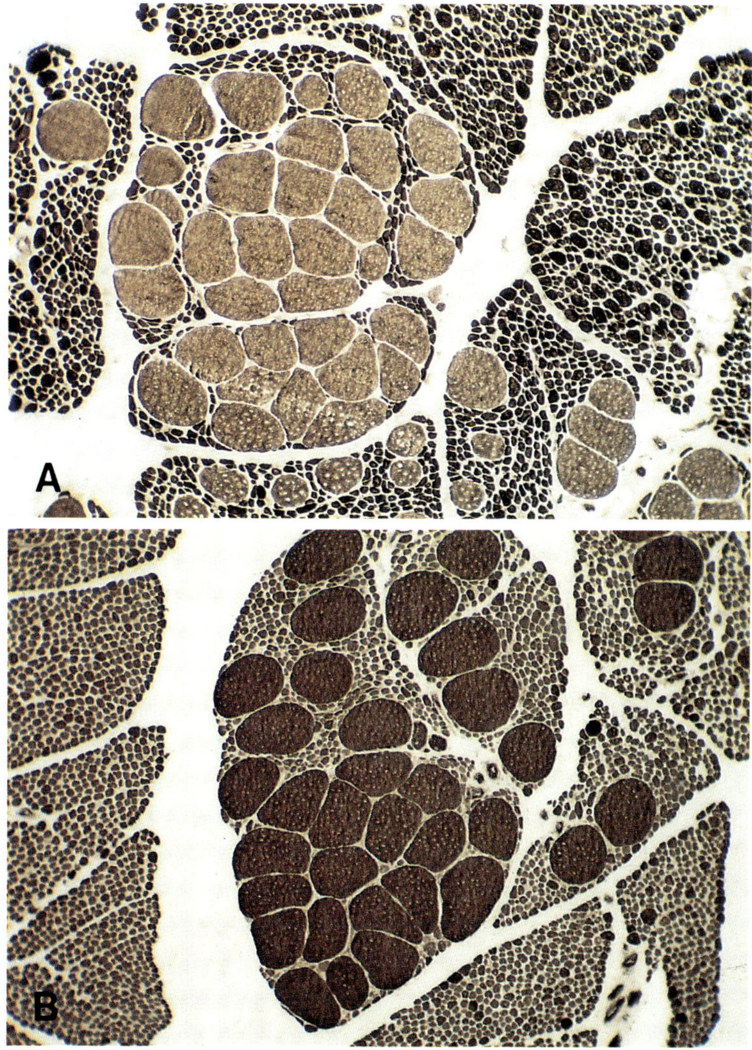

Figure 2–36. Type grouping in spinal muscular atrophy. Hypertrophied type 1 fibers are grouped together in one fascicle surrounded by fascicles composed of small, atrophic fibers. (*A*) ATPase pH 9.4. (*B*) ATPase pH 4.2.

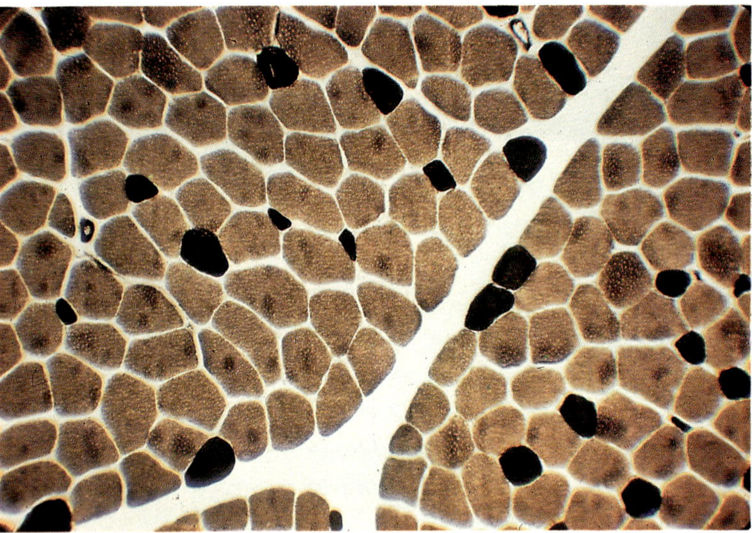

Figure 2-37. Type predominance. Muscle biopsy shows predominantly type 1 fibers, with only scattered type 2 fibers. ATPase pH 9.4.

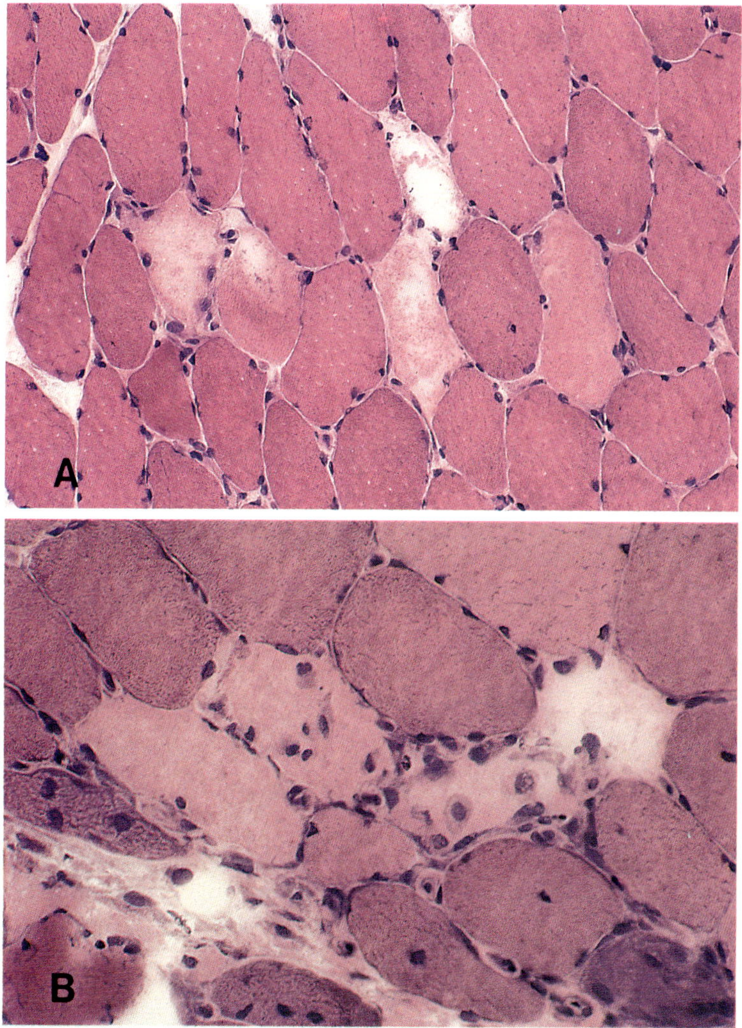

Figure 2–38. Myopathy. (*A*) Necrotic muscle fibers show loss of staining (H&E). (*B*) Pale muscle fibers infiltrated by macrophages (H&E).

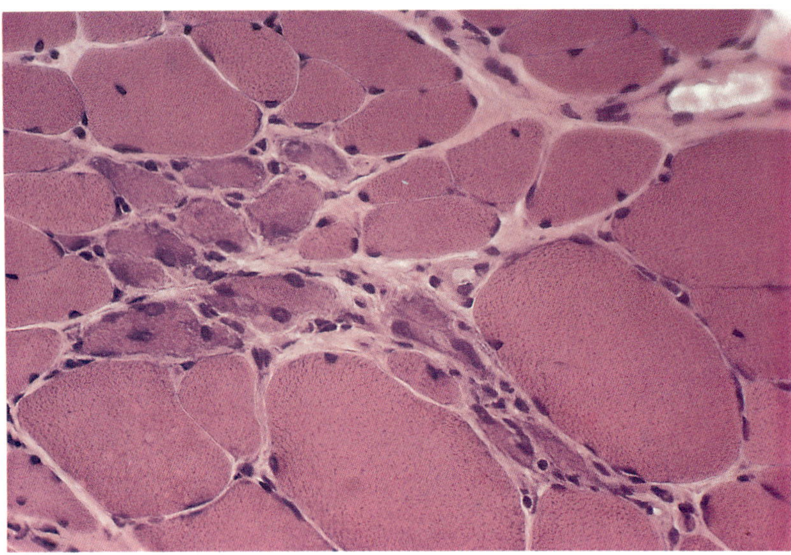

Figure 2–39. Muscle fiber regeneration. Small group of basophilic, regenerating muscle fibers (H&E).

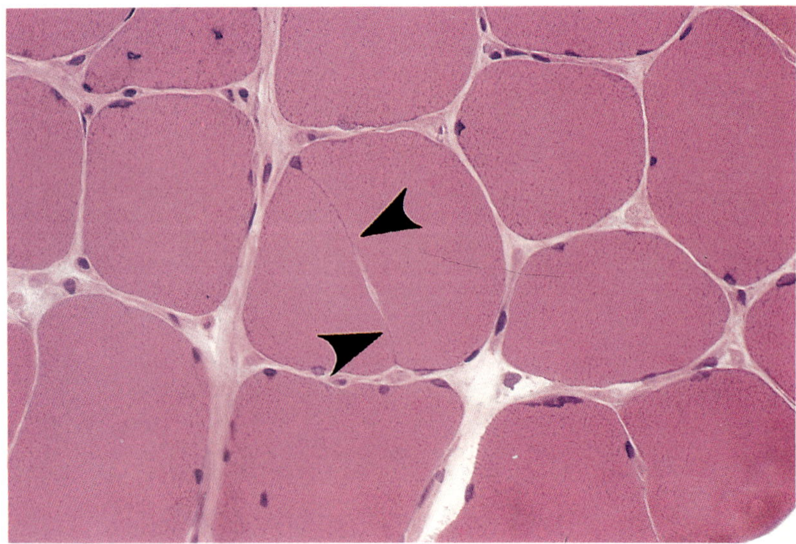

Figure 2–40. Muscle fiber splitting. Interposed sarcolemmal membrane (*arrowheads*) shows line of fiber splitting (H&E).

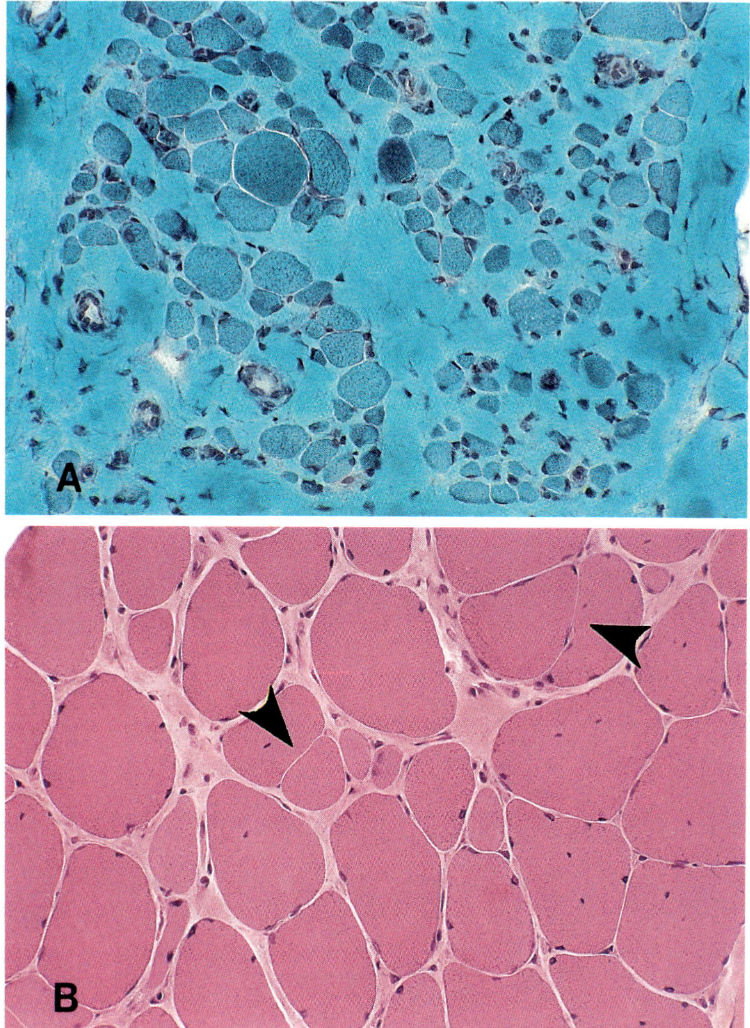

Figure 2–41. Chronic myopathy. Muscle biopsies demonstrate variability in fiber size, fiber splitting (*arrowheads*), loss of fibers, internal nuclei, and endomysial connective tissue proliferation. (*A*) Modified trichrome. (*B*) H&E.

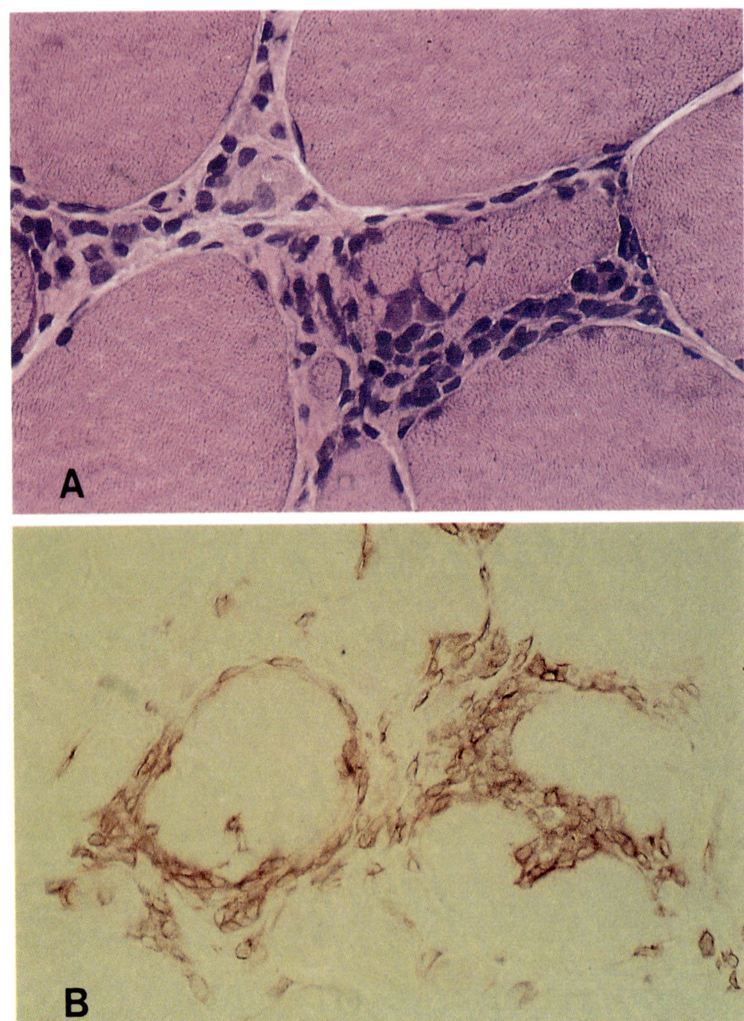

Figure 2–42. Cell infiltration in polymyositis. (*A*) Nonnecrotic muscle fiber invaded by mononuclear cells (H&E). (*B*) Mononuclear antibody stain demonstrates CD8-positive inflammatory cells invading muscle fibers.

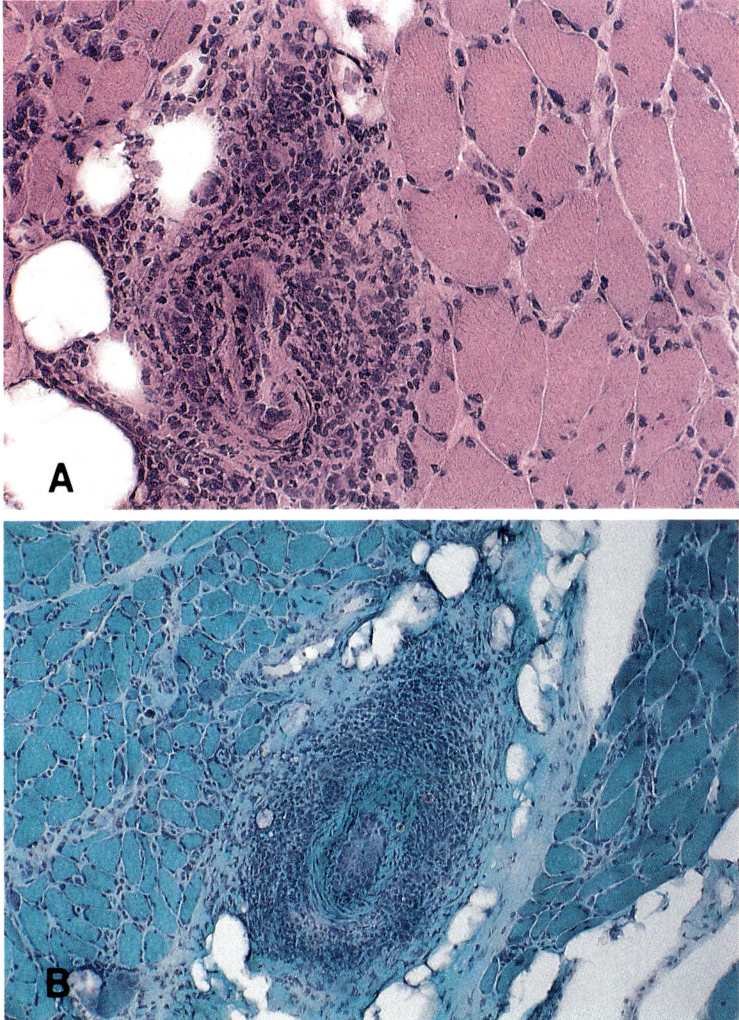

Figure 2–43. Vasculitis of muscle. Medium-size arteries show invasion by mononuclear inflammatory cells. (*A*) H&E. (*B*) Modified trichrome.

source for vasculitis; mononuclear cells can be seen invading the walls of small and medium-sized arteries (Fig. 2–43).

Preferential Fiber Type Involvement

Preferential atrophy of muscle fiber types occurs in certain conditions

Table 2–23 CAUSES OF SELECTIVE MUSCLE FIBER-TYPE ATROPHY

Type 1	Type 2
Myotonic dystrophy	Corticosteroids
Centronuclear myopathy	Hyperthyroidism
	Disuse
	Cachexia
	Central nervous system disease

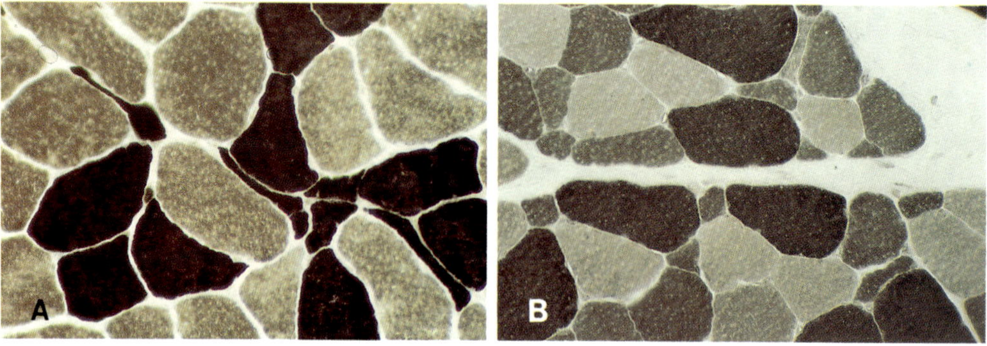

Figure 2–44. Type 2 muscle fiber atrophy. (*A*) Scattered, severely atrophic type 2 muscle fibers. ATPase pH 9.4. (*B*) Selective atrophy of type 2B muscle fibers (intermediate staining). ATPase pH 4.6.

(Table 2–23). The type 2 fibers, particularly type 2B, are selectively affected in hyperthyroidism, corticosteroid excess (endogenous or exogenous), disuse, cachexia, and upper motor neuron disease (Fig. 2–44). Type 1 fiber atrophy (Fig. 2–45) is less common but is prominent in myotonic dystrophy and in infants and children with centronuclear myopathy and congenital fiber type disproportion.

Certain cytoarchitectural abnormalities also have a fiber-type predilection, usually involving type 1 fibers. *Target fibers*, which affect mainly type 1 fibers, have already been discussed as a cardi-

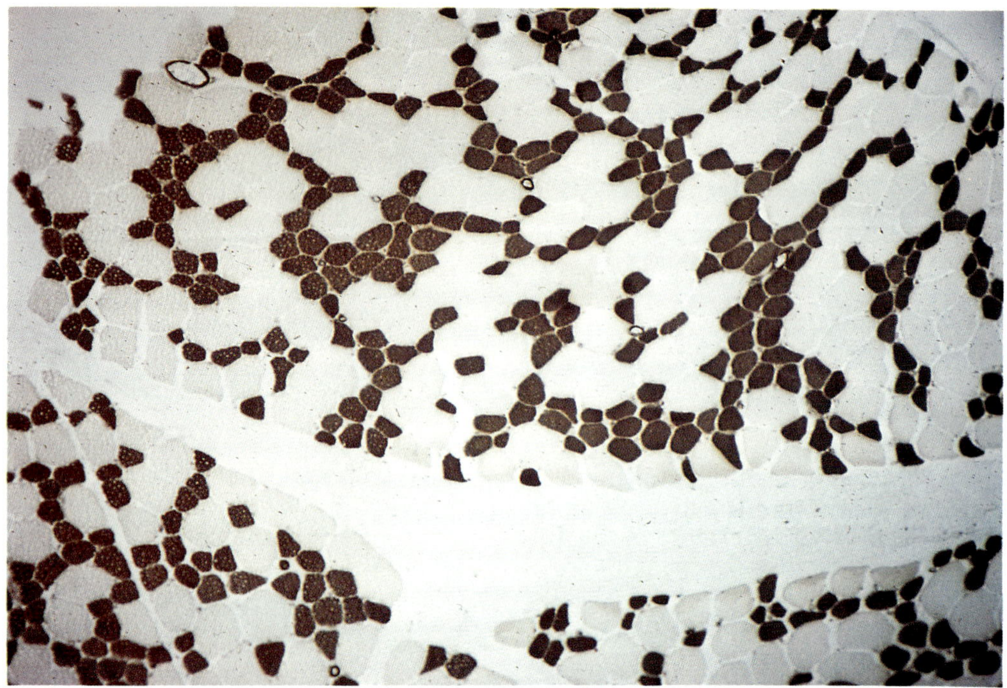

Figure 2–45. Type 1 muscle fiber atrophy. The type 1 fibers are uniformly smaller than type 2 fibers in this biopsy. ATPase pH 4.2.

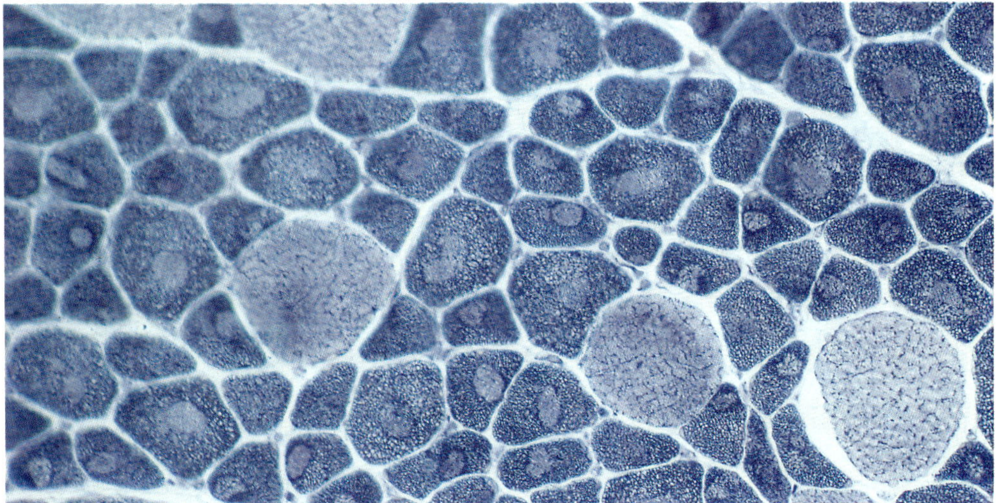

Figure 2–46. Central core disease. Muscle fibers show central regions devoid of oxidative enzymes in all type 1 fibers (NADH-TR).

nal feature of neurogenic disorders (see Fig. 2–34). *Central cores* resemble target fibers and are the diagnostic feature of a congenital myopathy, central core disease. Central cores (Figs. 2–46 and 6–1), like target fibers, affect mainly type 1 fibers and have a central zone unreactive with any NADH-TR; they do not have the densely stained zone surrounding the central region. In nemaline myopathy, *rod bodies*, originating from the Z disc, accumulate predominantly in type 1 fibers. Rod bodies appear as dark, red, or purple structures in the modified trichrome stain (Fig. 2–47). Ultrastructural examination dem-

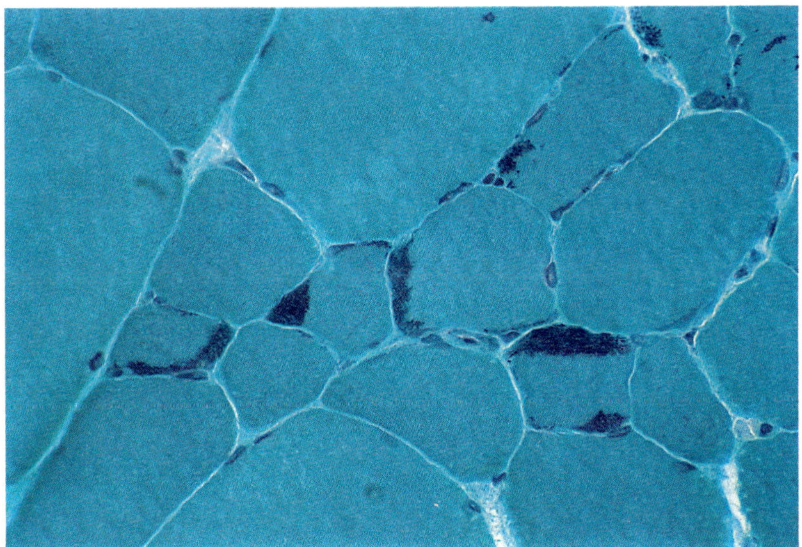

Figure 2–47. Nemaline myopathy. Muscle fibers show subsarcolemmal accumulations of rods (modified trichrome).

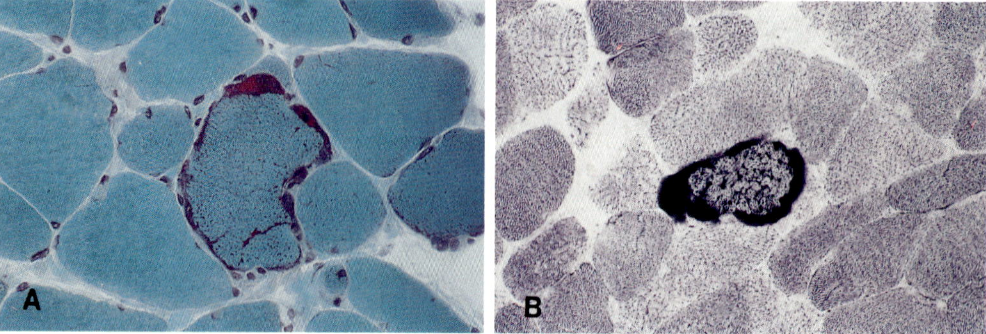

Figure 2–48. Ragged red fibers. (*A*) Muscle fibers show subsarcolemmal accumulation of red staining material and coarse red granules in sarcoplasm. Modified trichrome. (*B*) NADH-TR–positive material in ragged red fiber.

onstrates an osmiophilic, latticelike appearance of Z-disc origin, into which thin filaments insert (see Fig. 6–3).

Mitochondrial abnormalities also preferentially affect type 1 fibers. Ragged red fibers are so named because of the clusters of red-staining material under the sarcolemma in the trichrome stain (Fig. 2–48). Electron microscopy of ragged red fibers demonstrates clusters of enlarged, often bizarrely shaped mitochondria, many of which have closely packed cristae with intramitochondrial inclusions (see Fig. 8–2). This type of fiber abnormality is extremely important to recognize in light of recent developments in the understanding of the molecular genetics of mitochondrial disorders.

Tubular aggregates are one of the few cytoarchitectural abnormalities preferentially affecting type 2 fibers. Tubular aggregates are clusters of tubular proliferation arising from the sarcoplasmic reticulum. They demonstrate positive staining with NADH-TR, a negative reaction for SDH, and a prominent red appearance in the trichrome stain (Figs. 2–49 and 6–16). They may be seen in periodic paralysis, especially the hyperkalemic variety, but are also present in other conditions and often confer little or no diagnostic specificity.

Sources of Diagnostic Error

In addition to the risk of overlooking multifocal disease because of sampling error, in many instances the results of the muscle biopsy may be misleading. Moreover, the range of normal for muscle fiber diameters varies widely within, and especially between, different muscles.[46]

NERVE BIOPSY

Indications for Biopsy

Nerve biopsy may be indicated for patients with myopathies, because both proximal and distal muscle diseases often include neuropathic disorders in their differential diagnosis. Because the repertoire of pathologic changes of the nerve is limited, the indications for nerve biopsy are more restricted than for muscle biopsy. The nerve biopsy is most valuable for identifying changes in

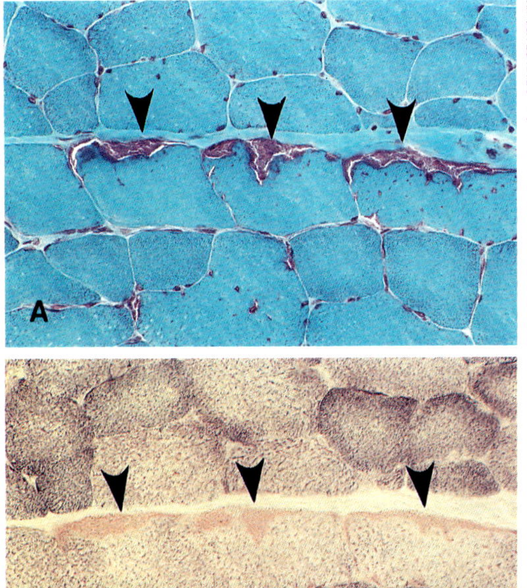

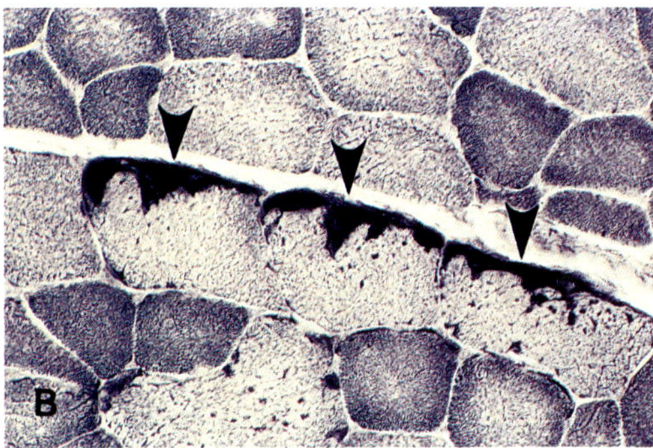

Figure 2–49. Tubular aggregates. (*A*) Muscle fibers (*arrowheads*) show subsarcolemmal red staining material that also is positive for NADH-TR (*B*) but not for SDH (*C*).

the blood vessels and in the supporting connective tissue elements of the nerve. The leading indication for nerve biopsy is a search for vasculitis.[41,75] Other indications include suspected amyloidosis, or granulomatous diseases such as sarcoidosis. A diagnosis of leprosy can also be made from a nerve biopsy.

In the acquired inflammatory demyelinating polyneuropathies, nerve biopsy is indicated only for patients with chronic disease; very few would advocate it in Guillain-Barré syndrome. In chronic inflammatory demyelinating polyneuropathy (CIDP), a nerve biopsy is often done to exclude other conditions, although an unequivocal diagnosis of CIDP is often impossible from nerve biopsy alone. In one series involving CIDP, inflammation in the nerve was found in only 10% of patients, whereas 21% had findings indicating an axonal rather than a demyelinating neuropathy, 40% had findings of de-

myelination, 12% had mixed features, and 17% had normal nerve biopsies.[8] For some immune-mediated neuropathies, the biopsy may help to identify IgM anti-myelin-associated glycoprotein antibody deposited in the myelin sheaths.[52] This finding is rare, however, because in most neuropathies associated with paraproteinemias, no antibody binding can be demonstrated.

In toxic neuropathies, very few specific changes are observed. Even in hexacarbon exposure, where neurofilament proliferation produces swollen axons,[53] the distribution of abnormalities and the time of biopsy in relation to exposure may preclude recognition by biopsy. The history of exposure and identification of toxic products in the serum or blood are far more specific. In endocrinopathies commonly affecting the nerve, including diabetes and hypothyroidism, diagnosis cannot be made on pathologic grounds.

Nerve biopsies are of very limited use in hereditary disorders. The abnormalities in hereditary motor sensory neuropathy type I (peripheral-nerve form of Charcot-Marie-Tooth disease) can be clearly demonstrated by the presence of demyelinated and remyelinated axons associated with onion-bulb formation, but an equally satisfactory diagnosis can be established by physical examination (pes cavus, hammer toes, hypertrophic nerves), slow nerve conduction velocities, and pedigree analysis. In other hereditary conditions, such as the lysosomal storage diseases, the biopsy can demonstrate the presence of certain storage products (for example, metachromatic granules), but a definitive diagnosis can only be established by biochemical assay of white blood cells or other appropriate tissue.

Selection of Biopsy Sites

SURAL NERVE

Biopsies are performed most commonly on the sural nerve. It may be reached through an incision over the calf or at the lateral malleolus. A convenient site for biopsy is in the lower leg, through an incision approximately 25 cm above the plantar surface of the heel, 1 cm lateral to the midline. The advantage of this site is that the nerve usually has not yet branched, and pressure-induced changes are unlikely. (At the level of the lateral malleolus, the nerve is chronically exposed to pressure from shoes.) In addition, the usual curvilinear incision at the ankle may heal slowly.

SUPERFICIAL PERONEAL NERVE

The next most accessible site for nerve biopsy is the anterior compartment of the lower leg, where the superficial peroneal nerve (a sensory branch of the common peroneal nerve) can be obtained. Biopsy of this nerve is done with the patient lying in a supine position, which is more comfortable than the prone position required for sural nerve biopsies. Positioning for sural nerve biopsy may be very difficult for some patients, such as those on a ventilator. When searching for vasculitis, the superficial peroneal nerve biopsy also offers the advantage of the close apposition of this nerve to the peroneus brevis muscle, facilitating a combined muscle/ nerve biopsy and avoiding a second incision.[75] Vasculitis is found in vessels in the peroneus brevis muscle at least as frequently as in the superficial peroneal nerve.[75]

The disadvantages of a biopsy of the superficial peroneal nerve are that fewer fascicles are found than in the sural nerve, and the nerve takes a more variable course, making the biopsy procedure potentially more difficult. In addition, potential pressure-induced changes of the common peroneal nerve at the fibular head may be reflected downstream at the site of the superficial peroneal nerve biopsy.

SUPERFICIAL RADIAL NERVE

A third nerve available for biopsy is the superficial radial nerve. The incision is made at the wrist; identification of the nerve may be difficult because of confusion with the surrounding tendons. In addition, the removal of this nerve results in a sensory loss over the thumb, which is disconcerting to some patients. Although it is a pure sensory nerve, biopsy is performed only as a last resort, such as in a patient who has a suspected vasculitis but has findings confined to the upper extremities.

Tissue Removal and Preparation

An important consideration for patient comfort at the time of nerve biopsy is direct infiltration of local anesthetic into the sheath of the nerve. Cutting the nerve without appropriate nerve block is very painful and should be avoided.

Removal of a specimen approximately 4 cm long is ideal.[71] A 1-cm segment of this specimen is separated, mounted on a chuck with gum tragacanth, and frozen for 10 to 15 seconds in isopentane cooled to $-160°C$. This procedure is identical to the method used for freezing muscle. Frozen sections are valuable for identification of immune deposits (immunoglobulin and complement) and for mononuclear cell typing (T cells, B cells, macrophages).[41] Another 1-cm segment of nerve is placed in buffered formalin and processed for paraffin sections, which are used to demonstrate vasculitis and connective tissue abnormalities such as inflammatory cells and granulomas. A portion of the remaining nerve is fixed at its in situ length (for example, attached to a tongue blade) in 3% phosphate-buffered glutaraldehyde for 30 minutes before dissection into 1- to 2-mm blocks, which are returned to the same fixative for 1.5 hours. These blocks are placed in 1% phosphate-buffered osmium tetroxide for 2 hours, followed by dehydration in graded alcohols and propylene oxide; they are subsequently embedded in a resin plastic media. Plastic sections 1 μm thick and stained with toluidine blue or paraphenylenediamine provide a basis for study by high-resolution light microscopy. For nerve fiber teasing, individual nerve fascicles are separated and put in 2% osmium tetroxide for 24 hours, then into 60% glycerol. Single nerve fibers are teased and placed on slides for further study. The combination of high-resolution light microscopy and nerve fiber teasing allows careful assessment of the type of nerve pathology: axonal versus demyelinating, and primary versus secondary demyelination. Electron microscopy is not necessary for most biopsies, but it is indicated in the rare cases in which a storage material is being sought.

SUMMARY

The most important step in the evaluation of a patient with myopathy is a critical analysis of the patient's symptoms. Whether the patient's major problem is exercise-induced (dynamic) symptoms, progressive proximal weakness, or fatigability requires precise definition. The clinical examination often helps to clarify these questions. Many myopathies have distinctive symptoms and signs that permit confident diagnosis without extensive laboratory testing. As discussed in the next chapter, it is frequently fruitful to examine the family history and, in many instances, family members themselves.

The laboratory evaluation, including serum muscle enzymes, electrodiagnosis, and muscle biopsy, may add substantial information. Electrodiagnostic studies are especially useful in clarifying whether the pathophysiologic basis of weakness is myogenic or neurogenic (for example, anterior horn cell disease, inflammatory polyradiculopathy, multifocal motor neuropathy). Especially important findings in myopathies include myotonic discharges, neuromyotonia (Isaac's syndrome), the abundant spontaneous discharges of acid maltase deficiency, and the fibrillations of inflammatory myopathy, all of which correlate with the activity of the disease. Electrodiagnostic studies of neuromuscular transmission are helpful in evaluating myotonic disorders, metabolic myopathies, periodic paralysis, and myasthenic syndromes. Muscle biopsies are particularly useful in evaluating inflammatory myopathy, congenital myopathy, dystrophin-deficient dystrophy, mitochondrial disorders, vasculitis, and metabolic defects. Nerve biopsy is less useful in evaluating the patient with suspected myopathy, although vasculitis, granulomatous disease, and inflammatory neuropathies may be clarified by nerve biopsy. For a number of hereditary myopathies, DNA analysis (discussed in detail in the next chapter) is becoming increasingly important as the definitive diagnostic approach. As the gene product is defined, it will be possible to diagnose hereditary disorders precisely by specific biochemical testing for missing or abnormal proteins.

REFERENCES

1. Adams RD, Shahani BT, and Young RR: Tremor in association with polyneuropathy. Transactions of the American Neurological Association 97:44, 1972.
2. Albers JW, Allen AA, Bastron JA, and Daube JR: Limb myokymia. Muscle Nerve 4:494, 1981.
3. Alevizos B, Spengos M, Vassilopoulos D, and Stefanis C: γ-glutamyl transpeptidase. Elevated activity in myotonic dystrophy. J Neurol Sci 28:225, 1976.
4. Arahata K and Engel AG: Monoclonal antibody analysis of mononuclear cells in myopathies, IV. Cell-mediated cytotoxicity and muscle fiber necrosis. Ann Neurol 23:168, 1988.
5. Askanas V, Engel WK, DiMauro S, Brooks BR, and Mehler M: Adult-onset acid maltase deficiency: Morphologic and biochemical abnormalities reproduced in cultured muscle. N Engl J Med 294:573, 1976.
6. Auger RG, Daube JR, Gomez MR, and Lambert EH: Hereditary form of sustained muscle activity of peripheral nerve origin causing generalized myokymia and muscle stiffness. Ann Neurol 15:13, 1984.
7. Barohn R, Miller R, and Griggs RC: Autosomal recessive distal dystrophy. Neurology 41:1365, 1991.
8. Barohn RJ, Kissel JT, Warmolts JR, and Mendell JR: Chronic inflammatory demyelinating polyradiculoneuropathy. Clinical characteristics, course and recommendations for diagnostic criteria. Arch Neurol 46:878, 1989.
9. Bastron JA: Myotonia and other abnormalities of muscle contraction arising from disorders of the motor unit. Res Publ Assoc Res Nerv Ment Dis 38:534, 1961.
10. Bigland-Ritchie B, Jones DA, and Woods JJ: Excitation frequency and muscle fatigue: Electrical responses during human voluntary and stimulated contractions. Exp Neurol 64:414, 1979.
11. Black HR, Quallich H, and Gareleck CB: Racial differences in serum creatine kinase levels. Am J Med 81:479, 1986.
12. Brooke MH, Fenichel GM, Griggs RC, et al: Clinical investigation in Duchenne dystrophy: II. Determination of the "power" of therapeutic trials based on the natural history. Muscle Nerve 6:91, 1983.
13. Buchthal F and Kamieniecka Z: The diagnostic yield of quantified electromyography and quantified muscle biopsy in neuromuscular disorders. Muscle Nerve 5:265, 1982.
14. Campbell SM, Clark S, Tindall EA, Forehand ME, and Bennett RM: Clinical characteristics of fibrositis. I. A "blinded," controlled study of symptoms and tender points. Arthritis Rheum 26:817, 1983.
15. Clark S, Campbell SM, Forehand ME, Tindall EA, and Bennett RM: Clinical characteristics of fibrositis. II. A "blinded," controlled study using standard psychological tests. Arthritis Rheum 28:132, 1985.
16. Costill DL: Sweating: Its composition and effects on body fluids. Ann N Y Acad Sci 301:160, 1977.
17. Daube J: Quantitative EMG in nerve-muscle disorders. In Stalberg E and Young R (eds): Clinical Neurophysiology. Butterworths, London, 1981, p 33.
18. Dubowitz V and Brooke MH: Muscle Biopsy: A Modern Approach. WB Saunders, Philadelphia, 1973.
19. Edwards R, Young A, and Wiles M: Needle biopsy of skeletal muscle in the diagnosis of myopathy and the clinical study of muscle function and repair. N Engl J Med 302:261, 1980.
20. Edwards RHT: Physiological and metabolic studies of the contractile machinery of human muscle in health

and disease. Phys Med Biol 24:237, 1979.

21. Edwards RHT and Hyde S: Methods of measuring muscle strength and fatigue. Physiotherapy 63:51, 1977.

22. Edwards RHT and Jones DA: Needle biopsy of skeletal muscle: A review of 10 years experience. Muscle Nerve 6:676, 1983.

23. Eisen A, Berry K, and Gibson G: Inclusion body myositis (IBM): Myopathy or neuropathy? Neurology 33:1109, 1983.

24. Engel AG: Congenital myasthenic syndromes. J Child Neurol 3:233, 1988.

25. Fenichel GM: Clinical syndromes of myasthenia in infancy and childhood. Arch Neurol 39:97, 1978.

26. Fleet WS and Watson RT: From benign fasciculations and cramps to motor neuron disease. Neurology 36:997, 1986.

27. Florence JM, Fox PT, Planer GJ, and Brooke MH: Activity, creatine kinase, and myoglobin in Duchenne muscular dystrophy: A clue to etiology? Neurology 35:758, 1985.

28. Florence JM, Pandya S, King WM, et al: Clinical trials in Duchenne dystrophy: Standardization and reliability of evaluation procedures. Phys Ther 64:41, 1984.

29. Griggs RC: Hypertrophy and cardiomyopathy in the neuromuscular diseases. Circ Res 34&35 (Suppl II):II-145, 1974.

30. Griggs RC, Forbes G, Moxley RT, and Herr BE: The assessment of muscle mass in progressive neuromuscular disease. Neurology 33:158, 1983.

31. Griggs RC, Pandya SP, Florence JM, et al: Randomized controlled trial of testosterone in myotonic dystrophy. Neurology 39:219, 1989.

32. Hallynck T, Soep HH, Thomis J, et al: Prediction of creatinine clearance from serum creatinine concentration based on lean body mass. Clin Pharmacol Ther 30:414, 1981.

33. Heymsfield SB, Arteaga C, McManus C, Smith J, and Moffitt S: Measurement of muscle mass in humans: Validity of the 24-hour urinary creatinine method. Am J Clin Nutr 37:478, 1983.

34. Howard JE, McGill KC, and Dorfman LJ: Properties of motor unit action potentials recorded with concentric and monopolar needle electrodes: ADEMG analysis. Muscle Nerve 11:1051, 1988.

34a. Jablecki CK: Myopathies. In Brown WF and Bolton CF (eds): Clinical Electromyography, ed 2. Butterworth-Heinemann, Boston, 1993, p 653.

35. Jockers-Wretou E, Grabert K, Müller E, and Pfleiderer G: Serum creatine kinase isoenzyme pattern in nervous system atrophies and neuromuscular disorders. Clin Chim Acta 73:183, 1976.

36. Kalyan-Raman UP, Kalyan-Raman K, Yunus MB, and Masi AT: Muscle pathology in primary fibromyalgia syndrome: A light microscopic, histochemical and ultrastructural study. J Rheumatol 11:808, 1984.

37. Karpati G, Carpenter S, Engel AG, et al: The syndrome of systemic carnitine deficiency: Clinical, morphologic, biochemical and pathophysiologic features. Neurology 26:16, 1975.

38. Kimura J: Electrodiagnosis in Diseases of Nerve and Muscle: Principles and Practice, ed 2. FA Davis, Philadelphia, 1989.

39. Kissel JT, Halterman RK, Rammohan KW, and Mendell JR: The relationship of complement-mediated microvasculopathy to the histologic features and clinical duration of disease in dermatomyositis. Arch Neurol 48:26, 1991.

40. Kissel JT, Mendell JR, and Rammohan KW: Microvascular deposition of complement membrane attack complex in dermatomyositis. N Engl J Med 314:329, 1986.

41. Kissel JT, Riethman JL, Omerza J, Rammohan KW, and Mendell JR: Peripheral nerve vasculitis: Immune characterization of the vascular lesions. Ann Neurol 25:291, 1989.

42. Koster JF, Slee RG, Van der Klei-Van Moorsel JM, Rietra PJGM, and Lucas CJ: Physico-chemical and immunological properties of acid α-glucosidase from various human tissues in relation

to glycogenosis type II (Pompe's disease). Clin Chim Acta 68:49, 1976.

43. Lambert EH: Neurophysiological techniques useful in the study of neuromuscular disorders. Res Publ Assoc Res Nerv Ment Dis 38:247, 1960.

44. Lance JW, Burke D, and Pollard J: Hyperexcitability of motor and sensory neurons in neuromyotonia. Ann Neurol 5:523, 1979.

45. Lang H and Würzburg U: Creatine kinase, an enzyme of many forms. Clin Chem 28/7:1439, 1982.

46. Mahon M, Toman A, Willan PLT, and Bagnall KM: Variability of histochemical and morphometric data from needle biopsy specimens of human quadriceps femoris muscle. J Neurol Sci 63:85, 1984.

47. Mawdsley RH and Knapik JJ: Comparison of isokinetic measurements with test repetitions. Phys Ther 62:169, 1982.

48. McComas AJ, Kereshi S, and Quinlan J: A method for detecting functional weakness. J Neurol Neurosurg Psychiatry 46:280, 1983.

49. Mechler F: Changing electromyographic findings during the chronic course of polymyositis. J Neurol Sci 23:237, 1974.

50. Medical Research Council. Aids to the Investigation of Peripheral Nerve Injuries. Her Majesty's Stationery Office, London, 1976.

51. Meltzer HY, Dorus E, Grunhaus L, Davis JM, and Belmaker R: Genetic control of human plasma creatine phosphokinase activity. Clin Genet 13:321, 1978.

52. Mendell JR, Sahenk Z, Whitaker JN, et al: Polyneuropathy and IgM monoclonal gammopathy: Studies on the pathogenetic role of anti-myelin-associated glycoprotein antibody. Ann Neurol 17:243, 1985.

53. Mendell JR, Saida K, Ganansia MF, et al: Toxic polyneuropathy produced by methyl n-butyl ketone. Science 185:787, 1974.

54. Deleted in proof.

55. Miller RG and Kuntz NL: Nerve conduction studies in infants and children. J Child Neurol 1:19, 1986.

56. Miller RG, Layzer RB, Mellenthin MA, Golabi M, Francoz RA, and Mall JC: Emery-Dreifuss muscular dystrophy with autosomal dominant transmission. Neurol 35:1230, 1985.

57. Mills KR and Edwards RHT: Investigative strategies for muscle pain. J Neurol Sci 58:73, 1983.

58. Mizusawa H, Takagi A, Sugita H, and Toyokura Y: Mounding phenomenon: An experimental study in vitro. Neurology 33:90, 1983.

59. Munsat TL, Baloh R, Pearson CM, and Fowler W: Serum enzyme alterations in neuromuscular disorders. JAMA 226:1536, 1973.

60. Myers GJ: Understanding the floppy baby. In Griggs RC and Moxley RT (eds): Advances in Neurology, Vol 17. Raven Press, New York, 1977, p 295.

61. Newham DJ, Jones DA, and Edwards RHT: Large delayed plasma creatine kinase changes after stepping exercise. Muscle Nerve 6:380, 1983.

62. Nomenclature Committee: A Glossary of Terms Used in Clinical Electromyography. American Association of Electromyography and Electrodiagnosis, Rochester, MN, 1980.

63. Osher RH and Griggs RC: Orbicularis fatigue: The "peek" sign of myasthenia gravis. Arch Ophthalmol 97:677, 1979.

64. Panayiotopoulos CP and Scarpalezos S: Dystrophia myotonica: Peripheral nerve involvement and pathogenetic implications. J Neurol Sci 27:1, 1976.

65. Partanen J and Lang H: EMG dynamics in polymyositis: A quantitative single motor unit potential study. J Neurol Sci 57:221, 1982.

66. Patel AN and Swami RK: Muscle percussion and neostigmine test in the clinical evaluation of neuromuscular disorders. N Engl J Med 281:523, 1969.

67. Pearson CM, Rimer DG, and Mommaerts WFHM: A metabolic myopathy due to absence of muscle phosphorylase. Am J Med 30:502, 1961.

68. Pickett JB: Late components of motor unit potentials in a patient with myoglobinuria. Ann Neurol 3:461, 1978.

69. Pleasure DE, Walsh GO, and Engel

WK: Atrophy of skeletal muscle in patients with Cushing's syndrome. Arch Neurol 22:118, 1970.

70. Pollock M and Dyck PJ: Peripheral nerve morphometry in myotonic dystrophy. Arch Neurol 33:33, 1976.

71. Ramirez JA, Mendell JR, Warmolts JR, and Griggs RC: Phenytoin neuropathy: structural changes in the sural nerve. Ann Neurol 19:162, 1986.

72. Roth G: The origin of fasciculations. Ann Neurol 12:542, 1982.

73. Roth G: Fasciculations and their F-response: Localisation of their axonal origin. J Neurol Sci 63:299, 1984.

74. Said G, Bathien N, and Cesaro P: Peripheral neuropathies and tremor. Neurology 32:480, 1982.

75. Said G, Lacroix-Ciaudo C, Fujimura H, Blas C, and Faux N: The peripheral neuropathy of necrotizing arteritis: A clinicopathological study. Ann Neurol 23:461, 1988.

76. Sanders DB: Acquired myasthenia gravis: In Brumback RA and Gerst JW (eds): The Neuromuscular Junction. Futura, Mount Kisco, NY, 1984, p 257.

77. Sanders DB and Howard JF: AAEE minimonograph #25: Single-fiber electromyography in myasthenia gravis. Muscle Nerve 9:809, 1986.

78. Shahani BT: Electromyography in CNS Disorders: Central EMG. Butterworth, Stoneham, MA, 1984.

79. Siegel AJ, Silverman LM, and Holman BL: Elevated creatine kinase MB isoenzyme levels in marathon runners: Normal myocardial scintigrams suggest noncardiac source. JAMA 246:2049, 1981.

80. Silverman LM, Mendell JR, Sahenk Z, and Fontana MB: Significance of creatine phosphokinase isoenzymes in Duchenne dystrophy. Neurology 26:561, 1976.

81. Sladky JT, Brown MJ, and Berman PH: Chronic inflammatory demyelinating polyneuropathy of infancy: A corticosteroid-responsive disorder. Ann Neurol 20:76, 1986.

82. Spiro AJ: Minipolymyoclonus. A neglected sign in childhood spinal muscular atrophy. Neurology 20:1124, 1970.

83. Stålberg E: Clinical electrophysiology in myasthenia gravis. J Neurol Neurosurg Psychiatry 43:622, 1980.

84. Stern LZ, Gruener R, Kirkpatrick JB, and Nemeth P: The fine structure of cortisone-induced myopathy. Exp Neurol 36:530, 1972.

85. Sunohara N, Takagi A, Nonaka I, Sugita H, and Satoyoshi E: Idiopathic hyperCKemia. Neurology 34:544, 1984.

86. Swift TR and Greenberg MK: Miscellaneous neuromuscular transmission disorders. In Brumback RA and Gerst JW (eds): The Neuromuscular Junction. Futura, Mount Kisco, NY, 1984, p 295.

87. Tripp ME, Katcher ML, Peters HA, et al: Systemic carnitine deficiency presenting as familial endocardial fibroelastosis: A treatable cardiomyopathy. N Engl J Med 305:385, 1981.

88. Trojaborg W and Buchthal F: Malignant and benign fasciculations. Acta Neurol Scand 41:(Suppl 13):251, 1965.

89. Tsung SH: Several conditions causing elevation of serum CK-MB and CK-BB. Am J Clin Pathol 75:711, 1981.

90. Uncini A, Lange DJ, Lovelace RE, Solomon M, and Hays AP: Long-duration polyphasic motor unit potentials in myopathies: A quantitative study with pathological correlation. Muscle Nerve 13:263, 1990.

91. Vincent A, Cull-Candy SG, Newsom-Davis J, Trautmann A, Molenaar PC, and Polak RL: Congenital myasthenia: End-plate acetylcholine receptors and electrophysiology in five cases. Muscle Nerve 4:306, 1981.

92. Warmolts JR: Electrodiagnosis in neuromuscular disorders. Ann Intern Med 95:599, 1981.

93. Watters GV and Williams TW: Early onset myotonic dystrophy: Clinical and laboratory findings in five families and a review of the literature. Arch Neurol 17:137, 1967.

94. Wei N, Pavlidis N, Tsokos G, Elin RJ, and Plotz PH: Clinical significance of low creatine phosphokinase values in patients with connective tissue diseases. JAMA 246:1921, 1981.

95. Weiner IH and Weiner HL: Nocturnal

leg muscle cramps. JAMA 244:2332, 1980.

96. Welch KMA and Goldberg DM: Serum creatine phosphokinase in motor neuron disease. Neurology 22:697, 1972.

97. Wettstein A: The origin of fascicula-tions in motoneuron disease. Ann Neurol 5:295, 1979.

98. Yunus MB and Masi AT: Juvenile pri-mary fibromyalgia syndrome: A clini-cal study of thirty-three patients and matched normal controls. Arthritis Rheum 28:138, 1985.

Chapter 3

GENETIC EVALUATION OF THE PATIENT AND FAMILY

CLINICAL EVALUATION
APPLICATION OF RECOMBINANT
  DNA TECHNOLOGY
USE OF GENETIC INFORMATION
  FOR DIAGNOSIS

The gene defect or chromosomal location of many inherited myopathies has been identified (Table 3–1). In many of the genetic muscle disorders, specific diagnosis now depends on demonstrating the gene defect or defective gene product. In still other muscle disorders, particularly the inflammatory myopathies, predisposing inherited factors may be important even though the disease also has an acquired rather than exclusively genetic cause. Evaluation of the patient with myopathy requires careful review of the family and, when appropriate, evaluation of the at-risk family members. In addition, for many muscle diseases, recombinant DNA technology provides specific information related to diagnosis that can be used for genetic counseling and prenatal diagnosis.

CLINICAL EVALUATION

Family history should be sought from the patient and family members but with a recognition that the family history may be unreliable. Factors contrib-uting to a misleading family history include denial of weakness for fear of job loss, failure to recognize mild manifestations, misinterpretation of facial features as part of family resemblance, and refusal to accept a genetic disease because of guilt or fear of losing a potential spouse. For all of these reasons, it is advisable to examine family members for signs of disease whenever possible. Myotonic dystrophy and facioscapulohumeral dystrophy are particularly likely to be overlooked despite obvious diagnostic features apparent to an examiner. The same is true for certain congenital and mitochondrial myopathies, in which extraocular motility abnormalities may be found. Characteristic facial and ocular features can also be detected on photographs of family members.

A positive family history may be helpful in diagnosis by defining the pattern of inheritance and identifying other at-risk family members. Asymptomatic, clinically normal siblings are at risk, particularly if younger than the age when the patient developed symptoms. In addition to the physical examination, certain laboratory tests may be helpful in identifying disease in at-risk family members. These tests include creatine kinase (CK) blood testing, electromyography, electrocardiography, and ophthalmologic evaluation. For many genetic disorders, however, recombinant DNA technology is the most direct and useful method of study.

Table 3–1 CHROMOSOMAL LOCALIZATION OF THE MYOPATHIES

Chromosome	Disease
1	Phosphofructokinase deficiency
	Carnitine palmitoyltransferase deficiency
	Adenosine monophosphate deaminase deficiency
	Nemaline myopathy
4	Facioscapulohumeral dystrophy
5	Limb-girdle dystrophy (autosomal dominant)
7	Myotonia congenita (autosomal recessive; Becker's disease)
	Myotonia congenita (autosomal dominant; Thomsen's disease)
	Phosphoglycerate mutase deficiency
9	Fukuyama congenital muscular dystrophy
11	Myophosphorylase deficiency (McArdle's disease)
	Lactate dehydrogenase deficiency
13	Severe childhood muscular dystrophy (autosomal recessive)
	Phosphoglycerate kinase deficiency
15	Limb-girdle dystrophy (autosomal recessive)
17	Hyperkalemic periodic paralysis
	Paramyotonia congenita
	Atypical myotonia congenita
	Acid maltase deficiency
19	Myotonic dystrophy
	Central core disease
	Malignant hyperthermia (Ryanodine receptor)
X	Duchenne and Becker dystrophies
	Emery-Dreifuss syndrome
	Centronuclear myopathy

APPLICATION OF RECOMBINANT DNA TECHNOLOGY

Many advances in molecular genetics are useful in everyday practice. The original isolation and cloning of disease-related genes depended on knowledge of well-defined proteins, such as in the hemoglobinopathies. More recently, an approach referred to as *reverse genetics* has defined the molecular basis of disorders for which the gene product is unknown. One of the best examples of defining a disease gene without prior knowledge of the gene product occurred in Duchenne and Becker muscular dystrophies (DMD/BMD) (see p. 104), leading to the discovery of the dystrophin gene defect.[12] Once a disease gene has been cloned, the use of genetic information becomes an integral part of diagnosis and carrier detection. Genetic information now defines Duchenne and Becker muscular dystrophy. In other diseases, even prior to characterization of a gene, linkage analysis defines its chromosomal localization; linkage information can then be used for carrier detection and prenatal diagnosis.[11] Table 3–1 lists some diseases in which linkage information is important for diagnosis.

Patient and Family Sampling

Disease genes can be detected by examination of patient DNA. For most disorders, the simplest and easiest source of DNA is peripheral blood leukocytes. The buffy coat of a sample of unclotted blood (using ethylenediaminetetraacetate acid [EDTA] or heparin) yields leukocytes from which DNA can be extracted. An advantage of using DNA for diagnosis, in contrast to identification of an abnormal gene product (e.g., dystrophin), is that all somatic cells of an individual contain the same DNA. In many instances expression of the gene product is confined to a target issue, which may require biopsy for analysis. Target tissue obtained any time during a patient's life can, however, serve as an alternative source of DNA and can be useful for families in whom the affected member is deceased. In the case of muscle disorders, samples of muscle are frequently stored in the fresh frozen state for indefinite periods; this tissue sample represents a valuable DNA reservoir.

FETAL SAMPLING

For prenatal diagnosis, two major sources of DNA are available. DNA can be extracted directly from cells in amniotic fluid samples, either at the time of amniocentesis or after culture of these cells for several weeks. A second source is from chorionic villus sampling (CVS). Because the outer layer of the chorionic plate is composed of cells originating in the fetus, biopsies of this placental layer through a transcervical or transabdominal approach at about 11 to 12 weeks gestation provides a direct source of fetal DNA. Opinion varies as to the risks of fetal mortality following CVS, but many believe that fetal mortality is not increased above the spontaneous abortion rate of the first trimester and that overall risks do not significantly differ from those of amniocentesis.[3]

Probes for DNA Analysis

Detection of disease genes requires the availability of suitable DNA probes to identify the gene of interest. Different types of probes are used. For genes with known sequences, chemically synthesized *oligonucleotide (single-stranded DNA) probes* are available. These probes hybridize either to a part of the gene, or, less often, to the entire gene. *Complementary DNA (cDNA) probes* are cloned fragments of copies of messenger RNA (mRNA). *Genomic DNA probes* are cloned fragments of natural DNA. These genomic DNA probes differ from cDNA probes in that genomic DNA probes include both coding regions (exons) and intervening sequences (introns) of the gene. Introns are spliced out of the transcript during mRNA processing. The resulting mRNA is spliced together and translated in the ribosomes to form the amino acid sequence of the protein gene product.

Genomic DNA probes are prepared through the use of restriction enzyme digestion of natural DNA. *Restriction enzymes* are obtained from bacteria and are named according to their bacterial source (for example, *Eco*RI derived from *E. coli*). Usually, restriction enzymes (also called endonucleases) recognize a specific sequence of between 4 and 6 base pairs and cut the DNA at every point where this target sequence occurs. These generated restriction fragments represent the probes for DNA analysis. Restriction endonuclease digestion of genomic DNA can also be used to identify inherited variations in DNA, known as polymorphisms, which usually have no phenotypic consequences. They are important, however, because they may result in restriction fragments of different sizes in different individuals or in differences in the fragment sizes between alleles in the same individual. These fragments of different lengths are called restriction fragment length polymorphisms (RFLPs). The RFLPs are especially useful as markers for establishing the position of genes to which they may be linked on a particular chromosome (see discussion on linkage analysis, p. 87).

Southern Blotting

The procedure known as Southern blotting (named for E. M. Southern) is a common method of DNA study for clinical genetic purposes (Fig. 3–1). The isolated DNA from any of the sources already mentioned is digested with restriction enzymes. The particular enzyme chosen depends on the gene or RFLP of interest. The digested DNA is loaded onto agarose gels, where differ-

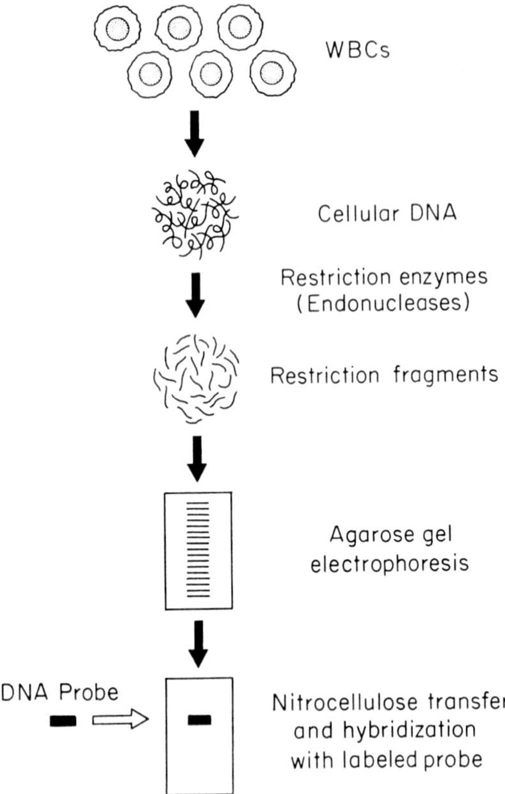

Figure 3–1. Southern blot analysis. DNA is extracted from white blood cells (WBCs), although other tissue sources of DNA may be used. The cellular DNA is digested by restriction enzymes, followed by electrophoresis on agarose gels, which separates the DNA according to the size of the fragments. The DNA is denatured by alkali treatment, and the fragments are transferred to a nitrocellulose filter, which is exposed to a labeled DNA probe. The probe will anneal to the complementary DNA, which can be identified by autoradiography or colorimetric methods.

ent size fragments are separated by electrophoresis. The term *Southern blotting* refers to the method of transferring DNA fragments from the agarose gel to a filter (nitrocellulose or other synthetic material) for hybridization using labeled DNA probes, which recognize complementary strands of DNA. In most cases the probes are labeled with radioisotopes and are visualized by means of autoradiography. An alternative technique employs avidin-biotin–labeled probes, which can be recognized by a colorimetric method.

Polymerase Chain Reaction

Polymerase chain reaction (PCR) is a powerful method of amplifying small amounts of DNA (Fig. 3–2). Picogram amounts of starting DNA can be amplified 1000-fold to microgram quantities of DNA. In clinical practice, this method is of great help for the study of disease

POLYMERASE CHAIN REACTION

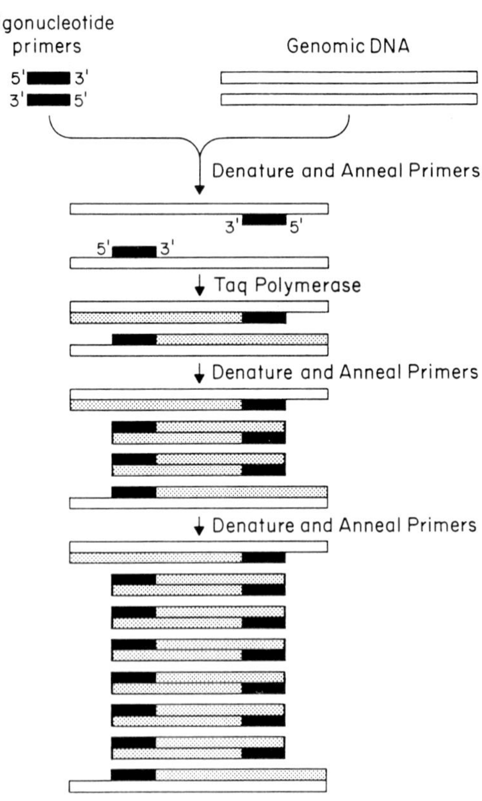

Figure 3–2. Polymerase chain reaction (PCR). A DNA preparation (usually genomic) is denatured and annealed to two short oligonucleotide primers complementary to sense and antisense strands flanking the target region. Taq (DNA) polymerase (see text) amplifies DNA beginning from the 3' ends of the primers. With repeat cycles of denaturing and annealing, the short products (dotted regions of DNA) can be preferentially amplified and will grow exponentially for 20 to 30 cycles until reaching a plateau.

genes that have been previously cloned and sequenced. A portion of the gene of interest (or less often, the entire gene) can be amplified for detection of a mutation. The technique of PCR employs a pair of oligonucleotide primers that consist of complementary sequences flanking a particular region of the gene of interest (see Fig. 3–2). The primers, chemically synthesized on the basis of a known sequence, anneal to the denatured (that is, single-stranded) DNA sample, and synthesis proceeds in a 5′ to 3′ direction after the addition of deoxyribonucleotide triphosphates (dNTPs). Development of this technique was markedly enhanced by the availability of a specific DNA polymerase derived from *Thermus aquaticus*, referred to as Taq polymerase. Following synthesis of the sense and antisense strands of genomic DNA, the products are denatured and allowed to reassociate again with the primers for further synthesis. The target sequence of DNA lying between the primers is preferentially amplified.

USE OF GENETIC INFORMATION FOR DIAGNOSIS

Detection of Disease Genes

Identification of a DNA mutation within a particular gene permits the unequivocal diagnosis of a specific disease; this ability has great importance in differentiating disorders with overlapping phenotypes, such as the muscular dystrophies. Mutation analysis is also very important for carrier detection and prenatal diagnosis. The common types of mutations are listed in Table 3–2. Deletions, duplications, and some point mutations are most readily detectable in clinical practice. Other types of mutations, such as splice-site and frame-shift mutations, often require more complex procedures such as isolation of mRNA from the target tissue.

Mutations causing *deletions and duplications* are the easiest to recognize (Fig. 3–3). DNA isolated from peripheral blood leukocytes can be analyzed using either of two methods. If cDNA probes are available for the coding region of the gene (as in DMD), a deletion can be seen using Southern blot analysis. If the gene has been sequenced, then PCR can be used to amplify DNA to detect the gene mutation. DMD deletions can be mapped to specific exon regions in approximately 65% of patients (Figs. 3–3 and 3–4).[5] Partial gene duplications, thought to arise by nonhomologous crossing over during meiosis, result in the increased intensity of a band of radioactivity corresponding to a specific DNA exon sequence, which can be identified on Southern blot analysis (see Fig. 3–3). Identifying such duplications requires careful quantitation of the amounts of DNA loaded in a gel,

Table 3–2 COMMON TYPES OF DNA MUTATIONS

Deletion	The loss of a sequence of DNA that results in regions on either side of the deletion being joined together; such defects result in the failure of transcription or production of abnormal gene products.
Duplication	A redundant DNA sequence that may represent any part of a gene or even an entire gene; such abnormalities usually impair transcription or translation of the gene product.
Insertion	The addition of one (a point mutation) or more base pairs, so that the coding sequence is altered.
Base substitution	Replacement of a single base, which alters the coding sequence (one type of point mutation).
Splice-site	Alterations of the base pair sequences at the exon-intron boundaries, which create errors in mRNA processing. If specific base pair relationships are altered, a new splice-site may be created.
Frame-shift	Any mutation altering the number of bases can change the reading frame of mRNA, which is read in triplets from a fixed starting point.

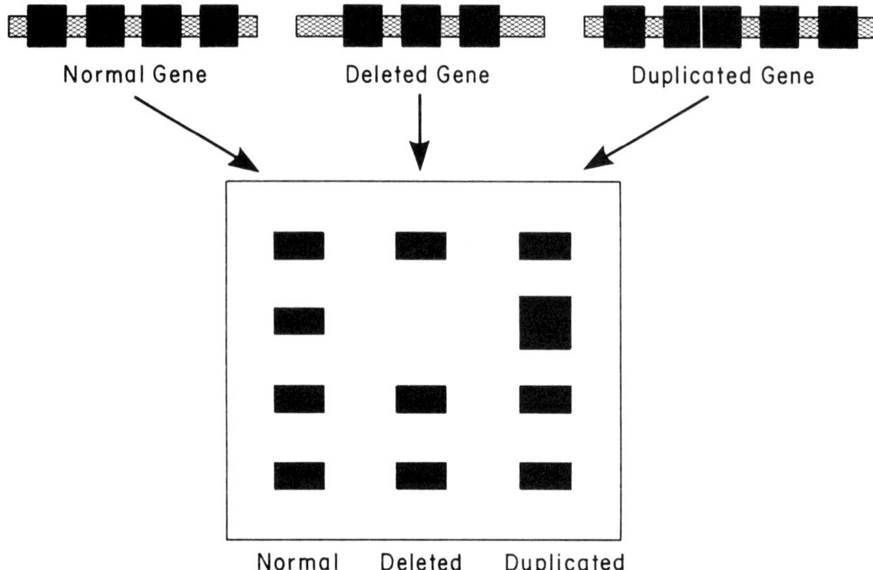

Figure 3–3. Southern blot of DNA from normal, deleted, and duplicated genes. The normal gene shows four exons (■), each represented on the gel. The deleted gene shows only three exons, with the specific exon deleted appearing as a blank region on the gel. The duplicated gene shows the specific duplication represented by twice the amount of DNA.

combined with scanning densitometric analysis.[10]

The tediousness of Southern blot analysis for recognizing deletions can be avoided by using PCR. A systematic approach to amplification of an entire coding region of a gene can be employed. For this method of determination, specific oligonucleotide primers are used to amplify regions of the gene. In fact, current methods (multiplex PCR) allow for simultaneously amplifying specific coding regions of the gene known to be hot spots for deletions.[1,4] This use of multiplex PCR is particularly valuable in DMD, where a complex of primers can be used to detect more than 98% of the deletions known to occur in the dystrophin transcript.[1] The PCR technique has also proved valuable in identifying increased numbers of trinucleotide repeats associated with X-linked bulbospinal muscular atrophy (Kennedy's syndrome),[13] myotonic dystrophy,[6,14] Huntington's disease,[10a] and spinocerebellar ataxia, type 1.[15a]

Disorders resulting from *point mutations*, either a *base substitution* or an *insertion*, are more difficult to recognize. Several approaches can now detect point mutations in patients. *Restriction enzyme mapping* is useful if a point mutation alters a base pair sequence, creating or removing a restriction enzyme site (Fig. 3–5). This approach has been used for sickle cell disease[18] and familial amyloidotic polyneuropathy.[2]

Allele-specific enzymatic amplification is another method of detecting point mutations. This PCR method employs a highly specific oligonucleotide primer, which will anneal only to the mutant DNA and not to the normal DNA copy[15] (Fig. 3–6). This technique provides for rapid diagnosis and is highly advantageous for carrier detection and prenatal diagnosis.

A third method, *chemical mismatch cleavage*, facilitates recognition of point mutations without the need for direct DNA sequencing of amplified PCR

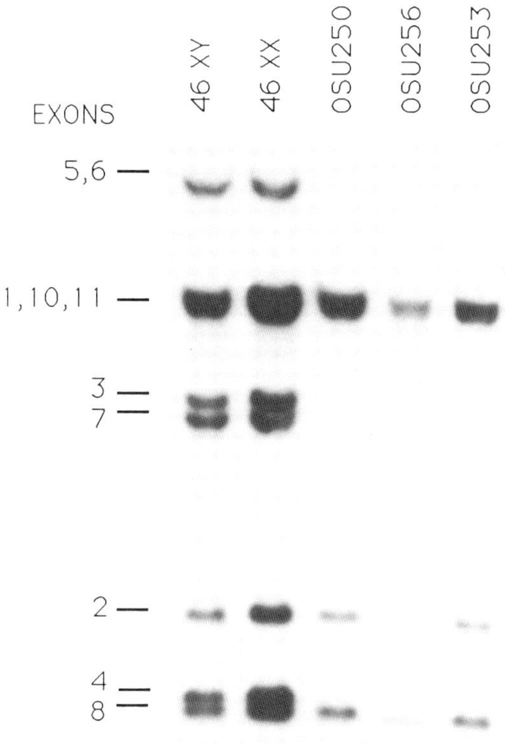

Figure 3–4. Southern blot analysis of genomic DNA from five patients: two normals (male = 46 XY, female 46 XX) and three Duchenne muscular dystrophy (DMD) patients (OSU250, OSU256, OSU253). The DNA has been digested with *Eco*RI, and deleted exons (5, 6 and 3, 7) can be seen in DMD lanes compared to normals. (Courtesy of Arthur Burghes, PhD, The Ohio State University.)

applications are limited. For example, *splice-site mutations* may occur in the processing of mRNA. The initial transcript of mRNA is a precursor corresponding to the entire gene, including introns and exons. Before leaving the nucleus to enter the cytoplasm, introns are removed and exons are spliced together. The potential for errors is apparent, especially in large genes, such as the dystrophin gene, which is estimated to have 75 or more exons. Removal of the introns and splicing of exons depends on the presence of a specific base pair sequence. At the 5′ exon-intron junction, the invariable sequence of bases, guanine and thymine, is referred to as the donor site (GT). At the 3′ junction, adenine and guanine compose the acceptor site (AG). Mutations causing abnormalities in donor and acceptor sites may induce splicing errors, resulting in a complete failure of RNA synthesis. In some instances, different species of abnormal mRNA are the result of new splice sites. Mutations occurring within an exon can mimic the acceptor site of the intron-exon boundary, resulting in a so-called *cryptic splice site* and causing the synthesis of an aberrant mRNA. Recognition of these types of mutations is possible by isolation of mRNA from the target tissue, followed by making a cDNA copy of the faulty message using reverse transcriptase and sequencing the DNA after PCR amplification.

The approach for studying splice-site mutations also has particular application for the interpretation of mutations affecting the reading frame of a nucleotide sequence. In the translation of mRNA, the genetic code is read in triplets from a fixed starting point at the 5′ end of the gene. A mutation that in any way changes the number of bases in a codon will alter the reading frame of the message. These *frame-shift mutations* often impair translation by producing a premature stop codon or by creating splice sites, permitting the production of an abnormal protein. Further understanding of these types of mutations also requires study of the mRNA and sequencing of the derivative cDNA. In the

products. After amplification of the normal and mutant DNA using PCR, the products are radiolabeled and allowed to anneal. At the site of the point mutation, the heteroduplexed DNA will be mismatched, and the DNA strands will be cleaved after exposure to osmium tetroxide (for thymine and cytosine mismatches) or hydroxylamine (for cytosine mismatches) following subsequent incubation with piperadine. This technique has been successfully used for detecting point mutations in ornithine transcarbamoylase deficiency, an X-linked recessive disease.[7]

Although it is appropriate to understand other types of mutations, clinical

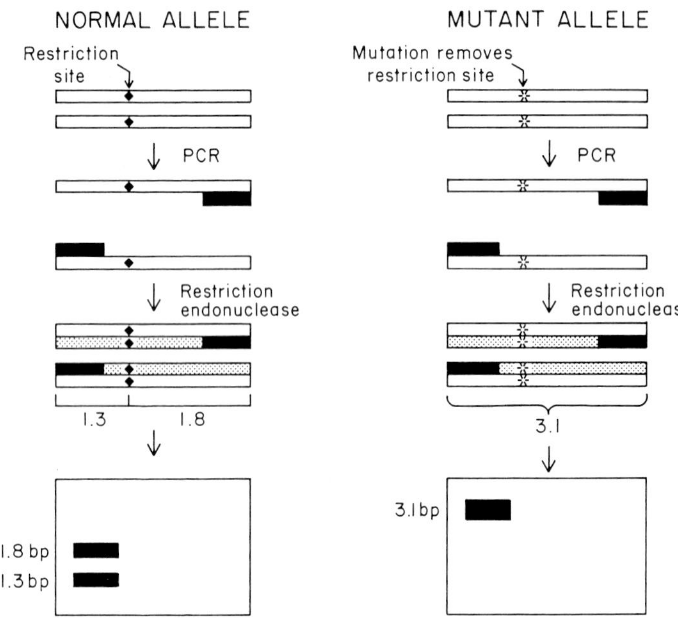

Figure 3–5. Restriction enzyme mapping. In the normal allele, a restriction site is shown (♦) related to a specific base pair (bp) sequence. In the mutant allele, a restriction site is removed by a point mutation (✺). After PCR amplification, the mutant allele is resistant to restriction endonuclease digestion, and only a 3.1 bp fragment can be seen. The normal site shows two DNA fragments of 1.8 bp and 1.3 bp.

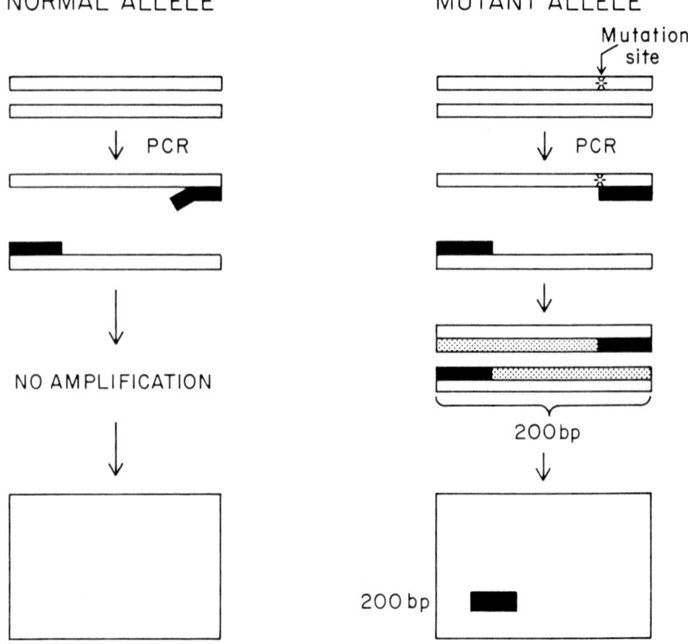

Figure 3–6. Allele-specific enzymatic amplification. Oligonucleotide primers for PCR are designed to anneal to the mutant allele at the site of the point mutation (✺). This will permit specific amplification only from the DNA of the mutant allele, which can be identified by gel electrophoresis. At the normal allele, the 3′ end of the primer will not be complementary, and thus no PCR amplification products will be found by gel electrophoresis.

future, rapid techniques of analysis will permit recognition of these types of mutations in clinical practice.

Carrier Detection and Prenatal Diagnosis

All of the methods described for mutation analysis can be applied to carrier detection and prenatal diagnosis. Once a specific mutation type has been defined in a proband, any one of the approaches outlined for detection of disease genes will be available. As noted previously, DNA derived from peripheral blood leukocytes is the best source to use for detection of carriers, whereas in prenatal diagnosis, DNA from amniotic cells or chorionic villus sampling is routinely used. These methods are currently being used in Duchenne dystrophy (see Chapter 4) and are applicable to many other myopathies (Table 3–1).

Linkage Analysis

For many muscle diseases, the gene product and the precise chromosomal localization are not yet known; to attain the goals of carrier detection and prenatal diagnosis, the reverse genetic approach becomes mandatory. The first objective is to define a locus on the chromosomal map for the disease gene of interest, using linkage analysis. The gene can be cloned and sequenced using sophisticated molecular techniques of chromosomal walking and jumping. This approach depends heavily on RFLPs, the DNA variations available because of inherited differences recognized by restriction enzymes. RFLPs are inherited as Mendelian codominant traits, but they are not confined to portions of the genome that express a phenotype and should not be confused with genes. Those RFLPs that lie close to genes are invaluable markers for following the inheritance of a gene through a family. Previously defined genes can

also be used as markers to help find the position of as-yet-unknown disease genes.

Linkage analysis is a systematic approach for finding disease genes. The principle is to establish the frequency of recombination (recombination fraction) between two loci as a measure of the distance separating them on the chromosome. Recombination is an event occurring during meiosis, in which two sister chromatids exchange DNA. For unlinked loci that are far apart on the same chromosome or on different chromosomes, the recombination fraction (that is, the proportion of recombinants occurring out of all of the opportunities available) is equal to 0.5 (50%). However great the distance between two loci, the recombination fraction will not exceed 0.5 because of multiple crossover events. For loci that are linked, the recombination fraction will vary between 0 and 0.5, depending on the distance. Chromosomal distance for linked loci is expressed in units known as Morgans (after T. H. Morgan), where a centimorgan (cM) corresponds to a distance between two loci with a 1% recombination frequency. It is important to understand the conceptual difference between distance on a linkage map and distance on a physical map of the human genome. Genetic distance defined by recombination may be inaccurate because of recombination hot spots and cold spots, variations between males and females, and differences in the position of chromosomes. For this reason, a major ongoing task of the international molecular biology community is to define a physical map of the human genome based on actual base sequencing.

To establish linkage between an inherited disease and an RFLP, DNA is obtained from family members. It is important to reemphasize that the RFLP is a random sequence, not coding for a gene, and usually is totally unrelated to the disease gene under study. If the chromosome on which the gene of interest is known, as in the case of an X-linked disease, the DNA probes can be specifically derived from that chromosome (see Table 3–1). This is possible through the use of fluorescence-activated cell sorters, which can isolate specific chromosomes. The first RFLP marker to be identified for a disease gene without an established gene product was associated with Huntington's disease.[8] Two large kindreds with many affected family members were studied. A battery of RFLPs was tested for linkage to the disease, and one marker, G8, was found to be linked to the Huntington's locus. In the case of Duchenne dystrophy, two RFLPs, RC8 and L1.28, were linked to the dystrophin gene several years before its cloning.[9,16] Analysis of a pedigree to establish linkage requires the use of a statistical method in which a *lod score* is derived. This word specifically refers to a ratio of the probability of linkage expressed as a logarithm and means the "log odd" or log of the odds of linkage. A lod score of +3.0 or greater is statistically significant evidence of linkage, whereas a score of less than −2.0 is evidence against linkage.

Once linkage has been established between a marker and a disease gene, not only is this information available to the molecular biologist attempting to clone the disease gene but the information may be very valuable for carrier detection and prenatal diagnosis. Thus in Duchenne dystrophy, approximately 65% of the mutations can be identified, leaving about 35% of cases in which the gene defect is still not apparent. For such a family, a host of linkage markers flanking the dystrophin gene have become available (see Fig. 4–16). Carrier detection studies or prenatal diagnoses using RFLPs require the availability of a minimum number of family members, including both parents and the proband, as well as the carrier suspect or fetus (see Fig. 4–17). Each family member must be evaluated with a battery of probes to find a probe or probes that will provide information necessary to trace the inheritance of the disease gene through the family. For a particular RFLP to be informative, individuals must be heterozygous for the polymorphism, so that restriction bands of different sizes can be identified and used as markers to follow the chromosome carrying the disease gene (see Figs. 4–16 and 4–17).

The major limitation of linkage analysis for diagnosis is the frequency of recombination. The greater the distance between the RFLP and the disease gene, the higher the risk for a recombination event. For example, an RFLP that is established to be 4 cM from the locus has a 4% recombination frequency. For disease genes in which flanking RFLPs are available, the statistical probability of error can be significantly reduced. If markers on either side of the locus are inherited together, for example, it is highly unlikely that a recombination event has occurred that would move the disease gene to the opposite chromosome and leave the flanking RFLPs intact. In the analysis of such a pedigree, in which flanking markers have been identified in parents and their offspring (where each of the markers is estimated to be 4 cM from the disease gene), the probability of a recombination event can be reduced from 4% for each linkage marker alone to 0.16% (4% × 4% = 0.16%) for the combined markers.

USE OF LINKAGE ANALYSIS IN SPECIFIC MYOPATHIES

The detailed use of linkage analysis is discussed in Chapter 4 under the specific diseases. Table 3–1 lists those conditions for which linkage analysis is applicable for genetic counseling and for prenatal diagnosis. For most of these disorders, the gene defect and abnormality of gene product will soon be defined. For all, the precision of linkage analysis will improve rapidly. An example of linkage analysis is presented in Chapter 4 (Figure 4–17).

One additional concept requiring a brief comment is *linkage dysequilibrium*, which implies that two loci are found in association more commonly than would be expected. For example, a mutation occurring at a particular locus may become separated from its original neighbors by recombination events. A state of equilibrium will finally be established so that the new mutation will be associated with a nearby locus according to the frequency of the allele in the population. In linkage dysequilibrium, the mutation is more often inherited with a specific locus. A well-known example of haplotypes in dysequilibrium occurs in the HLA complex between the genes encoding A1 and B8 in North Europeans. A1 has a frequency of 0.17, and B8, a frequency of 0.11, resulting in an expected frequency of 0.0187 (0.17×0.11); however, the observed frequency of this haplotype's being inherited together is 0.09.[17] The basis of linkage dysequilibrium is unknown. One possibility is a "founder effect," which implies that the mutation resulting in linkage dysequilibrium is a relatively recent event that has not passed through the number of generations necessary to reach a state of equilibrium. The founder effect therefore suggests that all cases in the population under study arose from a single mutation or from similar mutations. For certain genetic diseases, linkage dysequilibrium is an important tool for carrier detection and prenatal diagnosis and may accelerate the finding of a gene by linkage analysis. Linkage dysequilibrium is present in the French-Canadian myotonic dystrophy population and was important in the effort to define the candidate gene in this myopathy.[6,14]

SUMMARY

Information about the molecular genetics of inherited myopathies has virtually exploded in a short time. This new information necessitates a fundamental understanding of the application of recombinant DNA technology for the management of patients with hereditary myopathies. This chapter reviews the basics of these techniques as applied to clinical practice. DNA analysis is particularly important for the study of Duchenne and Becker dystrophy, mito-

chondrial myopathies, periodic paralyses, and some of the myotonias, and it seems likely that the gene lesions for many more hereditary myopathies will be defined in the very near future.

REFERENCES

1. Beggs AH, Koenig M, Boyce FM, and Kunkel LM: Detection of 98% of DMD/BMD gene deletions by polymerase chain reaction. Hum Genet 86:45, 1990.
2. Benson MD and Wallace MR: Amyloidosis. In Scriver CR, Beaudet AL, Sly WS, and Valle D (eds): The Metabolic Basis of Inherited Disease. McGraw-Hill, New York, 1990, p 2439.
3. Canadian Collaborative CVS-Amniocentesis Clinical Trial Group: Multicentre randomised clinical trial of chorion villus sampling and amniocentesis. Lancet 1:1, 1989.
4. Chamberlain JS, Gibbs RA, Ranier JE, Nguyen PN, and Caskey CT: Deletion screening of the Duchenne muscular dystrophy locus via multiplex DNA amplification. Nucleic Acids Res 16:11141, 1988.
5. Forrest SM, Cross GS, Flint T, Speer A, Robson K JH, and Davies KE: Further studies of gene deletions that cause Duchenne and Becker muscular dystrophies. Genomics 2:109, 1988.
6. Fu Y-H, Pizzuti A, Fenwick RG, et al: An unstable triplet repeat in a gene related to myotonic muscular dystrophy. Science 255:1256, 1992.
7. Grompe M, Muzny DM, and Caskey CT: Scanning detection of mutations in human ornithine transcarbamoylase by chemical mismatch cleavage. Proc Natl Acad Sci USA 86:5888, 1989.
8. Gusella JF, Wexler NS, Conneally PM, et al: A polymorphic DNA marker genetically linked to Huntington's disease. Nature 306:234, 1983.
9. Harper PS: DNA markers and Duchenne muscular dystrophy. Arch Dis Child 59:195, 1984.
10. Hu X, Burghes AHM, Ray PN, Thompson MW, Murphy EG, and Worton RG: Partial gene duplication in Duchenne

and Becker muscular dystrophies. J Med Genet 25:369, 1988.

10a. Huntington's Disease Collaborative Research Group: A novel gene containing a trinucleotide repeat that is expanded and unstable on Huntington's disease chromosomes. Cell 72:971, 1993.

11. Hyser CL, Griggs RC, Mendell JR, et al: Use of serum creatine kinase, pyruvate kinase, and genetic linkage for carrier detection in Duchenne and Becker dystrophy. Neurology 37:4, 1987.

12. Koenig M, Hoffman EP, Bertelson CJ, Monaco AP, Feener C, and Kunkel LM: Complete cloning of the Duchenne muscular dystrophy (DMD) cDNA and preliminary genomic organization of the DMD gene in normal and affected individuals. Cell 50:509, 1987.

13. La Spada AR, Wilson EM, Lubahn DB, Harding AE, and Fischbeck KH: Androgen receptor gene mutations in X-linked spinal and bulbar muscular atrophy. Nature 352:77, 1991.

14. Mahadevan M, Tsilfidis C, Sabourin L, et al: Myotonic dystrophy mutation: An unstable CTG repeat in the 3′ untranslated region of the gene. Science 255:1253, 1992.

15. Mendell JR, Jiang XS, Warmolts JR, Nichols WC, and Benson MD: Diagnosis of Maryland/German familial amyloidotic polyneuropathy using allele-specific, enzymatically amplified, genomic DNA. Ann Neurol 27:553, 1990.

15a. Orr HT, Chung MY, Banji S, et al: Expansion of an unstable trinucleotide CAG repeat in spinocerebellar ataxia type 1. Nature Genet 4:221, 1993.

16. Pembrey ME, Davies KE, Winter RM, et al: Clinical use of DNA markers linked to the gene for Duchenne muscular dystrophy. Arch Dis Child 59:208, 1984.

17. Thompson JS and Thompson MW: Genetics in Medicine, ed 3. WB Saunders, Philadelphia, 1980.

18. Trent RJ, Davis B, Wilkinson T, and Kronenberg H: Identification of β variant hemoglobins by DNA restriction endonuclease mapping. Hemoglobin 8:443, 1984.

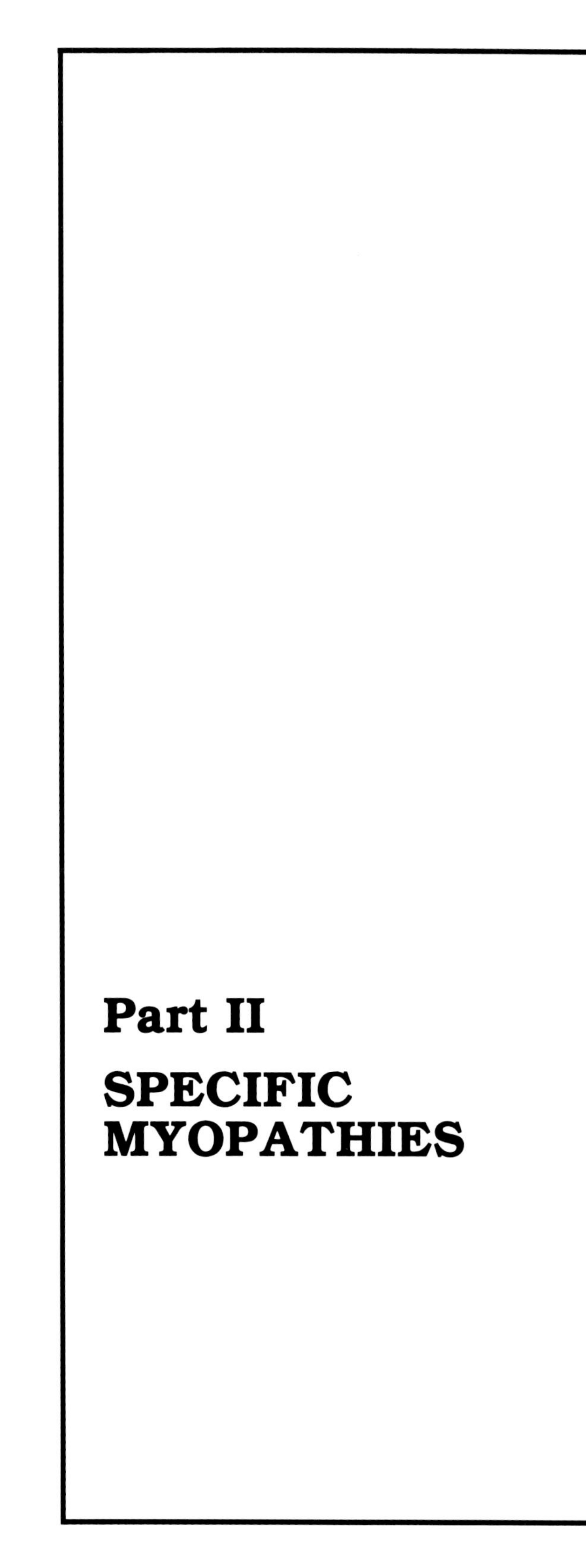

Part II

SPECIFIC MYOPATHIES

Chapter 4

THE MUSCULAR DYSTROPHIES

**DYSTROPHIN-DEFICIENT
  DYSTROPHIES
EMERY-DREIFUSS MUSCULAR
  DYSTROPHY
MYOTONIC MUSCULAR DYSTROPHY
FACIOSCAPULOHUMERAL
  MUSCULAR DYSTROPHY
SCAPULOPERONEAL SYNDROMES
LIMB-GIRDLE DYSTROPHY
OCULOPHARYNGEAL MUSCULAR
  DYSTROPHY
CONGENITAL MUSCULAR
  DYSTROPHY
DISTAL MYOPATHIES**

As a group, the muscular dystrophies can be defined as hereditary diseases that cause progressive muscle weakness. The term's implications — an unknown cause and a lack of effective treatment — are fading as our grasp of molecular defects continues to expand.

DYSTROPHIN-DEFICIENT DYSTROPHIES

Duchenne Muscular Dystrophy

Duchenne muscular dystrophy (DMD) (Table 4-1), less commonly referred to as pseudohypertrophic muscular dystrophy, occurs with an incidence of about 30 per 100,000 live male births.[143] The disease carries the name of the French neurologist, Duchenne, who established diagnostic criteria and accurately described muscle biopsy features. Molecular genetic studies led to the discovery of muscle dystrophin defi-

ciency,[88,89,234] which permits an unequivocal diagnosis of DMD and related phenotypes.

CLINICAL FEATURES

Although DMD can be diagnosed at birth on the basis of elevated serum creatine kinase (CK) activity and muscle biopsy, clinical manifestations are uncommon at that age. Some, but not all, boys with DMD exhibit delayed motor milestones, especially walking. Running and jumping prove particularly difficult and call attention to the muscle weakness. During the early stage of illness (ages 3–6), affected boys develop a broad-based waddling gait with an exaggerated lumbar lordosis (Fig. 4–1). To get up from the floor, the boys turn to face the floor, spread their legs, elevate their butts, and climb up their thighs using the hands (Gowers' sign, Fig. 4–2). Muscles often feel firm and rubbery, and certain muscle groups such as the calves, quadriceps, gluteals, and deltoids may be enlarged. Muscle fibers in these enlarged muscle groups undergo true hypertrophy early in the course of the disease. Later, when fat and connective tissue completely replace muscle, the term "pseudohypertrophy" is appropriate.

Muscle weakness follows a stereotyped pattern. The poor strength of the neck flexor group often goes unnoticed, but inability to lift the head against gravity occurs at all stages of the disease (see Fig. 2–2D and E). This neck flexor weakness distinguishes boys with typical DMD from those with a milder phenotype, termed outliers,[32] and from

Table 4–1 DYSTROPHIN-DEFICIENT DYSTROPHIES

Types	Musculoskeletal Features	Other Systems	Molecular Defect
Duchenne	Onset before age 5, progressive weakness of girdle muscles, calf hypertrophy, inability to walk after age 12, scoliosis, respiratory failure in second–third decade	Cardiomyopathy, mental retardation, gastric dilatation, intestinal pseudoobstruction	Severely reduced or absent dystrophin
Becker	Onset after age 5, progressive weakness of girdle muscles, calf hypertrophy, ability to walk after age 15, respiratory failure after fourth decade	Cardiomyopathy, mental retardation	Decreased or altered dystrophin
Outliers	Intermediate between Duchenne and Becker; neck flexors able to lift head against gravity; ability to walk after age 12 (but not age 15)	Cardiomyopathy, mental retardation	Decreased or altered dystrophin
Familial X-linked myalgia and muscle cramps	Muscle pain syndrome, calf hypertrophy, nonprogressive course	None	Altered dystrophin

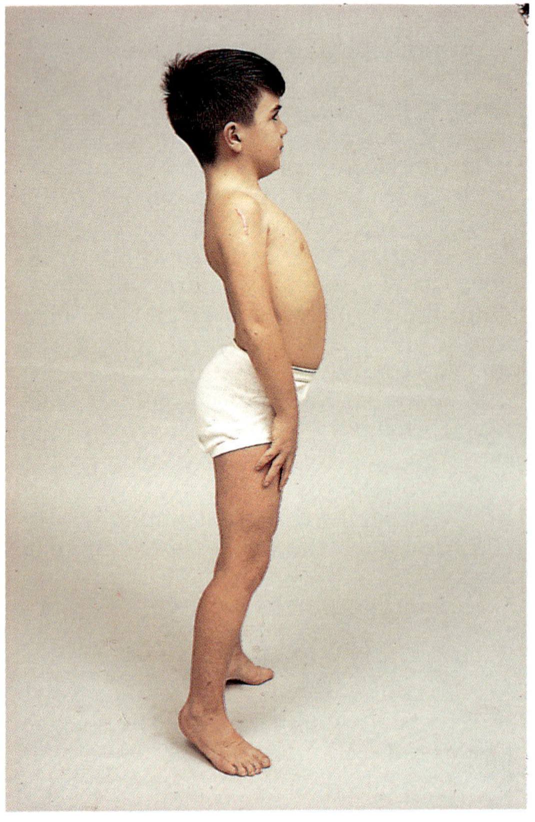

Figure 4–1. A 7-year-old boy with Duchenne dystrophy demonstrating lordotic posture and heel cord tightness (standing on toes).

those with Becker muscular dystrophy (see p. 102). The proximal lower-extremity muscles are involved earlier than upper-extremity muscles, and their weakness progresses more rapidly. The ankle plantar flexor and ankle invertor muscle groups remain remarkably strong throughout the entire illness. Except for the tongue, which often enlarges (see Fig. 2–18C), musculature innervated by cranial nerves remains relatively unaffected.

Functional ability, like overall strength, follows a relatively predictable pattern of deterioration.[32] Although boys between ages 3 and 6 often show transient improvement in performance of functional motor tasks such as climbing stairs, running, and getting up from the floor, by age 8 years they usually begin to lose the ability to walk and climb stairs. Most patients become dependent on long leg braces at about age 10 and become wheelchair-dependent around age 12.

Joint contractures are an important clinical manifestation. By age 6, most patients have contractures at the iliotibial bands, hip joints, and heel cords. Iliotibial band contractures severely

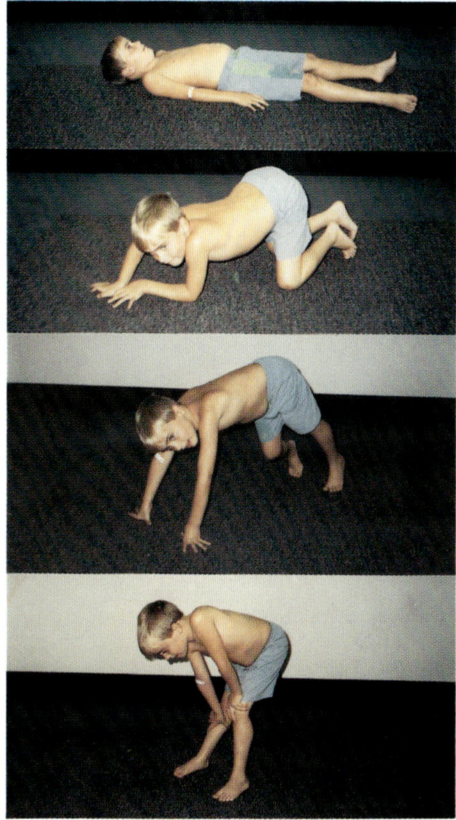

Figure 4–2. A 6-year-old boy with Duchenne dystrophy. In successive scenes (*top to bottom*) he demonstrates classic Gowers' sign in arising from the floor.

of contractures, particularly at the elbows and knees, correlates with decreasing ambulation and accelerates with increased wheelchair use. Contractures of shoulder joints do not occur until late in the disease.

Many boys with Duchenne dystrophy develop scoliosis requiring medical intervention.[31] The problem rarely occurs before age 11; severe curvatures usually evolve after wheelchair confinement. Increasing scoliosis, coupled with weakening of respiratory muscles, compromises pulmonary function. Unless patients receive respiratory support, death usually ensues around age 20, most commonly due to respiratory insufficiency and pneumonia.

Involvement of Other Organ Systems. The expression of dystrophin in tissues other than skeletal muscle, especially in cardiac and smooth muscle and brain,[88,89,234] may explain the involvement of these other organ systems.

Cardiac. As many as 90% of patients with DMD demonstrate electrocardiogram (ECG) abnormalities.[61,77] Tall right precordial R waves with an increased R/S amplitude ratio in V_1, and deep, narrow Q waves in left precordial leads are the most common and distinctive changes (Fig. 4–3). Intraatrial conduction-system defects are more common than atrioventricular and infranodal disturbances. Atrioventricular nodal block seldom occurs. Most patients demonstrate labile or persistent sinus tachycardia or other sinus arrhythmias. Ectopic rhythms, including atrial and ventricular premature beats, arise less frequently; ectopic tachyarrhythmias occur rarely.

limit hip flexion because of the fibrosis connecting the ileum with the tibia. Heel-cord contractures produce "toe walking" even in early childhood. Knee, elbow, and wrist extensor contractures occur at about age 8. The development

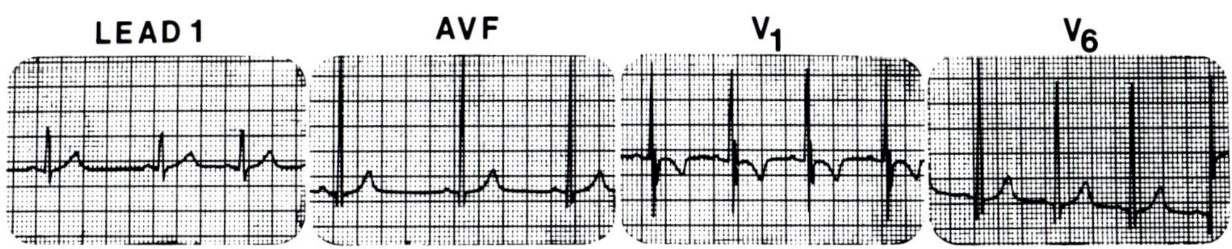

Figure 4–3. ECG leads in DMD showing tall precordial R waves, increased R/S ratio in V_1, and deep, narrow Q waves in V_6.

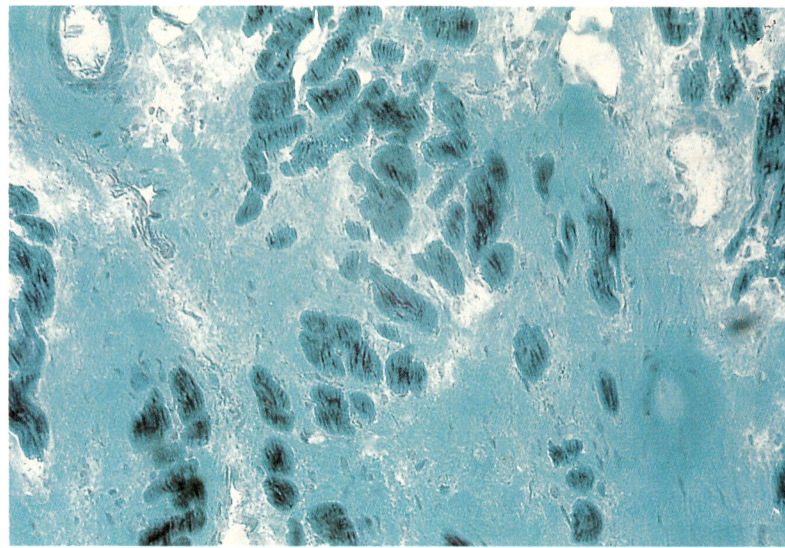

Figure 4–4. Severe myocardial fibrosis and loss of cardiac muscle from left ventricle of Duchenne dystrophy patient dying at age 21 (modified trichrome).

Autopsy studies of the hearts of patients with DMD show the initial and most extensive sites of myocardial fibrosis to be in the posterobasal portion and surrounding region of the left ventricular wall (Fig. 4–4). In contrast, the ventricular septum and the right ventricular and atrial mycoardium have much less involvement.[77] The conduction system seldom shows degenerative changes.

Most patients with DMD remain surprisingly free of cardiovascular symptoms. Congestive heart failure and cardiac arrhythmias usually occur only in the late stages, especially during times of stress from intercurrent infections. Rarely, however, patients have overt signs of congestive heart failure and, in fact, may die of cardiac failure with relative sparing of respiratory muscle function.[31]

Gastrointestinal. Clinical and pathologic involvement of smooth muscle of the gastrointestinal tract, although frequently overlooked, can be an important manifestation. A syndrome of acute gastric dilatation, also referred to as intestinal pseudo-obstruction, consists of sudden episodes of vomiting, associated with abdominal pain and distention, and may lead to death.[11,40] The acute gastric dilatation probably results from gastric hypomotility, which can be demonstrated by delayed gastric emptying using a standard radiolabeled meal of oatmeal.[11] Patients dying of this syndrome show degeneration of the outer, longitudinal, smooth-muscle layer of the stomach (Fig. 4–5).[11,123] Dystrophin deficiency leads to degeneration of smooth muscle.

Central Nervous System. The average intelligence quotient (IQ) of patients with DMD is approximately 1 standard deviation below the mean.[122] This impairment of intellectual function seems nonprogressive and affects the verbal ability more than the performance.[122] The mental subnormality in DMD cannot be attributed solely to physical limitations, as similarly disabled patients with spinal muscular atrophy do not have impaired intelligence.[46b] A neuropathologic correlate for mental retardation in DMD has not been established. Disordered neuronal cytoarchitecture and subcortical heter-

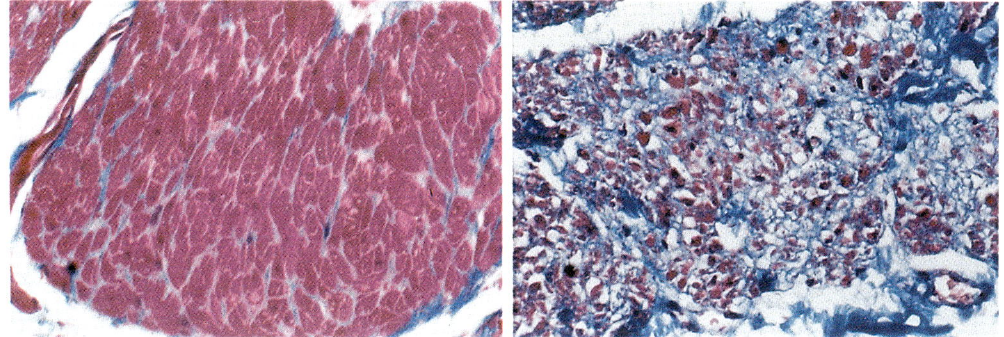

Figure 4–5. Outer layer of smooth muscle of stomach from normal patient (*left*) and patient with Duchenne dystrophy (*right*). Severe loss of muscle with connective tissue replacement is seen in Duchenne. Paraffin sections of formalin fixed stomach, Masson's trichrome. (Reprinted by permission of The New England Journal of Medicine 319:16,1988.)

otopias have been reported,[173] but such changes are not consistently demonstrable. A recent computerized tomography study revealed cerebral atrophy that appeared to increase with age but did not correlate with IQ.[229] The relationship of central nervous system abnormalities to dystrophin deficiency requires further studies, because the localization and function of brain dystrophin have not been determined.

LABORATORY FEATURES

In past years, serum CK, electromyography (EMG), and muscle biopsy were the most useful diagnostic tools in DMD. Now the basis for diagnosis rests on dystrophin analysis in skeletal muscle biopsies.[89]

Creatine Kinase. CK is the most important serum enzyme in the diagnosis of both DMD and other myopathies (see Chapter 2). Striking CK elevation may be observed in DMD even in the first years of life and often precedes obvious clinical manifestations. Levels of CK that are 50 times normal to greater than 100 times normal can be expected up to about age 3; thereafter, CK levels drop approximately 20% per year (Fig. 4–6).[32] A CK elevation that is less than 10 times normal, at any age (except very late in the course), is strong evidence against the diagnosis of Duchenne dystrophy.

Electromyography. The typical EMG findings indicate a myopathy characterized by early recruited, short-duration, low-amplitude, polyphasic motor unit potentials. As many as 50% of motor unit potentials may be polyphasic in weak proximal muscles, compared with 10% in normal muscle.[46] The short-duration potentials (3–7 milliseconds duration) appear more frequently in proximal muscles, and polyphasia appears more often in the distal muscles. The amplitude of the full recruitment pattern is reduced to 0.4 to 1.8 mV, compared with the normal of 1.5 to 4.5 mV.[46] Fibrillations and positive sharp waves, as well as complex repetitive discharges, may occur in all stages of the disease, probably because muscle fibers are separated from their innervation by segmental necrosis.[46] Reinnervation of the muscle fibers by axonal sprouts results in late components (satellite potentials), which follow the corresponding motor unit potentials by 15 to 25 milliseconds or longer. In late stages of the disease, when muscle has largely been replaced by fat and connective tissue, the number of motor units decreases, and some areas of the muscle may be electrically silent.

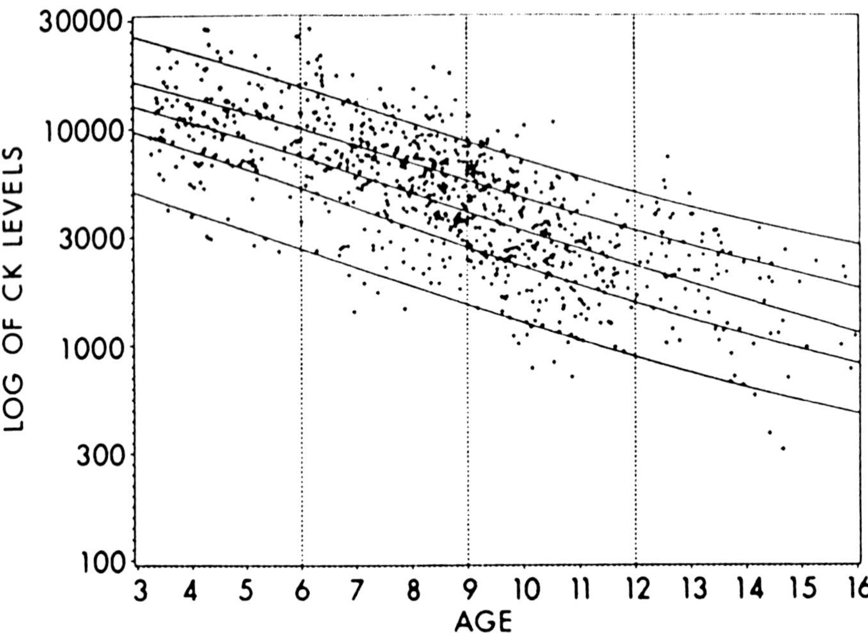

Figure 4–6. Creatine kinase (CK) gradually drops approximately 20% per year in Duchenne dystrophy. (From Brooke et al: Clinical investigation in Duchenne dystrophy: 2. Determination of the "power" of therapeutic trials based on the natural history. Musc Nerv 6:91, 1983. Copyright © 1983 John Wiley & Sons, Inc. Reprinted by permission of John Wiley & Sons, Inc.)

Muscle Biopsy. *Histology.* Distinctive biopsy features characterize Duchenne dystrophy (Fig. 4–7). These include increased variability in fiber size, with both small and hypertrophied fibers, and an alteration in fiber-type distribution consisting of type 1 fiber predominance and type 2B fiber deficiency. Type 2C fibers frequently appear. Small groups of basophilic regenerating and necrotic fibers are an important feature of DMD muscle biopsies (Fig. 4–8). Mononuclear cells, commonly seen in the endomysial connective tissue and occasionally in the invading necrotic fibers, consist of 80% cytotoxic T cells and 20% macrophages (Fig. 4–9).[3] Large, opaque, darkly stained fibers are very frequent and most likely result from segmental hypercontraction. These fibers often show small tears in the plasma membrane.[141] Proliferation of endomysial connective tissue (fibrosis) is a consistent feature that progresses over time. Fat will also gradually replace lost muscle fibers. Internal nuclei and split fibers occur less often than in the other muscular dystrophies.

Dystrophin Analysis. The definitive diagnosis of DMD must be made by demonstrating abnormalities in dystrophin, the gene product of the DMD locus. Dystrophin is a cytoskeletal protein found on the inner surface of the sarcolemma, which is demonstrable by immune staining using dystrophin antibodies (Fig. 4–10).[234] In DMD, absence of dystrophin can be demonstrated in the fresh-frozen sections typically used for routine histologic diagnosis (Fig. 4–11). Approximately 1% of the muscle fibers in DMD biopsies will demonstrate sarcolemmal staining. These dystro-

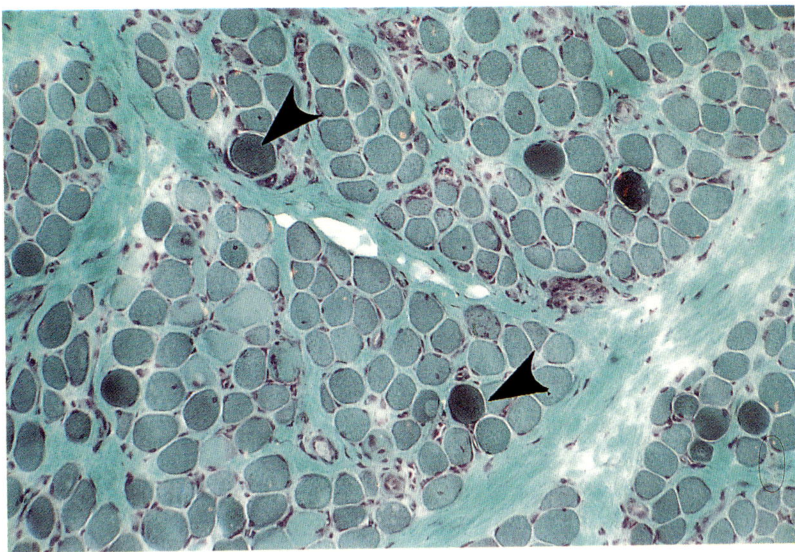

Figure 4–7. Typical muscle biopsy of Duchenne dystrophy, showing marked variability in fiber size, connective tissue surrounding many individual muscle fibers, and scattered, dark-staining, hypercontracted fibers (*arrowheads*) (modified trichrome).

phin-positive fibers are called revertants (Fig. 4–12). They arise spontaneously by a mutation superimposed on the underlying disease-causing mutation. This new mutation restores the reading frame and allows dystrophin expression. Western blot analysis, a technique by which electrophoresis of muscle components permits precise determination of proteins with specific molecular weights, is the best method to detect reduced amounts, or variants of dystrophin[89] with lower molecular weights (Fig. 4–13).

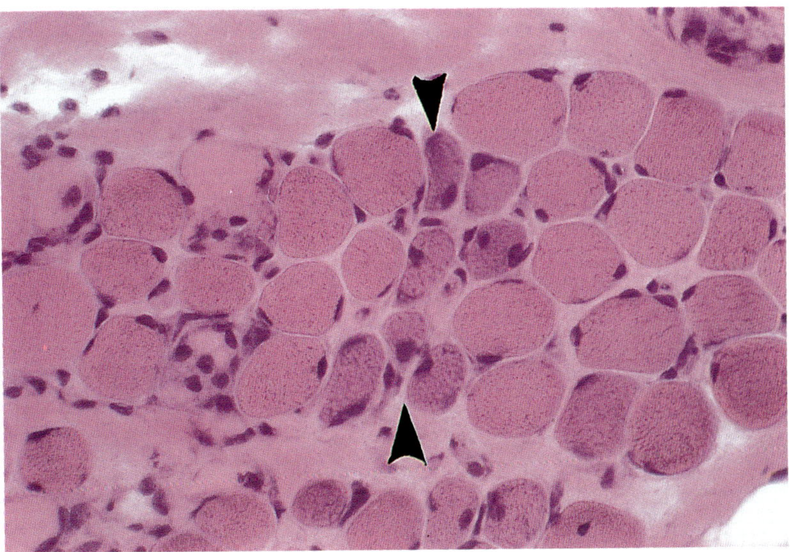

Figure 4–8. Muscle biopsy of Duchenne dystrophy shows a small group of regenerating muscle fibers (*between arrowheads*) amongst fibers with increased variability in size (H&E).

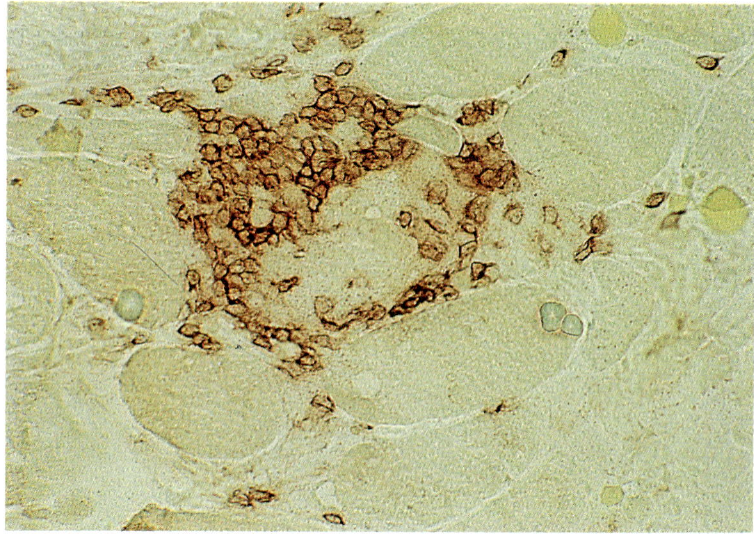

Figure 4–9. Immunostaining shows CD8 + cytotoxic cells invading a muscle fiber in Duchenne dystrophy.

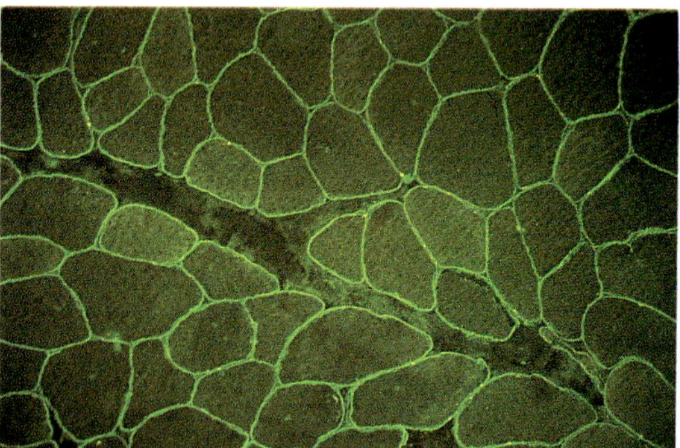

Figure 4–10. Normal muscle showing membrane localization of antibody directed against the 3′ end of dystrophin.

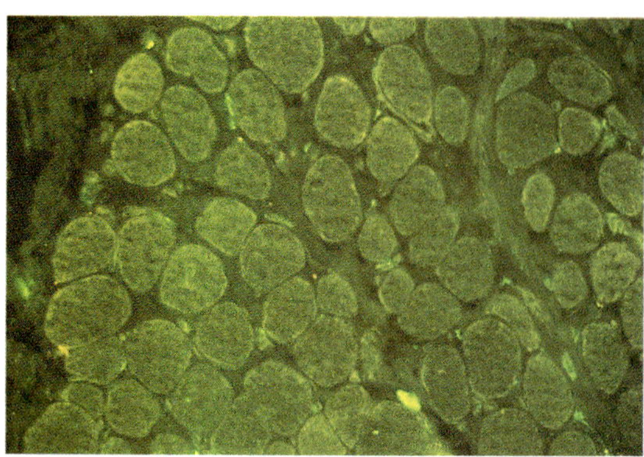

Figure 4–11. Absence of dystrophin on the membranes of muscle fibers in Duchenne dystrophy, using the same antibody as in Figure 4–10.

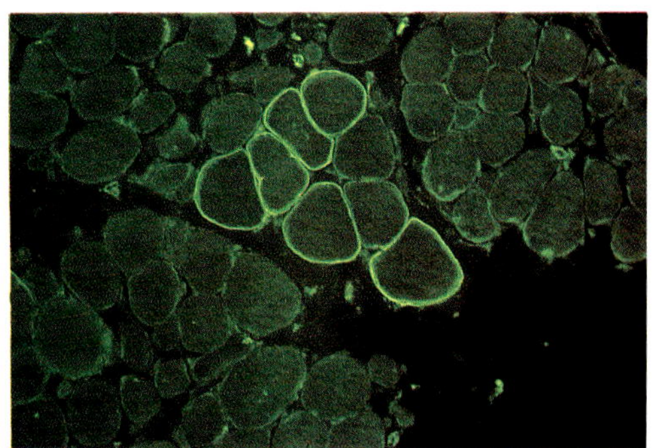

Figure 4–12. Cluster of revertant (dystrophin-positive) fibers amongst dystrophin-negative muscle fibers in Duchenne dystrophy biopsy using antibody directed against the 3′ end of dystrophin.

DNA Analysis. DNA isolated from peripheral blood leukocytes will identify deletions and duplications in approximately 65% of patients with DMD.[65] (See Chapter 3, Detection of Disease Genes, p. 83.) The deletions do not occur uniformly but are more frequent near the middle and the 5′ end of the gene.[225] The predilection for deletions in these areas of the gene remains poorly understood. The size of the deletion does not correlate with the severity of clinical manifestations. Approximately 25% of the nondeleted/nonduplicated DMD cases will have demonstrable point mutations in the dystrophin gene.[163a] Search for point mutations is more difficult, more time consuming, and more expensive compared to deletion/duplication analysis; the latter is more readily available in commercial laboratories. Because mutation analysis will not detect abnormalities in all patients with DMD, dystrophin analysis of muscle biopsies remains the diagnostic test of choice for DMD. Mutation analysis is

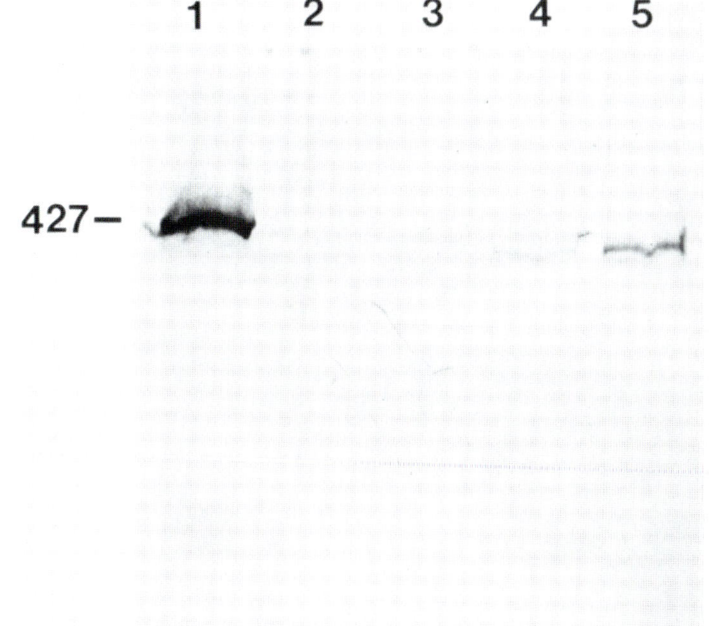

Figure 4–13. Western blot of skeletal muscle. Row 1 demonstrates normal dystrophin band (427Kd). Rows 2 and 3 are completely absent for dystrophin (typical of Duchenne dystrophy). In row 4, a faint band of dystrophin can be seen. Row 5 demonstrates a dystrophin band of reduced amount and slightly lower molecular weight (i.e., a band slightly below 427 Kd). The band in row 5 is characteristic of Becker muscular dystrophy.

important, however, because the detection of gene abnormalities has implications for family members with regard to carrier detection and prenatal diagnosis (see Chapter 3, p. 87).

Becker Muscular Dystrophy

The existence of a form of X-linked recessive muscular dystrophy more benign than DMD was first proposed by Becker and Kiener in 1955.[13] A number of families with similar clinical features soon were described, and the disorder was called Becker muscular dystrophy (BMD).[19] Despite differences in disease severity, DMD and BMD have many similarities. Until recently, however, it was not established whether they were genetically different disorders, distinct alleles, or extremes of a continuum. Recent investigations indicate that both DMD and BMD result from defects of a single gene. BMD has been estimated to occur approximately one tenth as frequently as DMD, with an incidence of around 3 per 100,000.[19,112]

CLINICAL FEATURES

The pattern of muscle wasting in BMD closely resembles that seen in DMD. The pelvic girdle and thigh muscles are prominently involved, with less involvement of anterior tibial and peroneal muscles. Proximal upper-extremity weakness develops after the onset of leg weakness. As the disease progresses, neck flexors become weak. Forearm muscles, hand intrinsics, and ankle plantar flexors remain strong until late in the illness. Patients with BMD have little or no facial muscle weakness. Calf muscles enlarge early in almost all patients. In contrast to patients with DMD, patients with BMD have only minor problems with contractures. Scoliosis also is less frequent, although it may develop after wheelchair confinement.

The natural history of the illness permits the distinction between DMD and BMD[170] (Table 4–1). The majority of patients with BMD initially experience difficulties between ages 5 and 15 years, although onset can occur in the third or fourth decade or even later. By definition, patients with BMD ambulate beyond age 15,[32] allowing for a clinical distinction between BMD and DMD. Patients with Becker dystrophy have a reduced life expectancy, but most survive at least into the fourth or fifth decade.

Mental retardation may be seen in BMD but not as frequently as in DMD.[170] Cardiac involvement occurs in BMD, and some patients develop features of cor pulmonale from respiratory failure.

LABORATORY FEATURES

Serum CK reaches values that are 20 to 100 times normal early in the disease. The EMG shows typical features of a myopathy. Muscle biopsy abnormalities are similar to those in DMD, with small groups of necrotic and regenerating fibers and hypercontracted fibers. In contrast to DMD, however, the proliferation of connective tissue is usually less. In BMD biopsies, split fibers and central nuclei appear more often, and small groups of atrophic fibers and pyknotic nuclear clumps may be seen. An unequivocal diagnosis of BMD requires Western blot analysis of muscle biopsy samples to demonstrate that dystrophin occurs in reduced amount or of abnormal size (Fig. 4–13).[90]

In Becker dystrophy, mutation analysis of DNA from peripheral blood leukocytes will recognize deletions and duplications of the dystrophin gene in approximately the same number (70%) of patients as in DMD.[114] Some of the nondeleted/nonduplicated BMD cases will be demonstrable point mutations, but the exact number has not been determined. Fewer BMD patients have point mutations compared with DMD patients.[163a] Because many patients with BMD do not have identifiable DNA abnormalities, dystrophin analysis is as important in diagnosis of BMD[114] as it is in DMD. The size of DNA deletions does not correlate with clinical severity, and sequences deleted in DMD patients (especially exons 3–7) may also be deleted in BMD.[129] Interestingly, however, about 95% of BMD patients show DNA deletions that do not alter the translational reading frame of messenger RNA (see Chapter 3, p. 85). This "in-frame" defect allows for production of some dystrophin and accounts for the presence of altered but not absent dystrophin on Western blot analysis.[90]

Phenotypic Variations of Dystrophin Deficiency

The availability of molecular diagnostic tools, particularly dystrophin testing of muscle biopsy samples, has expanded our recognition of the phenotypic expression of diseases occurring at the DMD/BMD gene locus. The preceding discussions imply a clear delineation between typical DMD and BMD patients, but a great heterogeneity of clinical presentation and course can be recognized, ranging from very severe to very mild. A well-recognized subgroup of patients, referred to as *outliers*, have clinical characteristics intermediate between DMD and BMD (see Table 4–1). Recognition of this subgroup was an outgrowth of the documentation of the natural history of DMD.[32] On Western blot studies of muscle biopsies, outliers resemble BMD and show dystrophin of reduced amounts or abnormal size (Fig. 4–13).[90] They can be identified clinically early in life by the relative preservation of strength of the neck flexors. Outliers maintain the ability to flex the neck against gravity (Fig. 4–14), whereas typical DMD patients lack this ability throughout their entire life. Outliers also retain the ability to climb stairs and walk longer (after age 12 years but not exceeding age 15), and have a greater forced vital capacity compared to typical DMD patients.

Dystrophin analysis permits the recognition of a milder form of dystrophin deficiency in certain patients who were previously classified as having limb-girdle dystrophy. These patients lack features otherwise typical of DMD. Even

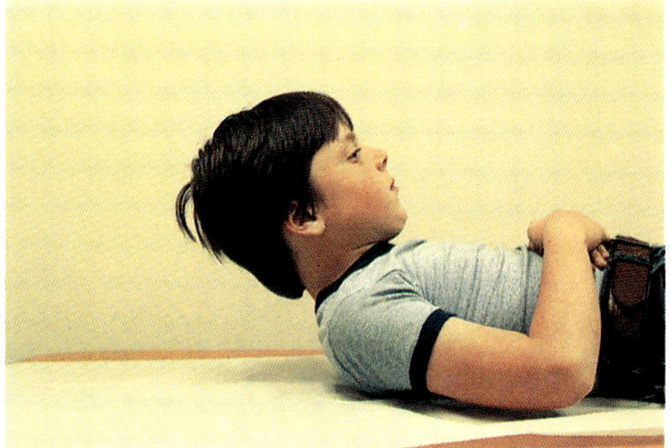

Figure 4–14. A 7-year-old boy with intermediate phenotype (an outlier) maintains the ability to flex his neck against gravity.

patients with a vastly different phenotype, including a nonprogressive myopathy with only myalgia and muscle cramps, have been found to have dystrophin abnormalities (abnormal in size without reduction in amount) (see Table 4–1).[69] At the other end of the spectrum, occasional patients that lack dystrophin present in the neonatal period with hypotonia and severe developmental delay. Dystrophin analysis in this neonatal group allows them to be distinguished from patients with congenital muscular dystrophies.

Genetics of Duchenne and Becker Muscular Dystrophies

The clinical manifestations of X-linked recessive disorders such as Duchenne dystrophy and Becker dystrophy are almost exclusively confined to males. Heterozygous females are usually asymptomatic carriers. Patients with DMD do not live to reproduce, so mutations carried by male patients will not be perpetuated in the family. New mutations must occur for the disease to continue in the population. According to Haldane,[78] assuming that mutation rates in male and female germ cells do not differ, one third of all DMD cases must represent new mutations. Mutation rates differing between the sexes would cause deviations from this figure.

Although some reports have indicated that less than one third of DMD patients represent new mutations,[172] such studies have been challenged on the basis of inadequate carrier testing methods.[20] Males with BMD may live to reproduce, although their relative fertility has been estimated at two thirds of normal. New mutations for BMD occur less frequently than for DMD and account for about 10% of cases.[170]

Early in female embryogenesis, random inactivation of one of the two X chromosomes occurs in somatic cells (Lyon hypothesis). Female relatives of DMD or BMD males occasionally demonstrate features of the disease if the X chromosome with the mutant gene remains active in a high percentage of muscle cells. A mild form of the disease usually occurs in these manifesting carriers, but a progressive limb-girdle syndrome may be encountered. The DMD or BMD phenotype has been observed in females in three rare circumstances: with an XO genotype (Turner's syndrome),[64] with a structurally abnormal X chromosome,[17] or with an X-autosome translocation.[24]

ISOLATION OF THE GENE AND GENE PRODUCT

The starting point for identifying the DMD/BMD gene on the X chromosome arose in the late 1970s from studies of rare females with myopathies comparable to DMD or BMD. In these cases, chromosomal studies demonstrated reciprocal translocations between an X chromosome and various autosomes.[125] A total of about 20 such cases have been reported and, repeatedly, the X-chromosomal breakpoints occur on the short arm within the Xp21 band, with variable sites for autosomal breakpoints. In these cases, the normal X chromosome becomes preferentially inactivated, demonstrating that disruption of a gene within the Xp21 band of the translocation results in the disease phenotype.

Independent studies, using restriction fragment length polymorphisms (RFLPs) as genetic markers (see Chapter 2), confirmed the DMD locus at Xp21.[44,149] Furthermore, studies in Becker dystrophy demonstrated linkage to the same RFLP markers, indicating that both diseases result from alterations of a single gene.[110]

Localization of the DMD locus at the Xp21 site accelerated the process leading to isolation of the gene causing Duchenne and Becker dystrophies. In 1985, Kunkel and colleagues studied the DNA from a male patient, BB, with DMD and three other X-linked conditions (retinitis pigmentosa, chronic granulomatous disease, and the McLeod red blood cell phenotype).[120] Cytogenetic studies of patient BB demonstrated a large deletion on the X chromosome. Using a unique strategy, Kunkel and coworkers[119] were able to isolate DNA clones (pERT 87) from BB that were deleted from the DNA of approximately 10% of DMD and BMD males. The same year, Worton and colleagues[165] cloned the DNA spanning a translocation junction in a female with a DMD phenotype having an X;21 translocation. The pERT 87 and the X J clones were subsequently shown to recognize messenger RNA and complementary DNA (see Chapter 3, p. 81) from muscle grown in culture[35,142]; thus, DNA from these clones represented possible candidate genes for DMD/BMD. As starting points for chromosomal walking, these clones later led to the complete cloning of the gene causing Duchenne and Becker dystrophies.[115]

The DMD/BMD gene has been estimated to be very large — 2000 kilobases (kb). Antibodies raised to polypeptides produced from cloned portions of the DMD/BMD gene were used by Hoffman and colleagues[88] to identify dystrophin, a 427-kd protein composed of 3685 amino acids. Furthermore, muscle biopsies of DMD patients demonstrated dystrophin deficiency.[89] These observations were confirmed by others,[104] and subsequent studies indicate that the extent of dystrophin deficiency correlates with disease severity.[90]

The functional role of dystrophin requires further studies for complete understanding. Dystrophin localizes to the sarcolemmal membrane (see Fig. 4–10), and the amino acid sequence suggests a cytoskeletal protein existing in a large oligomeric complex with four sarcolemmal glycoproteins as integral components.[59] The N-terminal portion of dystrophin has a similar amino acid sequence to the actin-binding domain of alpha-actinin.[18] Recent studies suggest that dystrophin may also bind actin.[87] Besides dystrophin, one of the four glycoproteins closely linked to it (a 156-kd constituent) has also been shown to be markedly reduced in DMD muscle.[59] This finding implies that a genetically determined deficiency of dystrophin could adversely affect other membrane proteins, and this combined loss contributes to muscle fiber breakdown.

CARRIER DETECTION AND PRENATAL DIAGNOSIS

Pedigree Analysis. Evaluation of pedigree data is the most important first step in establishing genetic risk. A woman with an affected son and at least one other affected male relative, in a pedigree consistent with X-linked recessive inheritance, has a carrier risk of 100% and can be considered an obligate carrier. Daughters of BMD males are also obligate carriers. Women with two or more sons with DMD or BMD (proven to be dystrophin deficient) can be considered obligate carriers even without other affected male relatives. Obligate carriers will transmit the diseased gene to 50% of their offspring; therefore, each male offspring has a 50% chance of being affected.

Mothers of isolated DMD or BMD patients and non–obligate-carrier females related to affected males may be carriers. Mothers of isolated DMD or BMD patients should not be considered obligate carriers, as one third of DMD cases and approximately 10% of BMD cases represent new mutants. A series of tests performed in conjunction with pedigree analysis will determine the carrier probability of possible carriers.

Creatine Kinase Determination. A variety of biochemical, histologic, and chemical tests have been used to identify carriers. The most widely employed has been the measurement of serum CK. When the CK level is elevated, it provides strong evidence in support of a carrier state, but it will not identify all carriers.[74] The determination of CK identifies less than 50% of the obligate carriers, with a false positive rate of 2.5%.[74] The rate of carrier detection using CK declines after the first two decades of life. Despite these limitations, an unequivocal CK elevation represents a positive test for the carrier state. CK testing of fetal blood cannot be used for identifying affected males in utero.

DNA Analysis. Two methods of DNA analysis, mutation analysis and RFLP linkage analysis, have application for carrier detection and prenatal diagnosis. Tests can be performed on DNA derived from peripheral blood leukocytes, chorionic villi, or amniotic fluid cells (see Chapter 3, p. 81).

Mutation Analysis. DNA analysis for carrier detection and prenatal diagnosis can be done only in DMD/BMD families with identifiable mutations (see Chapter 2). For this reason, DNA analysis should be done for all DMD/BMD patients. DNA can be screened by either Southern blot analysis or the polymerase chain reaction (PCR) (see Chapter 3, p. 82).

Southern blots reveal deletions as absent bands; at times, a band of abnormal size (junction fragment) can appear (Fig. 4–15) due to the joining together of normally noncontiguous segments of DNA as a result of the deletion. Partial gene duplications appear as an increased intensity of bands. Recognition of these gene duplications requires careful densitometric analysis of the blots.[93]

PCR offers advantages for mutation analysis. Amplification of specific deletion-prone "hot spot" regions of the dystrophin gene can detect approximately 98% of the deletions in patients with Duchenne or Becker dystrophies, using a multiplex PCR-based

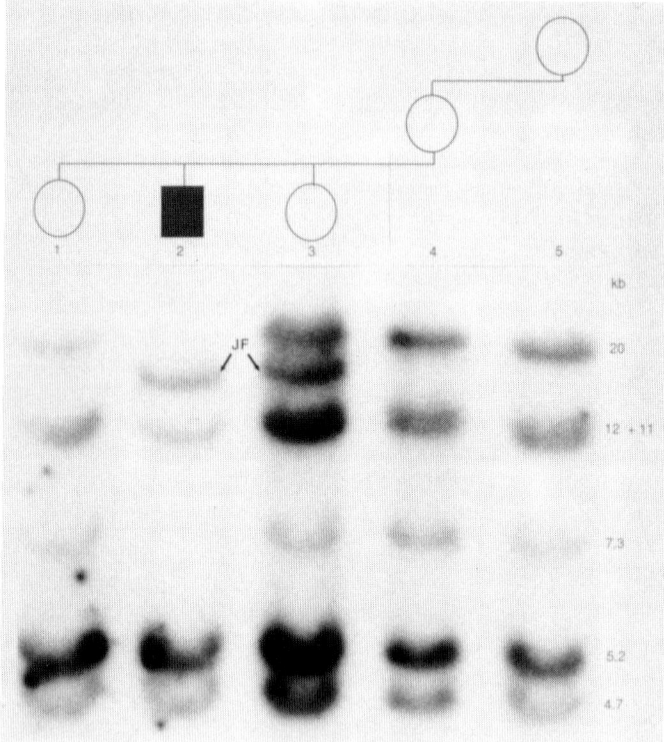

Figure 4–15. DNA from each family member was isolated from leukocytes. After a *Hind*III restriction enzyme digestion, cDNA probe 4-5a was hybridized by Southern blotting, revealing a junction fragment (JF) in the proband and his sister (lane 3). The mother (lane 4) is not carrying the mutation in her somatic DNA but has transmitted the mutation twice. The mother is a germinal mosaic carrier. Restriction fragment sizes are indicated in kilobases (Kb). (From Prior TW, et al: Germline mosaicism in carriers of Duchenne muscular dystrophy. Muscle & Nerve 15:960, 1992. Copyright© 1992 by John Wiley & Sons, Inc. Reprinted by permission of John Wiley & Sons, Inc.)

assay.[15,163] Furthermore, PCR-based assays may be completed in a fraction of the time required for Southern blot analysis. Thus, the status of an at-risk male fetus can be determined very rapidly, using DNA derived from chorionic villus sampling or amniotic cells.

The phenomenon of germline mosaicism must be considered in counseling for prenatal diagnosis.[7,41] Mothers without detectable deletions in DNA from peripheral blood leukocytes have produced more than one affected or carrier offspring in whom demonstrable deletions were identified (see Fig. 4–15).[163] In such cases, evidence suggests that the somatic cell lines (e.g., leukocytes used as a source for DNA analysis) have no abnormalities, but nevertheless, a mutation exists in the germline from which the ovum arises. Thus, if DNA analysis on peripheral blood leukocytes demonstrates a mutation in an affected boy, his mother still has a definite carrier risk even if she has no demonstrable mutation in DNA derived from peripheral blood. In this situation, prenatal diagnosis should be considered for subsequent pregnancies.

Restriction Fragment Length Polymorphism Linkage Analysis. RFLPs refer to inherited variations in the sizes of DNA fragments recognized by restriction enzyme digestion (see Chapter 3, pp. 81 and 87). These RFLPs occur frequently in the human genome, and their analysis is important for the genetic evaluation of families without an identifiable mutation.

Many RFLP probes (Fig. 4–16) that are closely linked to the DMD/BMD locus permit accurate determination of carrier status or prenatal genotype in DMD/BMD families,[23,149] but this approach does have shortcomings. First, to track the disease reliably, many family members must be available for blood drawing. Second, each family member must be individually evaluated with a

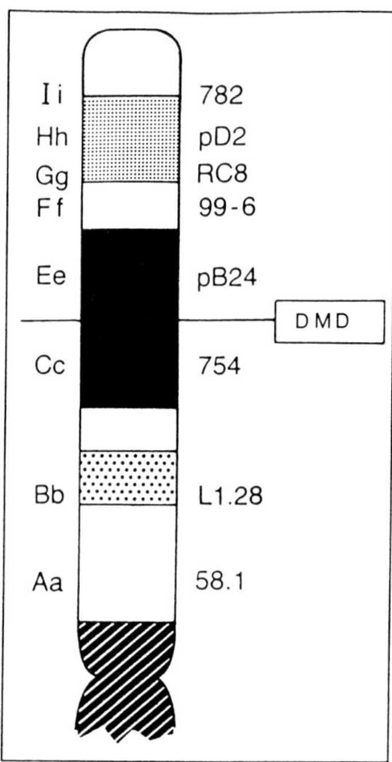

Figure 4–16. Short arm of the X chromosome showing approximate locations of eight DNA Duchenne dystrophy probes used for linkage analysis in families in which no deletion or duplication can be found. Each probe recognizes a restriction fragment length polymorphism (RFLP). The DMD locus is indicated. Upper-case letters on the left indicate the more frequent RFLP alleles of the marker loci indicated on the right; lower case letters, the less frequent RFLP alleles. (From Hyser C, et al: Use of serum creatine kinase, pyruvate kinase, and genetic linkage of carrier detection in Duchenne and Becker dystrophy. Neurology 37:4–10, 1987, with permission.)

battery of probes to find one or more combinations that provide enough information to trace the inheritance of the disease gene through the family. Finally, because these are linked markers, genotype prediction will always be less than 100% accurate; meiotic recombinations can disturb the relationship between the disease gene and the marker locus.

Case History

A 22-year-old woman came for genetic counseling to determine her carrier status for DMD. Her pedigree (Fig. 4–17) included an affected brother, who by DNA analysis had no identifiable deletion or mutation. Blood was obtained from her sister, both parents, and grandparents. After checking several RFLP probes (see Fig. 4–16), the family was found to be informative for probes 99-6 and 58.1. These flanking probes were used to track the Duchenne locus on the X chromosome through several generations. Both grandmother (with an affected grandson) and mother (with an affected son) were obligate carriers. Neither probe 99-6 nor 58.1 demonstrated recombination in generation II, III, or IV, making it highly unlikely that the Duchenne gene would recombine independently of these flanking markers.

The 22-year-old woman seeking knowledge of her carrier status must be advised that she carries the Duchenne gene with a high degree of certainty ($< 1\%$ error).

In summary, if an identifiable mutation can be detected in a DMD/BMD patient, carrier detection and prenatal diagnosis can be done reliably and rapidly using PCR. If the gene defect cannot be found, RFLP linkage studies are necessary, and more family members must be studied, some of whom may not be polymorphic for appropriate markers (see Chapter 3, p. 87).

Treatment

PHYSICAL THERAPY, BRACING, AND SURGERY

The management of patients with DMD requires a multidisciplinary approach. Early in the disease process, emphasis must be placed on stretching the heel cords, iliotibial bands, and hips. Contractures begin early, and stretching programs should be carried out by parents and school physical therapists. Heel-cord tightness can be delayed by night splints.[31]

By the age of 9 years, most boys with DMD require long leg braces. Double-upright metal braces were used for many years, but these have been replaced by lightweight, plastic, molded braces, which permit the lower portion

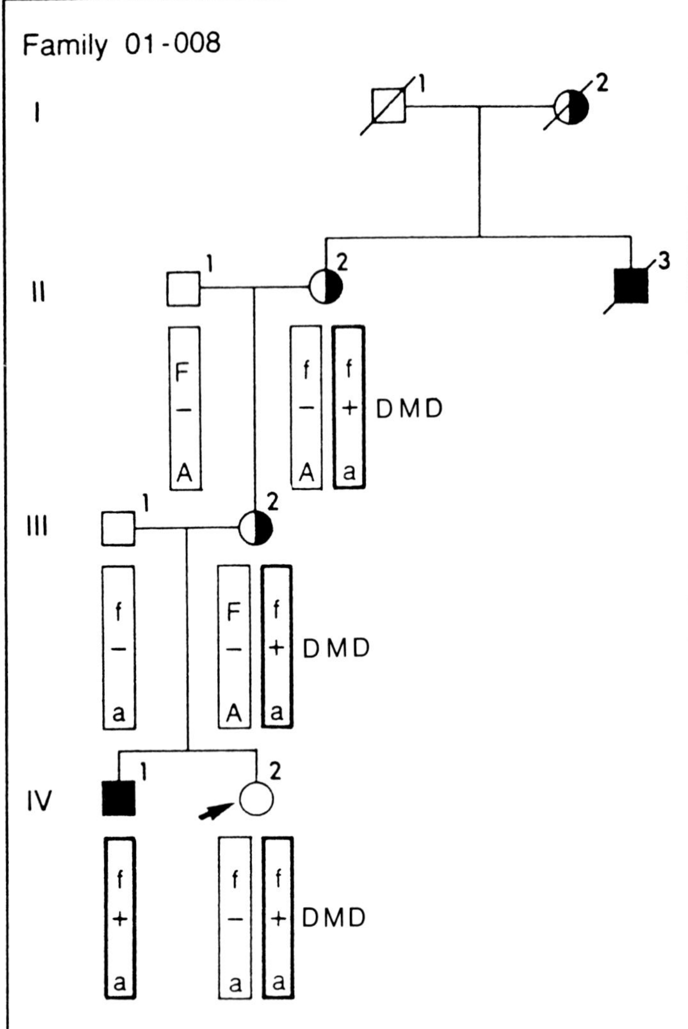

Figure 4-17. Pedigree of a four-generation Duchenne dystrophy family. The DMD locus is shown by the +. In this family, RFLPs recognized by probes 99-6 and 58.1 were informative and helped to establish with a high degree of certainty that IV-2 was a carrier (see Case History).

to fit inside a shoe. For some patients, surgical release of heel cords and iliotibial bands becomes necessary to fit braces. Tightness of the iliotibial bands may keep the braced leg in forced abduction, which can be counterproductive. Posterior tibial tendon transplantation adds very little function but may be necessary if the foot is persistently inverted. Surgical releases should be performed early to preserve ambulation, but the child and family must be motivated to accomplish the objective. Following surgical releases, long leg braces may be necessary. Prior to surgery, plans should be made for properly fitted, lightweight braces to be used immediately upon removal of the cast applied at the time of surgery.

Paraspinal muscle weakness results in scoliosis. This life-threatening complication reduces lung capacity and predisposes patients to atelectasis and pneumonia. Scoliosis can also be disfiguring and painful. Ambulation, or even standing (without necessarily walking in long leg braces), delays its onset. Wheelchair confinement promotes scoliosis, particularly if the patient slumps to one side, highlighting the need for proper wheelchair fitting. The proper use of a wheelchair with a reclining back and a neck extender, however, may retard scoliosis by promoting an extensor posture. The scoliosis-limiting effects of molded wheelchair inserts and various types of body jackets, referred to as thoracic-lumbar-sacral orthoses, have been disappointing. Once present, scoliosis inevitably progresses.

Major advances in spinal stabilization procedures permit correction of scoliosis.[127,189] The technique of segmental spinal stabilization described by Luque[127] has become the surgical method of choice (Fig. 4–18). Patients demonstrating progressive curvatures measuring 35° to 45° should be considered surgical candidates. A forced vital capacity greater than 35% of predicted is usually required for a successful postoperative course. Patients with vital capacity below this level are prone to more postoperative complications, including pneumonia or difficulty in extubating and weaning the patient from the ventilator. Anesthesia for patients with DMD should not include halogenated inhalational anesthetics or neuromuscular depolarizing agents such as succinylcholine. Adverse anesthetic reactions, similar but not identical to those of malignant hyperthermia, occur in patients with DMD.[106]

DRUG THERAPY

Attempts at drug intervention go back many decades; dramatic effects have been frequently reported but rarely sub-

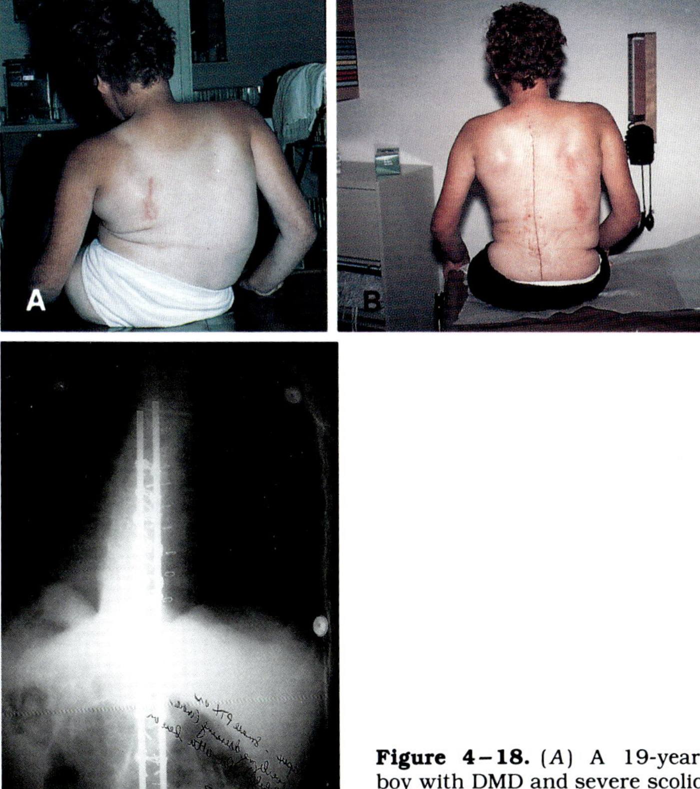

Figure 4–18. (A) A 19-year-old boy with DMD and severe scoliosis. (B) The same patient after surgical correction of scoliosis. (C) Radiograph of spine showing Luque rods in place.

stantiated. Two potentially important drugs, mazindol and prednisone, merit discussion.

Mazindol. Interest in mazindol, a presumed growth hormone inhibitor, developed from several observations. In 1981, Zatz and associates[231] described a unique 13-year-old boy with DMD and growth hormone deficiency, who had a remarkably benign course compared to his siblings. A tendency for a slower rate of progression was substantiated in a follow-up description of the same patient at age 18.[232] Zatz and colleagues[233] later reported benefit from 1 year of mazindol treatment in monozygotic twins with DMD.[233] Subsequently, a 12-month, randomized, double-blind study was performed with a large cohort of DMD boys. No beneficial effect was seen.[75] This disappointing result does not resolve issues related to growth hor-mone. At best, mazindol represents a weak growth hormone inhibitor, if, in fact, it has any significant effect on growth hormone secretion.[75] Further studies using more specific growth hor-mone inhibitors will be of interest.

Prednisone. Two separate random-ized, controlled trials have shown that prednisone produces a significant in-crease in muscle strength, pulmonary function, and functional ability in pa-tients with DMD.[76,136] Rapid improve-ment can be demonstrated within 10 days of drug administration (Fig. 4–19). Maximal improvement occurs within 3 months of the initiation of treatment. A prednisone dosage of 0.75 mg/kg per day produces the maximum increase in strength. Daily prednisone is more ef-fective than alternate-day treatment.[63] A prednisone dose of 0.65 mg/kg per day will maintain long-term improvement

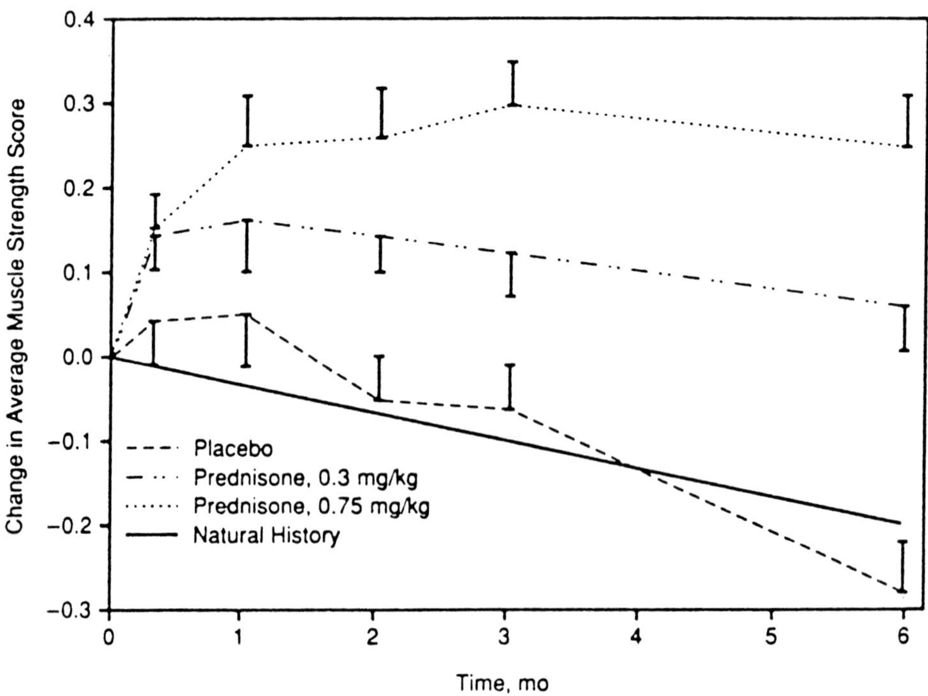

Figure 4–19. The results of a controlled trial of prednisone in Duchenne dystrophy. A dose of 0.75 mg/kg per day (n = 34) is more effective than 0.3 mg/kg per day (n = 33). The placebo group showed no improvement and paralleled the natural history rate of deterioration. The initial improvement occurred as early as 10 days after beginning treatment. (From Griggs RC, et al: Prednisone in Duchenne dys-trophy: A randomized, controlled trial defining the time course and dose response. Arch Neurol 48:383, 1991. Copyright © 1991, American Medical Association.)

Figure 4–20. The results of long-term treatment with prednisone of Duchenne dystrophy patients. Ninety-one boys were studied at 2 years and 87 boys at 3 years. During the maintenance period, the rate of decline in muscle strength differed very significantly from the natural-history rate of decline. During the initial treatment period, patients were divided into two groups for daily treatment with placebo versus prednisone. Only the prednisone group improved. During the next phase, patients received alternate-day prednisone, which was not as effective as daily prednisone. During the long-term maintenance period, all patients received a daily dose of 0.65 to 0.75 mg/kg of prednisone, and their muscle strength showed sustained improvement. (From Fenichel GM et al,[63] p 1875, with permission.)

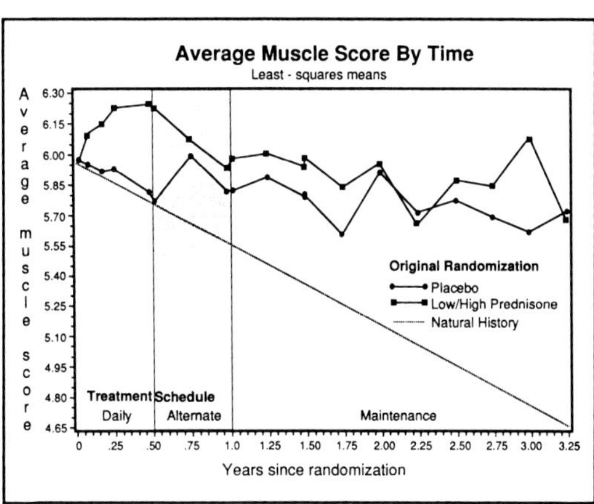

(Fig. 4–20). Significant side effects include growth retardation, weight gain, changes in facial appearance, growth of excessive body hair, and behavioral changes.[76,136]

Prednisone increases strength by increasing muscle mass[136] and decreasing muscle degradation.[147] The decrease in muscle degradation may be the result of an antiinflammatory effect related to a reduction in total T cells and cytotoxic-suppressor T cells.[111] Prednisone does not change dystrophin levels in muscle.[36]

In view of the side effects of prednisone, as well as the possibility that specific gene replacement treatment may be possible in the forseeable future, prednisone treatment for DMD should be reserved for those boys experiencing a major functional decline. A new corticosteroid, deflazacort, has fewer side effects than prednisone[50a]; studies comparing its efficacy with that of prednisone are in progress.

GENE THERAPY

Gene therapy has not yet become available for BMD or DMD. Strategies for introducing genes into tissue using viral vectors or direct gene transfer require more research for applicability to the dystrophin gene.[224]

In contrast to direct gene therapy, a method of cell therapy has been shown to be partially effective in genetic strains of mice with muscular dystrophies (Fig. 4–21).[105,158] The technique employs the use of myoblasts, the counterpart of resting or mononuclear cells, called satellite cells. These mononuclear cells adhere to the surface of normal muscle fibers and play a role in regeneration following muscle injury. Myoblasts can be harvested from muscle tissue by enzymatic dissociation of normal muscle. When injected directly into muscle, they fuse with host fibers; the donor nuclei express their own genotype in the host fiber. In the dystrophin-deficient mdx mouse animal model, the injected donor precursor cells convert dystrophin-negative fibers to dystrophin-positive fibers.[105,158] Despite suggestions from animal studies that myoblast transfer might help patients,[105,158] randomized, controlled clinical trials have met with little success.[77b,104a,135a] In one study, it was estimated that 1% of dystrophin-negative fibers became dystrophin-positive.[71a] In two other controlled trials, no expression of donor dystrophin was observed.[104a,135a] None of the three studies found evidence for improved strength in muscles undergoing myoblast transfer.

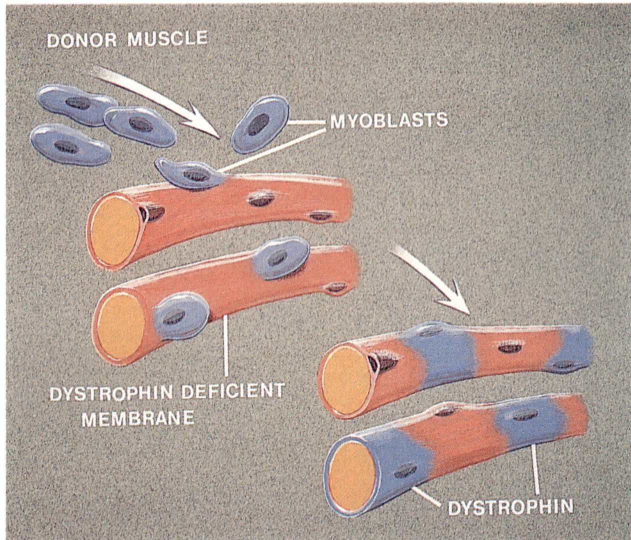

Figure 4–21. Diagram of cell therapy by myoblast transfer. Dystrophin-competent myoblasts (blue) are injected adjacent to multinucleated dystrophin-negative muscle fibers. After myoblast fusion, muscle fibers express dystrophin (blue) in the domain of the dystrophin-competent nuclei.

EMERY-DREIFUSS MUSCULAR DYSTROPHY

Emery-Dreifuss muscular dystrophy (Table 4–2) was initially recognized as an entity distinct from Duchenne and Becker dystrophies in 1966.[57] Dreifuss and Hogan had identified many of its typical features in 1961,[46a] and subsequent reports have further emphasized its unique profile.[91,174,175,202,215]

Clinical Features

The condition affects only males, although some females have shown a similar clinical picture. Prominent contractures can be recognized in early childhood or teenage years, often preceding muscle weakness. The contractures persist through the course of the disease and occur especially at the elbows and neck, with shortening of the Achilles tendon (Fig. 4–22). In the upper extremities, humeral muscle weakness affects the biceps and triceps, sparing the scapular muscles. In the legs, peroneal muscle weakness exceeds the involvement of proximal muscles. This distribution accounts for the name *humeroperoneal dystrophy*. Many patients also have pes cavus. Even severely affected patients are able to walk until the third decade, and some are so mildly affected as to have virtually no symptoms throughout life.

Cardiac involvement is an important and potentially life-threatening feature of Emery-Dreifuss muscular dystrophy,

Table 4–2 EMERY-DREIFUSS MUSCULAR DYSTROPHY

Inheritance	X-linked recessive linked to distal long arm at Xq27-28
Onset	Early childhood or teenage years
Clinical features	
Musculoskeletal	Prominent contractures at elbows and neck
	Weakness in humeroperoneal distribution
Other systems	Cardiac conduction defects, especially atrial arrhythmias
Laboratory features	No specific abnormalities:
	CK mild elevations ($<$10-fold)
	EMG myopathic
	Muscle biopsy shows myopathy (may have neurogenic atrophy)

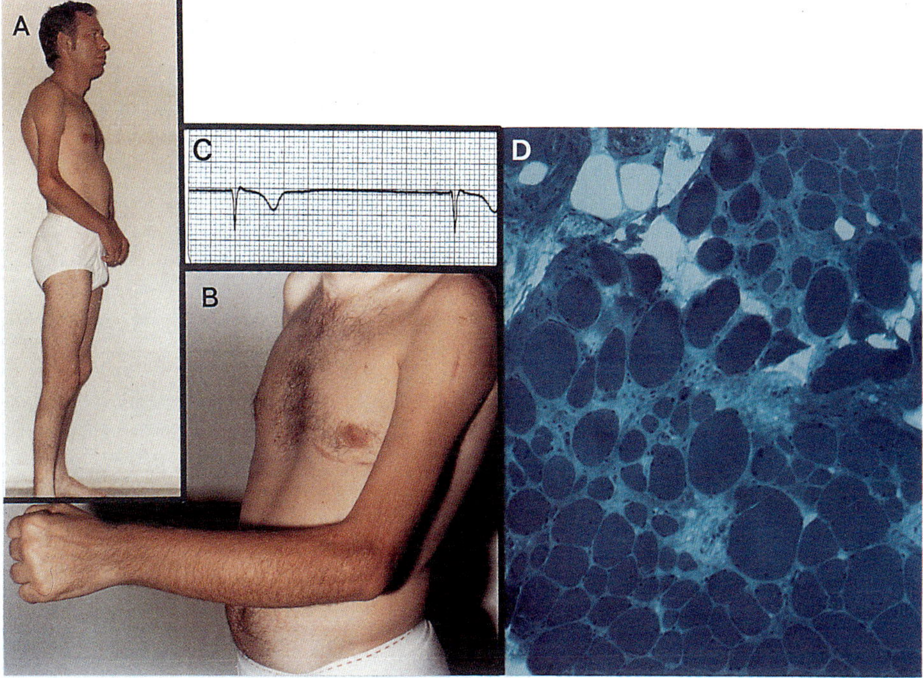

Figure 4–22. Emery-Dreifuss humeroperoneal muscular dystrophy: (*A, B*) marked wasting of humeral muscles, peroneal wasting, and elbow contractures. (*C*) ECG shows junctional rhythm with a heart rate of 34 per minute. (*D*) Muscle biopsy shows variability in fiber size, increased internal nuclei, and increased connective tissue (modified trichrome). (From Hopkins et al,[91] p 234. Reprinted with permission from Annals of Neurology 10:230–237, 1981.)

however, and affects even patients with minimal limb involvement.[57,175,215] The spectrum of atrial rhythm and conduction disturbances includes atrial fibrillation and atrial paralysis, as well as atrioventricular heart block varying from first-degree to complete. Profound bradycardia of prolonged duration may lead to a dilated cardiomyopathy.[215] Secondary complications include cerebral emboli, syncope, and sudden death.

Laboratory Features

Serum CK is mildly elevated. Conflicting EMG findings may indicate both myopathy and neuropathy.[175] Muscle biopsies have also shown a spectrum of changes ranging from preferential type 1 fiber atrophy to a more typically dys-

trophic pattern with some features indicating neurogenic atrophy.[91]

Electrocardiographic abnormalities range from abnormal P waves to permanent atrial paralysis, and from first-degree atrioventricular to complete heart block.

Genetics

From the earliest descriptions, pedigree analysis showed X-linked inheritance.[57] Linkage to deutan color blindness, a known X-linked trait, was unequivocally established in subsequent reports.[202] More recently, localization has been refined to the distal long arm of the X chromosome at regions q27-28,[22,201] with close linkage to the Factor VIII gene.[228] These linkage markers allow carrier detection and prenatal diagnosis using RFLPs.[162a] A small number of patients with a similar phenotype appear to have autosomal dominant transmission.[138]

Treatment

Treatment of Emery-Dreifuss muscular dystrophy must focus on maintaining mobility and function through stretching exercises. The muscle weakness progresses slowly. Respiratory failure can occur late in the course of the disease. Cardiac function must be monitored. Many patients eventually need permanent ventricular pacing, and prognosis depends, to a great extent, on preventing cardiac complications and sudden death.[138]

MYOTONIC MUSCULAR DYSTROPHY

Myotonic dystrophy, originally described by Steinert in 1909,[192] is the most common adult muscular dystrophy. Its prevalence is approximately 5 per 100,000 in most American and European populations, and the incidence is 13.5 per 100,000 live births.[30] Males and females are equally involved. In certain regions such as Quebec, Canada, the disease reaches an incidence of almost 1 in 500.[133a] The clinical expression of myotonic dystrophy varies widely, affecting many systems other than muscle.

Clinical Features (Table 4-3)

MUSCULOSKELETAL SYSTEM

The appearance of myotonic dystrophy patients can be so characteristic that a diagnosis becomes evident at first glance. Temporalis muscle wasting, hollow cheeks from masseter muscle atrophy and facial weakness produce a "hatchet-faced" appearance (Fig. 4-23). Frontal baldness and ptosis contribute to the typical appearance. Neck muscles, including the flexors and sternocleidomastoids, become involved early, as do the distal limb muscles. Hand function is impaired by weakness of the wrist extensors, finger extensors, and intrinsic hand muscles. Ankle dorsiflexor weakness may produce foot drop, which can be mistaken for a peripheral neuropathy. The proximal

Table 4-3 MYOTONIC DYSTROPHY

Inheritance	Autosomal dominant, linked to chromosome 19q13.2
Onset	Any decade including neonatal period
Clinical features	
Musculoskeletal	Onset any decade; slowly progressive muscle weakness of face, pharynx, masseter, temporalis, tongue, sternocleidomastoid; distal > proximal limbs; myotonia
Other systems	
Heart	Conduction system disorders in majority; mitral valve prolapse. Heart failure rare except from cor pulmonale
Respiratory	Diaphragm and intercostal muscle weakness; impaired ventilatory drive
Gastrointestinal	Dysphagia; aspiration; megacolon
Central nervous system	Personality changes of apathy; indifference and paranoia; hydrocephalus; retardation (congenital cases); hypersomnia
Endocrine	Hypogonadism; insulin resistance
Ocular	Cataracts; retinal and macular pigmentary degeneration, meibomian cysts; ptosis and ophthalmoparesis
Bone	Frontal bossing, small sella turcica, hyperostosis, high-arched palate
Laboratory features	CK normal to threefold increased
	EMG shows myotonia and myopathic changes. Muscle biopsy changes include fiber atrophy (50% preferential type 1), central nuclei, ring fibers, sarcoplasmic masses; ECG shows conduction system defects in majority

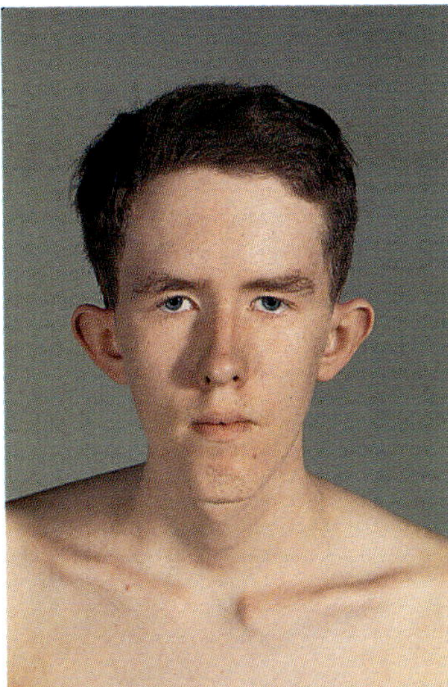

Figure 4–23. Typical facial features of myotonic dystrophy in a 22-year-old patient with maternally transmitted disease. Both this patient and his sister have moderate mental retardation.

muscles remain stronger than the distal throughout the course, although the quadriceps muscles may undergo preferential atrophy and weakness at any time. The combination of weakness in knee extension and ankle dorsiflexion causes "back kneeing" (genu recurvatum). Palatal, pharyngeal, and tongue involvement produce a dysarthric speech, a nasal voice, and swallowing problems. Tongue atrophy can be severe (see Fig. 2–18C). Some patients have respiratory insufficiency because of diaphragm and intercostal muscle weakness.

Myotonia. In myotonic dystrophy patients, myotonia seldom causes complaints but has considerable diagnostic importance. Myotonia can be easily detected by percussion of thenar, wrist extensor, and lingual muscles or by evaluation of grip release (see Figs. 2–6 and 2–7). Tongue myotonia can be demonstrated by percussion of a tongue blade placed perpendicularly across the tongue, producing a sustained contraction ("napkin ring sign"; see Fig. 2–8). As the disease progresses, myotonia becomes difficult to detect because of

muscle wasting. Myotonia may not develop until after age 5.

CARDIAC INVOLVEMENT

Cardiac disturbances occur in a majority of patients with myotonic dystrophy. Approximately 90% show electrocardiographic abnormalities,[145] including first-degree heart block or more extensive conduction-system involvement. Left anterior hemiblock or right bundle branch block signifies abnormalities of all three fascicles of the cardiac conduction system (Fig. 4–24).[72] Serious complications of myotonic dystrophy include complete heart block and sudden death, but predictive criteria indicating the proper time for pacemaker insertion have not been established. Pacemaker implantation is wise in patients having unexplained syncope or when second-degree heart block is demonstrated by Holter monitoring. Pacing should also be considered for patients who have evidence of trifascicular conduction disturbance and marked prolongation of the P-R interval (>270 milliseconds).

In myotonic dystrophy, ventricular and atrial ectopic beats occur frequently, more often than tachyarrhythmias. Antiarrhythmic agents must be used with caution, because drugs suppressing cardiac conduction pose considerable hazard. Digitalis should be avoided because it may precipitate complete or second-degree heart block. Quinidine, procainamide, and tocainide also should be avoided. In most instances, patients with conduction disturbances requiring antiarrhythmic therapy should have prophylactic pacemaker implantation. If myotonia requires treatment, phenytoin is the safest agent to use.[72]

Manifestations of congestive heart failure occur far less frequently than conduction disturbances. Heart failure, if present, usually results from cor pulmonale secondary to respiratory failure and hypoxia. Despite the infrequency of congestive heart failure, myocardial contractility may be abnormal[85]; the

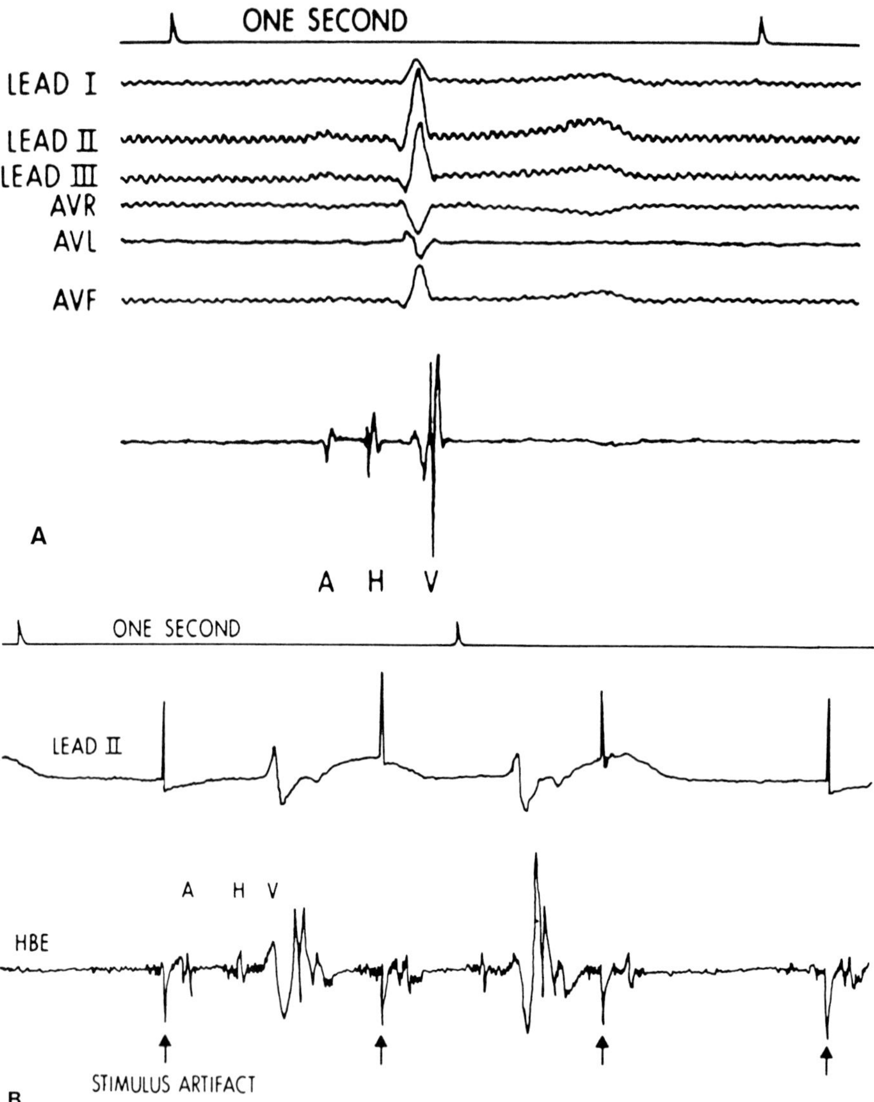

Figure 4–24. Cardiac abnormalities in a patient with myotonic dystrophy. (*A*) A His bundle ECG (*bottom trace*) indicates the intervals assessed. The A wave reflects atrial depolarization; the H wave, His bundle depolarization; and V, the ventricular depolarization, all measured by the His bundle electrode. (*B*) A His-bundle ECG (from a different patient) shows first-degree A-V block, left anterior hemiblock, and right bundle branch block. During atrial tachypacing, the Wenckebach phenomenon developed. At a higher rate of pacing, a 2:1 A-V block developed. (From Griggs et al,[72] p 38, with permission.)

lack of overt cardiac failure may, in part, reflect a diminished demand resulting from the physical inactivity common in these patients.

The incidence of mitral valve prolapse is increased,[71,166] but in most patients, echocardiograms do not show the redundant leaflets that account for an in-creased risk of infection or emboli. Consequently, there is no need for prophylactic antibiotics before dental or surgical procedures.[166] Furthermore, the myxomatous degeneration associated with mitral valve prolapse was not seen at autopsy in a myotonic dystrophy patient in whom clinical and echocardiographic evidence indicated prolapse of the mitral valve.[166]

RESPIRATORY SYSTEM

Myotonic dystrophy patients often have respiratory difficulties at a time in their illness when limb weakness is modest. Besides diaphragm and intercostal muscle weakness, additional factors important in respiratory compromise include a decreased response to hypoxia and hypercapnia, even in the face of relatively normal pulmonary function and blood gases. This lack of response indicates an abnormality in brainstem neuroregulatory mechanisms.[81] In addition, myotonic dystrophy patients demonstrate debilitating degrees of hypersomnia, especially in the daytime, and these symptoms may be misdiagnosed as narcolepsy. Many patients also gain excessive weight because of declining activity, further compromising respiratory capacity. Finally, their sensitivity to sedative drugs may predispose these patients to complications following general anesthesia.[21,26]

GASTROINTESTINAL SYSTEM

Symptoms affecting many regions of the gastrointestinal tract occur in as many as 80% of myotonic dystrophy patients. Impaired swallowing, posing a risk of aspiration, can be due to delayed relaxation of pharyngeal muscles.[92] Dysphagia may result from diminished esophageal motility associated with dilatation of the esophagus.[92,153] Reduced colonic activity leads to megacolon and fecal impaction, and the anal sphincter may undergo reflex myotonic contractions.[80]

CENTRAL NERVOUS SYSTEM

Mental aberrations occur in many patients with myotonic dystrophy. Prominent symptoms include apathy and indifference, with a lack of motivation leading to unemployment, even in patients with only mild weakness. A suspicious, paranoid, or frankly hostile personality is common. Mental retardation is an important feature, almost exclusively affecting those with the congenital form of the disease.[161,162] Intellectual function does not progressively decline. Prominent structural changes in the brain are infrequent, but generalized atrophy and ventricular dilatation have been observed.[169,230]

ENDOCRINE FUNCTION

Testicular atrophy associated with fibrosis of the seminiferous tubules is a common manifestation of myotonic dystrophy.[133] Many patients have reduced circulating androgen levels, with an associated increase of gonadotropins.[83] As the disease progresses, infertility occurs in both male and female patients. Women may have a high rate of fetal loss.[188] Male patients with impotence often have decreased plasma testosterone levels; androgen administration may restore potency. No evidence, however, suggests that androgen deficiency contributes to muscle weakness.[73]

Despite hyperinsulinemia following a glucose challenge, patients with myotonic dystrophy usually do not have glucose intolerance.[146] The frequency of diabetes mellitus is not increased, and the clinical complications of insulin resistance seen in adult-onset diabetics do not develop. The low basal metabolic rate observed in myotonic dystrophy is not accounted for by hypothyroidism, and the myotonia seen with hypothyroidism is not related in any way to myotonic dystrophy.

The frequent occurrence of cranial hyperostosis in myotonic dystrophy may be mistaken, especially in men, for an underlying brain tumor such as meningioma.

OCULAR SYSTEM

Posterior subcapsular cataracts are common in adults with myotonic dystrophy. Most can be seen by direct ophthalmoscopy, although some will be appreciated only by slit lamp evaluation. Less common ocular abnormalities include retinal pigmentary degeneration (peripheral or involving the macula),[86] low intraocular pressure, extraocular muscle myotonia, and extraocular muscle weakness. Meibomian cysts occur often and may require surgical drainage.

Congenital Myotonic Dystrophy

Typically, a pregnancy complicated by polyhydramnios and poor fetal movements precedes the birth of a hypotonic infant with congenital myotonic dystrophy (Table 4–4), which may be overlooked as a cause for hypotonia (see Table 5–2). In all cases of congenital myotonic dystrophy, the mother is the parent affected. Facial and jaw muscle weakness in the infant produces a "tented" upper lip accompanied by feeding and sucking difficulties. Severe respiratory distress is common. Clubfeet and generalized joint contractures also may occur. In congenital myotonic dystrophy, the muscle biopsy will show nonspecific features of increased variability in fiber size, sometimes with preferential type 1 fiber atrophy. Myotonia will not be present in the neonatal period and may not appear until age 5 or older. Even in the absence of problems in the neonatal period, developmental delay is common, as is mental retardation. The hatchet-faced appearance of adult myotonic dystrophy is usually more exaggerated because of more severe facial weakness combined with poor development of the jaw muscles.

The cause of congenital myotonic dystrophy affecting the offspring of affected mothers has not been determined. Genetic imprinting is thought to represent the most suitable explanation.[79] Early in fetal development, either the X or Y chromosome has a differential effect on a particular expressed trait. Analogies also have been made to neonatal myasthenia gravis, but in myotonic dystrophy no transmissible serum factors have been identified. Furthermore, no method of distinguishing mothers prone to have children with congenital myotonic dystrophy has emerged. At least 50% of siblings of affected offspring appear entirely normal.[1,84]

Laboratory Features

The diagnosis of myotonic dystrophy usually can be made on clinical grounds alone. Serum CK levels may be normal or mildly elevated. EMG evidence of myotonia will be found readily in most cases with typical clinical features and is helpful in identifying affected family members who have no definite signs of myotonic dystrophy. Local cooling of the muscle and sampling of multiple muscles (especially facial, shoulder girdle, and paraspinal muscles) will increase the diagnostic sensitivity of the EMG evaluation.[98,195] Myopathic features with low-amplitude, short-duration, polyphasic motor unit potentials will usually be present in affected patients. In evaluating a floppy infant for congenital myotonic dystrophy, however, myotonia will not be present, and the mother should be examined. If a diag-

---

Table 4–4 CONGENITAL MYOTONIC DYSTROPHY

Inheritance	Occurs in 25% of offspring of affected myotonic dystrophy mothers
Clinical features	Hypotonia, respiratory distress, poor suck and swallowing, facial and jaw weakness (tented upper lip), clubfeet, joint contractures, hydrocephalus, mental retardation
Laboratory features	No specific abnormalities: CK level normal EMG often does not show myotonia (mother always abnormal) Muscle biopsy shows only fiber-size variability

nosis of myotonic dystrophy cannot be established in the mother on the basis of clinical features, an EMG may be necessary to look for myotonia.

Modest slowing of motor nerve conduction velocities has been demonstrated in myotonic dystrophy patients.[98] Furthermore, some studies have demonstrated an increase in the latency of F waves and delay or absence of H reflexes.[157] Sural nerve biopsies in myotonic dystrophy patients have been shown to be mildly abnormal in some,[39] but not all, studies.[160] These electrophysiologic and morphologic findings of neuropathy appear to have little clinical importance.

Muscle biopsy findings in myotonic dystrophy patients include a wide variety of changes. No single feature is diagnostic, but the collective picture distinguishes these patients from those with other neuromuscular diseases (Figs. 4–25, 4–26, 4–27). Muscle atrophy, selectively involving type 1 fibers, occurs in about 50% of cases. Increased numbers of central nuclei are typical. Fiber atrophy may be so severe that only nuclear clumps remain. Ring fibers and sarcoplasmic masses (homogeneous areas of disorganized myofibrillar material) occur with increased frequency. Necrosis of muscle fibers and increased connective tissue, common in other muscular dystrophies, are uncommon in myotonic dystrophy.

Genetics

Myotonic dystrophy is an autosomal dominant disorder. Evidence indicates that new mutations do not contribute to the pool of affected individuals. An intriguing aspect of the disease has been the marked variation in clinical severity and the evidence that anticipation occurs within families[164]; that is, the disease increases in severity with succeeding generations. Initially, anticipation was explained by the possibility of observer ascertainment bias, but it now has a clear basis in the molecular defect of the disease. The occurrence of congenital cases as the offspring of mothers but not of fathers with myotonic dystrophy remains incompletely understood, but it has been found that anticipation resulting from a greater number of trinucleotide repeats is characteristic

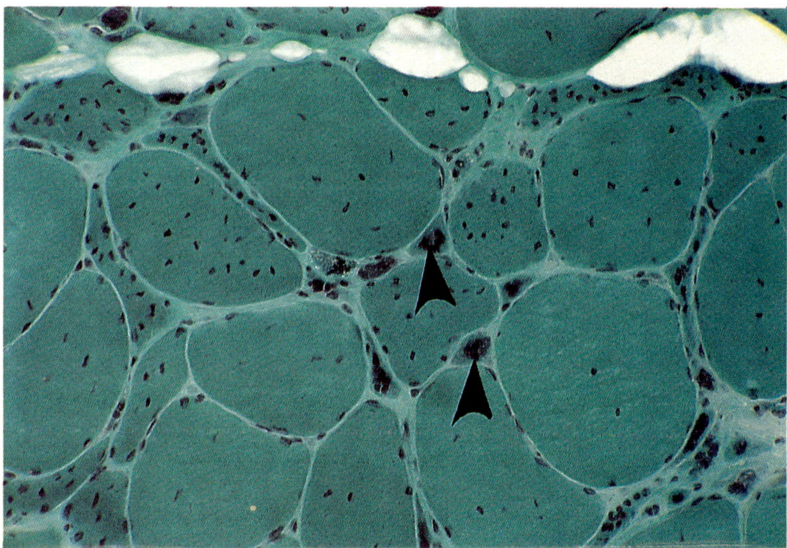

Figure 4–25. Muscle biopsy typical of myotonic dystrophy, showing muscle fibers with excessive numbers of central nuclei, small angular fibers, and severely atrophic fibers with nuclear clumps (*arrowheads*) (modified trichrome).

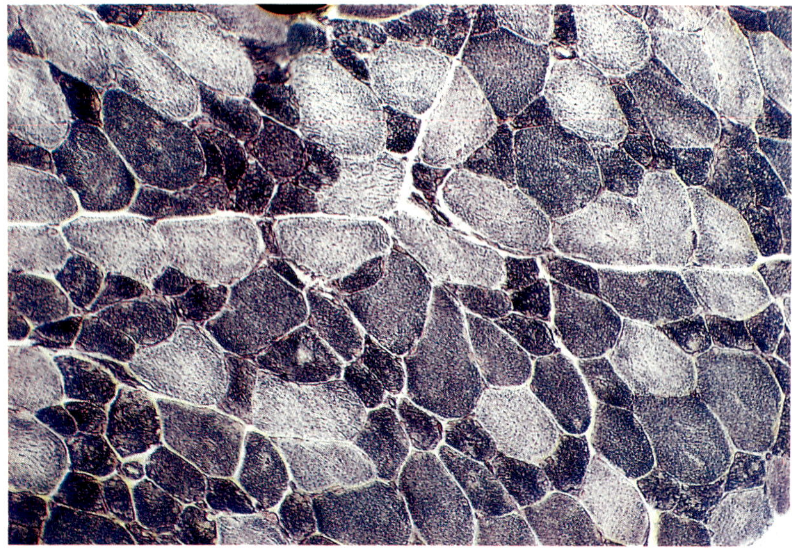

Figure 4–26. Biopsy from myotonic dystrophy showing type 1 fiber atrophy (dark fibers). Some fibers show focal areas of loss of oxidative enzymes (moth-eaten fibers) (NADH-tetrazolium reductase).

of maternally transmitted myotonic dystrophy (see below).

Myotonic dystrophy was the first human disorder to show genetic linkage, as demonstrated in 1954 by Mohr.[140] Linkage was shown with the Lewis blood group system. Subsequently the gene for myotonic dys-trophy was linked to the long arm of chromosome 19 using markers that include the C3 complement locus, peptidase D, secreter, and Lutheran blood groups.[43,55,154,219] Further work demonstrated a series of even more tightly linked markers to the region of chromosome 19q13.2, including B cell lym-

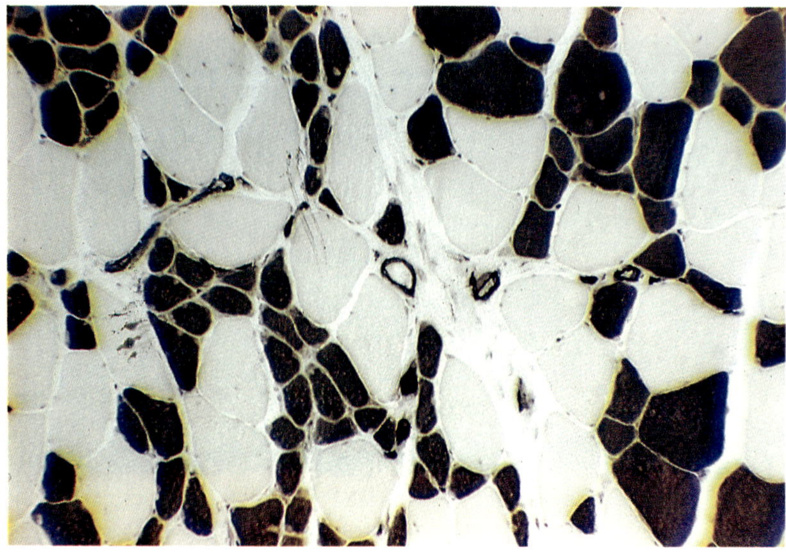

Figure 4–27. Type 1 fiber atrophy (dark fibers) in myotonic dystrophy. ATPase stain pH 4.2. The acid preincubation renders type 1 fibers dark and accentuates the presence of atrophy.

phoma 3 (BCL3),[116] apolipoprotein C2 (APOC2),[159,186] CK skeletal muscle isoenzyme (CKMM),[34] and the anonymous DNA fragment LDR152.[12] Recombination events placed all linkage markers on the proximal (centromeric) side of the myotonic dystrophy gene.[227]

The use of a series of somatic cell hybrids culminated in the isolation of a probe distal to the locus and very tightly linked to the disease gene.[100] The proximal and distal markers defined the limits of the gene. The intervening region containing the myotonic dystrophy gene was then isolated as a series of overlapping cosmid and yeast artificial chromosome (YAC) clones. YACs are 100- to 1000-kb segments of human DNA that have been cloned in yeast cells. Using radiation hybrids of the myotonic region of chromosome 19, new probes were mapped in the region of the gene.[28] These new probes detected strong linkage disequilibrium between the myotonic dystrophy gene and specific alleles detected by the probes, indicating that they were very close to the gene. The YAC clones containing the myotonic dystrophy region were used to screen complementary DNA (cDNA) from patients with myotonic dystrophy, and one clone detected a patient-specific band.[4,37,82] Other groups confirmed the initial finding, and it was then shown that the mutation in myotonic dystrophy results in an expansion of a trinucleotide (CTG) repeat in the 3′ untranslated region of the gene.[27,66,128] The number of repeats was shown to increase progressively in kindreds showing anticipation: normal-appearing individuals carrying the gene have a normal or minimal increase in the number; those with mild disease have a moderate increase; and those with severe disease, a marked increase.

There are a number of cases with clinical features of myotonic dystrophy that do not have an expansion of CTG repeats.[203a] It is not known whether these cases represent mutations within the gene or occur by other mechanisms. Certain families with an atypical, proximal weakness are not linked to chromosome 19q35.[147a]

The myotonic dystrophy gene codes for a protein that has an amino acid composition strikingly homologous to a serine-threonine-specific, (cAMP) cyclic adenosine monophosphate-dependent protein kinase and has been termed myotonin-protein kinase.[66] Kinases phosphorylate and thereby modulate ion channel function, so that an abnormal kinase may explain the abnormal excitability of muscle, the abnormal phosphorylation of erythrocytes, the abnormality of insulin action, and other tissue defects.[164] The development of antibodies to this protein can be expected to shed considerable light on the molecular basis for the disease.

The greater severity of the disease in the affected children of affected mothers than in affected children of affected fathers reflects the greater number of trinucleotide repeats seen in maternally transmitted cases. The reason for this difference may be the impaired function or survival of sperm containing a larger number of repeats.[3a] Other possible mechanisms include a circulating factor toxic to the fetus, mitochondrial inheritance of nongenomic DNA, or genetic imprinting. The mother with one severely affected infant is more likely to have other such infants.[84] At this time, mitochondrial inheritance appears unlikely because the mitochondrial DNA of congenital cases has been sequenced and is normal.[204] Genetic imprinting can explain differential effects of maternal versus paternal transmission and has been well documented in other diseases.[79] On the other hand, congenital cases typically improve in 4 to 6 weeks, suggesting the presence of a toxic, circulating factor from the mother. The time-course of improvement is reminiscent of that seen in antibody-mediated, transient, neonatal myasthenia gravis.

Treatment

Molded ankle-foot orthoses, which control foot drop and stabilize the ankle, help prevent falling. The quadriceps weakness common in many myotonic dystrophy patients, which causes the knee to give way suddenly, can be difficult to treat. For severe quadriceps weakness, an extension above the knee may be added to the standard ankle-foot orthoses, but most patients will not tolerate these modified long leg braces.

Myotonia rarely warrants aggressive treatment. Hand weakness rather than myotonia causes difficulties for most myotonic dystrophy patients. Furthermore, the most effective antimyotonia drugs, including quinine and procainamide, can impair cardiac conduction. Quinine and procainamide lengthen the P-R interval; phenytoin notably shortens it. Considering the choices, phenytoin appears to be the preferred agent for the occasional patient who requires treatment. Acetazolamide, effective as an antimyotonia agent in certain patients with other myotonic disorders, has proven ineffective in myotonic dystrophy. The efficacy of tocainide and calcium channel blocking agents in treating myotonia has not been firmly established, but these may prove useful as alternative drugs.

Many patients with myotonic dystrophy require lens replacement for posterior subcapsular cataracts. Corrective surgery for ptosis should be avoided, because facial weakness following ptosis surgery may cause incomplete eye closure and lead to corneal ulcerations. Surgical drainage may be necessary for meibomian cysts.

The respiratory complications of myotonic dystrophy require attention. An intense program of pulmonary hygiene can be helpful. This program includes incentive spirometry, coughing and deep-breathing exercises, postural drainage, and prompt antibiotic therapy for respiratory infections. Patients should be encouraged to lose weight; sedative drugs should be avoided.

The natural history of cardiac conduction disturbances has not been well characterized. It is not clear which patients need prophylactic cardiac pacemaker insertion. We recommend careful follow-up of asymptomatic individuals with early conduction-system abnormalities. Pacemaker insertion is strongly considered for patients with unexplained syncope or advanced conduction-system abnormalities, including evidence of second-degree heart block or trifascicular conduction disturbances with marked prolongation of the P-R interval.

FACIOSCAPULOHUMERAL MUSCULAR DYSTROPHY

In the revised classification of Walton and Nattrass in 1954,[213] facioscapulohumeral (FSH) dystrophy, sometimes referred to as Landouzy-Dejerine dystrophy, was assigned as one of three major forms of dystrophy, in addition to Duchenne and limb-girdle types (Table 4–5). This position as a distinct nosologic entity has often been challenged because of the heterogeneity of clinical and laboratory features of FSH dystrophy, but molecular studies have es-

Table 4–5 FACIOSCAPULOHUMERAL DYSTROPHY

Inheritance	Autosomal dominant; linked to distal chromosome 4q
Onset	First to fifth decade
Clinical features	
Musculoskeletal	Weakness usually of muscles of face, shoulder girdle, and anterior compartment of legs; 20% have pelvic girdle weakness; slow progression
Other systems	Labile hypertension; sensorineural hearing loss; Coats' disease (retinal telangiectasia, exudation and detachment)
Laboratory features	No specific abnormalities:
	CK level normal or elevated (usually less than fivefold)
	EMG myopathic
	Myopathic muscle biopsy with variable inflammation

tablished it as a distinct, genetically homogeneous disorder. Families without facial weakness, in which weakness is confined to scapuloperoneal muscles, may have other neuromuscular diseases, including spinal muscular atrophy,[101,102] Davidenkow's syndrome of scapuloperoneal neuropathy,[95,101] or a form of muscular dystrophy with weakness in a scapuloperoneal distribution without facial involvement.[155] The spectrum of scapuloperoneal syndromes is further discussed below.

Clinical Features

When fully developed, FSH dystrophy has a characteristic facial appearance and pattern of muscle weakness.[156,190,199,208,235] Typical onset occurs in childhood or young adult years, although some patients are not affected until middle life.[156] Facial weakness is the initial manifestation in most cases. A glum, expressionless facial appearance develops, accompanied by inability to smile, whistle, or fully close the eyes (Fig. 4–28). Patients appear mildly exophthalmic, and many sleep with partially open eyes. The weakness of the shoulder girdle, rather than of the facial muscles, usually brings the patient to medical attention.

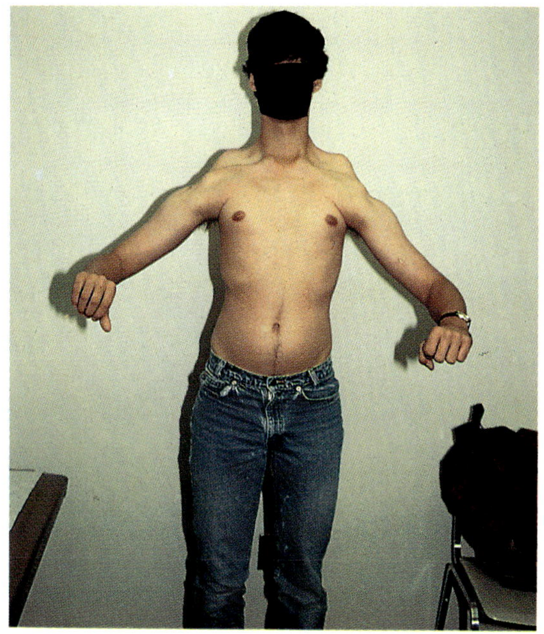

Figure 4–29. Difficulty with arm elevation in facioscapulohumeral dystrophy.

Loss of strength of scapular stabilizer muscles makes arm elevation difficult (Fig. 4–29). Scapular winging becomes apparent with attempts at abduction and forward movement of the arms (Fig. 4–30). The involved scapular stabilizer muscles include the lower portion of the

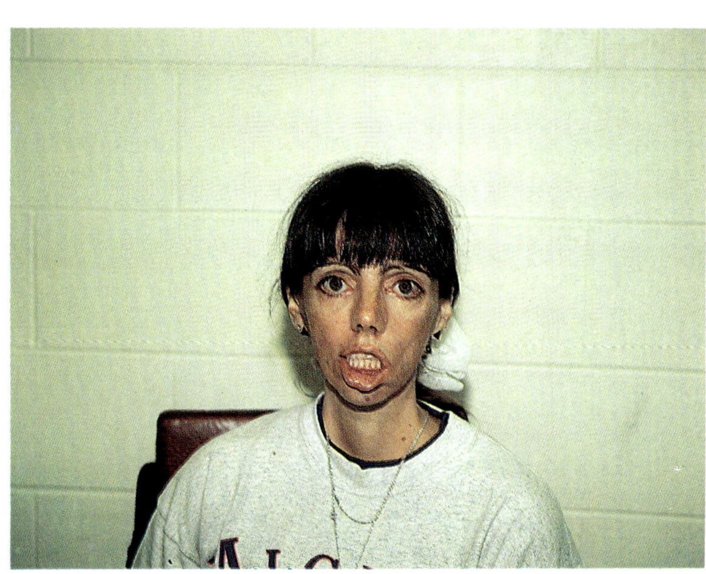

Figure 4–28. Marked facial weakness in facioscapulohumeral muscular dystrophy. Severe weakness of the orbicularis oris allows the lower lip to fall away from the teeth. Weakness of orbicularis oculi produces a pseudoexophthalmic appearance.

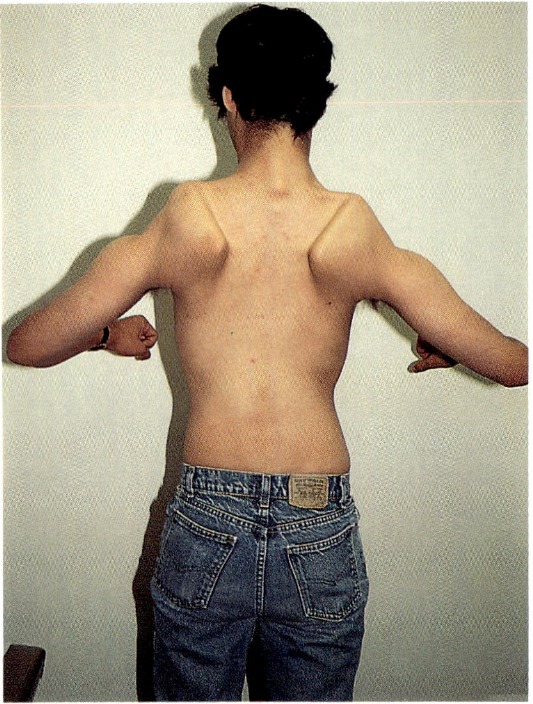

Figure 4–30. Prominent scapular winging in facioscapulohumeral dystrophy.

trapezius, the rhomboid, and the serratus anterior. The sternocostal head of the pectoral muscle is often atrophic and weak. These findings produce a distinctive posture with the shoulders thrust forward and a flattened appearance of the chest wall. In the arms, the triceps and biceps muscles may be severely affected. The deltoid muscles usually remain strong, although they appear weak unless tested with the scapula mechanically fixed against the chest wall by placing the patient in a supine position or holding the scapula in place. Wrist extension weakness invariably exceeds that of wrist flexion. Weakness of the anterior compartment muscles of the legs is another early manifestation; patients may present with foot drop. Abdominal muscle weakness often produces a Beevor's sign. When the patient is supine and relaxed, head flexion results in movement (usually upward) of the umbilicus.

In more than half of patients, life expectancy is normal, and the weakness will remain confined to facial, upper-extremity, and distal lower-extremity muscles. Patients usually can adjust their lifestyle to compensate. On the other hand, in about 20% of patients the disease will progress to involve the muscles of the pelvic girdle. These patients may experience wheelchair confinement and, rarely, respiratory insufficiency.

Characteristically, other organ systems are not involved in FSH dystrophy. Occasional involvement of heart muscle[194] is usually the result of an unrelated, coincidental illness. Labile hypertension, however, is a frequent accompaniment, the cause of which is unknown.

Patients with FSH dystrophy have an increased incidence of sensorineural hearing loss. Coats' disease, a disorder consisting of telangiectasia, exudation, and detachment of the retina, also occurs.[190,199,226] Coats' disease, apart from any association with muscular dystrophy, causes blindness in children.[130] Mental retardation[199] and corticospinal tract signs[226] have been reported in patients with muscular dystrophy and Coats' disease. Retinal abnormalities detectable by fluorescein angiography may be present in some FSH dystrophy patients, but neither the hearing nor eye abnormalities are useful in diagnosis.

The diagnosis of FSH dystrophy depends on the clinical picture and the exclusion of other disorders that can occasionally simulate this picture, including nemaline myopathy, inclusion body myositis, and polymyositis. Muscle biopsy is more useful in excluding such disorders than in demonstrating specific features of FSH dystrophy.

Laboratory Features

Serum CK may be normal or mildly elevated. EMG usually indicates a myopathic pattern. Occasional neuropathic findings are related in most instances to

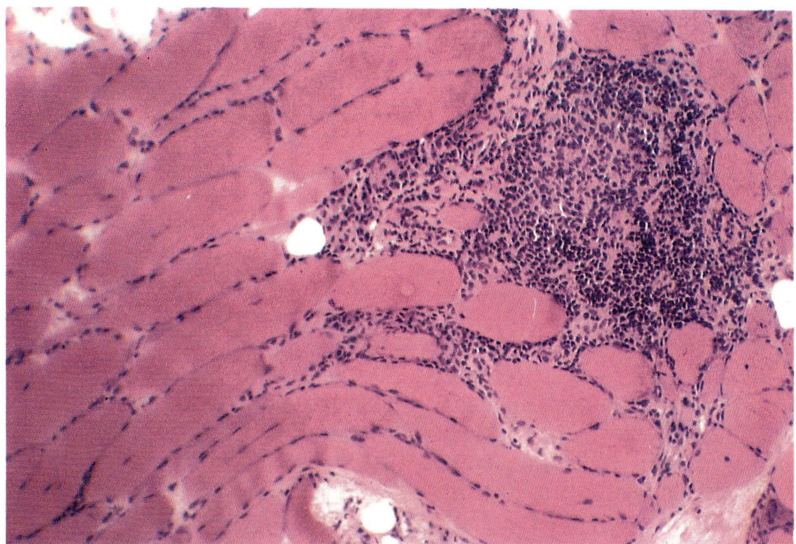

Figure 4–31. Muscle biopsy from patient with facioscapulohumeral dystrophy, showing prominent focal collection of inflammatory cells. (H&E).

secondary nerve injuries from stretching of the brachial plexus, or to focal compression neuropathies of branches of the radial, median, or ulnar nerves.

The muscle biopsy shows isolated, angular, and necrotic fibers; moth-eaten fibers; and moderate endomysial connective tissue proliferation. Histologic abnormalities show a multifocal distribution. One region of a biopsy may be severely affected, while an adjacent area shows minor abnormalities (Figs. 4–31 and 4–32). At one time, the finding of a prolific inflammatory infiltrate in some muscle biopsies raised the possibility of a disorder overlapping with

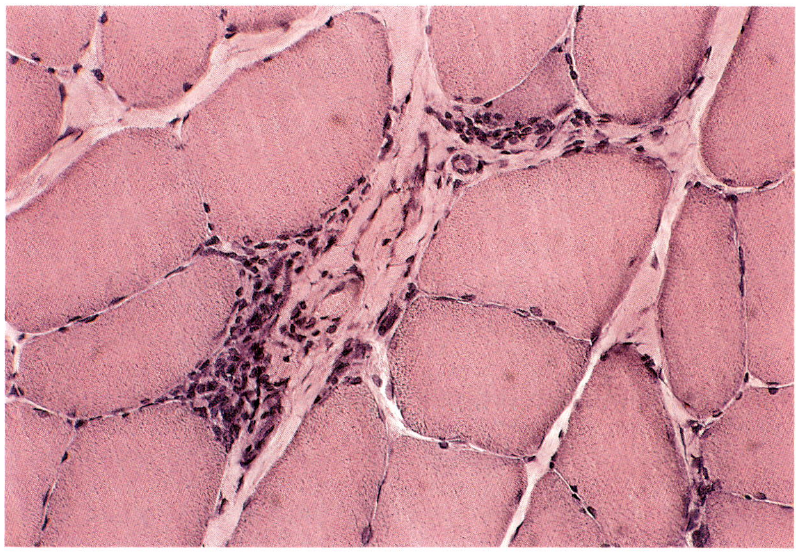

Figure 4–32. Muscle biopsy from patient with facioscapulohumeral dystrophy, showing mononuclear cells immediately adjacent to, but not invading, muscle fibers (H&E).

the inflammatory myopathies.[148] The presence of inflammation in the muscle biopsy specimen is no longer considered to have that implication. Furthermore, muscle inflammation on muscle biopsy does not alter the natural history of FSH dystrophy.

Genetics

The estimated incidence of FSH dystrophy is 1 in 20,000.[56] An autosomal dominant inheritance pattern with almost complete penetrance has been established, but requires examination of each family member for confirmation, since approximately 30% of those affected will be unaware of involvement.[156] The variability of disease expression, ranging from nonprogressive facial weakness to severe wheelchair confinement, suggests that a second, modifying gene may influence the course of the illness.

Linkage studies using RFLPs have localized the FSH dystrophy gene to the distal portion of the long arm of chromosome 4.[216,220–222] Within families that have clinical evidence for autosomal dominant inheritance, there is evidence for disease heterogeneity.[68a] A probe that appears to be within the FSH locus has recently been discovered. Studies with this probe have already shown that sporadic cases usually represent new mutations.[77a,198,221] There is evidence that the FSH gene is adjacent to telomeric heterochromatin; deletions of this heterochromatin may alter FSH gene expression by a process termed "position effect variegation."[223a]

Treatment

In certain individuals with FSH dystrophy, surgery may be indicated to treat scapular winging. If the deltoid muscle has good strength, the range of motion of the shoulder can be improved by fixing the scapula to the thorax. Surgical techniques for scapulothoracic fixation employ strips of fascia, synthetic material,[108] or wire plates.[124] Surgery should be restricted to patients with mild disease and should be done on the side of dominant hand function.

In severely affected patients, abdominal and truncal muscle weakness, combined with weakness of the hip girdle, leads to a protuberant abdomen and accentuated lumbar lordosis. In ambulatory patients, this posture compensates for weakness, but in patients confined to a wheelchair, a corset or brace may provide comfort. Nonambulatory patients will be helped by a motorized chair with an adjustable height control; some patients find a hospital bed useful. Weakness of the anterior compartment muscles of the leg may be helped by ankle-foot orthoses.

SCAPULOPERONEAL SYNDROMES

Many case studies and literature reviews have attempted to clarify the heterogeneous group of disorders referred to as "scapuloperoneal syndromes." Brossard[33] was the first to describe a syndrome of weakness confined to the shoulder girdle and distal lower-extremity muscles. Scapuloperoneal syndromes have been reported with disorders of skeletal muscle,[107,126,167,203] spinal motor neurons,[2,102,103,168,213] and peripheral nerve.[42,95,101,151,171]

Muscular Dystrophy with Scapuloperoneal Distribution

Several reports document the occurrence of a primary muscle disorder with clinical weakness in a scapuloperoneal distribution and sparing facial muscles.[107,126,167,203] At least some scapuloperoneal dystrophy families represent a separate nosologic entity, distinct from FSH dystrophy, in which the disorder is not transmitted by a gene at the 4q35 locus (R.T. Tawil, unpublished data).

CLINICAL FEATURES

The age of onset of muscular dystrophy confined to a scapuloperoneal distribution has varied from childhood to young adult or middle life.[126,167,203] The symptoms may begin in the distal lower extremities,[126,203] or in the shoulder girdle and scapular muscles.[167] The muscle weakness will either ascend or descend to involve the muscle groups not initially affected. Lower-extremity weakness causes difficulty in walking because of foot drop, and shoulder weakness limits the range of motion of the arms. Scapuloperoneal dystrophy has been slowly progressive and does not ordinarily result in severe disability or wheelchair confinement.

LABORATORY FEATURES

The CK level is mildly elevated, and EMG changes indicate myopathy. The muscle biopsy shows variability in fiber size, increased central nuclei, muscle fiber splitting, and increased connective tissue and fat.[203]

GENETICS

The inheritance pattern has usually been autosomal dominant,[167,203] although sporadic cases occur.[126,203]

Sparing of facial muscles should differentiate scapuloperoneal dystrophy from FSH dystrophy. Nevertheless, clear distinction may not always be possible, as indicated by reports of "scapuloperoneal dystrophy" with mild facial weakness.[203] The confusion is furthered by reports of a kindred followed for more than 40 years.[107] Kazakov and colleagues[107] personally examined patients belonging to four generations of the family originally reported by Oransky.[155] Early in the course, muscles of the shoulder girdle and peroneal group were affected, a pattern preserved for many years; but facial muscle weakness later developed, and the clinical picture was indistinguishable from FSH

dystrophy. Genetic studies will clarify the diagnosis in such families.

Emery-Dreifuss muscular dystrophy resembles scapuloperoneal dystrophy, but the X-linked recessive inheritance, cardiomyopathy, contractures of elbows and neck, and humeroperoneal weakness (sparing scapular muscles) clearly distinguish it from scapuloperoneal dystrophy.

Spinal Muscular Atrophy with Scapuloperoneal Distribution

Several well-documented families with a scapuloperoneal distribution of spinal muscular atrophy have been reported.[2,102,168,213] The reports include autopsy confirmation of anterior horn cell and bulbar motor nuclei degeneration.[102]

CLINICAL FEATURES

The onset of this condition occurs between ages 30 and 50, with weakness and atrophy always starting in the distal leg muscles. In contrast to scapuloperoneal dystrophies, all muscles below the knee become affected. Subsequently, the shoulder muscles become affected and, late in the course, usually the pelvic girdle muscles. The condition progresses slowly and leads to severe weakness and wheelchair confinement.

LABORATORY FEATURES

Laboratory findings may be confusing. CK levels can be mildly elevated, and the muscle biopsy may show mixed myopathic and neuropathic features. Ideally, features of reinnervation will be present, especially type grouping. The EMG should provide the clearest differentiation, with abundant fibrillation potentials, positive sharp waves, and reduced interference pattern on maximal voluntary effort. Fasciculations will be variable. Unfortunately, in some muscle groups the EMG will also have some myopathic features.

GENETICS

An autosomal dominant pattern was clearly established in three families.[2,101,168] In additional patients having a less well defined scapuloperoneal distribution, patterns have been sporadic or possibly autosomal recessive.[58]

Peripheral Neuropathy with Scapuloperoneal Distribution (Davidenkow's Syndrome)

In 1939, Davidenkow published his experience with an entity he described as having features overlapping but distinct from the "amyotrophy of Charcot and Marie" and the "myopathy of Landouzy and Dejerine."[42] Subsequent reports have confirmed the existence of a peripheral nerve disorder that presents with a scapuloperoneal distribution.[95,103,151,171]

CLINICAL FEATURES

Scapuloperoneal neuropathy may appear in either childhood or adult years. Weakness usually begins in the distal lower extremities, with subsequent involvement of the scapular stabilizer and muscles of the shoulder girdle. These patients have an accompanying sensory loss in a stocking-glove distribution. Tendon reflexes are depressed throughout and usually absent at the ankles. The condition progresses slowly and may affect the pelvic girdle muscles, but it does not usually lead to severe disability or wheelchair confinement. Pes cavus is an early sign of the disorder.[171]

LABORATORY FEATURES

The CK level will be normal or mildly elevated. Electrodiagnostic studies indicate a peripheral neuropathy, with mildly[95] or moderately[171] slowed conduction velocities and absent sensory-nerve action potentials. The EMG shows fibrillation potentials, positive sharp waves, and pathologically enlarged motor unit potentials, as well as a reduction in motor unit recruitment. Sural nerve biopsies have demonstrated findings indicative of a primary axonal neuropathy with secondary demyelination and remyelination.[95]

GENETICS

The inheritance pattern has generally been autosomal dominant,[151,171] but sporadic cases occur.[95,103]

LIMB-GIRDLE DYSTROPHY

Limb-girdle dystrophy (Table 4–6) refers to a heterogeneous group of clinical disorders that includes several types of inherited muscle diseases. The term "limb-girdle dystrophy" was given credibility by the revised classification

---

Table 4–6 LIMB-GIRDLE DYSTROPHY

Inheritance	Autosomal recessive
	Autosomal dominant (may be linked to Pelger-Huët anomaly of peripheral blood leukocytes)
Onset	Early childhood to adult years
Clinical features	
Musculoskeletal	Slowly progressive pelvic and shoulder-girdle weakness
Other systems	Cardiomyopathy (10% have heart failure)
Laboratory features	No specific abnormalities:
	CK level elevated (< 10-fold)
	EMG myopathic
	Myopathic muscle biopsy

of Walton and Natrass, introduced in 1954.[213] They proposed that limb-girdle was a major form of dystrophy, along with Duchenne and FSH. From the outset, it became apparent that limb-girdle dystrophy represented more than one disorder. In fact, even the clinical features outlined by Walton and Natrass included heterogeneity. The characteristics of limb-girdle dystrophy, as defined, included a muscle condition expressed in both males and females, with onset ranging from late in the first decade to the fourth decade. Patients had both autosomal recessive and autosomal dominant inheritance, weakness beginning in either the shoulder or pelvic girdle muscles, and a variable rate of progression.

The heterogeneity of limb-girdle dystrophy has been documented by the finding that genes code for the disorder in at least two different loci: one on 5q[191] and one on 15q.[14] From a practical viewpoint, limb-girdle dystrophy refers to patients not fitting into one of the better defined groups: that is, after excluding other forms of neuromuscular disease accounting for weakness, a label of limb-girdle dystrophy becomes acceptable for an inherited, progressive myopathy.

Clinical Features

In limb-girdle dystrophy, the initial symptoms of weakness of the proximal leg muscles usually begin in the second or third decade. Upper-limb involvement, with scapular winging, appears later. In certain instances the onset may be delayed until the third or fourth decade. Muscle weakness progresses slowly, and some patients advance to a stage of wheelchair dependency. Chronic alveolar hypoventilation from severe diaphragm weakness may be seen. Approximately 10% of patients have clinically significant cardiac involvement accompanied by heart failure. The variation in distribution of weakness and rate of progression will be dictated by individual familial characteristics.

Table 4-7 LIMB-GIRDLE SYNDROMES—SUBTYPES

Severe childhood muscular dystrophy with autosomal recessive inheritance
Juvenile (scapulohumeral) dystrophy of Erb
Pelvifemoral dystrophy of Leyden-Mobius
Adult-onset muscular dystrophy with autosomal dominant inheritance
Myopathy limited to quadriceps (certain such cases have been dystrophin-deficient)

In discussions of limb-girdle dystrophy, five subtypes or variants have been described (Table 4-7).[187,211] In the autosomal recessive form of severe childhood muscular dystrophy, clinical features overlap with those of Duchenne dystrophy, but the involvement of both males and females indicates a different inheritance pattern.[16,49,96,97,113,193] This form of childhood dystrophy has been described in two large Amish kindreds,[193] and in families from Tunisia.[96] A 50-kd protein, one of the components of the dystrophin-associated glycoprotein complex, has been found to be deficient in some but not all patients with this severe form of childhood muscular dystrophy.[133b,185a] Another autosomal recessive variant of limb-girdle dystrophy, the juvenile (scapulohumeral) dystrophy of Erb, begins in teenage years with involvement of shoulder girdle muscles and progresses slowly.[25,144] A third subtype of limb-girdle dystrophy, referred to as pelvifemoral dystrophy of Leyden-Mobius, affects pelvic girdle muscles initially, with later spread to upper extremities. Onset of this slowly progressive condition occurs from the first to the fifth decade. Pelvifemoral dystrophy has been described with autosomal recessive and X-linked inheritance.[25,144] Some of these cases probably represent phenotypic variants of dystrophin deficiency. A fourth variant, adult-onset limb-girdle dystrophy with autosomal dominant inheritance, presents in early adult life (third to fourth decade) with shoulder and pelvic girdle weakness.[6,180] In one family, the dystrophy was linked to the Pelger-Huët anomaly of white blood cells (hyposegmented neutrophils with rodlike, dumbbell, peanut-shaped, or spectacle-like nuclei and increased coarseness of chromatin of all white blood cells).[180] The final reported subtype of limb-girdle dystrophy is a myopathy limited to the quadriceps muscles.[45,212] The disorder has been described in families with an autosomal dominant pattern of inheritance,[60] and in another with two affected brothers.[223] Review of these reports reveals more extensive involvement of weakness. A paucity of subsequent reports suggests that myopathy limited to quadriceps muscles does not represent a specific entity. The cases probably represent other conditions, particularly spinal muscular atrophy or inclusion body myositis, a disorder with predilection for quadriceps muscles (see Chapter 5) and dystrophin deficiency.

Laboratory Features

Elevated CK, a myopathic EMG, and muscle biopsy features indicative of myopathy characterize limb-girdle dystrophy. In accord with its heterogeneity, the changes in these laboratory studies will vary greatly. Nevertheless, a certain range of findings can be expected, and attention to variations outside these limits will prevent mistaken diagnoses. For example, in limb-girdle dystrophy, the CK levels should be in the range of 5 to 10 times normal; elevations of greater than 10-fold suggest a sporadic case of Becker dystrophy. On the other hand, CK levels typically do not rise more than threefold in spinal muscular atrophy. EMG studies demonstrating mixed myopathic and neuropathic changes raise the possibility of inclusion body myositis (see Chapter 4). The presence of abundant spontaneous activity (complex repetitive discharges or myotonia), especially in the lumbar paraspinal and abdominal muscles, suggests a glycogen storage disease such as acid maltase deficiency.

The muscle biopsy in limb-girdle dys-trophy will show a spectrum of changes including muscle fiber atrophy and hypertrophy, increased connective tissue, muscle fiber necrosis, and a wide range of architectural changes including split, whorled, moth-eaten, and ring fibers. The finding of such nonspecific features in sporadic cases of Becker muscular dystrophy emphasizes the need for dystrophin analysis as part of muscle biopsy assessment.

Electrocardiographic changes accompany some variants of limb-girdle dystrophy. Nonspecific ST-T wave abnormalities, inverted T waves, or loss of anterior wall forces may be seen. Such changes do not occur in other muscular dystrophies or in spinal muscular atrophy and are infrequent in polymyositis.

Genetics

Either autosomal recessive or autosomal dominant inheritance may be seen, depending on the individual family. Identifying the molecular basis for limb-girdle dystrophy has proved to be more difficult than it was for Duchenne and Becker dystrophy. Genetic linkage studies have thus far defined an autosomal recessive form linked to chromosome 15q,[14] and an autosomal dominant form linked to chromosome 5q.[191] It has been postulated that a cytoskeletal protein (the gene product of a locus on chromosome 6) related to the dystrophin complex[59] might be abnormal in limb-girdle dystrophy. Despite the clinical similarities of limb-girdle and Becker dystrophy, the latter has not been linked to chromosome 6.

Treatment

Supportive care, but not specific treatment, can be offered. Long leg braces are seldom helpful, because adults do poorly with orthotic devices extending above the knee. In occasional patients, the physiologic and psychologic benefits of therapeutic standing may justify their use. Some patients may be candidates for a modified long leg brace designed to bend during ambulation, as opposed to the usual locked-knee position of long leg braces. Use of a wheelchair for shopping or recreational activities will help to preserve the patient's energy.

Cardiac or respiratory muscle involvement may need specific treatment, as in patients with other neuromuscular diseases (see Chapter 10). Ankle and leg edema may develop from dependency and stasis, and its prevention can be important in improving mobility and avoiding the induration of skin that increases susceptibility to infection from minor trauma. Edema does not necessarily indicate heart failure. A program of intermittent leg elevation, supportive stockings, and judicious use of diuretics will usually alleviate edema, but agents such as phenylbutazone, nifedipine, or propranolol may exacerbate it in wheelchair-bound patients.

OCULOPHARYNGEAL MUSCULAR DYSTROPHY
(Table 4–8)

Three important and distinct disorders present with features of progressive external ophthalmoplegia (PEO). One of these disorders, centronuclear or myotubular myopathy, an important congenital myopathy, is discussed with that group of conditions (see Chapter 6). A second disorder with PEO represents a mitochondrial myopathy with ragged red fibers (see Chapter 6). The discussion here is restricted to oculopharyngeal muscular dystrophy.[8,9,29,179,200,209]

Oculopharyngeal muscular dystrophy, described by Taylor in 1915,[200] was thought to represent a neuronal disorder. Kiloh and Nevin were the first to recognize this as a form of muscular dystrophy (ocular myopathy),[109] and the term oculopharyngeal muscular dystrophy was introduced later by Victor and associates.[209]

Clinical Features

Oculopharyngeal muscular dystrophy most often presents in the fourth to sixth decade with ptosis, usually asymmetric early in the course (see Fig. 2–18). As ptosis worsens, patients must contract the frontalis muscle in order to raise the upper eyelids, or retroflex the head, resulting in an "astronomist's posture." Dysphagia is another early symptom. The swallowing problems may become debilitating and result in pooling of secretions in the nasopharynx, with repeated episodes of aspiration resulting in coughing and occasionally leading to pulmonary infections. Extraocular muscle impairment varies in degree, but it usually does not progress to complete ophthalmoplegia. Laryngeal weakness may cause dysphonia. Mild neck and extremity weakness occur, seldom leading to functional disability. In one variant of the disease described in Japan, oculopharyngodis-

Table 4–8 OCULOPHARYNGEAL MUSCULAR DYSTROPHY

Inheritance	Autosomal dominant
Onset	Fourth to sixth decade
Clinical features	
Musculoskeletal	Ptosis, dysphagia
	Mild limb weakness
	Variable extraocular motility loss
Other systems	Aspiration and repeated pulmonary infections
Laboratory features	CK level normal to elevated threefold
	EMG myopathic
	Muscle biopsy shows rimmed vacuoles and tubular filaments
	(8.5 nm diameter) within nuclei

tal myopathy, weakness, and wasting of the distal muscles accompanies ptosis and extraocular muscle weakness.[179] Cardiac conduction-system abnormalities have also been described in the Japanese variant,[179] the only involvement of an organ system outside of skeletal muscle.

only in oculopharyngeal dystrophy. These unbranched tubular filaments may reach 0.5 μm in length, often show striations with a periodicity of 7 to 7.5 nm,[205] and differ from the larger, 15- to 18-nm intranuclear and extranuclear filaments seen in inclusion body myositis (see Chapter 5).

Laboratory Features

In oculopharyngeal dystrophy, CK elevations reach two to three times normal. A myopathic EMG is typical. The histologic findings differentiate this condition from other disorders associated with progressive external ophthalmoplegia. Characteristically, small, often subsarcolemmal, rimmed vacuoles lined with granular material (Fig. 4–33) can be found associated with fibers showing increased variability in size. Electron microscopy shows the rimmed vacuoles to contain membranous whorls, accumulations of glycogen, and other nonspecific debris, some of which seems to be of lysosomal origin. Tubular filaments (8.5 nm in diameter) within muscle nuclei are seen

Genetics

Oculopharyngeal muscular dystrophy has an autosomal dominant inheritance pattern with complete penetrance. French Canadians are the most commonly affected ethnic group,[8,9] and are related by a common ancestor emigrating to Quebec in 1634.[8] The disorder also occurs with increased frequency in Spanish-American families in southern Colorado, northern New Mexico, and Arizona,[8] and in large kindreds of Jewish families of Eastern European background.[209] The unique involvement of the distal muscles and the heart in Japanese cases raises questions about the relationship of this variant to more typical oculopharyngeal muscular dystrophy.

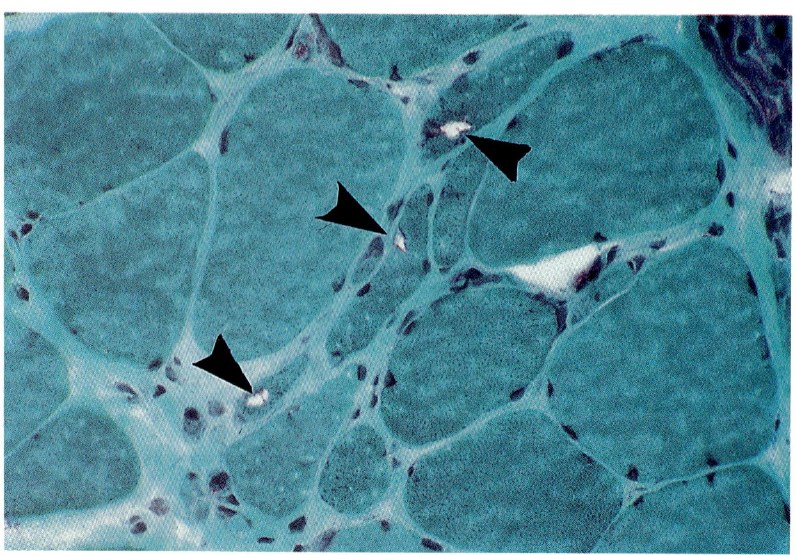

Figure 4–33. Muscle biopsy from a patient with oculopharyngeal muscular dystrophy. Three small fibers show vacuoles (*arrowheads*) (modified trichrome).

Treatment

The progressive dysphagia that leads to inanition and aspiration makes oculopharyngeal muscular dystrophy a potentially life-threatening disease. Manometric studies reveal low pharyngeal pressures and abnormalities in relaxation and coordination of the pharyngoesophageal sphincter. Aperistaltic muscle contractions occur in the proximal esophagus. Distal esophageal motility changes exacerbate the dysphagia. Pharyngoesophageal sphincter abnormalities may benefit from cricopharyngeal myotomy (see Chapter 10).[70] The lower esophageal involvement may improve with metoclopramide hydrochloride.

Eyelid crutches can improve vision obstructed by ptosis. Ptosis surgery is appropriate if orbicularis oculi muscle strength will allow unimpaired eyelid closure postoperatively.

CONGENITAL MUSCULAR DYSTROPHY

Congenital muscular dystrophy, Duchenne dystrophy, and myotonic dystrophy are the three forms of muscular dystrophy that present at birth or in the first year of life. It has not been determined whether congenital muscular dystrophy includes one or more genetic disorders, but cases can be divided clinically into a group with associated central nervous system involvement and one with only skeletal muscle disease (Table 4–9).*

Congenital Muscular Dystrophy without Cerebral Involvement

CLINICAL FEATURES

In the Western world, a form of congenital muscular dystrophy presents at

---

*References 67, 68, 121, 134, 135, 176, 183, 207.

birth or in the first few months of life.[121,134,207] Manifestations include hypotonia, proximal limb weakness, and joint contractures affecting elbows, hips, knees, and ankles. The contractures of congenital muscular dystrophy, referred to as arthrogryposis when present at birth, set this disease apart from Duchenne and myotonic dystrophy. Congenital hip dislocation may be present in occasional patients. About one third of patients have weakness of facial muscles, but other cranial nerve musculature is spared. The finding of full extraocular motility excludes centronuclear myopathy (see Chapter 6). The severity of congenital muscular dystrophy varies greatly. Roughly one half remain severely disabled, never achieving the ability to stand independently. Rarely, patients die of respiratory insufficiency during the first few years of life; the reported mortality of 15%[183] may be an overestimate. Some patients have delayed motor milestones but learn to walk, although difficulties in running and stair-climbing persist.

LABORATORY FEATURES

The laboratory features of congenital muscular dystrophy reflect disease heterogeneity. Most patients have CK elevations in the range of three to four times normal, but rare patients with proven non-Duchenne dystrophy have 10-fold to 20-fold elevations. The EMG demonstrates a myopathic pattern. Electrophysiologic studies are essential to exclude other causes of hypotonia in the newborn, especially forms of spinal muscular atrophy, congenital peripheral neuropathy, and neuromuscular transmission disorders (see Chapter 5, Table 5–2). Muscle biopsy abnormalities are nonspecific, in most cases demonstrating variability of fiber size, increased connective tissue, varying numbers of necrotic and regenerating muscle fibers, and increased central nuclei. All muscle biopsies from patients with suspected congenital muscular dystrophy must have dystrophin analysis because of the rare patient

Table 4–9 CONGENITAL MUSCULAR DYSTROPHIES

Type	Inheritance	Musculoskeletal Features	Other Systems
Congenital muscular dystrophy without cerebral involvement	Autosomal recessive	Onset at birth; hypotonia, contractures, delayed milestones, variable course	None
Fukuyama congenital muscular dystrophy	Autosomal recessive	Onset at birth; hypotonia, contractures, delayed milestones, progressive weakness, death by 10–12 years	Seizures, microcephaly
Cerebro-ocular-dysplasia muscular dystrophy	Autosomal recessive	Similar to Fukuyama type	Macrocephaly, hydrocephalus, ocular abnormalities leading to blindness, mental retardation
Congenital muscular dystrophy with cerebral hypomyelination	Autosomal recessive	Similar to congenital muscular dystrophy without cerebral involvement; delayed speech in some	Hypomyelination of cerebral white matter

with Duchenne dystrophy presenting in early infancy with hypotonia and developmental delay.[135]

Congenital Muscular Dystrophy with Cerebral Involvement

An important group of congenital muscular dystrophy patients have central nervous system and ocular involvement.[67,68] The central nervous system abnormalities can be attributed to an arrest in the migration and differentiation of neurons, leading to micropolygyria of the cerebral and cerebellar hemispheres, lissencephaly, diffuse or focal hypomyelination of the cerebral white matter, neuronal ectopias, ventricular enlargement, and hypoplastic or absent pyramidal tracts.

CLINICAL FEATURES

Fukuyama Congenital Muscular Dystrophy. A well-defined form of congenital muscular dystrophy associated with cerebral involvement was described by Fukuyama and colleagues in 1960.[68] This disorder presents at birth with generalized hypotonia, weak cry, poor suck; and facial, truncal, and limb weakness, more marked in proximal muscles. Calf muscle hypertrophy is common. Mild contractures at the elbows and knees worsen with time. Central nervous system involvement includes generalized tonic-clonic seizures and developmental delay in both motor and verbal spheres. Microcephaly and enlarged ventricles (hydrocephalus ex vacuo) often occur. Some children with Fukuyama congenital muscle (FCMD) may learn to sit or crawl, but few can stand. The condition leads to cachexia and death by the end of the first decade.

Cerebro-Ocular-Dysplasia Muscular Dystrophy. Another variant of congenital muscular dystrophy occurs in association with cerebro-ocular dysplasia.[67,176] This disorder combines the features of cerebro-ocular dysplasia of

Walker[206,210] (also called Warburg's syndrome[214]), and Fukuyama congenital muscular dystrophy. The clinical neuromuscular features parallel FCMD, but patients with cerebro-ocular-dysplasia muscular dystrophy (COD-MD) also have ocular pathology including corneal abnormalities, cataracts, immature anterior chamber angle ciliary body abnormalities, retinal dysplasia (with or without retinal detachment), abnormal retinal pigment epithelium, abnormal retinal vascularization, and hypoplasia of the optic nerve.[176] Hydrocephalus and macrocephaly have been more common in COD-MD than in FCMD.[176]

Congenital Muscular Dystrophy with Hypomyelination. In another variant of congenital muscular dystrophy, computed tomography (CT) or magnetic resonance imaging (MRI) scans show varying degrees of hypomyelination of the cerebral white matter, but most cases have no apparent clinical signs of central nervous system disease except for delayed verbal development.[54] Ocular abnormalities do not occur. In our own series of patients with congenital muscular dystrophy, none of whom had features of FCMD or COD-MD, we identified radiologic evidence of hypomyelination in one third. The relationship of these cases to FCMD and COD-MD has not been well defined.

LABORATORY FEATURES

Neither the CK, EMG, or muscle biopsy will distinguish congenital muscular dystrophies occurring with or without cerebral involvement. The CK values range from normal to fourfold to five times normal, although we have observed 20-fold increases in non-Duchenne dystrophy patients. The EMG shows a myopathic pattern. Nonspecific muscle biopsy features include increased variability in muscle fiber size, loss of muscle fibers with infiltration of fat and connective tissue, and scattered muscle fibers undergoing degeneration and regeneration with increased central nuclei. Dystrophin analysis must be done in all cases of congenital muscular dystrophy. The importance of this test cannot be overemphasized, because Duchenne dystrophy patients with severe hypotonia and markedly delayed motor and verbal milestones present a picture similar to congenital muscular dystrophy. The importance of recognizing Duchenne dystrophy in the neonatal period cannot be overemphasized because of the possibility for carrier detection and prenatal diagnosis.

In congenital muscular dystrophy with central nervous system disease, hypomyelination will be highlighted by CT or MRI. The distribution of low-density areas may be either diffuse and symmetric, or focal. In some, the hypodensity diminishes or disappears with time, suggesting a correlation with delay in myelination. Other findings include dilatation of the ventricular system, broadening of cortical gyri, and prominence of the cisterna magna and interhemispheric and sylvian fissures.

GENETICS

Sporadic occurrences account for most of the cases of congenital muscular dystrophy without central nervous system involvement, although autosomal recessive inheritance has been reported. In FCMD, a 25% incidence of consanguinity was observed, and autosomal recessive inheritance has been established as the major mode of transmission.[67] The prevalence of FCMD in Japan has lead to speculation about a possible environmental factor. The high spontaneous abortion rate also supports a possible environmental factor.[67] The inheritance pattern for COD-MD also appears to be autosomal recessive.[206] The dysplasia affecting eye and brain raises the possibility of an intrauterine insult occurring before the seventh week of gestation.

An entity referred to as *rigid spine syndrome* has clinical features that overlap with congenital muscular dystrophy.[5,47,48,50,52,150,183] Patients have limitation in flexion of the neck and trunk, scoliosis, contractures of the elbows and knees, and mild, nonprogressive muscle weakness. A characteristic posture occurs, with neck hyperextension, forward tilting of the trunk, and flexion at the hips. Some patients have delayed motor milestones, and recognition of the condition usually occurs in early childhood. The CK level may be mildly elevated, and the EMG is myopathic. Muscle biopsy features differ[50,150,183] but typically show increased variability in fiber size and proliferation of endomysial and perimysial connective tissue. No consistent pattern of inheritance has been observed in the rigid spine syndrome. Most cases have been sporadic, although rare familial examples have been reported.[5,52]

Documentation of the rigid spine syndrome as a distinct nosologic entity awaits further proof. Some cases may represent variants of congenital muscular dystrophy, but conclusions will require precise criteria or identification of a specifically abnormal gene product upon which to base a diagnosis. Although Emery-Dreifuss muscular dystrophy and the rigid spine syndrome have contractures in common, the X-linked recessive inheritance and cardiomyopathy of Emery-Dreifuss are distinguishing features.

Treatment

Treatment of all subvarieties of congenital muscular dystrophy patients requires stretching to improve joint range of motion. The functional capabilities of infants and very young children can be maximized by special wheelchair modifications and adaptive seating. Anticonvulsant medications will be necessary for some patients.

DISTAL MYOPATHIES

Four groups of distal myopathies can be distinguished on the basis of clinical criteria (Table 4–10). Although the term "muscular dystrophy" has not

Table 4–10 DISTAL MYOPATHIES

Type	Inheritance	Musculoskeletal Features	Laboratory Studies	Other Systems
Late-adult-onset Welander myopathy type I	Autosomal dominant (predominantly Scandinavian)	Onset in midlife; begins in hands, spreads to distal leg muscles; slowly progressive	CK level normal or slightly increased. Biopsy—variable; vacuolar myopathy in some cases	None
Markesbery myopathy type II	Autosomal dominant (non-Scandinavian)	Onset in midlife; begins in distal leg muscles; spreads to hand muscles; slowly progressive	CK level normal or slightly increased Biopsy—vacuolar myopathy	Cardiomyopathy
Early-adult-onset Type I (Nonaka)	Autosomal recessive or sporadic	Onset in legs (anterior compartment)	CK level increased, usually $<10\times$ normal. Biopsy—vacuolar myopathy	None
Type II (Miyoshi)	Autosomal recessive or sporadic	Onset second–third decade; begins in distal leg muscles, spreads to hand muscles; slowly progressive	CK level increased, usually $>10\times$ normal. Biopsy—dystrophy without vacuoles; gastrocnemius often "end stage"	None

been used consistently in reference to these conditions, they fulfill the definition because of their hereditary nature and progressive course.

Because most patients presenting with distal weakness have denervating disorders, especially peripheral neuropathies, the distal myopathies require careful confirmatory EMG and muscle biopsy studies in order to establish the diagnosis. Moreover, distal weakness occurs in many other muscle conditions, including myotonic dystrophy (p. 114), FSH dystrophy (p. 123), inclusion body myositis (p. 171), debranching enzyme deficiency (p. 266), carnitine deficiency (p. 269), and phosphorylase *b* kinase deficiency (p. 262).

Welander Myopathy (Late-Adult-Onset – Type I)

CLINICAL FEATURES

In 1951, Welander[218] described a late-adult-onset distal myopathy (type 1) in 249 patients in 72 Swedish pedigrees with a mean age of onset of 47 years (range 20–77 years). Weakness develops in the small muscles of the hands, particularly the thumb and index finger, before spreading to other fingers. The distal limb muscles of the legs become involved later in most patients, causing a steppage gait. Proximal muscles are involved in less than one quarter of patients. About one half of patients lose the distal muscle stretch reflexes. The disease usually progresses slowly. In the small percentage with rapid progression, proximal muscle involvement and distal lower-extremity weakness occur earlier in the course. Patients with Welander myopathy have a normal life expectancy.

LABORATORY FEATURES

The CK level may be normal or increased twofold to threefold. EMG studies demonstrate a chronic myopathy with occasional fibrillations and positive sharp waves. The muscle biopsy

features include the nonspecific changes of excessive variability in fiber size, increased central nuclei, endomysial connective tissue proliferation, and fat deposition.

GENETICS

An autosomal dominant inheritance pattern has been well demonstrated in the large pedigrees described by Welander.[217,218] In the variant of Welander myopathy with more rapid progression, homozygosity for the gene may account for the altered phenotype.[217]

Another form of distal myopathy of Scandinavian ethnic background, also with autosomal dominant inheritance, has a different clinical course.[53] Distal hand muscle involvement occurs early in the course, but the group is distinguished from those with Welander myopathy by involvement of the hand flexors rather than extensors and subsequent evolution to involve proximal and distal muscles with respiratory compromise. A further distinguishing feature is the presence of cytoplasmic bodies. (Cytoplasmic body myopathy is discussed in Chapter 6).

Late-Onset Distal Myopathy Type II (Markesbery)

CLINICAL FEATURES

A distal myopathy with features distinctly different from Welander's cases has been recognized.[94,131,132,196] In these patients, weakness of the distal leg muscles is the initial symptom, with onset in the fifth decade. Weakness spreads to involve intrinsic hand and wrist extensor muscles. Late in the course, the proximal limb and trunk muscles become involved. This subvariety of distal myopathy further differs from Welander myopathy because of potentially life-threatening cardiomegaly, congestive heart failure, and intractable tachyarrhythmias resulting from diffuse interstitial fibrosis and

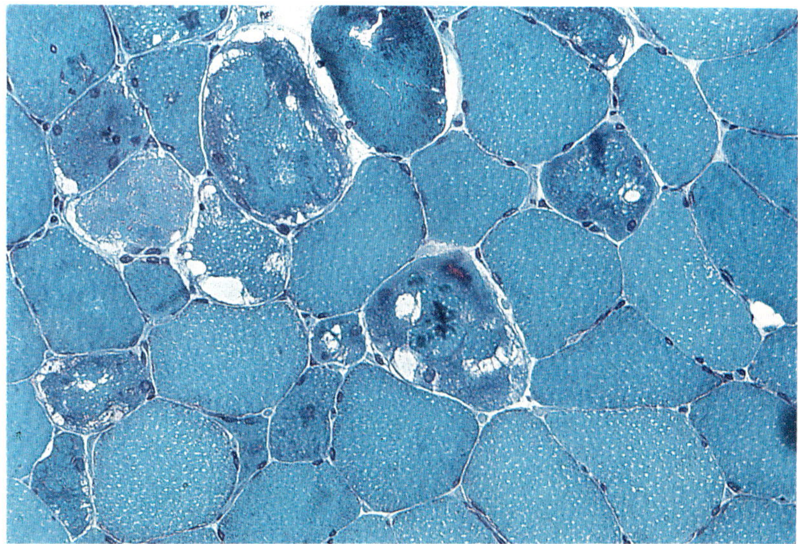

Figure 4–34. Muscle biopsy from dominantly inherited late-onset distal myopathy, illustrating multiple vacuoles in fibers (modified trichrome).

degenerative changes of cardiac muscle.[132] Recently, cases with similar distal weakness and histopathology have been identified in Finland.[208a]

LABORATORY FEATURES

A normal or mildly elevated CK is accompanied by myopathic EMG findings. The muscle biopsy shows a spectrum of changes including variation in fiber size, increased central nuclei, endomysial connective tissue proliferation, and muscle fiber necrosis. In addition, muscle fibers demonstrate single or multiple rimmed vacuoles (Fig. 4–34) with basophilic (H&E) or purplish-red (modified trichrome) granular material, which by electron microscopy shows features typical of autophagia (Fig. 4–35).[131,132]

GENETICS

A French-English background and an unequivocal pattern of autosomal dominant inheritance was documented in the Markesberg late-onset distal myopathy.[131,196] The Finnish cases described by Udd et al.[208a] are also autosomal dominantly inherited.

Early-Adult-Onset Distal Myopathy

There are two distinct forms of distal myopathy that begin in adolescence or early adulthood. One form initially involves the anterior compartment of the legs (type I) and the other, the posterior compartment (type II — Miyoshi) (Table 4–10).

TYPE I

Clinical Features. Weakness usually begins in the anterior compartment and manifests as foot drop. Rarely, it can begin in the hands. Type I disease is relatively benign and only slowly progresses. Spread to proximal muscles can occur late in the course of illness.[118,152,197]

Laboratory Features. The CK level tends to be moderately elevated. Muscle

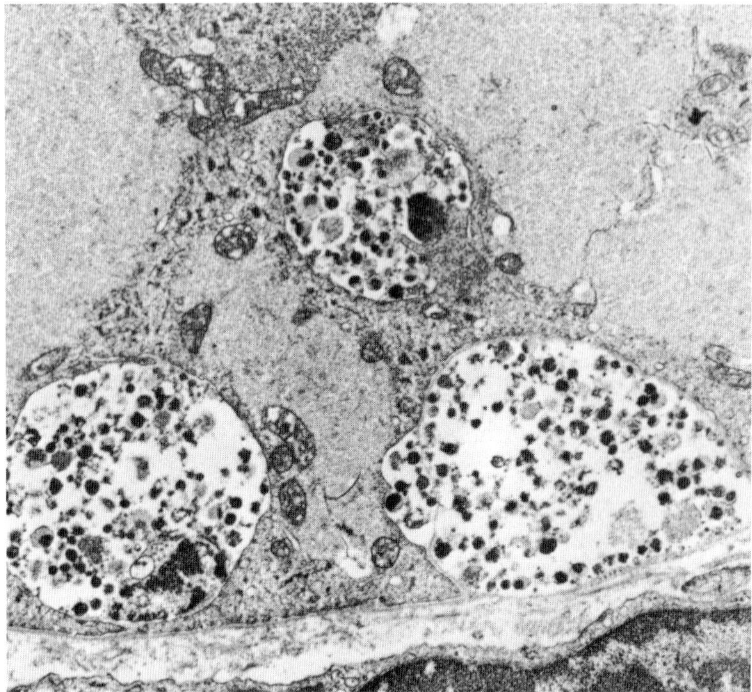

Figure 4–35. Electron micrograph from dominantly inherited late-onset distal myopathy, showing membrane-bound vacuoles containing vesicles and granular cytoplasmic debris. (From Markesbery WR: Pathology of muscular dystrophy and related disorders. Advances in Neurology 17:182, 1977, with permission.)

biopsy reveals a vacuolar myopathy; endomysial connective tissue is only moderately increased.

Genetics. Both autosomal recessive and sporadic cases have been reported. The disorder may be similar, if not identical to, certain cases of hereditary inclusion body myositis (see Chapter 5, pp. 171–176).

TYPE II—MIYOSHI

The myopathy described by Miyoshi[139] is characterized by early weakness and atrophy of the gastrocnemius (Fig. 4–36). Usually there is sparing of the intrinsic muscles of the feet (Fig. 4–37), and symptoms progress to involve the anterior compartment and then more proximal leg muscles. The condition is often progressive and results in severe disability with loss of ambulation.[10,117,131,137]

Laboratory Features. In Miyoshi distal myopathy, CK elevations are in the range of 10 times normal, higher than for other distal myopathies. EMG studies show a myopathic pattern with fibrillations and positive sharp waves and excessively recruited small motor unit potentials. The biopsy is dystrophic without vacuoles.

Genetics. An autosomal recessive pattern has been established for the Miyoshi distal myopathy.[10,139] Sporadic cases have been reported but these could also be examples of autosomal recessive inheritance.[118,137,152] Gene linkage to chromosome 2 has recently been established.[15a]

TREATMENT

No specific forms of treatment benefit patients with either type I or II distal myopathy. Trials of corticosteroids and

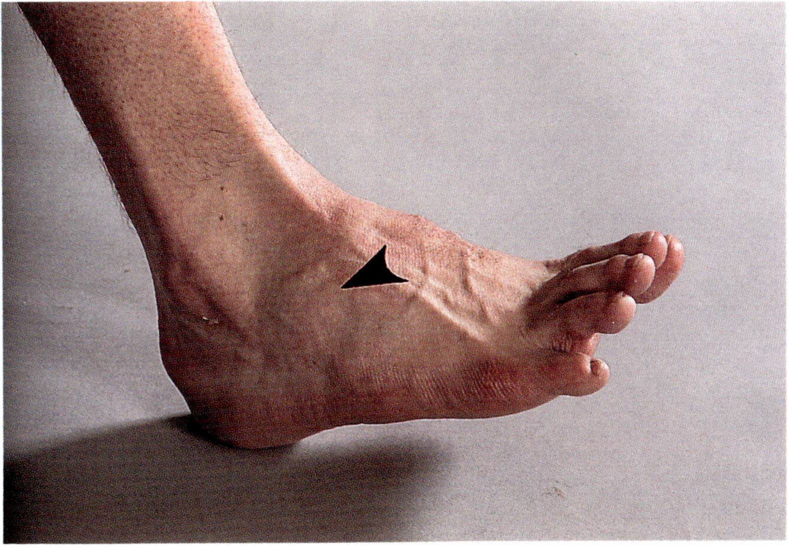

Figure 4–36. Type II early-adult-onset distal myopathy (Miyoshi myopathy). The extensor digitorum brevis muscle (*arrowhead*) is spared.

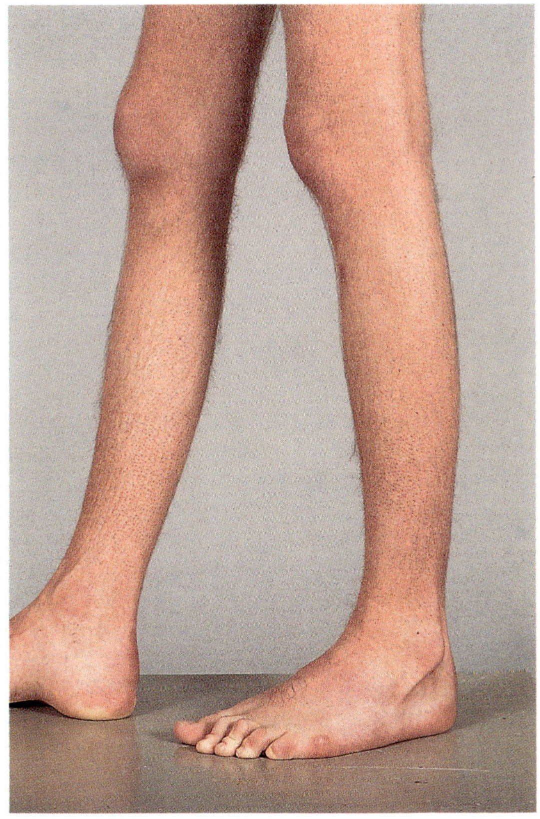

Figure 4–37. Gastrocnemius muscle wasting in type II early-adult-onset distal myopathy.

azathioprine have been unsuccessful in Miyoshi myopathy.[10] Ankle-foot orthoses can be helpful for patients with major leg weakness of the anterior compartment.

SUMMARY

The new term, dystrophin-deficient dystrophies, illustrates the sweeping change in our understanding of Duchenne and Becker muscular dystrophies. The young boy with large calves, proximal muscle weakness, and markedly elevated serum CK as well as a dystrophic-appearing muscle biopsy may have Duchenne, Becker, or an autosomal recessive form of muscular dystrophy. The diagnosis now hinges on the determination of dystrophin, a situation which indicates the rapid integration of molecular genetic advances in this clinical field. The diagnostic information has important implications for prognosis, family planning, and possibly therapeutic intervention in the future. The identification of carriers and prenatal diagnosis of the fetus through analysis of DNA have been important practical benefits from these recent developments.

Similar advances are emerging for myotonic muscular dystrophy, FSH muscular dystrophy, and Emery-Dreifuss muscular dystrophy. Precise localization of the gene is at hand for each of these disorders, although the underlying biochemical defect remains unknown. By contrast, the other major forms of muscular dystrophy are still defined by their clinical features, which permit relatively firm diagnosis of the scapuloperoneal syndromes, oculopharyngeal dystrophy, congenital muscular dystrophy, and the distal myopathies. The remarkable phenotype variation in the dystrophin-related dystrophies suggests that one or more of these clinically distinct disorders will be allelic and represent different disorders of the same gene.

Finally, the limb-girdle muscular dystrophies remain the most ambiguous clinical category. Here, some patients may be identified with an underlying metabolic defect or inflammatory myopathy, whereas others have an autosomal recessive form of muscular dystrophy with uncertain genetic localization. The identification of a treatable disorder that can masquerade as limb-girdle muscular dystrophy, such as carnitine deficiency or inflammatory myopathy, is of paramount importance in evaluating such patients.

REFERENCES

1. Aicardi J, Conti D, and Goutieres F: Aspects cliniques et genetriques des formes precoces de la dystrophie myotonique de Steinert. J Genet Hum (Suppl) 23:146, 1975.
2. André JM, et al: Les amyotrophies scapulo-peroneales. (A propos de deux cas de syndrome de Stark-Kaeser). Ann Med 11:925, 1972.
3. Arahata K and Engel AG: Monoclonal antibody analysis of mononuclear cells in myopathies, I. Quantitation of subsets according to diagnosis and sites of accumulation and demonstration and counts of muscle fibers invaded by T cells. Ann Neurol 16:193, 1984.
3a. Ashizawa T, Anvret M, Baiget M, et al: Characteristics of intergenerational contractions of the CTG repeat in myotonic dystrophy. Am J Hum Genet 54:414, 1994.
4. Aslanidis C, Jansen G, Amemiya C, et al: Cloning of the essential myotonic dystrophy region and mapping of the putative defect. Nature 355:548, 1992.
5. Aver'ianov IuN, Il'ina NA, Vinogradova NV, et al: Rigid spine syndrome. Zhurnal Nevropatologii I Psikhiatrii Imeni 81:1457, 1981.
6. Bacon PA and Smith B: Familial muscular dystrophy of late onset. J Neurol Neurosurg Psychiatry 34:93, 1971.
7. Bakker E, VanBroeckhoven C, Bonten EJ, et al: Germline mosaicism and Duchenne muscular dystrophy mutations. Nature 329:554, 1987.
8. Barbeau A: The syndrome of hereditary late onset ptosis and dysphagia in French Canada. In Kuhn E (ed): Symposium uber Progressive Muskeldystrophie, Myotonie, Myasthenie. Springer-Verlag, Berlin, 1966, p 102.
9. Barbeau A: Oculopharyngeal muscular dystrophy in French Canada. In Burnette JR, and Barbeau A (eds): Progress in Neuro-Ophthalmology. Excerpta Medica, Amsterdam, 1967, p 3.
10. Barohn R, Miller RG, and Griggs RC: Autosomal recessive distal dystrophy. Neurology 41:1365, 1991.
11. Barohn RJ, Levine EJ, Olson JO, and Mendell JR: Gastric hypomotility in Duchenne's muscular dystrophy. N Engl J Med 319:15, 1988.
12. Bartlett RJ, Pericak-Vance MA, Yamaoka L, et al: A new probe for the diagnosis of myotonic muscular dystrophy. Science 235:1648, 1987.
13. Becker PE and Kiener F: Eine neue X-chromosomale muskeldystrophie. Arch Psychiatr Z Neurol 193:427, 1955.

14. Beckman JS, Richard I, Hillaire D, et al: A gene for limb-girdle muscular dystrophy maps to chromosome 15 by linkage. C R Acad Sci III 312:141, 1991.

15. Beggs AH, Koenig M, Boyce FM, and Kunkel LM: Detection of 98% of DMD/BMD gene deletions in PCR. Hum Genet 86:45, 1990.

15a. Bejaoui K, Hirabayashi K, Hentati F, et al: Linkage of Miyoshi myopathy (distal autosomal recessive muscular dystrophy) locus to chromosome 2 p 12–14. Nat Genet, submitted 1994.

16. Ben Hamida M, and Fardeau M: Severe autosomal recessive, limb-girdle muscular dystrophies frequent in Tunisia. In Angelini C, Danieli GA, and Fontanari D (eds): Muscular Dystrophy Research: Advances and New Trends. Excerpta Medica, Amsterdam, 1980, p 143.

17. Berg BO and Conte F: Duchenne muscular dystrophy in a female with a structurally abnormal X-chromosome [abstract]. Neurology 24:356, 1974.

18. Blanchard A, Ohanian V, and Critchley D: The structure and function of alpha-actinin. J Muscle Res Cell Motil 10:280, 1989.

19. Blythe H and Pugh RJ: Muscular dystrophy in childhood: The genetic aspect: A field study in the Leeds region of clinical types and their inheritance. Ann Hum Genet 23:127, 1958.

20. Bobrow M, Walker A, and Walton J: The parental origin of mutations causing Duchenne muscular dystrophy. Arch Neurol 45:85, 1988.

21. Boheimer N, Harris JW, and Ward S: Neuromuscular blockade in dystrophia myotonica with atracurium besylate. Anaesthesia 40:872, 1985.

22. Boswinkel E, Walker A, Hodgson S, et al: Linkage analysis using eight DNA polymorphisms along the length of the X chromosome locates the gene for Emery-Dreyfuss muscular dystrophy to distal Xq. Cytogenet Cell Genet 40:586, 1985.

23. Botstein D, White RL, Skolnick M, and Davis RW: Construction of a genetic linkage map in man using restriction fragment length polymorphisms. Am J Hum Genet 32:314, 1980.

24. Boyd Y, Buckle V, Holt S, Munro E, Hunter D, and Craig I: Muscular dystrophy in girls with X: Autosome translocations. J Med Genet 23:484, 1986.

25. Bradley WG: The limb-girdle syndromes. In Vinken PJ and Bruyn GW (eds): Handbook of Clinical Neurology. North Holland, Amsterdam, 1979, p 433.

26. Bray RJ and Inkster JS: Anaesthesia in babies with congenital dystrophia myotonica. Anaesthesia 39:1007, 1984.

27. Brook JD, McCurrach M, Harley H, et al: Molecular basis of myotonic dystrophy: Expansion of a trinucleotide (CTG) repeat at the 3' end of a transcript encoding a protein kinase family member. Cell 68:799, 1992.

28. Brook JD, Zemelman B, Haddingham K, et al: Radiation reduced hybrids for the myotonic dystrophy locus. Genomics 13:243, 1992.

29. Brooke MH: A Clinician's View of Neuromuscular Diseases. Williams & Wilkins, Baltimore, 1986, p 123.

30. Brooke MH: A Clinician's View of Neuromuscular Diseases. Williams & Wilkins, Baltimore, 1986, p 194.

31. Brooke MH, Fenichel GM, Griggs RC, et al: Duchenne muscular dystrophy: Patterns of clinical progression and effects of supportive therapy. Neurology 39:475, 1989.

32. Brooke MH, Fenichel GM, Griggs RC, et al: Clinical investigation in Duchenne dystrophy. 2. Determination of the "power" of therapeutic trials based on the natural history. Muscle Nerve 6:91, 1983.

33. Brossard J: Etude clinique sur une forme hereditaire d'atrophie musculaire progressive debutant par les membres inferieurs (type femoral avec griffe des orteils). Steinheil, Paris, 1886, p 174.

34. Brunner HG, Korneluk RG, Coerwinkel-Driessen M, et al: Myotonic dystrophy is closely linked to the gene for muscle-type creatine kinase (CKMM). Hum Genet 81:308, 1989.

35. Burghes AHM, Logan C, Hu X, Belfall B, Worton RG, and Ray PN: A cDNA clone from the Duchenne/Becker muscular dystrophy gene. Nature 328:434, 1987.

36. Burrow KL, Coovert DD, Klein CJ, et al: Dystrophin expression and somatic reversion in prednisone-treated and untreated Duchenne dystrophy. Neurology 41:661, 1991.

37. Buxton J, Shelbourne P, Davies J, et al: Detection of an unstable fragment of DNA specific to individuals with myotonic dystrophy. Nature 355:547, 1992.

38. Carpenter S and Karpati G: Pathology of skeletal muscle. Churchill Livingstone, New York, 1984.

39. Cros D, Harnden P, Pouget J, Pellissier JF, Gastaut JL, and Serratrice G: Peripheral neuropathy in myotonic dystrophy: A nerve biopsy study. Ann Neurol 23:470, 1988.

40. Crowe CG: Acute dilatation of stomach as a complication of muscular dystrophy. Br M J 1:1371, 1961.

41. Darras BT and Francke U: A partial deletion of the muscular dystrophy gene transmitted twice by an unaffected male. Nature 329:556, 1987.

42. Davidenkow S: Scapuloperoneal amyotrophy. Arch Neurol Psych 41:694, 1939.

43. Davies KE, Jackson J, Williamson R, et al: Linkage analysis of myotonic dystrophy and sequences on chromosome 19 using a cloned complement 3 gene probe. J Med Genet 20:259, 1983.

44. deMartinville B, Kunkel LM, Bruns G, et al: Localization of DNA sequences in the region Xp21 of the human X chromosome: search for molecular markers close to the Duchenne muscular dystrophy locus. Am J Hum Genet 37:235, 1985.

45. Denny-Brown D: Myopathic weakness of quadriceps. Proc R Soc Med 32:867, 1939.

46. Desmedt JE and Borenstein S: Regeneration in Duchenne muscular dystrophy. Arch Neurol 33:642, 1976.

46a. Dickey RP, Ziter FA, and Smith RA: Emery-Dreifuss muscular dystrophy. J Pediatr 104:555, 1984.

46b. Dubowitz V: Intellectual impairment in muscular dystrophy. Arch Dis Child 40:296, 1965.

47. Dubowitz V: Some unusual neuromuscular disorders. In Walton JN, Canal N, and Scarlato G (eds): International Congress on Muscle Diseases. Excerpta Medica, Amsterdam, 1969, p 568.

48. Dubowitz V: Recent advances in neuromuscular disorders. Rheumatol Phys Med 11:126, 1971.

49. Dubowitz V: Rapidly progressive limb girdle muscular dystrophy in childhood. In Angelini C, Danieli GA, and Fontanari D (eds): Muscular Dystrophy Research: Advances and New Trends. Excerpta Medica, Amsterdam, 1980, p 129.

50. Dubowitz V and Brooke MH: Muscle Biopsy. A Modern Approach. WB Saunders, London, 1973, p 368.

50a. Dubrovsky AL, Mesa L, Marco P, et al: Deflazacort treatment in Duchenne muscular dystrophy. Neurology 41 (Suppl 1):136, 1991.

51. Echenne B, Arthuis M, and Billard C: Congenital muscular dystrophy and cerebral CT scan anomalies. Results of a collaborative study of the Société de Neurologie Infantile. J Neurol Sci 75:7, 1986.

52. Echenne B, Astruc J, Brunel D, Pages M, Baldet P, and Martinazzo G: Congenital muscular dystrophy and rigid spine syndrome. Neuropaediatrics 14:97, 1983.

53. Edstrom L, Thornell LE, and Eriksson A: A new type of hereditary distal myopathy with characteristic sarcoplasmic bodies and intermediate (skeletin) filaments. J Neurol Sci 47:171, 1980.

54. Egger J, Kendall BE, Erdohazi M, Lake BD, Wilson J, and Brett EM: Involvement of the central nervous system in congenital muscular dystrophies. Dev Med Child Neurol 25:32, 1983.

55. Eiberg H, et al: Linkage relationship between the locus for C3 and 50 polymorphic systems: Assignment of C3

to the DM-SE-LU linkage group; confirmation of C3-LES linkage; support of LES-DM synteny. In Proceedings of the Sixth International Congress on Human Genetics. Alan Liss, New York, 1983.

56. Emery AEH: Population frequencies of inherited neuromuscular diseases: A world survey. Neuromuscular Disorders 1:19, 1991.

57. Emery AEH and Dreifuss FE: Unusual type of benign X-linked muscular dystrophy. J Neurol Neurosurg Psychiatry 29:338, 1966.

58. Emery ES, Fenichel GM, and Eng G: A spinal muscular atrophy with scapuloperoneal distribution. Arch Neurol 18:129, 1968.

59. Ervasti JM, Ohlendieck K, Kahl SD, Gaver MG, and Campbell KP: Deficiency of a glycoprotein component of the dystrophin complex in dystrophic muscle. Nature 345:315, 1990.

60. Espir MLE and Matthews WB: Hereditary quadriceps myopathy. J Neurol Neurosurg Psychiatry 36:1041, 1973.

61. Farah MG, Evans EB, and Vignos PJ: Echocardiographic evaluation of left ventricular function in Duchenne's muscular dystrophy. Am J Med 69:248, 1980.

62. Feigenbaum JA and Munsat TL: A neuromuscular syndrome of scapuloperoneal distribution. Bull Los Angeles Neurol Soc 35:47, 1970.

63. Fenichel GM, Florence JM, Pestronk A, et al: Long term benefit from prednisone therapy in Duchenne muscular dystrophy. Neurology 41:1874, 1991.

64. Ferrier P, Bamatter F, and Klein D: Muscular dystrophy (Duchenne) in a girl with Turner's syndrome. J Med Genet 2:38, 1965.

65. Forrest SM, Cross GS, Flint T, Speer A, Robson KJ, and Davies KE: Further studies of gene deletions that cause Duchenne and Becker muscular dystrophies. Genomics 2:109, 1988.

66. Fu YH, Pizzuti A, Fenwick R, et al: An unstable triplet repeat in a gene related to myotonic muscular dystrophy, myotonin protein kinase. Science 255:1256, 1992.

67. Fukuyama Y, Osawa M, and Suzuki H: Congenital progressive muscular dystrophy of the Fukuyama type: Clinical, genetic and pathological considerations. Brain Dev 3:1, 1981.

68. Fukuyama Y, Kawazura M, and Haruna H: A peculiar form of congenital progressive muscular dystrophy. Report of fifteen cases. Paediatr Univ Tokyo 4:5, 1960.

68a. Gilbert JR, Stajich JM, Wall S, et al: Evidence for heterogeneity in facioscapulohumeral muscular dystrophy (FSHD). Am J Hum Genet 53:401, 1993.

69. Gospe SM, Lazaro RP, Lava NS, Grootscholten PM, Scott MO, and Fischbeck KH: Familial X-linked myalgia and cramps: A nonprogressive myopathy associated with a deletion of the dystrophin gene. Neurology 39:1277, 1989.

70. Goto I, Kanazawa Y, Kobayashi T, Murai Y, and Kuroiwa Y: Oculopharyngeal myopathy with distal and cardiomyopathy. J Neurol Neurosurg Psychiatry 40:600, 1977.

71. Gottdiener JS, Hawley RJ, Gay JA, DiBianco R, Fletcher RD, and Engel WK: Left ventricular relaxation, mitral valve prolapse, and intracardiac conduction in myotonia atrophica: assessment by digitized echocardiography and noninvasive His bundle recording. Am Heart J 104:77, 1982.

72. Griggs RC, Davis RJ, Anderson DC, and Dove JT: Cardiac conduction in myotonic dystrophy. Am J Med 59:37, 1975.

73. Griggs RC, Kingston W, Herr BE, Forbes G, and Moxley RT: Myotonic dystrophy: Effect of testosterone on total body potassium and on creatinine excretion. Neurology 35:1035, 1985.

74. Griggs RC, Mendell JR, Brooke MH, et al: Clinical investigation in Duchenne dystrophy, V. Use of creatine kinase and pyruvate kinase in carrier detection. Muscle Nerve 8:60, 1985.

75. Griggs RC, Moxley RT, Mendell JR, et al: Randomized, double-blind trial of

mazindol in Duchenne dystrophy. Muscle Nerve 13:1169, 1990.

76. Griggs RC, Moxley RT, Mendell JR, et al: Prednisone in Duchenne dystrophy: A randomized, controlled trial defining the time course and dose response. Arch Neurol 48:383, 1991.

77. Griggs RC, Reeves W, and Moxley RT: The heart in Duchenne dystrophy. In Rowland, LP (ed): Pathogenesis of Human Muscular Dystrophies. Excerpta Medica, Amsterdam, 1977, p 661.

77a. Griggs RC, Tawil R, Storvick D, Mendell JR, and Altherr MR: Genetics of facioscapulohumeral muscular dystrophy: New mutations in sporadic cases. Neurology 43:2369, 1993.

77b. Gussoni E, Paulath G, Lanctot AM, et al: Normal dystrophin transcripts detected in Duchenne muscular dystrophy patients after myoblast implantation. Nature 356:435, 1992.

78. Haldane JBS: The rate of spontaneous mutation of a human gene. J Genet 321:317, 1935.

79. Hall JG: Genomic imprinting and its clinical implications. N Engl J Med 326:827, 1992.

80. Hamel-Roy J, Devroede G, Arhan P, Tetreault JP, and Lemieux B: Functional abnormalities of the anal sphincters in patients with myotonic dystrophy. Gastroenterology 86:1469, 1984.

81. Hansotia P and Frens D: Hypersomnia associated with alveolar hypoventilation in myotonic dystrophy. Neurology 31:1336, 1981.

82. Harley HG, Brook JD, Rundle SA, et al: Expansion of an unstable DNA region and phenotypic variation in myotonic dystrophy. Nature 355:545, 1992.

83. Harper P, Penny R, Foley TP Jr, Migeon CJ, and Blizzard RM: Gonadal function in males with myotonic dystrophy. J Clin Endocrinol Metab 35:852, 1972.

84. Harper PS: Congenital myotonic dystrophy in Britain. II. Genetic basis. Arch Dis Child 50:514, 1975.

85. Hartwig GB, Rao KR, Radoff FM, Coleman RE, Jones RH, and Roses AD: Radionuclide angiocardiographic analysis of myocardial function in myotonic muscular dystrophy. Neurology 33:657, 1983.

86. Hayasaka S, Kiyosawa M, Katsumata S, Honda M, Takase S, and Mizuno K: Ciliary and retinal changes in myotonic dystrophy. Arch Ophthalmol 102:88, 1984.

87. Hemmings L, Kuhlman PA, Critchley DR: Analysis of the actin-binding domain of α-actinin by mutagenesis and demonstration that dystrophin contains a functionally homologous domain. J Cell Biol 116:1369, 1992.

88. Hoffman EP, Brown RH, and Kunkel LM: Dystrophin: The protein product of the Duchenne muscular dystrophy locus. Cell 51:919, 1987.

89. Hoffman EP, Fischbeck KH, Brown RH, et al: Characterization of dystrophin in muscle-biopsy specimens from patients with Duchenne's or Becker's muscular dystrophy. N Engl J Med 318:1363, 1988.

90. Hoffman EP, Kunkel LM, Angelini C, Clarke A, Johnson M, and Harris JB: Improved diagnosis of Becker muscular dystrophy by dystrophin testing. Neurology 39:1011, 1989.

91. Hopkins LC, Jackson JA, and Elsas LJ: Emery-Dreifuss humeroperoneal muscular dystrophy: An X-linked myopathy with unusual contractures and bradycardia. Ann Neurol 10:230, 1981.

92. Horowitz M, Maddox A, Maddern GJ, Wishart J, Collins PJ, and Shearman DJ: Gastric and esophageal emptying in dystrophia myotonica: Effect of metoclopramide. Gastroenterology 92:570, 1987.

93. Hu X, Burghes AH, Ray PN, Thompson MW, Murphy EG, and Worton RG: Partial gene duplication in Duchenne and Becker muscular dystrophies. J Med Genet 25:369, 1988.

94. Huhn VA: Über distale myopathien, insbesondere die myopathia distalis tarda (hereditaria). Fortschr Neurol Psychiatr 34:589, 1966.

95. Hyser CL, Kissel JT, Warmolts JR, and Mendell JR: Scapuloperoneal

neuropathy: A distinct clinicopathologic entity. J Neurol Sci 87:91, 1988.

96. Ionasescu V and Zellweger H: Duchenne muscular dystrophy in young girls? Acta Neurol Scand 50:619, 1974.

97. Jackson CE and Strehler DA: Limb-girdle muscular dystrophy: Clinical manifestations and detection of preclinical disease. Pediatrics 41:495, 1968.

98. Jamal GA, Weir AI, Hansen S, and Ballantyne JP: Myotonic dystrophy: A reassessment by conventional and more recently introduced neurophysiological techniques. Brain 109:1279, 1986.

99. Jansen G, Mahadevan M, Amemiya C, et al: Characterization of the myotonic dystrophy region predicts multiple protein isoform-encoding mRNAs. Nature Genetics 1:261, 1992.

100. Johnson K, Shelbourne P, Davies J, et al: A new polymorphic probe which defines the region of chromosome 19 containing the myotonic dystrophy locus. Am J Hum Genet 46:1073, 1990.

101. Kaeser HE: Die familiare scapuloperoneale muskelatrophie. Dtsch Z. Nervenheilk 186:379, 1964.

102. Kaeser HE: Scapuloperoneal muscular atrophy. Brain 88:407, 1965.

103. Kaeser HE: Scapulo-peroneal syndrome. In Vinken PJ and Bruyn GW (eds): Handbook of Clinical Neurology. North-Holland, Amsterdam, New York, Oxford, 1975, p 57.

104. Kao L, Krstenansky J, Mendell J, Rammohan KW, and Gruenstein E: Immunological identification of a high molecular weight protein as a candidate for the product of the Duchenne muscular dystrophy gene. Proc Nat Acad Sci USA 85:4491, 1988.

104a. Karpati G, Ajdukovic D, Arnold D, et al: Myoblast transfer in Duchenne muscular dystrophy. Ann Neurol 34:8, 1993.

105. Karpati G, et al: Implantation of non-dystrophic allogeneic myoblasts into dystrophic muscles of mdx mice produces "mosaic" fibers of normal microscopic phenotype. In Kedes LH and Stockdale FE (eds): Cellular and Molecular Biology of Muscle Development. Alan Liss, New York, 1989, p 973.

106. Karpati G and Watters GV: Adverse anaesthetic reactions in Duchenne dystrophy. In Angelini C, Danielli GA, and Fontanari D (eds): Muscular Dystrophy Research: Advances and New Trends. Excerpta Medica, Amsterdam, 1980, p 206.

107. Kazakov VM, Bogorodinsky DK, and Skorometz AA: Myogenic scapuloperoneal syndrome-muscular dystrophy in the K. kindred: Reexamination of the K. family described for the first time by Oransky in 1927. Eur Neurol 13:350, 1975.

108. Ketenjian AY: Scapulocostal stabilization for scapular winging in facioscapulohumeral muscular dystrophy. J Bone Joint Surg 60A:476, 1978.

109. Kiloh LG and Nevin S: Progressive dystrophy of the external ocular muscles (ocular myopathy). Brain 74:9, 1951.

110. Kingston HM, Sarfarazi M, Thomas NS, and Harper PS: Localisation of the Becker muscular dystrophy gene on the short arm of the X chromosome by linkage to cloned DNA sequences. Hum Genet 67:6, 1984.

111. Kissel JT, Burrow KL, Rammohan KW, Mendell JR, and CIDD Study Group: Mononuclear cell analysis of muscle biopsies in prednisone-treated and untreated Duchenne muscular dystrophy. Neurology 41:667, 1991.

112. Kloepfer HW and Emery AEH: Genetic aspects of neuromuscular disease. In Walton JN (ed): Disorders of Voluntary Muscle. J. & A. Churchill LTD, London, 1969.

113. Kloepfer HW and Talley C: Autosomal recessive inheritance of Duchenne-type muscular dystrophy. Acta Genet 7:314, 1957.

114. Koenig M, Beggs AH, Moyer M, et al: The molecular basis for Duchenne versus Becker muscular dystrophy:

Correlation of severity with type of deletion. Am J Hum Genet 45:498, 1989.

115. Koenig M, Hoffman EP, Bertelson CJ, Monaco AP, Feener C, and Kunkel LM: Complete cloning of the Duchenne muscular dystrophy (DMD) cDNA and preliminary genomic organization of the DMD gene in normal and affected individuals. Cell 50:509, 1987.

116. Korneluk RG, MacLeod HL, McKeithan TW, Brooks JD, and MacKenzie AE: A chromosome 19 clone from a translocation breakpoint shows close linkage and linkage disequilibrium with myotonic dystrophy. Genomics 4:146, 1989.

117. Kuhn E and Schroder JM: A new type of distal myopathy in two brothers. J Neurol 226:181, 1981.

118. Kumamoto T, Fukuhara N, Nagashima M, Kanda T, and Wakabayashi M: Distal myopathy: Histochemical and ultrastructural studies. Arch Neurol 39:367, 1982.

119. Kunkel LM, Hejtmancik JF, Caskey CTH, et al: Analysis of deletions in DNA from patients with Becker and Duchenne muscular dystrophy. Nature 322:73, 1986.

120. Kunkel LM, Monaco AP, Middlesworth W, Ochs HD, and Latt SA: Specific cloning of DNA fragments absent from the DNA of a male patient with an X chromosome deletion. Proc Natl Acad Sci USA 82:4778, 1985.

121. Lazaro RP, Fenichel GM, and Kilroy AW: Congenital muscular dystrophy: Case reports and reappraisal. Muscle Nerve 2:349, 1979.

122. Leibowitz D and Dubowitz V: Intellect and behaviour in Duchenne muscular dystrophy. Dev Med Child Neurol 23:577, 1981.

123. Leon SH, Schuffler MD, Kettler M, and Rohrmann CA: Chronic intestinal pseudoobstruction as a complication of Duchenne's muscular dystrophy. Gastroenterology 90:455, 1986.

124. Letournel E, Fardeau M, Lytle JO, Serrault M, and Gosselin RA: Scapulothoracic arthrodesis for patients who have fascioscapulohumeral muscular dystrophy. J Bone Joint Surg 72:78, 1990.

125. Lindenbaum RH, Clarke G, Patel C, and Moncrieff M: Muscular dystrophy in an X;1 translocation female suggests that Duchenne locus is on X chromosome short arm. J Med Genet 16:389, 1979.

126. Lovelace RE and Menken M: The scapulo-peroneal syndrome: Dystrophic type. Excerpta Med Int Cong Series 193:247, 1969.

127. Luque ER: Segmental correction of scoliosis with rigid internal fixation: Preliminary report in orthopaedic transactions. J Bone Joint Surg 2:136, 1977.

128. Mahadevan M, Tsilfidis C, Sabourin L, et al: Myotonic dystrophy mutation: An unstable CTG repeat in the 3' untranslated region of the gene. Science 245:1253, 1992.

129. Malholtra SB, Hart KA, Klamut HJ, et al: Frame-shift deletions in patients with Duchenne and Becker muscular dystrophy. Science 242:755, 1988.

130. Manschot WA and De Bruijn WC: Coats's disease: Definition and pathogenesis. Br J Ophthalmol 51:145, 1967.

131. Markesbery WR, Griggs RC, and Herr B: Distal myopathy: Electron microscopic and histochemical studies. Neurology 27:727, 1977.

132. Markesbery WR, Griggs RC, Leach RP, and Lapham LW: Late onset hereditary distal myopathy. Neurology 24:127, 1974.

133. Marshall J: Observations on endocrine function in dystrophia myotonica. Brain 82:221, 1959.

133a. Mathieu J, De Braekeleer M, and Prévost C: Genealogical reconstruction of myotonic dystrophy in the Saguenay–Lac Saint Jean area (Quebec, Canada). Neurology 40:839, 1990.

133b. Matsumura K, Tomé FMS, Collin H, et al: Deficiency of the 50 k dystrophin-associated glycoprotein in severe childhood autosomal recessive muscular dystrophy. Nature 359:320, 1992.

134. McMenamin JB, Becker LE, and Murphy EG: Congenital muscular dystrophy: A clinicopathologic report of 24 cases. J Pediatr 100:692, 1982.

135. Mendell JR, Iannaccone ST, Burrow KW, et al: Dystrophin analysis in congenital muscular dystrophy. Ann Neurol 28:170, 1990.

135a. Mendell JR, Kissel JT, Stevens R, et al: Prospective, controlled trial of six monthly myoblast transfers in Duchenne dystrophy [abstract]. Neurology 44:A268, 1994.

136. Mendell JR, Moxley RT, Griggs RC, et al: Randomized, double-blind six-month trial of prednisone in Duchenne's muscular dystrophy. N Engl J Med 320:1592, 1989.

137. Miller RG, Blank NK, and Layzer RB: Sporadic distal myopathy with early adult onset. Ann Neurol 5:220, 1979.

138. Miller RG, Layzer RB, Mellenthin MA, Golabi M, Francoz RA, and Mall JC: Emery-Dreifuss muscular dystrophy with autosomal dominant transmission. Neurology 35:1230, 1985.

139. Miyoshi K, Iwasa M, Kawa H, et al: Autosomal recessive distal muscular dystrophy: A new type of distal muscular dystrophy observed characteristically in Japan. Nippon Rinsho 35:3922, 1977.

140. Mohr J: A Study of Linkage in Man. Munskgaard, Copenhagen, 1954.

141. Mokri B and Engel AG: Duchenne dystrophy: Electron microscopic findings pointing to a basic or early abnormality in the plasma membrane of the muscle fiber. Neurology 25:1111, 1975.

142. Monaco AP, Neve RL, Colletti-Feener C, Bertelson CJ, Kurnit DM, and Kunkel LM: Isolation of candidate cDNAs for portions of the Duchenne muscular dystrophy gene. Nature 323:646, 1986.

143. Monckton G, Hoskin V, and Warren S: Prevalence and incidence of muscular dystrophy in Alberta, Canada. Clin Genet 21:19, 1982.

144. Moser H, Wiesmann U, Richterich R, and Rossi E: Progressive muscle dystrophy, VIII. Occurrence, clinical aspects and genetics of types I and II. Schweiz Med Wochenschr 96:169, 1966.

145. Motta J, Guilleminault C, Billingham M, Barry W, and Mason J: Cardiac abnormalities in myotonic dystrophy: Electrophysiologic and histopathologic studies. Am J Med 67:467, 1979.

146. Moxley RT, Griggs RC, and Goldblatt D: Decreased insulin sensitivity of forearm muscle in myotonic dystrophy. J Clin Invest 62:857, 1978.

147. Moxley RT, Lorenson M, Griggs RC, et al: Decreased breakdown of muscle protein after prednisone therapy in Duchenne dystrophy. J Neurol Sci (Suppl) 98:419, 1990.

147a. Moxley RT, Ricker K, Koch M, Heine R, and Lehmann-Horn F: Families with "myotonic dystrophy" showing no CTG repeat expansion of the myotonic dystrophy allele [abstract]. Neurology 44(Suppl):A268, 1994.

148. Munsat TL, Piper D, Cancilla P, and Mednick J: Inflammatory myopathy with facioscapulohumeral distribution. Neurology 22:335, 1972.

149. Murray JM, Davies KE, Harper PS, Meredith L, Mueller CR, and Williamson R: Linkage relationship of a cloned DNA sequence on the short arm of the X chromosome to Duchenne muscular dystrophy. Nature 300:69, 1982.

150. Mussini JM, Gray F, Hauw JJ, Piette AM, and Prost A: Rigid spine syndrome: histological examinations of male and female cases. Acta Neuropathol (Berl) (Suppl 7):331, 1981.

151. Nakahara K, Higa S, Nishihira T, et al: A new type of hereditary motor sensory neuropathy in Okinawa Island: Clinical and pathological study [abstract]. Muscle Nerve 9(Suppl):126, 1986.

152. Nonaka I, Sunohara N, Ishiura S, and Satoyoshi E: Familial distal myopathy with rimmed vacuole and lamellar (myeloid) body formation. J Neurol Sci 51:141, 1981.

153. Nowak TV, Anuras S, Brown BP, Ionasescu V, and Green JB: Small intestine motility in myotonic dystrophy

patients. Gastroenterology 86:808, 1984.

154. O'Brien T, Ball S, Sarfarazi M, Harper PS, and Robson EB: Genetic linkage between the loci for myotonic dystrophy and peptidase D. Ann Hum Genet 47:117, 1983.

155. Oransky W: Uber einen hereditaren typus progressiver muskeldystrophie. Deutsch Z Nervenheilk 99:147, 1927.

156. Padberg G: Facioscapulohumeral disease. Doctoral thesis, University of Leiden, Intercontinental Graphics, 1982.

157. Panayiotopoulos CP and Scarpalezos S: Dystrophia myotonica: Peripheral nerve involvement and pathogenetic implications. J Neurol Sci 27:1, 1976.

158. Partridge TA, Morgan JE, Coulton GR, Hoffman EP, and Kunkel LM: Conversion of mdx myofibres from dystrophin-negative to -positive by injection of normal myoblasts. Nature 337:176, 1989.

159. Pericak-Vance MA, Yamaoka LH, Assinder RIF, et al: Tight linkage of apolipoprotein C2 to myotonic dystrophy on chromosome 19. Neurology 36:1418, 1986.

160. Pollock M and Dyck PJ: Peripheral nerve morphometry in myotonic dystrophy. Arch Neurol 33:33, 1976.

161. Portwood MM, Wicks JJ, Lieberman JS, and Duveneck MJ: Intellectual and cognitive function in adults with myotonic muscular dystrophy. Arch Phys Med Rehabil 67:299, 1986.

162. Portwood MM, Wicks JJ, Lieberman JS, and Fowler WM: Psychometric evaluation in myotonic muscular dystrophy. Arch Phys Med Rehabil 65:533, 1984.

162a. Poustka A, Dietrich A, Langenstein G, Toniolo D, Warren ST, and Lehrach H: Physical map of human Xq27-qter: Localizing the region of the fragile X mutation. Proc Natl Acad Sci USA 88:8302, 1991.

163. Prior TW, Friedman KJ, Highsmith WE, Perry TR, and Silverman LM: Molecular probe protocol for determining carrier status in Duchenne and Becker muscular dystrophies. Clin Chem 36:441, 1990.

163a. Prior TW, Papp AC, Snyder PJ, et al: Identification of new mutations in the dystrophin gene. Am J Hum Genet 53:1217, 1993.

164. Ptacek LJ, Johnson KJ, and Griggs RC: Mechanisms of disease: Genetics of the myotonic muscle disorders. N Engl J Med 328:482, 1993.

165. Ray PN, Belfall B, Duff C, et al: Cloning of the breakpoint of an X;21 translocation associated with Duchenne muscular dystrophy. Nature 318:672, 1985.

166. Reeves WC, Griggs R, Nanda NC, Thomson K, and Gramiak R: Echocardiographic evaluation of cardiac abnormalities in Duchenne's dystrophy and myotonic muscular dystrophy. Arch Neurol 37:273, 1980.

167. Ricker K and Mertens HG: The differential diagnosis of the myogenic (facio)-scapulo-peroneal syndrome. Eur Neurol 1:275, 1968.

168. Ricker K, Mertens HG, and Schimrigk K: The neurogenic scapulo-peroneal syndrome. Eur Neurol 1:257, 1968.

169. Riggs JE, Rubenstein MN, and Gutmann L: Myotonic dystrophy and normal-pressure hydrocephalus. Neurology 35:1535, 1985.

170. Ringel SP, Carroll JE, and Schold SC: The spectrum of mild X-linked recessive muscular dystrophy. Arch Neurol 34:408, 1977.

171. Ronen GM, Lowry N, Wedge JH, Sarnat HB, and Hill A: Hereditary motor sensory neuropathy type I presenting as scapuloperoneal atrophy (Davidenkow syndrome), electrophysiological and pathological studies. Can J Neurol Sci 13:264, 1986.

172. Roses AD: Mutants in Duchenne muscular dystrophy: Implications for prevention. Arch Neurol 45:84, 1988.

173. Rosman NP and Kakulas BA: Mental deficiency associated with muscular dystrophy: A neuropathological study. Brain 89:769, 1966.

174. Rotthauwe HW, Mortier W, and Beyer H: New type of recessive X-linked

muscular dystrophy: Scapulo-humeral-distal muscular dystrophy with early contractures and cardiac arrhythmias. Humangenetik 16:181, 1972.

175. Rowland LP, Fetell M, Olarte M, Hays A, Singh N, and Wanat FE: Emery-Dreifuss muscular dystrophy. Ann Neurol 5:111, 1979.

176. Santavuori P, Leisti J, and Kruss S: Muscle, eye and brain disease: A new syndrome. Neuropaediatrie 8:550, 1977.

177. Sanyal SK and Johnson WW: Cardiac conduction abnormalities in children with Duchenne's progressive muscular dystrophy: Electrocardiographic features and morphologic correlates. Circulation 66:853, 1982.

178. Sarnat HB, O'Connor T, and Byrne PA: Clinical effects of myotonic dystrophy on pregnancy and the neonate. Arch Neurol 33:459, 1976.

179. Satoyoshi E and Kinoshita M: Oculopharyngodistal myopathy. Arch Neurol 34:89, 1977.

180. Schneiderman LJ, Sampson WI, Schoene WC, and Haydon GB: Genetic studies of a family with two unusual autosomal dominant conditions: Muscular dystrophy and Pelger-Huet anomaly. Am J Med 46:380, 1969.

181. Schotland DL and Rowland LP: Muscular dystrophy: Features of ocular myopathy, distal myopathy, and myotonic dystrophy. Arch Neurol 10:433, 1964.

182. Schwartz MS and Swash M: Scapuloperoneal atrophy with sensory involvement: Davidenkow's syndrome. J Neurol Neurosurg Psychiatry 38:1063, 1975.

183. Seay AR, Ziter FA, and Petajan JH: Rigid spine syndrome: A type I fiber myopathy. Arch Neurol 34:119, 1977.

184. Serratrice G, Cros D, Pellissier JF, Gastaut JL, and Pouget J: Dystrophie musculaire congénitale. Rev Neurol (Paris) 136:445, 1980.

185. Serratrice G, et al: Scapuloperoneal myopathies, myelopathies, and neuropathies. In Serratrice G and Roux H (eds): Peroneal atrophies and related disorders. Masson, New York, 1979, p 233.

185a. Sewry CA, Sansome A, Matsumura K, et al: Deficiency of the 50 KDA dystrophin-associated glycoprotein and abnormal expression of utrophin in two South Asian cousins with variable expression of severe childhood autosomal recessive muscular dystrophy. Neuromuscul Disord 4:1, 1993.

186. Shaw DJ, Meredith AL, Sarfarazi M, et al: The apolipoprotein CII gene: subchromosomal localization and linkage to the myotonic dystrophy locus. Hum Genet 70:271, 1985.

187. Shields RW: Limb girdle syndromes. In Engel AG and Banker BQ (eds): Myology. McGraw-Hill, New York, 1986, p 1349.

188. Shore RN: Myotonic dystrophy: Hazards of pregnancy and infancy. Dev Med Child Neurol 17:356, 1975.

189. Siegel IM: Spinal stabilization in Duchenne muscular dystrophy: Rationale and method. Muscle Nerve 5:417, 1982.

190. Small RG: Coats' disease and muscular dystrophy. Trans Am Acad Ophthalmol Otolaryngol 72:225, 1968.

191. Speer MC, Yamaoka LH, Gilchrist JH, et al: Confirmation of genetic heterogeneity in limb-girdle muscular dystrophy: Linkage of an autosomal dominant form to chromosome 5q. Am J Hum Genet 50:1211, 1992.

192. Steinert H: Myopathologische beiträge. I. Über das klinische und anatomische bild des muskelschwunds der myotoniker. Dtsch Ztschrf Nervenh 37:58, 1909.

193. Stern LM: Four cases of Duchenne-type muscular dystrophy in girls. Med J Aust 2:1066, 1972.

194. Stevenson WG, Perloff JK, Weiss JN, and Anderson TL: Facioscapulohumeral muscular dystrophy: Evidence for selective, genetic electrophysiologic cardiac involvement. J Am Coll Cardiol 15:292, 1990.

195. Streib EW and Sun SF: Distribution of electrical myotonia in myotonic

muscular dystrophy. Ann Neurol 14:80, 1983.

196. Sumner D, Crawfurd MD'A, and Harriman DGF: Distal muscular dystrophy in an English family. Brain 94:51, 1971.

197. Sunohara N, Nonaka I, Kamei N, and Satoyoshi E: Distal myopathy with rimmed vacuole formation. A follow-up study. Brain 112:65, 1989.

198. Tawil R, Storvick D, Weiffenbach B, Altherr MR, Feasby TE, and Griggs RC: Chromosome 4q DNA rearrangements in monozygotic twins discordant for facioscapulohumeral muscular dystrophy. Hum Muta 2:492, 1993.

199. Taylor DA, Carroll JE, Smith ME, Johnson MO, Johnston GP, and Brooke MH: Facioscapulohumeral dystrophy associated with hearing loss and Coats syndrome. Ann Neurol 12:395, 1982.

200. Taylor EW: Progressive vagus-glossopharyngeal paralysis with ptosis. A contribution to the group of family diseases. J Nerv Ment Dis 42:129, 1915.

201. Thomas NST, Williams H, Elsas LJ, Hopkins LC, Sarfarazi M, and Harper PS: Localisation of the gene for Emery-Dreifuss muscular dystrophy to the distal long arm of the X chromosome. J Med Genet 23:596, 1986.

202. Thomas PK, Calne DB, and Elliott CF: X-linked scapuloperoneal syndrome. J Neurol Neurosurg Psychiatry 35:208, 1972.

203. Thomas PK, Schott GD, and Morgan-Hughes JA: Adult onset scapuloperoneal myopathy. J Neurol Neurosurg Psychiatry 38:1008, 1975.

203a. Thornton CA, Griggs RC, and Moxley RT: Myotonic dystrophy with no trinucleotide repeat expansion. Ann Neurol 35:269, 1994.

204. Thyagarajan D, Byrne E, Noer S, et al: Mitochondrial DNA sequence analysis in congenital myotonic dystrophy. Ann Neurol 30:724, 1991.

205. Tomé FMS and Fardeau M: Nuclear inclusions in oculopharyngeal dystrophy. Acta Neuropathol 49:85, 1980.

206. Towfighi J, Sassani JW, Suzuki K, and Ladda RL: Cerebro-ocular dysplasia: Muscular dystrophy (COD-MD) syndrome. Acta Neuropathol (Berl) 65:110, 1984.

207. Turner JWA and Lees F: Congenital myopathy: A fifty-year follow-up. Brain 85:733, 1962.

208. Tyler FH and Stephens FE: Studies in disorders of muscles. II. Clinical manifestations and inheritance of facioscapulohumeral dystrophy in a large family. Ann Intern Med 32:640, 1950.

208a. Udd B, Partanen J, Halonen P, et al: Tibial muscular dystrophy: Late adult-onset distal myopathy in 66 Finnish patients. Arch Neurol 50:604, 1993.

209. Victor M, Hayes R, and Adams RD: Oculopharyngeal muscular dystrophy: A familial disease of late life characterized by dysphagia and progressive ptosis of the eyelids. N Engl J Med 267:1267, 1962.

210. Walker AE: Lissencephaly. Arch Neurol Psychol 48:13, 1942.

211. Walton JN: Clinical examination of the neuromuscular system. In Walton JN (ed): Disorders of Voluntary Muscle. Churchill Livingstone, New York, 1981, p 448.

212. Walton JN: Two cases of myopathy limited to the quadriceps. J Neurol Neurosurg Psychiatry 19:106, 1956.

213. Walton JN and Nattrass FJ: On the classification, natural history and treatment of the myopathies. Brain 77:12, 1954.

214. Warburg M: Hydrocephaly, congenital retinal nonattachment, and congenital falciform fold. Am J Ophthalmol 85:88, 1978.

215. Waters DD, Nutter DO, Hopkins LC, and Dorney ER: Cardiac features of an unusual X-linked humeroperoneal neuromuscular disease. N Eng J Med 293:1017, 1975.

216. Weiffenbach B, Bagley R, Falls K, et al: Linkage analyses of five chromosome 4 markers localizes the facioscapulohumeral muscular dystrophy (FSHD) gene to distal 4q35. Am J Hum Genet 51:416, 1992.

217. Welander L: Homozygous appearance of distal myopathy. Acta Genet 7:321, 1957.

218. Welander L: Myopathia distalis tarda hereditaria. Acta Medica Scand (Suppl 265) 141:1, 1951.

219. Whitehead AS, Solomon E, Chambers S, Bodmer WF, Povey S, and Fey G: Assignment of the structural gene for the third component of human complement to chromosome 19. Proc Natl Acad Sci USA 79:5021, 1982.

220. Wijmenga C, Frants RR, Brouwer OF, Moerer P, Weber JL, and Padberg GW: Location of facioscapulohumeral muscular dystrophy gene on chromosome 4. Lancet 336:651, 1990.

221. Wijmenga C, Hewitt JE, Sandkuijl LA, et al: Chromosome 4q DNA rearrangements associated with facioscapulohumeral muscular dystrophy. Nat Genet 2:26, 1992.

222. Wijmenga C, Padberg GW, Moerer P, et al: Mapping of facioscapulohumeral muscular dystrophy gene to chromosome 4q35-qter by multipoint linkage analysis and in situ hybridization. Genomics 9:570, 1991.

223. Wijngaarden GK, Hagen CJ, Bethlem J, and Meijer AE: Myopathy of the quadriceps muscles. J Neurol Sci 7:201, 1968.

223a. Winokur ST, Bengtsson U, Feddersen J, et al: The DNA rearrangement associated with facioscapulohumeral muscular dystrophy involves a heterochromatin-associated repetitive element: Implications for a role of chromatin structure in the pathogenesis of the disease. Chromosome Research, in press, 1994.

224. Wolff JA, Malone RW, Williams P, et al: Direct gene transfer into mouse muscle in vivo. Science 247:1465, 1990.

225. Worton RG and Thompson MW: Genetics of Duchenne muscular dystrophy. Annu Rev Genet 22:601, 1988.

226. Wulff JD, Lin JT, and Kepes JJ: Inflammatory facioscapulohumeral muscular dystrophy and Coats syndrome. Ann Neurol 12:398, 1982.

227. Yamaoka LH, Pericak-Vance MA, Speer MC, et al: Tight linkage of creatine kinase (CKMM) to myotonic dystrophy on chromosome 19. Neurology 40:222, 1990.

228. Yates JRW, Affara NA, Jamieson DM, et al: Emery-Dreifuss muscular dystrophy: Localisation to Xq27.3→qter confirmed by linkage to the factor VIII gene. J Med Genet 23:587, 1986.

229. Yoshioka M, Okuno T, Honda Y, and Nakano Y: Central nervous system involvement in progressive muscular dystrophy. Arch Dis Child 55:589, 1980.

230. Young RSK, Gang DL, Zalneraitis EL, and Krishnamoorthy KS: Dysmaturation in infants of mothers with myotonic dystrophy. Arch Neurol 38:716, 1981.

231. Zatz J, Betti RTB, and Levy JA: Benign Duchenne muscular dystrophy in a patient with growth hormone deficiency. Am J Med Genet 10:301, 1981.

232. Zatz J and Betti RTB: Benign Duchenne muscular dystrophy in a patient with growth hormone deficiency: A five year follow-up. Am J Med Genet 24:567, 1986.

233. Zatz M, Betti RTB, and Frota-Pessoa O: Treatment of Duchenne muscular dystrophy with growth hormone inhibitors. Am J Med Genet 24:549, 1986.

234. Zubrzycka-Gaarn EE, Bulman DE, Karpati G, et al: The Duchenne muscular dystrophy gene product is localized in sarcolemma of human skeletal muscle. Nature 333:466, 1988.

235. Zundel WS and Tyler FH: The muscular dystrophies. N Engl J Med 273:537, 1965.

Chapter 5

INFLAMMATORY MYOPATHIES

DERMATOMYOSITIS
POLYMYOSITIS
INCLUSION BODY MYOSITIS
MYOPATHIES ASSOCIATED WITH
  OTHER CONNECTIVE-TISSUE
  DISEASES
GIANT-CELL AND
  GRANULOMATOUS MYOSITIS
EOSINOPHILIC SYNDROMES AND
  MYOSITIS
MYOSITIS AND MYOPATHIES
  CAUSED BY INFECTIOUS AGENTS
GRAFT VERSUS HOST DISEASE

The term "inflammatory myopathy" denotes muscle diseases in which inflammatory cells are a conspicuous histopathologic feature. For most inflammatory myopathies, although etiology remains uncertain, clinical, histologic, electromyographic, and serologic criteria now permit definition and clinical classification (Table 5–1). Three diseases, dermatomyositis, polymyositis, and inclusion body myositis, affect muscle much more than other organ systems. On the other hand, collagen-vascular and connective-tissue diseases, as well as a large number of infectious diseases, often involve muscle but usually do not present as a myopathy because of the conspicuous involvement of other organ systems.

Dermatomyositis, polymyositis, and inclusion body myositis have recently become readily distinguishable by clinical and laboratory diagnostic criteria (Table 5–2). They should no longer be lumped together by terms such as "polydermatomyositis."[84]

DERMATOMYOSITIS

Dermatomyositis is the most easily recognized inflammatory myopathy. Childhood and adult forms overlap in clinical and laboratory features but differ in prognosis and treatment.

Clinical Features

SKIN

A highly characteristic rash distinguishes dermatomyositis (Fig. 5–1).[167] Erythema and scaling and telangiectatic lesions occur over the malar region of the face, usually involving the eyelids, which often have a violaceous (heliotrope) appearance. Similar lesions may be seen in sun-exposed areas at the hairline of the neck, the dorsum of the hands (particularly the metacarpophalangeal and interphalangeal joints), the extensor surfaces of the knees and elbows, and the medial and lateral malleoli. Papular, erythematous changes over the knuckles, referred to as Grottron's papules, are highly characteristic (see Fig. 5–1D). Periorbital edema is common, and necrotizing vasculitis of the skin can occur in severe cases in both children and adults. Rarely, patients with sarcoidosis,[101] lupus erythematosus, or mixed connective-tissue disease may have similar skin manifestations, but few other conditions present diagnostic confusion.

Evaluation of nailfold capillaries often reveals enlarged and deformed capillary loops surrounded by avascular

Table 5–1 INFLAMMATORY MYOPATHIES

PRIMARY
Dermatomyositis
Polymyositis
Inclusion body myositis

OCCURRING IN OTHER DISEASES
Connective-tissue diseases: Mixed connective-tissue disease; progressive systemic sclerosis; systemic lupus erythematosus; rheumatoid arthritis; Sjögren's syndrome; polyarteritis nodosa and other forms of systemic vasculitis; Behçet's syndrome
Giant-cell and granulomatous myositis: Giant-cell myositis; sarcoidosis; inflammatory bowel disease
Eosinophilic syndromes and myositis: Eosinophilic polymyositis; diffuse fasciitis with eosinophilia (Shulman's syndrome); eosinophilia-myalgia syndrome associated with tryptophan; toxic-oil syndrome
Infectious agents: Viral; protozoal; helminthic (trichinosis, cysticercosis, echinococcosis); bacterial; fungal

---

areas (Fig. 5–2).[163,215] Abnormal capillaries also occur in systemic vasculitis, in progressive systemic sclerosis, and in mixed connective-tissue disease.[134] The changes in the capillaries are usually best seen by nailfold capillary microscopy (Fig. 5–3).

MUSCLE WEAKNESS

Myalgias are seldom the chief complaint of adults with dermatomyositis. When questioned, however, children often report muscle pain and tenderness. Muscle weakness usually develops subacutely (over weeks) but may be either insidious (months) or fulminant (days). The weakness initially affects proximal muscles, including neck flexors, hip flexors and extensors, trunk, and shoulder-girdle muscles. Weakness may progress to involve distal muscles. Dysphagia occurs in at least one third of patients.[98] Inflammation and muscle fiber degeneration cause abnormalities of esophageal motility in both the upper (skeletal muscle) and lower (smooth muscle) portion of the esophagus.[55,98,105a] Even gastric emptying may be impaired.[98] Weakness only rarely progresses to involve respiratory muscles; ventilatory failure is uncommon. Muscle stretch reflexes are usually preserved and may seem hyperactive considering the degree of muscle weakness.

Table 5–2 DISTINGUISHING CLINICAL FEATURES OF IDIOPATHIC INFLAMMATORY MYOPATHIES

	Childhood Dermatomyositis	Adult Dermatomyositis	Polymyositis	Inclusion Body Myositis
Weakness	Proximal; dysphagia	Proximal; dysphagia	Predominantly proximal weakness; dysphagia	Proximal and distal; dysphagia
Muscle pain	>50%	<25%	<10%	None
Skin	Periorbital edema; erythematous rash; calcinosis	Periorbital edema; erythematous rash	None	None
Joint involvement	Contractures	Contractures; effusions	Uncommon	None
Other systems	Rarely involved; occasional infarcts of bowel, kidney, retina	Arrhythmias; interstitial lung disease	Arrhythmias; heart failure; interstitial lung disease	None
Risk of malignancy	Minimal	Increased	Increased	None

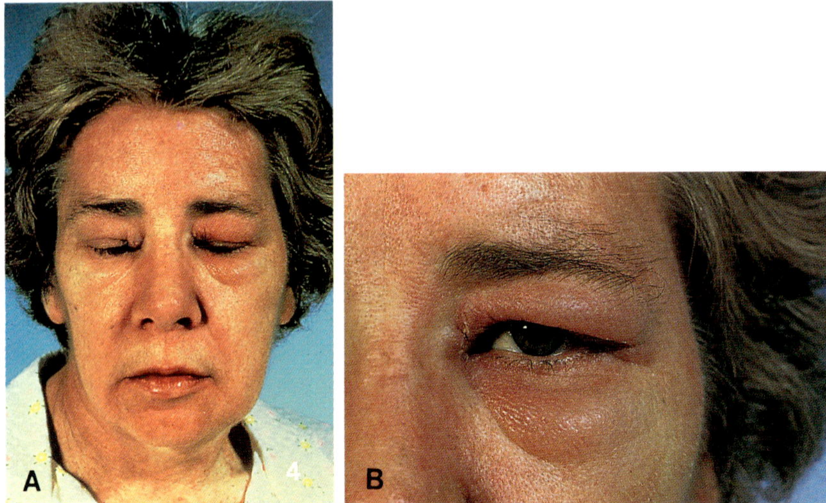

Figure 5–1. Severe skin rash in dermatomyositis. (*A*) The rash involves the forehead, neck, and eyelids (heliotrope). (*B*) Periorbital edema may be seen in severe cases.

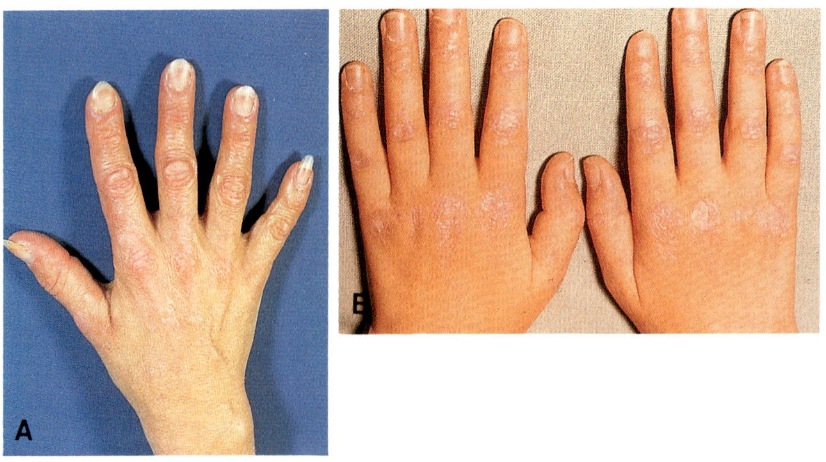

Figure 5–2. (*A*, *B*) Rash on hands in dermatomyositis.

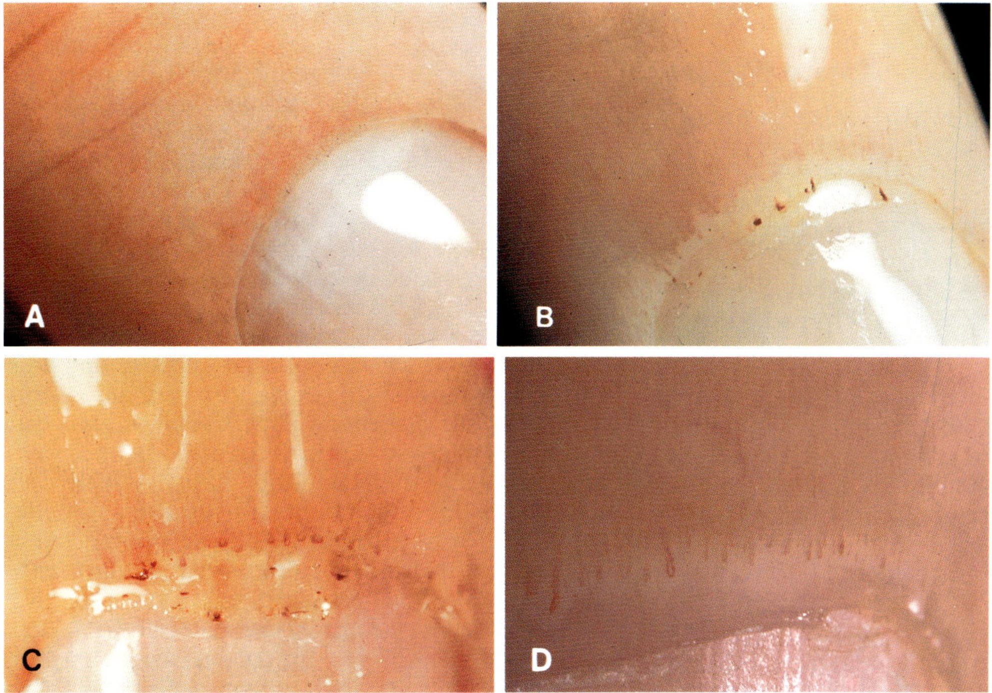

Figure 5–3. Nailfold capillary microscopy. Capillary loops can be visualized by using the +40 objective of the ophthalmoscope. Immersion oil must be dropped on the nailfold to prevent (defract) the light from shining in the eye of the examiner. (*A*) Normal capillary loops. (*B*) Nailfold thrombi in a patient with features of dermatomyositis and progressive systemic sclerosis. (*C*) Nailfold hemorrhage in a patient with systemic vasculitis. (*D*) Dilated loops in a patient with scleroderma.

OTHER MANIFESTATIONS

Joints.   Contractures are a frequent and early complication of dermatomyositis. Even prior to diagnosis, limitation of motion may occur at the elbows, wrists, and shoulders. Arthralgias are frequent, and joint effusions may be seen.[31]

Heart.   Overt clinical cardiac manifestations are rare, but cardiomegaly, dyspnea, and congestive heart failure all may result from focal areas of myocardial inflammation.[6,7,219] Cardiac abnormalities include atrioventricular and bundle branch block; frequent premature ventricular beats; and tachycardia of either ventricular or supraventricular origin.[7,219] In addition, defects in ventricular and septal wall motion can be detected by echocardiography or radionuclide scintigraphy.[7,95]

Lungs.   Patients with significant pharyngeal and upper-esophageal motility impairment may develop aspiration pneumonia. Aspirated materials include not only food substances but also bacteria-laden oropharyngeal secretions and regurgitated gastric contents.[60]

Interstitial lung disease affects 5% to 10% of adult patients with dermatomyositis.[123,196] A fulminant and sometimes fatal form of this complication presents with acute fever, dyspnea, productive cough, and a diffuse "ground glass" appearance on chest radiographs. Other patients have an insidious form of interstitial lung disease with dyspnea and a diffuse reticulonodular infiltration on chest film. Some patients with interstitial lung disease have few clinical manifestations. Pulmonary artery hypertension can accompany dermatomyositis, but it usually occurs in patients with an overlapping connective tissue disease.[123]

Vasculitis. Necrotizing vasculitis may affect several organs, particularly the skin, muscle, and gastrointestinal tract (leading to visceral perforations), especially in the childhood form of dermatomyositis.[11,135] This vasculitis has been called the "systemic angiopathy of childhood."[11] In rare patients, other affected tissues may include the retina, kidneys, and lung.

Cancer. Many clinicians believe that patients with dermatomyositis and polymyositis have an increased risk of cancer. The estimates of risk, especially with dermatomyositis, have been reported to be 5 to 11 times greater than for the population at large, and even higher for men more than age 50.[13,32] No prospective longitudinal study has addressed these issues. Investigators disagree about the relationship of inflammatory myopathies to cancer,[120,133] but we believe that a definite association exists between myositis and malignancy, particularly in patients more than age 40 with dermatomyositis.[13,32,120,133] Severity of myositis does not correlate with the presence of neoplasm. Most malignancies are discovered before or concurrently with the inflammatory myopathy.[133] An extensive workup for cancer seldom increases the identification of occult neoplasms in these patients and is not cost-effective. The appropriate evaluation includes a thorough physical examination, analysis of stool for occult blood, a chest roentgenogram, and mammography in women.

Laboratory Features

BLOOD STUDIES

Serum creatine kinase (CK) is elevated in more than 90% of dermatomyositis patients; levels do not correlate with severity of weakness or rate of progression. The CK level may be normal even with marked limb weakness. The erythrocyte sedimentation rate (ESR) is usually normal; an elevated ESR suggests an associated illness such as a collagen-vascular disease.

Autoantibodies to a variety of nuclear antigens (antinuclear antibodies [ANA]) are found in patients with connective tissue diseases[4,15,21,24,92,175,223] (Table 5–3). Most autoantibodies do not help in the diagnosis of inflammatory myopathies except that certain antibodies suggest an overlapping collagen-vascular disorder or mixed connective-tissue disease. Four autoantibodies, however, may help to define subsets of myositis. The most important is the antibody to Jo-1 antigen, which is present in one third of patients with inflammatory myopathies. Jo-1 is a cytoplasmic enzyme (histidyl-transfer RNA synthetase).[175] The antibody occurs in a genetically distinct group with HLA-DR3 or HLA-DRw6 haplotypes in the setting of a polymyositis syndrome with interstitial lung disease, arthritis, and Raynaud's phenomenon.[175] Antibodies to PM-1 and Ku antigens are more common in the overlap syndrome of polymyositis and progressive systemic sclerosis.[92,223] The antibody to SS-A (Ro) is associated with Sjögren's syndrome and may be a marker for myocardial involvement in the inflammatory myopathies.[15] Thus, these autoantibodies may subcategorize patients and provide prognostic information.

ELECTRODIAGNOSTIC STUDIES

During the initial phase of acute dermatomyositis, insertional activity is increased, with trains of fibrillations and positive waves accompanied by complex repetitive discharges and myopathic motor units. The amount of spontaneous activity correlates with the degree of disease activity. Weak muscles usually show early recruitment of small units.

In addition to brief, small, polyphasic motor units, studies in patients with chronic or relapsing inflammatory my-

Table 5-3 AUTOANTIBODIES IN CONNECTIVE TISSUE DISEASE

Target Antigen	Disease
DNA	
Double-stranded	SLE
Native	SLE, rarely other CTD
Single-stranded	SLE, other CTD, nonrheumatic diseases
HISTONES	Drug-induced lupus, RA, SLE
RIBONUCLEOPROTEINS	
RNP*	MCTD
SM	SLE
SS-A (Ro)	SLE, MCTD, Sjögren's
SS-B (La)	SLE, MCTD, Sjögren's
CHROMATIN-ASSOCIATED	
Centromere	PSS, CREST
Sci-70	PSS
KU	PM/PSS overlap
OTHER NUCLEAR PROTEINS	
Jo-1	PM > DM with ILD
PM-1	PM/PSS overlap
Mi-2	DM > PM

SLE = systemic lupus erythematosus; CTD = connective tissue disease; RA = rheumatoid arthritis; MCTD = mixed connective-tissue disease; PSS = progressive systemic sclerosis; CREST = calcinosis, Raynaud's, esophageal dysmotility, sclerodactyly, telangiectasia; ILD = interstitial lung disease.
*(U_2) RNP is more accurate designation.

opathies often show increased numbers of long-duration, high-amplitude polyphasic potentials. The enlarged motor unit potentials presumably reflect sprouting and reinnervation of regenerating muscle fibers and subsequent enlargement of motor unit territory.

With very advanced disease, probably as a result of extensive fibrosis in markedly weak muscles, the recruitment pattern may be decreased. The finding of reduced recruitment and long-duration motor units can be erroneously interpreted as a neurogenic process. In fact, such long-duration motor units may characterize any severe, long-standing muscle disease.

HISTOLOGIC STUDIES

Perifascicular muscle fiber atrophy (Fig. 5-4) is a highly specific finding for dermatomyositis and occurs in nearly 75% of patients. The term "atrophy" is misleading, however, because the small fibers at the periphery of the fascicle are selectively damaged because of microvascular insult.* During early stages of injury, muscle fibers exhibit focal myofibrillar and oxidative enzyme loss. Features typical of regeneration, including basophilic cytoplasm and internal nuclei, appear later. The microvasculature (especially the capillary network) is selectively lost at the periphery of fascicles in the region of perifascicular muscle-fiber damage.[34,58] The histologic changes in dermatomyositis are multifocal and vary in severity in different regions of the same muscle biopsy. Fascicles with very severe damage may show only remnants of very small (atrophic) fibers at the periphery. In fulminant cases, muscle infarction produces wedge-shaped or contiguous areas of muscle fiber necrosis.

The inflammatory component in dermatomyositis differs from that of polymyositis and inclusion body myo-

---

*References 11,34,58,104,115,117,233.

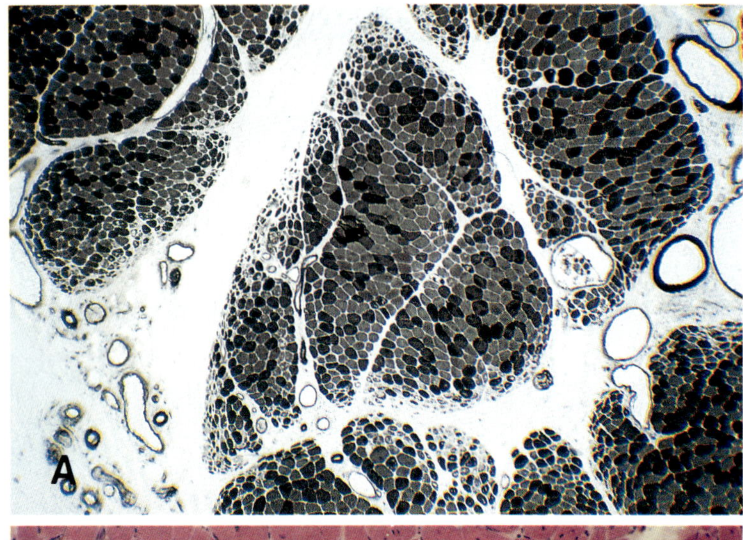

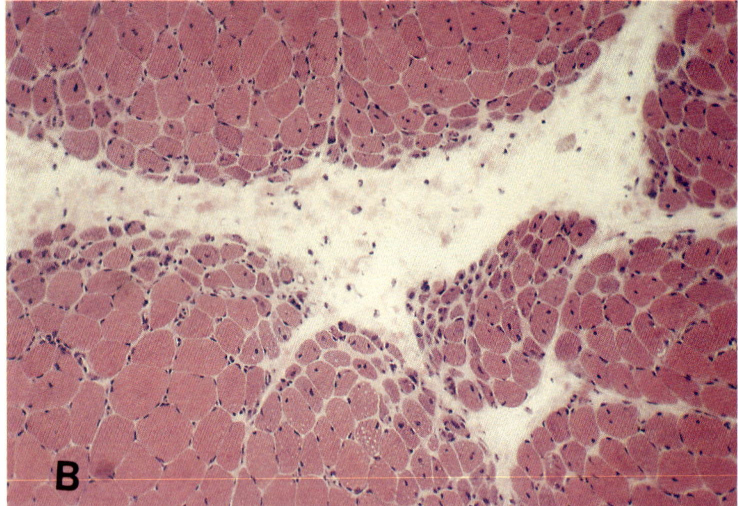

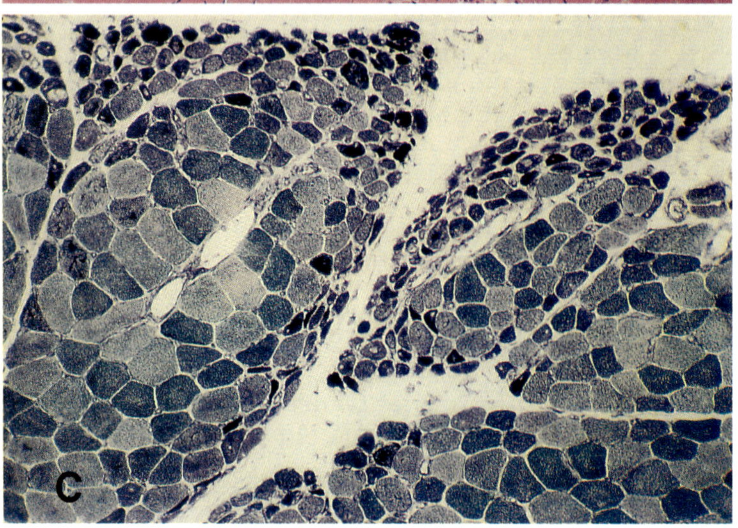

Figure 5–4. Perifascicular muscle fiber damage in dermatomyositis. (*A*) ATPase stain pH 9.4 shows atrophy and fiber loss at the periphery of the fascicles. Both type 1 (light) and type 2 (dark) fibers are affected. (*B*) Small fibers are seen at the periphery of the fascicles. The presence of one or more internal nuclei within the muscle fibers indicates previous or ongoing muscle fiber regeneration (H&E stain). (*C*) The muscle fiber damage is highlighted in this oxidative enzyme stain demonstrating atrophic and dark-staining fibers in the perifascicular region. NADH-tetrazolium reductase stain.

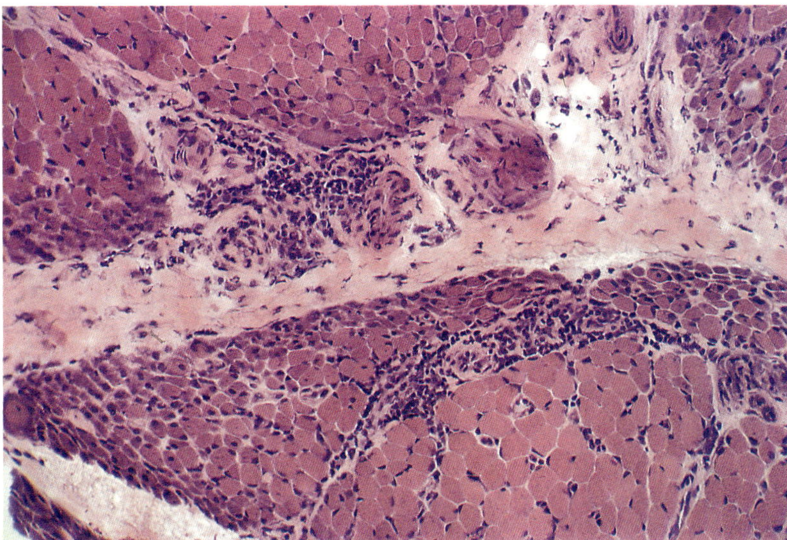

Figure 5–5. Inflammation in dermatomyositis is prominent in the perimysial connective tissue and in a perivascular distribution (H&E).

sitis.[2,67] Focal invasion of muscle fibers by inflammatory cells is infrequent. Instead, inflammatory cells collect in the perimysial connective tissue and in perivascular locations (Fig. 5–5). In dermatomyositis, the proportion of B cells and CD4+ (T helper) cells in the inflammatory cell infiltration is higher, whereas in polymyositis and inclusion body myositis, CD8+ (cytotoxic suppressor T cells) make up a greater percentage of cells. Macrophages comprise one fourth to one third of the inflammatory cells in both dermatomyositis and polymyositis.[67]

Immune deposits in blood vessels[115,117,233] are another characteristic feature of muscle biopsies in dermatomyositis (Fig. 5–6). These microvascular deposits consist of IgM, less often IgG, and complement components, including C3, C9, and neoantigens of the C5b-9 complement membrane attack complex (MAC).[115,117,233] Strong evidence suggests that these immune deposits are important in the pathogenesis of the vascular lesion discussed below. Similar immune deposits may be seen in the affected areas of the skin at the dermal-epidermal junction.[50,167]

Skeletal-muscle capillaries show distinctive ultrastructural changes.[10,58] Endothelial cells appear swollen and contain microvacuoles and inclusions (Fig. 5–7). These endothelial inclusions are not seen in polymyositis or inclusion body myositis.[10,34,58,162] They appear in the earliest stages of dermatomyositis, preceding muscle fiber necrosis and inflammation.[58]

Management

CHILDHOOD DERMATOMYOSITIS

The therapy and prognosis of childhood dermatomyositis differ from that of adult dermatomyositis. Corticosteroids are effective in virtually 100% of patients with the childhood disease, and remission with eventual complete withdrawal of medication can be anticipated. As discussed below, adults usually respond to corticosteroids but often require other agents and seldom remain in remission if medication is stopped.

Opinions vary about appropriate regimens of corticosteroid treat-

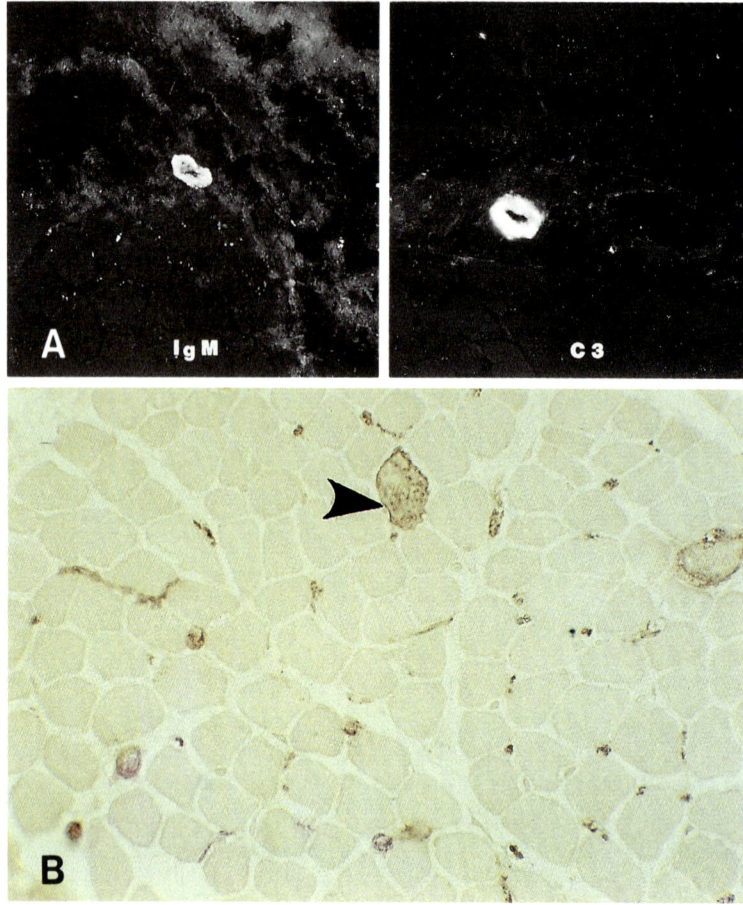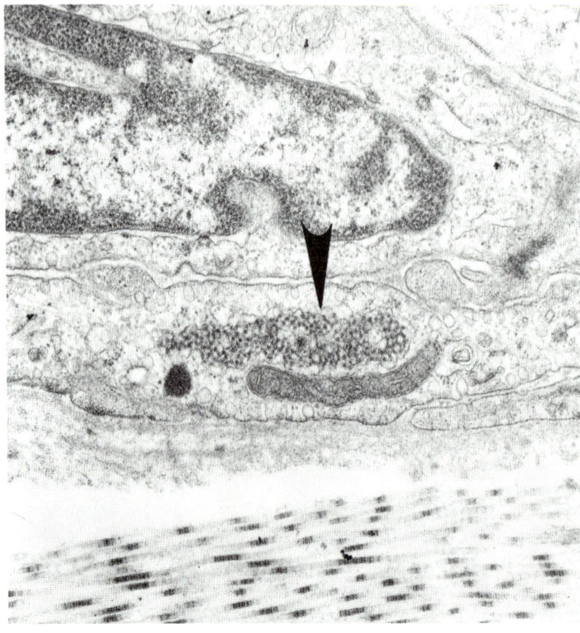

Figure 5–6. Immune deposits in dermatomyositis, demonstrated by peroxidase-labeled antibody to the neoantigens of C5b-9 membrane attack complex (MAC). (*A*) IgM and C_3 deposits in perimysial blood vessels. (*B*) MAC is deposited throughout the microvasculature. MAC also participates in the process of muscle fiber necrosis (*arrowhead*).

Figure 5–7. Electron micrograph of capillary in dermatomyositis showing endothelial inclusion composed of undulating tubules (*arrowhead*).

ment.[62,118,214,221] Disease tempo and severity are key factors in decision making. A recommended treatment protocol is listed in Table 5–4. Prednisone should be administered daily until unequivocal improvement occurs in muscle strength. Patients with severe weakness may need longer daily treatment. As strength improves, a gradual dose reduction and conversion to an alternate-day regimen is possible in most patients and results in less adrenal suppression and fewer side effects.[70] Most patients continue treatment for at least 1 year after improvement or for a total of 2 years (see Table 5–4). Elevations of CK levels during steroid tapering may signal a recurrence, but if CK changes conflict with clinical findings, muscle strength is a better measure of response to therapy. CK levels can rise with exercise and fall with decreased activity.

Table 5–4 MANAGEMENT OF DERMATOMYOSITIS

INITIAL TREATMENT
Prednisone 1.0–1.5 mg/kg/per day (maximum 100 mg) (before breakfast)
Dietary counseling: low sodium, low free sugar (complex carbohydrates preferable), caloric limitation
Eye evaluation for cataracts, glaucoma
Supplemental calcitriol 0.5 μg daily (1, 25-dihydroxyvitamin D_3) and elemental calcium 1000 mg daily
Exercise and range of motion
Follow strength and serum CK at 2- to 4-week intervals
Monitor serum electrolytes, glucose, hematocrit, at 1- to 2-month intervals

AFTER DEFINITE IMPROVEMENT AND RECOVERY OF AMBULATION
Alternate-day therapy: change to twice the daily dose of prednisone (maximum 120 mg) before breakfast on alternate days
Continue until function much better, then taper
Tapering of prednisone: reduce dosage (10%–20%) at 4- to 8-week intervals. Do not reduce dosage if there are signs or symptoms of decreasing strength.

---

*Severely ill patients often benefit from intravenous methylprednisolone 500 mg twice daily for 3 days.

Adults over 50 and other severely weak patients are often given azathioprine (2–3 mg/kg/per day) 3 to 7 days after beginning prednisone.

Conversely, a fall in CK level may be misleading as a prognostic sign because corticosteroids may lower CK levels in a variety of muscle diseases without necessarily producing an increase in strength.[73]

Cytotoxic agents such as azathioprine, cyclophosphamide, and methotrexate may be required for patients who experience dose-limiting side effects of corticosteroids. It is best to avoid their use in children, however, because of the medication's possible long-term carcinogenic and teratogenic effects.[30,43,116,140,145,212] Until recently, azathioprine has been considered to be the best alternative to prednisone as an immunosuppressant drug, whether used alone or as a corticosteroid-sparing agent.[140] A controlled trial of intravenous immune globulin infusions showing significant benefit in treatment-resistant dermatomyositis suggests that this agent may have a place in the treatment of dermatomyositis.[51a] More experience will be required, especially in children, but it is entirely appropriate to employ intravenous immune globulin infusions prior to cytotoxic agents. We would not as yet recommend immune globulin prior to a trial of prednisone. Immune globulin infusions are extraordinarily expensive, require continued maintenance therapy for an unknown period, and can have major side effects.[224a]

The use of high doses of corticosteroids has changed the natural history of childhood dermatomyositis. The disabling complications of immobility, muscle atrophy, and contractures, which previously affected as many as half of the patients, have nearly disappeared. In addition, cutaneous calcinosis is less frequent and less severe, although it may occur after several months of active disease. Furuncle-like lesions, which are palpably indurated or rock hard, tend to develop over pressure points and extrude caseous or chalky material. These lesions can be painful but improve with surgical or spontaneous drainage. They often leave disfiguring scars. Cutaneous calcinosis may persist and progress for many years after other signs of disease activity have resolved. Agents that are reported to have helped in individual cases include colchicine,[222] diphosphonates,[49] and systemic or local corticosteroids,[29] but there is not enough information to recommend one or another of these treatments.

ADULT DERMATOMYOSITIS

Nearly all patients with adult dermatomyositis respond to corticosteroids. We recommend prednisone 1.0 to 1.5 mg/kg in a single daily dose (maximum 100 mg). For most, but not all, patients the dosage may be tapered to an alternate-day schedule once improvement begins (see Table 5–4). High doses of corticosteroids should be maintained until patients improve substantially, after which a slowly tapering schedule can be initiated. It is seldom possible to discontinue treatment completely. Most patients require a dosage of 10 to 30 mg every other day for many years. As indicated above for childhood dermatomyositis, there may be a role for intravenous immune globulin in adult dermatomyositis,[51a] but more clinical experience will be required before specific recommendations can be made.

PREVENTION OF CORTICOSTEROID SIDE EFFECTS

The long-term use of corticosteroids is a potentially serious cause of morbidity. Alternate-day therapy clearly diminishes cosmetic and other side effects and partially preserves adrenal responsivity.[70] Patients must be advised about, and monitored for, side effects such as cataracts, glaucoma, hypertension, sodium retention, diabetes, hypokalemia, osteopenia, and aseptic necrosis of the hip. Approximately 10% of patients develop glaucoma as an idiosyncratic sensitivity to corticosteroids[23]; patients should be periodically screened for elevated intraocular pressure.

The routine use of calcitriol (1,25-dihydroxyvitamin D3) and calcium supplementation has proven benefit in the prevention of corticosteroid osteoporosis.[87,191a] We routinely recommend calcitriol 0.5 µg per day and 1000 mg of elemental calcium daily. The calcium can be given as either calcium carbonate or calcium gluconate. Patients on this regimen should have serum calcium checked periodically to avoid hypercalcemia. The dose of calcitriol can be adjusted by 0.25-µg increments if necessary. The relationship between corticosteroids and peptic ulcer disease has not been clearly defined.[46] Cimetidine and ranitidine (histamine H_2-receptor antagonists) may be useful in acute stressful situations in which endogenous corticosteroids are elevated,[173] but these drugs are not necessary for routine use.

Severe side effects from corticosteroids are an indication for adding azathioprine.[30,116,140] Azathioprine reduces the amount of corticosteroids necessary to achieve or maintain remission,[43] but it takes more than 3 months to produce a major effect.[30] We start with 50 mg/d and gradually increase to 2 to 3 mg/kg per day in divided doses with food. The drug has significant toxicity, including a 10% incidence of acute systemic reactions (more common in women) consisting of fever, nausea, or rash.[116] This reaction or acute pancreatitis precludes further use and has no relation to dose. Bone marrow suppression and hepatotoxicity are dose-related side effects; blood counts and liver function studies must be monitored at 1- to 2-week intervals initially. After treatment is well established, monitoring can be reduced to 4- to 6-week intervals. Concurrent use of allopurinol is dangerous because it interferes with metabolism of azathioprine and thereby potentiates its toxicity.[116] Methotrexate[145,212] or cyclophosphamide are alternative immunosuppressive drugs, but we prefer azathioprine except in refractory disease.

The rash in dermatomyositis may persist after resolution of skeletal muscle manifestations. The rash, however, is not an indication for adjunctive immunosuppressant treatment.

Because the risk of side effects is substantial for each of the agents used to treat dermatomyositis, the clinician must fully inform patients about potential toxicity. Table 5–5 provides a list that can be used.

Pathogenesis

Current evidence suggests that dermatomyositis has a different pathogenesis than other inflammatory

Table 5–5 INFORMING PATIENTS REGARDING RISKS OF CORTICOSTEROIDS AND CYTOTOXIC DRUGS

The following agent(s) — prednisone, azathioprine, or cyclophosphamide — are being used to treat your disease. The major risks or side effects and some preventive measures are listed below. Side effects may occur even with efforts at prevention, but keeping the dosage as low as possible reduces the risks of side effects.

PREDNISONE (AND OTHER CORTICOSTEROIDS)

Side Effects	*Prevention*
FLUID AND ELECTROLYTE DISTURBANCES	
Sodium retention	Low sodium diet
Fluid retention	Low sodium diet
Potassium loss	Potassium replacement (if indicated)
Hypertension	Monthly checks; treatment
MUSCULOSKELETAL	
Steroid atrophy with muscle weakness	Exercise program
Osteoporosis and bone fractures	Supplemental calcium
Hip necrosis	
GASTROINTESTINAL	
Peptic ulcer	Antacids; H_2 blockers
Nausea	
Abdominal distention	
Weight gain	Caloric restriction
DERMATOLOGIC	
Impaired wound healing	
Thin, fragile skin	
Bruising	
Increased sweating	
Change in facial appearance	
Skin striae	
Increase in face and body hair	
Acne	
NEUROLOGIC	
Dizziness	
Headache	
Disturbed thinking or hallucinations	
Personality change	
Insomnia	
ENDOCRINE	
Menstrual irregularities	
Suppression of growth in children	
Diabetes	Diet low in sugar
IMMUNE	
Reduced resistance to infection	
OPHTHALMIC	
Cataracts	
Glaucoma	

Continued

Table 5–5 INFORMING PATIENTS REGARDING RISKS OF CORTICOSTEROIDS AND CYTOTOXIC DRUGS (*Continued*)

AZATHIOPRINE

General guidelines for use of azathioprine: Introduce gradually, starting with 50 mg/day for 3–7 days; 100 mg/day for 3–7 days; then full dose. Obtain complete blood cell count and test liver function weekly for 6 weeks, then at least monthly. A therapeutic response requires 3–6 months, and any toxicity resolves slowly.

Side Effects	*Prevention*
HYPERSENSITIVITY REACTION	
Nausea, vomiting, fever, flulike symptoms within 1 month of starting drug	Introduce drug gradually
HEMATOLOGIC	
Leukopenia	Monitoring of blood counts (weekly initially, then monthly)
Anemia	
GASTROINTESTINAL	
Loss of appetite	Take in divided doses with food
Hepatic dysfunction	Monitoring of liver function
OTHER	
Hair loss	
Pancreatitis	
Lowered resistance to cancer (possible)	
Effect on fetus	Contraceptive measures advisable
Allopurinol (gout medication) contraindicated	

CYCLOPHOSPHAMIDE

Side Effects	*Prevention*
GASTROINTESTINAL	
Loss of appetite	Take in divided doses with food
Nausea or vomiting	Monitoring of liver function
HEMATOLOGIC	
Lowering of white blood count	Monitoring of blood counts (weekly initially, then monthly)
Anemia	
GENITOURINARY	
Cystitis	Ample fluid intake and frequent voiding
Bladder cancer	
DERMATOLOGIC	
Impaired wound healing	
Hair loss	
Skin and fingernails may become darker	
OTHER	
Lowered resistance to cancer	
Lung fibrosis	
Effect on fetus	Contraceptive measures mandatory

myopathies.[2,58,67,115,117] The microvasculature appears to be a primary site of injury in this disease, and studies indicate that a complement-mediated vasculopathy is the primary immunopathogenic event in the evolution of muscle lesions (see Fig. 5–6). Both immunoglobulin and complement, with activation of C5b-9 complement membrane attack complex (see Fig. 5–6), can be found in the microvasculature as an accompaniment to early muscle fiber damage.[58,115,117] In addition, ultrastructural studies show that capillary abnormalities precede other structural changes in muscle.[58]

Several features distinguish those mononuclear cell infiltrates seen in the muscle biopsies of dermatomyositis patients from features in other inflammatory myopathies. More B cells infiltrate the biopsy, whereas the invasion of muscle fibers by cytotoxic T cells is uncommon.[2,67] In addition, the inflammatory infiltrate shows a more abundant perivascular and perimysial distribution, rather than the endomysial cell location characteristic of other inflammatory myopathies.

Factors responsible for initiating vascular damage in dermatomyositis have not been uncovered. The presence of tubular structures resembling viruses within capillaries has suggested a viral cause to some investigators, but the only conclusive evidence is a single well-documented case of childhood dermatomyositis associated with influenza virus.[76] Preliminary but unsubstantiated evidence suggests that picornavirus is present in muscle in a small number of patients[126,188]; further work is necessary to determine if this virus plays a role in pathogenesis.

POLYMYOSITIS

Polymyositis is not merely a variant of dermatomyositis without the rash. Although some similar clinical features may be present in both disorders, recent evidence indicates a different underlying pathogenesis (see p. 170). As discussed in detail below, the differential diagnosis of polymyositis is long, and it is difficult to define specific criteria for the disorder. Unlike dermatomyositis, it has neither a highly characteristic feature such as a rash, nor a distinctive muscle histology like perifascicular atrophy. Nevertheless, by applying rigid criteria (Table 5–6) one can define a group of patients likely to have polymyositis. Cases failing to meet all of these criteria are common, however, and a definite diagnosis cannot be made in many such patients.

Clinical Features

MUSCLE WEAKNESS

Polymyositis rarely presents before age 20, although childhood and even infantile cases have been reported.[25,27,28,57,200,224] Muscle weakness usually develops subacutely or insidiously; rarely the disorder may have a fulminant presentation. Proximal limb and neck flexor muscles are weakened; distal muscle involvement varies. Absolutely normal distal muscle strength and function should raise suspicion of an alternative muscle disorder such as a muscular dystrophy. Dysphagia is common in polymyositis. As in dermato-

---

Table 5–6 CRITERIA FOR DIAGNOSIS OF POLYMYOSITIS

Clinical:	Symmetrical proximal weakness; slight but definite distal weakness is usually present
CK:	Elevated (commonly at least 10X normal)
EMG:	Fibrillations, early recruitment and small, polyphasic motor unit potentials
Biopsy:	Endomysial inflammation with focal muscle fiber invasion; muscle fiber necrosis; perivascular mononuclear inflammation

Differential Diagnosis	Criteria for Exclusion
Dermatomyositis	Rash and biopsy
Inclusion body myositis	Severe distal weakness; biopsy
Other collagen vascular diseases	Usual criteria
Sarcoidosis	Biopsy
Metabolic myopathies	Biopsy
Toxic, infectious	History, specific diagnostic study
Endocrine	Appropriate hormone studies
Limb-girdle muscular dystrophy	Family history; biopsy; EMG

myositis, impaired mobility can be demonstrated in the pharyngeal muscles and the upper and lower esophagus.[55,98,105a] Ventilatory failure resulting from muscle weakness is uncommon but occurs more often than in dermatomyositis or inclusion body myositis.[26,230]

As many as one third of patients with polymyositis have muscle pain, but it is rarely the chief complaint. Prominent myalgia should suggest other disorders, particularly polymyalgia rheumatica, joint disorders, or diffuse fasciitis.

OTHER MANIFESTATIONS

The cardiac and pulmonary complications resemble those of adult dermatomyositis.[60,83,109,193,196,230] Cardiac symptoms from inflammatory lesions of the myocardium, congestive heart failure, atrial and ventricular arrhythmias, and the sick sinus syndrome[83,109,193] may precede skeletal-muscle symptoms. Interstitial lung disease complicates polymyositis with the same frequency as in dermatomyositis.[60,196] Patients may also have aspiration pneumonia related to dysphagia.

Retrospective studies suggest a small but definite increase in the risk of cancer with polymyositis.[13,32,120,133] Better, prospective studies are needed to define this association.

Laboratory Features

BLOOD STUDIES

Elevated CK levels, at least 5 to 10 times normal, are one criterion for the diagnosis of polymyositis.[27,28] The levels of other muscle enzymes, including alanine aminotransferase, aspartate aminotransferase (AST), and lactate dehydrogenase (LDH), are often elevated, and this should not be misinterpreted as a sign of liver involvement. Autoantibodies of value in the diagnosis of polymyositis include Jo-1, PM-1, and Mi-2.[4,21,24,175]

ELECTRODIAGNOSTIC STUDIES

Electromyography is usually abnormal in polymyositis. Characteristic findings include small, polyphasic, early recruited motor unit potentials. Fibrillations and positive sharp waves tend to correlate with activity of the disease and are usually most numerous in paraspinal muscles.

HISTOLOGIC STUDIES

Scattered muscle fiber necrosis and inflammatory infiltration are the hallmarks of polymyositis (Fig. 5–8).[2,67] The degree of inflammation varies: The endomysial connective tissue (especially nonnecrotic muscle fibers) may

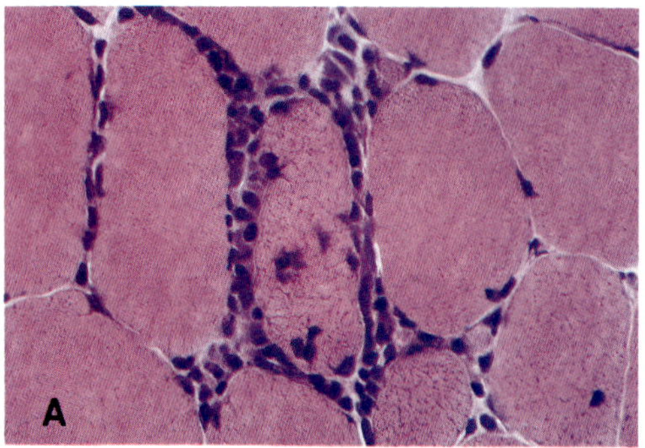
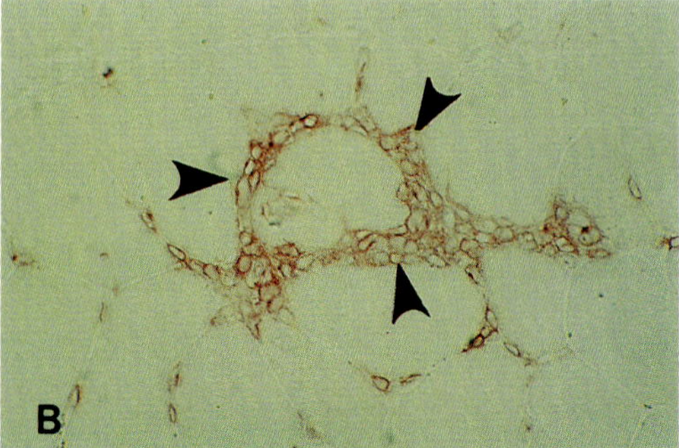

Figure 5–8. Focal invasion of nonnecrotic muscle fibers in polymyositis. (*A*) Mononuclear cells are seen invading a muscle fiber (H&E). (*B*) CD8+ mononuclear cells (*arrowheads*) surround and invade a muscle fiber.

contain focal collections of inflammatory cells, which may also be found within perimysial connective tissue as well as in relation to blood vessels. The major components of the inflammatory infiltrate are CD8+ cytotoxic/suppressor T cells and macrophages.[2,67] The CD8+ cells use the common α/β T-cell receptor for recognition of antigen. A single case of polymyositis has been reported, which was mediated by CD8-T cells expressing the γ/δ receptor.[97a] Less specific histologic changes include variability in muscle fiber size and the replacement of muscle fiber by connective tissue. Neither perifascicular atrophy nor muscle infarcts are observed, and immunofluorescent studies do not show the MAC deposition characteristic of dermatomyositis.

Differential Diagnosis

A diagnosis of polymyositis relies on a thorough search to exclude other causes of weakness (see Table 5–5). Muscular dystrophies of various types usually have distinctive clinical features, although patients with a limb-girdle syndrome often present a challenging problem. Magnetic resonance imaging (MRI) or computed tomography (CT) scans may demonstrate extensive fatty infiltration of muscle in muscular dystrophy, an uncommon finding in polymyositis (Fig. 5–9).[226] Slowly evolving metabolic myopathies, particularly carnitine deficiency and glycogen storage diseases like acid maltase deficiency, may be indistinguishable clinically from polymyositis, but the muscle

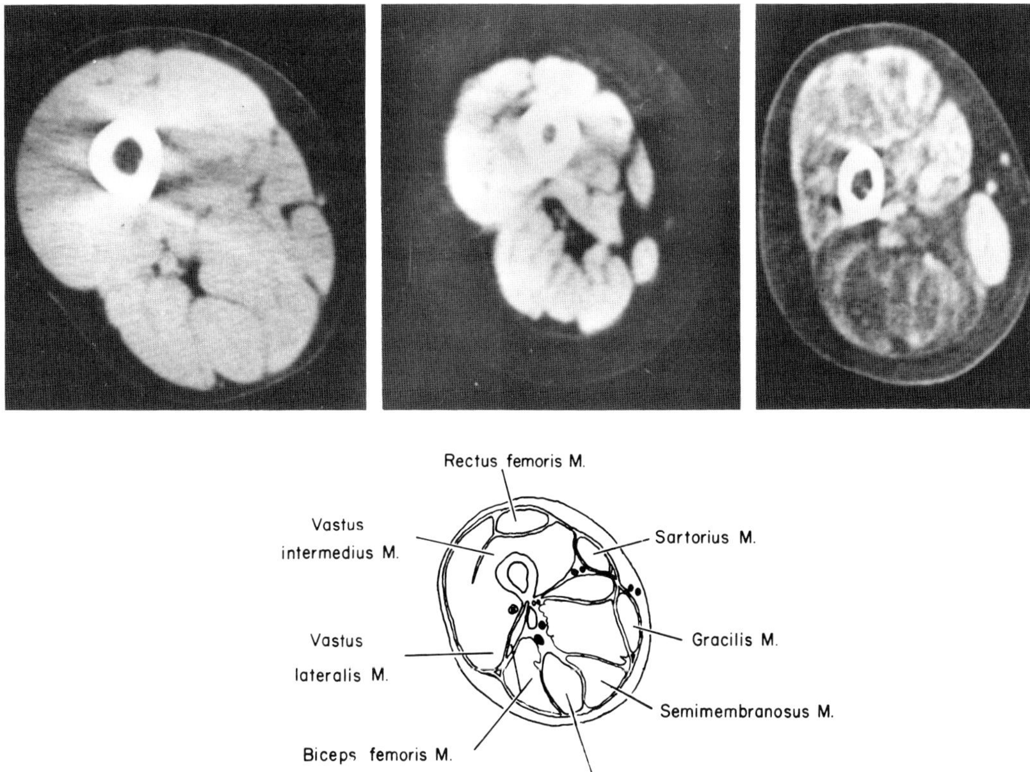

Figure 5–9. Computerized tomography of the thigh. (*Left*) Normal muscle appears homogeneous. (*Center*) In early polymyositis, the muscle remains relatively homogeneous but is atrophic. (*Right*) In muscular dystrophy, selected homogeneous muscles are replaced by fat.

biopsy should provide differentiation. (See pp. 263–266 for discussion of acid maltase deficiency and pp. 269–272 for carnitine deficiency.)

An unequivocal diagnosis of polymyositis requires the presence of all of the following: symmetric, proximal weakness; electromyographic abnormalities as described above; CK elevation; and necrosis and inflammatory cell infiltration on muscle biopsy. None of these individual criteria are diagnostic, however, as each may be seen in other neuromuscular diseases. Even the appearance of inflammatory cells in the muscle biopsy can be misleading. As these cells may be recruited in response to muscle fiber breakdown from any cause, such as defects in energy metabolism associated with rhabdomyolysis (Chapter 7), or the muscular dystrophies, especially facioscapulohumeral and Duchenne types (Chapter 4).

Distinguishing Polymyalgia Rheumatica from Polymyositis

Although polymyalgia rheumatica is a disease of joints rather than muscle (see Chapter 11), it is occasionally mistaken for polymyositis. The presenting symptoms suggest a muscle disease to patient and physician alike. Typically the polymyalgia patient is more than 60 years of age and has the insidious onset of "muscle" pain, stiffness, and weakness in the shoulders and thighs. Both atrophy and weakness develop as a consequence of pain. Polymyositis is suspected because of the distribution of wasting and weakness. Because slight elevations of CK may occur in polymyalgia rheumatica, the unwary may conclude that major muscle damage is present. *Polymyalgia rheumatica should be suspected if pain is a dominant complaint* and if strength seems better than the degree of atrophy suggests. Usually the ESR is elevated in polymyalgia rheumatica and normal in polymyositis. If corticosteroids are instituted, the patient with polymyalgia

rheumatica improves within a matter of 1 to 3 days, whereas a response in polymyositis usually takes weeks or months. Lowering of the sedimentation rate by corticosteroids or nonsteroidal anti-inflammatory agents (including aspirin) may obscure the diagnosis of polymyalgia rheumatica.

Management

Treatment of polymyositis is the same as for dermatomyositis (see Table 5–4). The goal of converting to alternate-day prednisone is important, in order to reduce steroid side effects. For patients refractory to corticosteroids, or those in whom steroid side effects demand a lowering of the dose despite clinical improvement, other immunosuppressive agents must be considered.[43] Azathioprine (in the doses outlined for dermatomyositis) is the drug of choice. Methotrexate or cyclophosphamide may also be considered.

Pain should not be the major indication for treatment with immunosuppressive drugs. Pain management should be approached through alternative measures, particularly nonsteroidal anti-inflammatory drugs.

Pathogenesis

The infiltration of inflammatory cells in the endomysial connective tissue with focal invasion of muscle fibers distinguishes polymyositis from dermatomyositis (see Figs. 5–5 and 5–8). The cell infiltration consists mainly of CD8+ cytotoxic/suppressor cells expressing the α/β T-cell receptor.[2,67,97a] A single case of polymyositis was mediated by CD8-γ/δ T cells.[97a] Macrophages are also a significant component of the endomysial inflammatory infiltrate. Nonnecrotic muscle fibers are often surrounded or invaded by activated lymphocytes demonstrating the major histocompatibility class antigen, IA.[67] Nonnecrotic but focally invaded muscle fibers also express major histocompatibility complex (MHC) class I receptor.[64] These findings appear to be an extension of earlier observations showing lymphocyte toxicity directed against cultured muscle fibers.[86] Unlike dermatomyositis, immune studies in polymyositis do not show deposits of immunoglobulin or complement in the microvasculature. In summary, the findings in polymyositis strongly favor a targeted, cell-mediated immune response directed against muscle fibers.

Case History

A 55-year-old teacher presented with a history of weakness progressive over the previous 12 months. She had dysphagia and proximal weakness with scapular winging. She was unable to sit up from a supine position, rise from a deep knee bend or from a low chair, or walk on her heels, and her gait was waddling. Manual muscle testing confirmed grade 4 strength in proximal arm and leg muscles. Sensation was normal and reflexes brisk. The CK level was elevated 12- to 15-fold, and AST and LDH levels were two times normal. The ESR and endocrine and immunologic studies were normal. Electromyography (EMG) demonstrated numerous fibrillations and early recruitment of brief, low-amplitude motor unit potentials. Muscle biopsy showed widespread muscle necrosis, with mononuclear inflammatory cells surrounding necrotic fibers and in perivascular accumulations. A diagnosis of polymyositis was made.

Because the patient remained ambulatory and able to work, no treatment was instituted. The patient remained weak for the next year but gradually improved. Ten years later, muscle strength and CK level were normal, and she was asymptomatic.

Comment: This patient showed evidence for an active, inflammatory myopathy as the cause of her proximal muscle weakness. The CK level, EMG, and muscle biopsy supported a diagnosis of polymyositis. Most patients with polymyositis, particularly when weakness limits function, should have corticosteroid treatment. Unlike dermatomyositis, however, the natural history of polymyositis is not well characterized, and weakness is not always progressive. In this woman, muscle strength and laboratory readings returned to normal without treatment.

INCLUSION BODY MYOSITIS

The term *inclusion body myositis* (IBM) was coined in 1971 by Yunis and Samaha.[239] The disorder resembles polymyositis but is differentiated by vacuolated muscle fibers and nuclear and cytoplasmic fibrillary inclusions. Controversy concerning the specificity of the histopathology of IBM delayed its general acceptance as a distinct order, but it is now unequivocally established as a well-defined entity separate from dermatomyositis and polymyositis.[33,130,186]

Clinical Features

The weakness associated with inclusion body myositis begins and progresses gradually but relentlessly, usually over many months or years. The disorder has a male preponderance and usually begins after age 50, although no age groups have been entirely excluded.[130,184] It has a distinctive pattern of muscle weakness, in which both proximal and distal muscles are usually affected. Typical findings include weakness of the wrist flexors and finger flexors, and relative preservation of wrist and finger extensors. Atrophy of the volar forearm muscles is characteristic. In the lower extremities, prominent weakness and atrophy of the quadriceps muscles, combined with varying degrees of proximal and distal muscle weakness, provide a characteristic picture. Dysphagia occurs in about one third of patients with inclusion body myositis, and findings on barium swallow indicate that the major dysfunction is in upper esophageal muscles.[130,186] Musculature innervated by the cranial nerves is otherwise spared in most cases. Facial muscle weakness (particularly orbicularis oculi) is present in a minority of patients. Muscle stretch reflexes are usually normal, although loss of quadriceps reflexes may accompany significant atrophy of this muscle group.[130]

Heart involvement has not been documented in inclusion body myositis, although it may be difficult to distinguish such involvement from other causes of cardiovascular abnormalities in this older group of patients. No association with malignancy has been documented, but inclusion body myositis has been seen in combination with various immune-mediated diseases, including idiopathic thrombocytopenic purpura, interstitial lung disease, diabetes mellitus, systemic lupus erythematosus, and Sjögren's syndrome.[36,130]

Laboratory Features

BLOOD STUDIES

The CK level may be normal, but is usually elevated twofold to fivefold. Exceptional patients may have levels reaching 10 times normal. Autoantibodies are generally absent, and the sedimentation rate is usually normal.

ELECTRODIAGNOSTIC STUDIES

In inclusion body myositis, EMG demonstrates increased insertional activity, often with fibrillations, accompanied by short-duration, polyphasic, early re-cruited motor unit potentials. The incidence of long-duration potentials is also commonly increased, and this mixed pattern of short- and long-duration potentials supports a diagnosis of inclusion body myositis, although it may also occur in other chronic inflammatory myopathies.

HISTOLOGIC STUDIES

The diagnosis of inclusion body myositis clearly rests on muscle biopsy findings.[33,130,186] Routine light microscopic sections stained with hematoxylin and eosin (H&E) or modified trichrome demonstrate single or multiple rimmed vacuoles lined with granular material (Fig. 5–10). In addition, varying degrees of endomysial inflammation may be present. The inflammatory cells consist of CD8+ T cells and some macrophages. Nonnecrotic muscle fibers are invaded by mononuclear cells (see Fig. 5–10).[2,67] The pattern of inflammation is similar to that of polymyositis, although perimysial and perivascular inflammatory infiltration occurs less often in inclusion body myositis. Small groups of atrophic fibers of mixed histochemical type are also commonly observed in this disorder, raising the possibility of a superimposed neurogenic component. Careful searching reveals eosinophilic cytoplasmic inclusions in some cases.

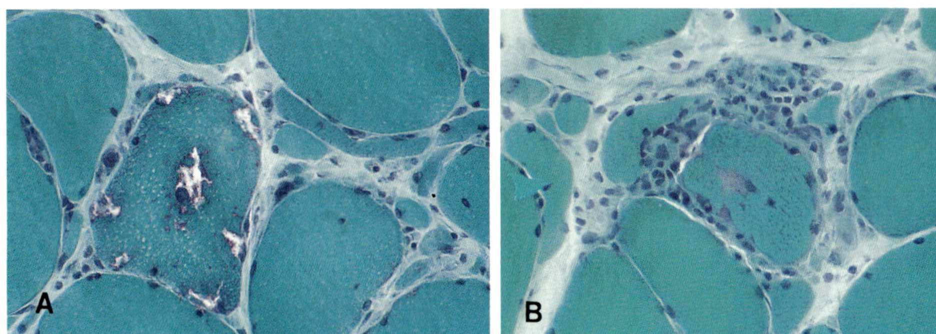

Figure 5–10. Inclusion body myositis. (*A*) Muscle fiber showing multiple rimmed vacuoles. Many small fibers, some angular in appearance, can be seen (modified trichrome). (*B*) Muscle fiber surrounded and invaded by mononuclear inflammatory cells (modified trichrome).

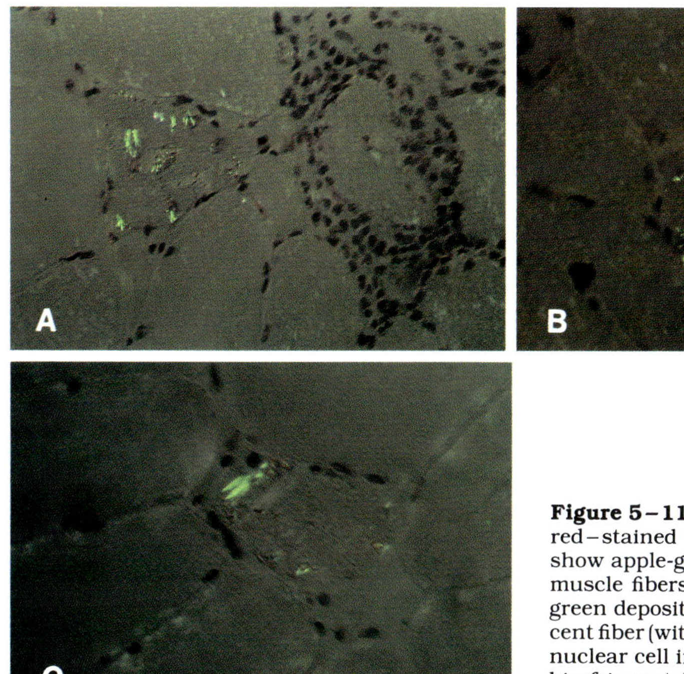

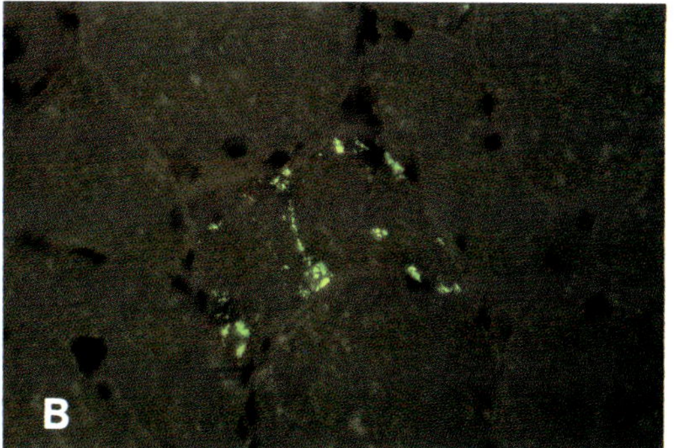

Figure 5–11. Inclusion body myositis: Congo red–stained sections under polarized light show apple-green birefringent deposits within muscle fibers. (*A*) Granular and wispy apple-green deposits within a muscle fiber. An adjacent fiber (without green deposits) shows mononuclear cell invasion. (*B*) and (*C*) Apple-green birefringent deposits. The amyloid deposits are variable, subtle, and often overlooked.

Demonstration of amyloid-positive material within muscle fibers can facilitate the diagnosis of inclusion body myositis.[144b] These highly specific apple-green birefringent deposits (Fig. 5–11) seen with polarized light are not found in other vacuolar myopathies. The diagnosis of inclusion body myositis can be confirmed by the electron microscopic demonstration of non-branching filaments[33,130,239] (also referred to as tubulofilaments) usually measuring 15 to 18 nm in diameter and varying in length from 1 to 5 nm (Fig. 5–12). These filaments occur in loose bundles, in parallel or random orientation, most often adjacent to rimmed vacuoles. Filaments also occur within the nucleus, usually surrounded by a thin rim of marginated chromatin. The rimmed vacuoles in inclusion body myositis have ultrastructural features of autophagia and are composed of whorls of membranous material and myelin figures as well as amorphous debris. These autophagic vacuoles are not specific for inclusion body myositis

and can also be seen in myopathies related to chloroquine,[132] colchicine,[136] vincristine,[41] acid maltase deficiency,[65] hypokalemic periodic paralysis, and oculopharyngeal muscular dystrophy.[225] In these disorders, however, the autophagic vacuoles do not have the associated filaments characteristic of inclusion body myositis. Additional studies demonstrate that vacuolated muscle fibers in inclusion body myositis contain strong ubiquitin immunoreactivity that by immunoelectronmicroscopy colocalizes to the cytoplasmic tubulofilaments.[5a,5b] The vacuolated fibers also contain immunoreactive inclusions positive for β-amyloid protein.[5c] By immunogold electronmicroscopy, β-amyloid protein localizes to clusters of loosely packed amyloid-like fibrils 6 to 8 nm in diameter. The significance of β-amyloid protein accumulation in a muscle disease, similar to that seen in Alzheimer's disease, Down's syndrome, and Dutch-type hereditary cerebrovascular amyloidosis, is not known.

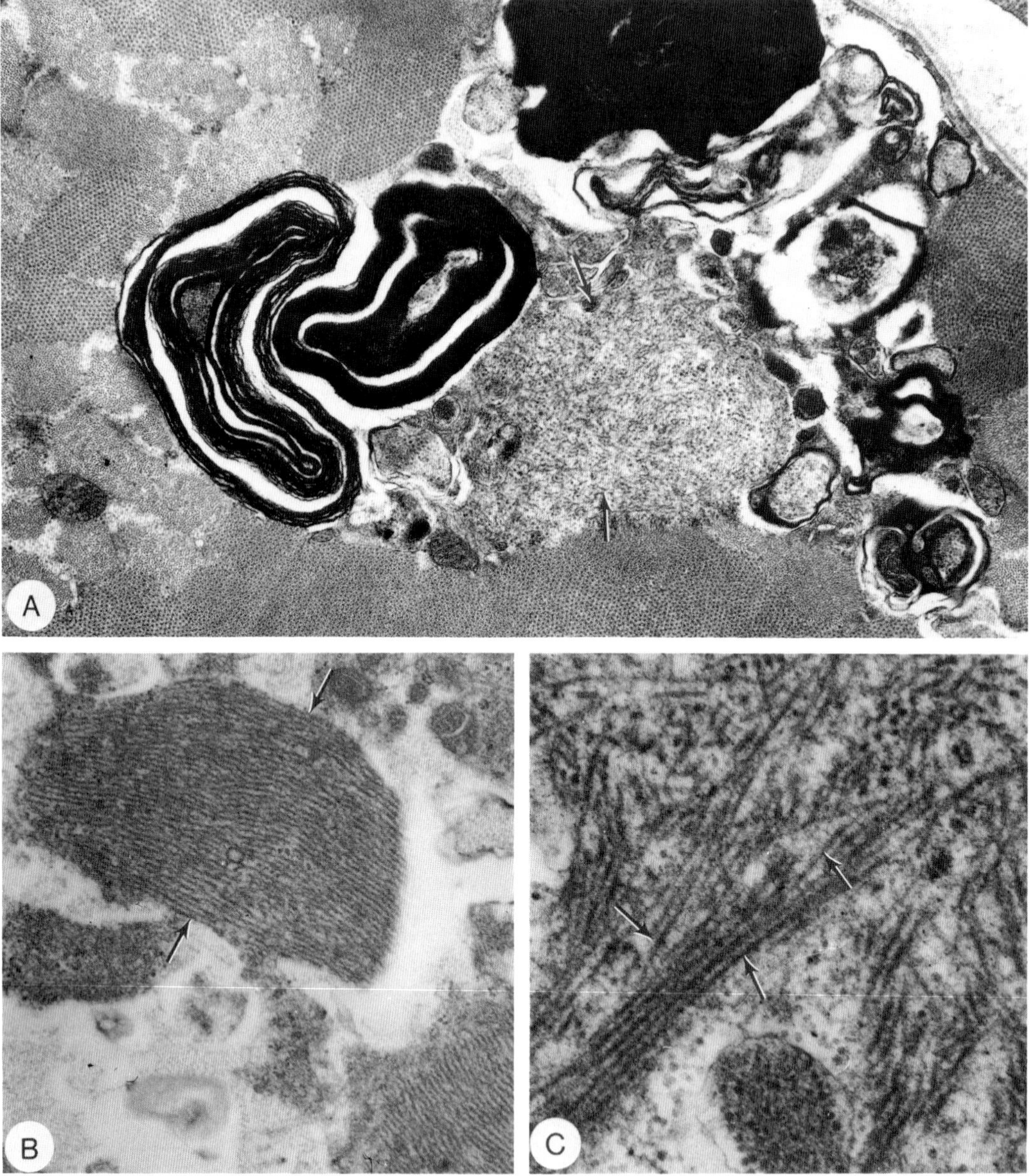

Figure 5–12. Electron micrograph of muscle fibers in inclusion body myositis. (*A*) Autophagic vacuole in a subsarcolemmal location showing a bundle of 15- to 18-nm filaments at the periphery of the vacuole (*arrows*). (*B*) Bundle of parallel 15- to 18-nm filaments (*arrows*). (*C*) Less compact array of 15- to 18-nm filaments (*arrows*).

Treatment

No effective therapy has been found for inclusion body myositis.[130] Modest transient improvement has been reported with corticosteroids, but a sustained response is lacking.[44] Patient numbers have been too small to assess the use of other immunosuppressive drugs alone or in combination with prednisone, but trials of azathioprine, cyclophosphamide, nitrogen mustard, cyclosporine, and plasma exchange have all been unsuccessful. No beneficial effect was observed following total body irradiation.[110] A preliminary report has suggested that intravenous immune globulin improves strength,[213] and controlled trials are under way.

Progression of the disease often leads to significant disability. The weakness of knee extensors predisposes patients to sudden falls. Long leg braces are generally not appropriate for this older group of patients, but the use of a cane, and for some patients, knee orthoses, may be helpful. In addition, ankle-foot orthoses may be used for ankle dorsiflexor weakness. Although most patients remain ambulatory, many benefit from use of a wheelchair or three-wheeled, motorized vehicle, particularly for long distances.

Pathogenesis

The cause of inclusion body myositis remains unknown. The significance of the filamentous inclusions is a subject of debate. Since the earliest observation of filaments by Chou in 1967,[39] a possible relation to myxovirus has been suggested. Antibody reactivity to mumps virus antigens has been shown in the area of the rimmed vacuoles.[40] Unfortunately the specificity for mumps antibody has not been confirmed.[160,179]

The inflammatory infiltrate parallels that seen in polymyositis and is characterized by invasion of nonnecrotic muscle fibers by CD8+ cytotoxic/suppressor T cells, suggesting an immune-mediated component.[2,67] Nevertheless, ascribing a primary or secondary role to the inflammation remains difficult. In addition, the inflammatory infiltrate varies significantly between cases, ranging from mild to florid.

Recently, a hereditary component has been suggested by the appearance of inclusion body myositis in families. A multigeneration family supported an autosomal dominant inheritance,[14] and in a sibship affecting five of six brothers, the muscle disease was associated with a periventricular leukoencephalopathy.[45] The inherited cases also demonstrate the Congo red positive inclusions,[144b] strong ubiquitin immunoreactivity,[5a,5b] and β-amyloid positive protein.[5c] Elucidation of these genetic factors will be important.

Case History

A 69-year-old retired personnel manager had a 20-month history of progressive, painless leg weakness that began during a flulike illness. Gradually he became unable to rise from a squat and to climb and descend stairs. Later his grip strength decreased. The patient had consumed alcoholic beverages containing a minimum of 90 mL ethanol (8 oz of hard liquor) daily for many years. No rash or dysphagia were noted, and cardiac and pulmonary function appeared normal. Examination showed normal cranial and bulbar strength, deltoid 5/5, biceps 4−/4−, wrist extensors 5/5, wrist flexors 4−/4−, iliopsoas 4/4, quadriceps 4/4, anterior tibialis 4/4, gastrocnemius 5/5. There was atrophy of proximal muscles and of wrist flexors and anterior tibial muscles. Sensation and reflexes were normal. The CK level was increased twofold to threefold and EMG showed numerous fibrillations and positive sharp waves as well as increased recruitment of small-amplitude, short-duration motor unit potentials.

The muscle biopsy showed widespread evidence of an active inflammatory myopathy, with necrotic fibers surrounded by inflammatory cells and with numerous perivascular collections of lymphocytes and macrophages. The patient discontinued alcohol intake for 6 months, but the weakness progressed. A 6-month trial of daily corticosteroids alone, followed by addition of azathioprine for more than 1 year did not improve strength. A repeat muscle biopsy again showed findings of active myopathy with the additional features typical of inclusion body myositis (see Figs. 5–10 to 5–12). Review of his earlier biopsy disclosed rare muscle fibers with rimmed vacuoles that had been overlooked. The patient remains ambulatory despite slow progression of weakness during 5 years. Pulmonary and cardiac function have been maintained.

Comment: The features of this patient's weakness were typical of inclusion body myositis. Both distal and proximal weakness were present. The lack of response to treatment prompted repeat studies leading to the diagnosis. Many patients with inflammatory myopathies that fail to respond to corticosteroids have inclusion body myositis. The initial biopsy may lack the distinctive biopsy findings of inclusion body myositis, which are more apparent on repeat sampling of muscle. In several reports, patients had a history of heavy alcohol use but did not improve with abstinence.

MYOPATHIES ASSOCIATED WITH OTHER CONNECTIVE-TISSUE DISEASES

Inflammatory myopathies rarely complicate other well-defined connective-tissue diseases. It is the exceptional patient with systemic lupus erythematosus, rheumatoid arthritis, or progressive systemic sclerosis who has inflammation of the muscle as an important component of the disease. Nevertheless, *overlap syndromes* do occur, in which two well-defined connective-tissue diseases affect the same patient. For example, a patient may have systemic lupus erythematosus and polymyositis or dermatomyositis. To clarify whether the diseases coexist by coincidence, each disorder must be evaluated using the respective American Rheumatologic Association Criteria.

Mixed Connective-Tissue Disease

A separate disorder referred to as *mixed connective-tissue disease* (MCTD), originally described and defined by Sharp and colleagues in 1972,[199] must be distinguished from overlap syndromes. MCTD has features of several connective-tissue diseases but does not fulfill their independent criteria. It has some features of systemic lupus erythematosus, progressive systemic sclerosis, polymyositis, and rheumatoid arthritis and is defined by the presence of high serum titers of antibody to ribonucleoprotein (RNP).

The original definition of MCTD has been challenged because the overlapping features of systemic lupus erythematosus, progressive systemic sclerosis, polymyositis, and rheumatoid arthritis may not all occur concurrently, and antibody to RNP can be seen in other conditions. Nonetheless, sufficient clinical and laboratory data exist to support the existence of MCTD as a distinct condition.

CLINICAL FEATURES

The inflammatory myopathy of MCTD presents with muscle weakness indistinguishable from isolated forms of polymyositis and dermatomyositis. Neck flexor and proximal limb weakness are predominant, and dysphagia with esophageal dysmotility may occur in some patients. Associated findings, however, distinguish MCTD from other inflammatory myopathies.[18,19,88,164,199] Striking cutaneous manifestations include especially the swollen, sausage-like fingers and sclerodactyly (Fig. 5–13), as well as erythematous patches over the knuckles, periungual telangiectasia, and heliotrope changes over the eyelids similar to dermatomyositis. Distinctive, "squarish" facial telangiectases are frequent (Fig. 5–14). Alo-

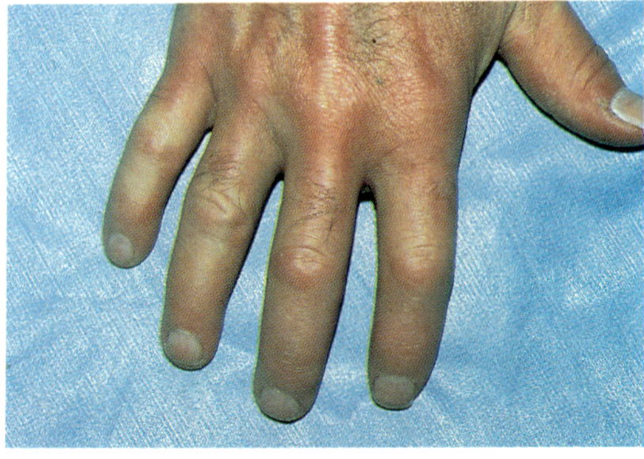

Figure 5–13. Hand of patient with mixed connective tissue disease, showing sausage like fingers and tight skin.

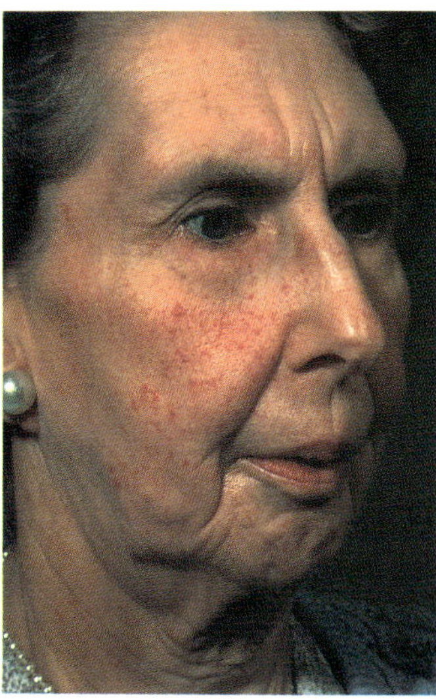

Figure 5–14. Facial telangiectasia in mixed connective tissue disease. The lesions often have a "squarish" shape.

pecia may also be present. Raynaud's phenomenon and nondeforming arthritis are present in most patients. Collectively these features resemble the CREST syndrome (calcinosis, Raynaud's phenomenon, esophageal dysmotility, sclerodactyly, telangiectasia).

Prognosis depends largely on the degree of involvement of major organs. Pulmonary hypertension, a life-threatening complication, results from a primary vascular abnormality caused by intimal proliferation of lung arterioles.[56,234] A few patients with pulmonary hypertension in MCTD have interstitial lung disease.[56,234] Pericarditis is the most common cardiac manifestation, although an inflammatory cardiomyopathy may also develop.[19,199] Renal involvement, especially membranous glomerulonephritis, affects approximately one fourth of patients and can lead to a nephrotic syndrome.[199] Sensory trigeminal neuropathy is a common, disconcerting but not life-threatening complication in MCTD.[5] This neuropathy often develops insidiously but may evolve over a matter of days or a few weeks. The condition involves one or more divisions of the trigeminal nerve, involving all sensory modalities and affecting one or both sides. Pain usually accompanies sensory loss. The complication also occurs with other connective tissue diseases including progressive systemic sclerosis, Sjögren's syndrome, systemic lupus erythematosus, and dermatomyositis.[5,81]

LABORATORY FEATURES

Autoantibodies aid in the diagnosis of MCTD[92,175,223]; high titers of ANA, speckled pattern, and antibody to RNP are characteristic (Table 5–3). These antibodies include those to an ENA, an extractable nuclear antibody. Specialized studies of antibody to RNP demonstrate the antigenic component to be a uridine-rich nucleotide (accounting for the more specific name of U_1RNP).[172] Serum rheumatoid factor is elevated in approximately one half of patients with MCTD.

The CK level is often 10 to 15 times normal, but may not be that elevated. The EMG abnormalities are identical to those seen in polymyositis and dermatomyositis.

The muscle biopsy changes in most cases of MCTD resemble those of dermatomyositis but tend to be more heterogeneous. Preferential perifascicular muscle fiber damage is associated with inflammation in a perimysial and perivascular distribution. Some cases of MCTD have scattered necrotic fibers focally invaded by inflammatory cells, but they do not reach the numbers found in polymyositis or inclusion body myositis. Immunoglobulin (Ig) and complement deposits in the microvasculature occur with less consistency than in dermatomyositis. IgG, IgM, and complement have been reported in muscle fibers and along the sarcolemma.[166] This suggests a primary, immunologically mediated attack directed against muscle fibers, but we have been unable to confirm these findings.

TREATMENT

Treatment of the inflammatory myopathy complicating MCTD should be approached with somewhat different expectations than treatment of dermatomyositis and polymyositis. Complete remission is rarely achieved. Treatment should be initiated with daily prednisone, 1.0 to 1.5 mg/kg, and then switched to an alternate-day regimen as soon as possible (Table 5–4). Suppression of the disease, as measured by increased strength and lower CK levels, is possible but often depends on long-term steroid dependence. The weakness with MCTD is rarely life-threatening, so that prognosis depends more on extramuscular organ system involvement, especially pulmonary, renal, and cardiac manifestations; the extent of this involvement often will determine the treatment strategy. For steroid-resistant cases, cytotoxic agents, including azathioprine or cyclophosphamide, are needed.[99]

PATHOGENESIS

The immunopathogenesis of MCTD remains poorly understood. The presence of anti-RNP antibodies, hypergammaglobulinemia,[19] immune-complex deposits in kidney,[19,207] circulating immune complexes,[51,61,89] and reduced complement levels[19,178] all suggest a role for the humoral immune system. Little direct proof exists, however, and the claims of direct muscle damage by autoantibodies have not been substantiated. The presence of inflammatory infiltrates in other organ systems[19,166] highlights the complexity of the underlying factors.

Progressive Systemic Sclerosis

A majority of patients with progressive systemic sclerosis develop debilitating weakness and fatigue. Most often the weakness results from poor nutrition and disuse rather than inflammation. Nevertheless, an overt inflammatory myopathy, either polymyositis or dermatomyositis, occurs in association with scleroderma in approximately 10%

to 15% of patients,[42,232] who have a true overlap syndrome. The diagnosis of polymyositis or dermatomyositis requires appropriate clinical and laboratory criteria: symmetric proximal muscle weakness, an elevated CK level, EMG features of inflammatory myopathy, and demonstration by muscle biopsy of inflammatory infiltration with focal invasion of muscle fibers. This picture contrasts with the features found in the usual muscle biopsy of scleroderma, in which the inflammatory component is minimal and confined to the perimysial connective tissue; and muscle fiber changes include only fiber size variability and atrophy of type 2 muscle fibers.

Treatment of muscle weakness in scleroderma requires careful attention to nutritional factors and physical therapy to increase range of motion and encourage ambulation. If the disease overlaps with polymyositis or dermatomyositis, then corticosteroid treatment identical to that outlined for the inflammatory myopathy is appropriate (see Table 5–3).

Systemic Lupus Erythematosus

Neuromuscular complications frequently complicate systemic lupus erythematosus and are often multifactorial. Less than 5% of patients have an overlap syndrome with polymyositis or dermatomyositis.[74,100,228] The most frequent causes of weakness in patients with systemic lupus erythematosus are listed on Table 5–7. Joint involvement commonly causes pain, leading in turn to disuse atrophy. The drugs used to treat lupus, including corticosteroids and chloroquine, often cause a myopathy; chloroquine produces a vacuolar myopathy (see p. 374).[132,165]

The laboratory features indicating an overlap syndrome with inflammatory myopathy are those already outlined. The muscle biopsy in systemic lupus erythematosus, when there is no inflammatory myopathy, shows an increased

Table 5–7 CAUSES OF WEAKNESS IN SYSTEMIC LUPUS ERYTHEMATOSUS

Central Nervous System Involvement including Myelopathy

Peripheral Neuropathy
   Inflammatory polyradiculoneuropathy
   Axonal polyneuropathy
   Mononeuritis multiplex

Myopathy
   Inflammatory myopathy
   Disuse atrophy from articular pain
   Medication toxicity: corticosteroids,
     chloroquine

variability in fiber size, particularly associated with atrophy of type 2 muscle fibers.

The approach to treatment for systemic lupus erythematosus overlapping with inflammatory myopathy is identical to that for dermatomyositis and polymyositis (see Table 5–4). Treatment of other neuromuscular manifestations depends on their specific cause.

Rheumatoid Arthritis

Patients with rheumatoid arthritis have many causes for weakness (Table 5–8) and commonly develop neuromuscular complications.[113] Most often, joint pain causes disuse atrophy and muscle weakness. Other common problems include joint involvement in the spine, in which vertebral subluxation damages the spinal cord and nerve roots; and the vasculitis of rheumatoid disease, which can be associated with severe peripheral nerve damage.[63] Occasionally, an overlap syndrome of polymyositis and rheumatoid arthritis may occur. Long-standing rheumatoid arthritis may be associated with a focal nodular myositis.[113] In addition, penicillamine (used to treat the arthritis) may induce an inflammatory myopathy (see p. 375).[154]

Laboratory features may be difficult to interpret in rheumatoid arthritis. The CK level is elevated with any associated inflammatory myopathy. Nerve root and peripheral nerve changes in rheumatoid arthritis are usually readily identified by EMG and nerve conduction studies. EMG screening of proximal muscles may be extremely helpful in identifying a myopathy. Many changes can be seen in the muscle biopsy. Atrophy of type 2 muscle fibers commonly accompanies joint pain, disuse, and corticosteroid treatment (see Fig. 2–44), and atrophy of neurogenic muscle fibers is common. One can diagnose an inflammatory myopathy complicating rheumatoid arthritis only on seeing

Table 5–8 DIFFERENTIAL DIAGNOSIS OF MUSCLE WEAKNESS IN THE PATIENT WITH CHRONIC RHEUMATOID ARTHRITIS

Spinal Cord and Radicular Disease
   Vertebral subluxation
   Odontoid dislocation
   Osteophytic compression of roots
Peripheral Neuropathy
   Inflammatory demyelinating neuropathy
   Axonal polyneuropathy
   Mononeuritis multiplex from nerve infarction
   Toxic: gold-induced
Neuromuscular Junction
   Myasthenia gravis: possibly increased
     frequency
   Penicillamine-induced myasthenia gravis
   Myasthenic syndrome: increased frequency
Myopathy
   Disuse atrophy
   Inflammatory myopathy including focal
     nodular myositis
   Sjögren's syndrome with inflammatory
     myopathy
   Waldenström's hyperglobulinemic purpura
     with inflammatory myopathy
   Toxic
     Corticosteroid atrophy
     Penicillamine — myositis
     Cimetidine — myositis
     Chloroquine — vacuolar myopathy
Coincidental Disease and Overlap Syndromes
   Systemic lupus erythematosus
   Dermatomyositis
   Mixed connective-tissue syndrome
Misdiagnosis (Diseases Resembling Rheumatoid
   Arthritis)
   Amyloidosis
   Cryoglobulinemia, heavy-chain disease, other
     dysglobulinemias
   Sarcoidosis
   Dermatomyositis with active synovitis

mononuclear cell infiltration in the endomysial connective tissue and focal invasion of muscle fibers. Focal nodular myositis produces distinctive changes with large, compact aggregates of mononuclear cells (lymphocytes and plasma cells) in the fascia and perimysial connective tissue.

When muscle weakness complicates rheumatoid arthritis, treatment must be directed specifically toward each possible cause. Clinically significant inflammatory myopathy should be treated with corticosteroids and cytotoxic drugs as needed (see Tables 5–4 and 5–5). Therapeutic regimens must be tailored to each individual and considered in the context of all medications being administered.[34a]

Sjögren's Syndrome

In Sjögren's syndrome, destruction of the lacrimal and salivary glands results in mucosal and conjunctival dryness (sicca syndrome). Primary Sjögren's syndrome occurs in isolation from other diseases; secondary Sjögren's syndrome is associated with other connective tissue disorders, particularly rheumatoid arthritis.

Myalgias or weakness commonly accompany Sjögren's syndrome, but polymyositis or dermatomyositis are infrequent,[170,185] and other processes must be considered in determining whether a myopathy is present. Weakness is often the result of joint pain and disuse atrophy. Peripheral neuropathy may also be present, most commonly a sensory polyneuropathy, often with a severe ataxic component suggesting involvement of the dorsal root ganglia.[82a,124] The systemic vasculitis complicating Sjögren's syndrome may be manifested as a mononeuritis multiplex.[143]

Inflammatory infiltration of the salivary gland, documented by biopsy of the lower lip, provides laboratory confirmation of Sjögren's syndrome. Autoantibodies, especially anti-SS-A (Ro), also are often present in these patients. An elevated CK level, along with EMG and muscle biopsy features typical of inflammatory myopathy, must be found to confirm a diagnosis of polymyositis or dermatomyositis.

A subset of patients with Sjögren's syndrome and myositis also have a distinctive, purpuric rash in dependent portions of the extremities.[185] When this rash accompanies a polyclonal gammopathy, the disorder is termed Waldenström's hyperglobulinemic purpura.[187]

Polyarteritis Nodosa and Other Forms of Systemic Vasculitis

Pain and weakness of the extremities are common in patients with polyarteritis nodosa. Clinical and laboratory findings almost always point to peripheral neuropathy as the cause of symptoms. Muscle biopsy often provides evidence for vasculitis, but widespread muscle necrosis and other features of myositis are usually absent. Some cases reported as "myositis" have not had elevation of the CK level or other evidence to point to myopathy.[72]

Patients with other forms of systemic vasculitis also experience limb pain and weakness (Table 5–9). Muscle biopsy may show evidence of vasculitis, but as in polyarteritis, nerve, not muscle, is usually the primary site of the lesion; however, muscle biopsy is often as use-

Table 5–9 SYSTEMIC DISEASES CHARACTERIZED BY VASCULITIS OF MUSCLE AND NERVE

Polyarteritis nodosa
Churg-Strauss syndrome
Wegener's granulomatosis
Rheumatoid vasculitis
Henoch-Schönlein purpura
Cryoglobulinemia
Angiitis related to methamphetamine, cocaine, and other recreational drugs
Takayasu's disease (rare)
Giant-cell arteritis (rare)

ful as nerve biopsy to establish the diagnosis of vasculitis. A random muscle biopsy will not be as productive as one guided by EMG abnormalities. The peroneus brevis muscle represents a biopsy site with a proven high yield for diagnosis of vasculitis.[117a]

Behçet's Syndrome

Adults and children with Behçet's syndrome can develop limb pain and swelling attributable to myositis.[3] Most patients present with a painful calf or thigh rather than muscle weakness.[124a] Thrombophlebitis and cutaneous vasculitis are much more common features of Behçet's syndrome than muscle weakness and must be excluded as a cause of limb pain before diagnosing myositis.

GIANT-CELL AND GRANULOMATOUS MYOSITIS

Giant-Cell Myositis

Giant-cell myositis can be identified in a small proportion of patients whose clinical picture resembles polymyositis. Muscle biopsy reveals granuloma formation. The inflammatory process usually includes giant cells (Fig. 5–15).

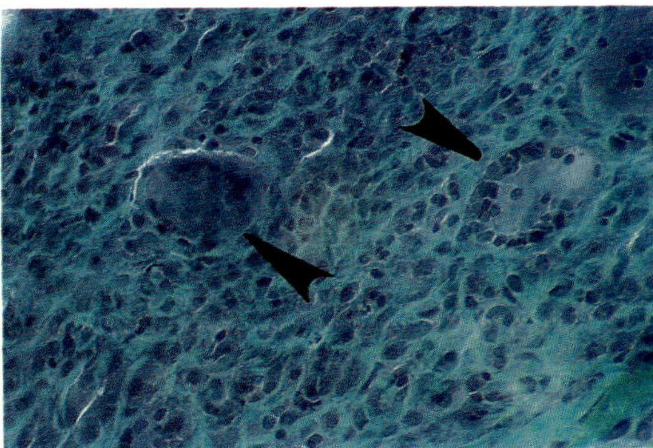

Figure 5–15. Giant cell myositis and thymoma. Muscle biopsy shows inflammation with giant cells (*arrowheads*) (modified trichrome).

Some of these patients have evidence for sarcoidosis, but in others no underlying diagnosis can be established.

Rare patients with myasthenia gravis and thymoma may develop severe giant-cell myositis and myocarditis.[158] The pathogenesis of this disorder is unknown. Thymectomy and prednisone treatment may be beneficial.

Sarcoidosis

Sarcoidosis may present as progressive weakness from an inflammatory myopathy without other features of typical sarcoidosis.[204] In addition, muscle involvement is common in biopsies of patients with sarcoidosis who have no muscular symptoms.[204,220] Muscle biopsy shows characteristic noncaseating granulomas in 20% to 70% of patients.[220]

FOCAL MYOSITIS

Sarcoidosis can occasionally present with localized masses in muscle.[204] These masses are often not tender and occur either singly or in small numbers in various limb muscles.[204] Lesions are common in biceps or gastrocnemius muscles and can result in pseudohypertrophy.[138] Histologically, the lesions consist of inflammatory cells with noncaseating granulomas (Fig. 5–16), and they can occur at any time during the course of the disease. Lesions improve with corticosteroids, but since they frequently produce few symptoms, treatment is usually dictated by other symptoms of sarcoidosis.

ASSOCIATION WITH DERMATOMYOSITIS

A rash highly suggestive of dermatomyositis was noted in a patient with sarcoidosis,[101] and more recently, a patient with all the cardinal manifestations of dermatomyositis was found also to have sarcoidosis. Whether the two disorders were coincidental is unclear.[129] An association between sar-

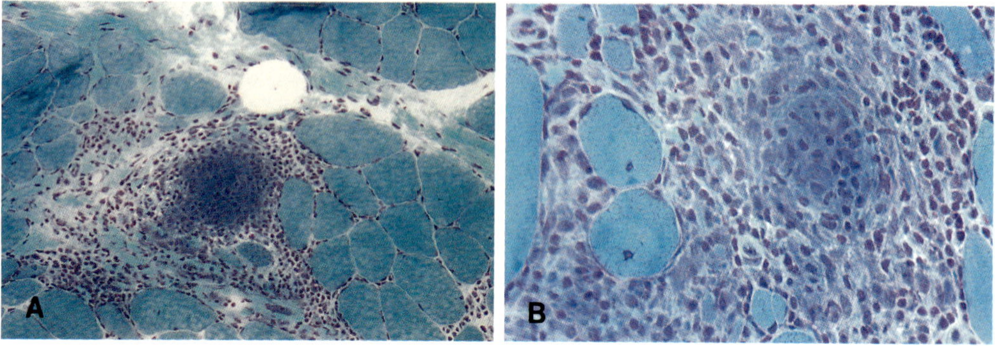

Figure 5–16. Sarcoid myopathy. Noncaseating granulomas at low (*A*) and high (*B*) magnifications (modified trichrome).

coid and other connective tissue disorders has been postulated.[144]

Case History

A 68-year-old woman developed progressive weakness approximately 6 to 8 weeks before admission. Weakness caused difficulty in arising from chairs and climbing stairs. Her muscles ached. She lost 20 lb but did not complain of diplopia, dysphagia, or dysarthria. Her medical history was significant for a thyroid goiter.

Examination demonstrated normal function of cranial nerve musculature. She had marked weakness of neck flexors and extensors, so that she could not raise her head against gravity, and she displayed similar weakness of the proximal arm and leg muscles, with a lesser degree of distal weakness. Muscle stretch reflexes were intact, as was the sensory exam.

The CK level was 2675 μg/L (normal < 215), sedimentation rate 72, ANA 1:320 diffuse pattern. The titer of acetylcholine receptor antibody was markedly elevated. CT showed a noninvasive tumor of the thymus in the anterior mediastinum.

Repetitive nerve stimulation did not reveal a decrementing response in the limbs or facial muscles. Attempts to improve strength with edrophonium were negative. Biopsy of the left biceps showed the invasion of nonnecrotic muscle fibers by mononuclear cells typical of polymyositis. A striking focal collection of mononuclear cells was also found, with scattered giant cells (see Fig. 5–15).

The patient was treated with high-dose prednisone, 100 mg daily. She initially worsened for approximately 2 weeks but then improved. Over many months she made a complete recovery. Her CK levels returned to normal. There were never any overt signs of myasthenia gravis. The titer of acetylcholine receptor antibody decreased, but she still had elevated titers (about ¼ the original level) after 1.5 years. Interestingly, the thymic mass gradually resolved on repeat CT scans without surgical removal.

Comment: Recognition of giant-cell myositis and thymoma has important implications for treatment.[158] Many patients have an associated myocarditis that can result in heart failure and arrhythmias. Others, unlike this patient, display overt symptoms of myasthenia gravis at some time. The resolution of this patient's thymic mass is of interest. No other reported cases have had spontaneous or steroid-induced thymic involution, which suggests that this thymic tumor was, in fact, benign thymic hyperplasia.

Inflammatory Bowel Disease

A granulomatous myositis has been reported in occasional patients with Crohn's disease. Sulfasalazine has produced a rapid improvement in muscle symptoms and a reduction in the CK level, supporting a causal rather than coincidental relationship between the disorders. Myositis is clearly rare, however, because one large series of 700 patients did not identify muscle disease in any patient.[85] Vasculitis has also been observed in the muscle of patients with Crohn's disease.[78]

Myositis is also a rare complication of patients with ulcerative colitis. Weakness in patients with inflammatory bowel disease is multifactorial, however, and corticosteroids used in severe cases of ulcerative colitis as well as in Crohn's disease can lead to steroid myopathy. Severely ill patients with both disorders also develop muscle wasting because of whole-body protein catabolism caused by the underlying disease.

EOSINOPHILIC SYNDROMES AND MYOSITIS

Eosinophilic syndromes associated with myositis are important causes of muscle pain and weakness.

Eosinophilic Polymyositis

Eosinophilic polymyositis usually occurs as part of the hypereosinophilic syndrome (HES),[71,125,216] a disorder of unknown cause. The syndrome is defined by persistent eosinophilia, with 1500 eosinophils/mm^3 for at least 6 months, or death within 6 months of onset; no evidence of parasitic, allergic, or other known causes of eosinophilia; and organ system dysfunction directly related to eosinophilia. Cardiac and neurologic manifestations are frequent, but polymyositis associated with HES is rare.[71]

CLINICAL FEATURES

Eosinophilic polymyositis causes muscle pain and varying degrees of proximal weakness. The muscle manifestations may be obscured by other neurologic complications, including cerebral infarction, diffuse encephalopathy, and peripheral neuropathy.[71] Eosinophilic polymyositis associated with HES carries a poor prognosis for long-

term survival. Cardiac complications cause many deaths, especially endocardial thrombosis, which predisposes to systemic embolization. Other cardiac manifestations include congestive heart failure, valvular disease, and arrhythmias. Pulmonary (fibrosis and bronchial asthma), gastrointestinal, and renal involvement also cause significant morbidity. Skin manifestations include generalized petechial rash, nailbed hemorrhages, and Raynaud's phenomenon.[71]

LABORATORY FEATURES

Varying degrees of hypereosinophilia, elevated sedimentation rate, hypergammaglobulinemia, and anemia are present in HES.[71] A mildly elevated CK and a myopathic EMG accompany the inflammatory myopathy.

The muscle biopsy findings simulate idiopathic polymyositis, but eosinophils make up a greater percentage of the infiltrating cells. Endomysial inflammation with focal muscle fiber invasion occurs in addition to the perivascular and perimysial infiltrate. Nodular granulomas, similar to the extravascular lesions described in Churg-Strauss syndrome, are often present.

TREATMENT

Despite the poor prognosis for polymyositis associated with HES, a very aggressive approach to treatment has been advocated, with claims of increased survival.[71,169] Treatment consists of prednisone, 1 mg/kg per day, switching to alternate-day therapy with signs of improvement. In refractory cases, hydroxyurea (0.5–1.5 g/d) has been added to maintain a leukocyte count less than 10,000/mm^3. Leukapheresis has also been used in patients with very high eosinophil counts. Aggressive medical and surgical management of cardiac complications improves survival. Included are treatment of congestive heart failure, systemic anticoagulation, and replacement of damaged heart valves when appropriate.[71]

DIFFERENTIAL DIAGNOSIS

Two uncommon disorders, *focal eosinophilic myositis*[1,208,237] and *eosinophilic perimyositis*,[121,197] have symptoms that overlap those of eosinophilic polymyositis. Muscle tenderness and pain, but not weakness, occur in both conditions. Localized areas of swelling may be seen in focal eosinophilic myositis. Usually these two disorders have no associated systemic manifestations, and their favorable prognosis contrasts dramatically with that of eosinophilic polymyositis. Asthma, however, has been associated with eosinophilic perimyositis.[197]

Laboratory findings in focal eosinophilic myositis and eosinophilic perimyositis overlap with other syndromes associated with myositis and eosinophilia: elevations of ESR and CK levels and peripheral blood eosinophilia. The muscle biopsy in focal eosinophilic myositis shows varying degrees of muscle fiber necrosis, with inflammation evidenced by the presence of mononuclear cells, plasma cells, and eosinophils. In eosinophilic perimyositis, the inflammatory infiltrate is confined to the perimysial connective tissue.

Both of these disorders have been reported to be self-limiting, but they may recur.[197] It is worth noting that one case of eosinophilic perimyositis[121] was associated with tryptophan ingestion (see below).[93] Some patients may need corticosteroid treatment, but it should be used sparingly because most cases resolve spontaneously.

PATHOGENESIS

Neither the mechanisms of tissue damage nor the stimulus for eosinophilia in these eosinophilic syndromes have been elucidated. The number of infiltrating eosinophils varies considerably and does not account for all of the observed tissue damage. Nevertheless, the tissue-damaging potential of the eosinophil has been well documented,[79] especially the eosinophil-granule major basic protein and eosinophil-derived neurotoxin, both found as components of the eosinophilic granules.[79]

Diffuse Fasciitis with Eosinophilia (Shulman's Syndrome)

The names *diffuse fasciitis with eosinophilia, eosinophilic fasciitis*, and *Shulman's syndrome* (acknowledging the author of the initial four cases), refer to the same disorder, which is characterized by fascial thickening and inflammation.[75,122,156a,189,201]

CLINICAL FEATURES

The condition affects men and women of all ages, but most often those between the ages 40 and 60. Edema of the extremities may be the initial symptom, although patients usually come to medical attention because of muscle pain and tenderness. Joint contractures, especially involving the elbows and wrists, may be prominent. Cutaneous manifestations include pitting edema, induration, and dimpling (so-called *peau d'orange*, or "skin like an orange," resembling that seen in infiltrating breast cancer). In contrast to progressive systemic sclerosis, the epidermis in diffuse fasciitis is neither thickened nor bound down, and Raynaud's phenomenon is absent. Localized morphea (circumscribed sclerosis of skin) has been observed in diffuse fasciitis.[122]

Proximal muscles may be weakened to varying degrees, but pain and tenderness make strength quantitation difficult. Polyarthritis and synovitis add to patient discomfort. The kidneys, lungs, and heart are not involved, but various rheumatologic disorders may occur.[189] A disproportionately high percentage of patients develop aplastic anemia.[22,97,202] Other hematologic complications include thrombocytopenic purpura,[231] myeloid leukemia,[148] myeloproliferative disorders,[148] preleukemia,[111] and Hodgkin's disease.[147]

LABORATORY FEATURES

Peripheral eosinophilia, hypergammaglobulinemia, and an elevated erythrocyte sedimentation rate are common but are not essential for diagnosis. In fact, eosinophilia occurs in about two thirds of patients.[122] The CK level is usually normal or mildly elevated. EMG may show a mild reduction in the size and amplitude of motor unit potentials; muscle membrane irritability is confined to superficial muscle layers just beneath the fascia. During the EMG examination, the electromyographer will often notice the thickened fascia, and patients will complain of pain because of inflammation in the fascial layers.

The diagnosis depends on a full-thickness biopsy extending from skin to muscle, to demonstrate that inflammation is mostly restricted to fascia. Although this aggressive tissue sampling has advantages, the effects may be disfiguring because of slow healing and possible infection in patients treated with immunosuppressive drugs. When the clinical features strongly favor diffuse fasciitis, an open biopsy of muscle and overlapping fascia may be preferable. Histologic sections reveal thickened fascia infiltrated by inflammatory cells, including mononuclear cells, plasma cells, and eosinophils (Fig. 5–17). Damage to the superficial layer of muscle fibers and perimysial connective tissue immediately adjacent to the fascia is common.

TREATMENT

According to Shulman, diffuse fasciitis had a more favorable prognosis than progressive systemic sclerosis.[201] Additional experience, however, has indicated a less satisfactory outcome for some patients.[122] Diffuse fasciitis should be treated with a single, daily dose of prednisone, 1.0 to 1.5 mg/kg, with change to an alternate-day schedule as soon as possible and subsequent slow tapering (see Table 5–4). For patients refractory to corticosteroids, other immunosuppressive drugs have been used, including azathioprine and hydroxychloroquine.[122] In one patient with persistent thrombocytopenia and diffuse fasciitis, prednisone in combination with cyclosporine achieved a favorable outcome. Controlled treatment trials or even data from large numbers of patients with Shulman's syndrome have not been reported and will be difficult to obtain because of the relatively small number of patients affected.

PATHOGENESIS

The cause of diffuse fasciitis with eosinophilia remains unknown. The condition does not appear to be a variant of

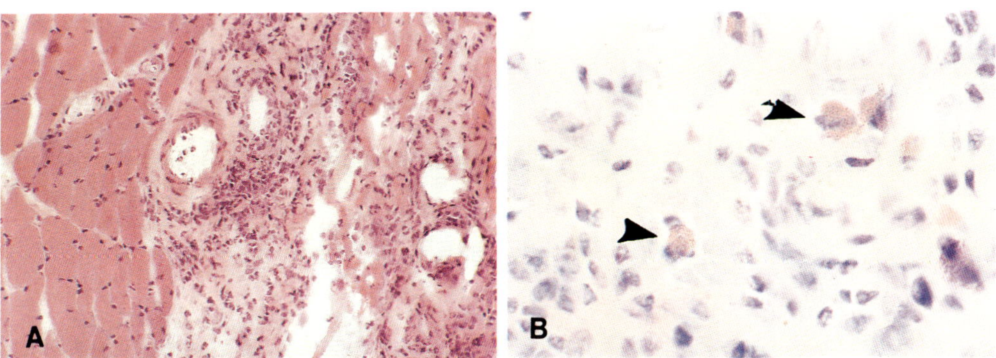

Figure 5–17. Diffuse fasciitis. (*A*) The layer of connective tissue overlying the muscle, usually very thin, is markedly thickened by fibrous tissue (H&E). (*B*) The inflammation is composed of mononuclear cells and scattered eosinophils (*arrowheads*) (Wright's stain).

scleroderma. Suggestions by Shulman and others of a relationship between diffuse fasciitis and exercise have not been substantiated.[201]

Several findings suggest an immune pathogenesis. While IgG, IgM, and C3 deposits have been observed in the fascia, this finding is not consistent.[75] Antiplatelet antibodies have been identified in some patients with combined fasciitis and thrombocytopenia.[231] In one case associated with aplastic anemia, an IgG serum fraction inhibited growth of erythroid and granulocytic progenitor cells.[96] Additional work is required to clarify the pathogenesis of this disorder.

Case History

A 47-year-old farmer had a 6-week history of elevated afternoon temperatures (100°F–101°F) accompanied by muscle aching and difficulty in walking and bending because of swollen, stiff, and painful extremities. His mother died of myasthenia gravis at age 40.

Physical examination demonstrated swollen arms and legs and tenderness of muscles in all extremities. Manual muscle strength testing was normal. Muscle stretch reflexes and sensory examination were normal.

On laboratory study the white blood cell (WBC) count was $4300/mm^3$, with 54% segmented neutrophils, 24% lymphocytes, 5% monocytes, and 17% eosinophils. The total eosinophil count was $1214/mm^3$ (normal $0–450/mm^3$), hemoglobin 12.3 g/dL, hematocrit 35%, platelets $44,000/mm^3$; Westergren ESR was 26; serum immunoelectrophoresis showed slight polyclonal hypergammaglobulinemia; the CK level was 14; and trichinosis serologic tests were negative. Bone marrow examination revealed a decrease in megakaryocytes but normal myeloid and erythroid series. Eosinophils were increased.

Muscle biopsy of the quadriceps muscle included overlying fascia. The fascia was infiltrated with mononuclear inflammatory cells and eosinophils (see Fig. 5–17). This inflammatory response extended into the superficial perimysial connective tissue, but the endomysium was free of infiltrate. No muscle fiber abnormalities were present.

A diagnosis of eosinophilic fasciitis (Shulman's syndrome) was established on the basis of clinical and histologic changes. The patient was treated with a high-dose prednisone, beginning with 100 mg daily. Within 3 months the myalgias and muscle swelling disappeared. During this time, however, he developed more severe thrombocytopenia (as low as $3000/mm^3$), and required repeated platelet transfusions. Erythroid and myeloid cells were also depressed, and at their nadir hemoglobin reached a level of 7.0 g/dL and the WBC count was $3.3/mm^3$. Because of persistent thrombocytopenia, the patient was maintained on prednisone therapy, to which cyclosporine was added (originally 10 mg/kg per day, followed by maintenance at 6 mg/kg per day). On this regimen, platelets increased to between 50,000 and $60,000/mm^3$, and platelet transfusions were no longer required. After 3 years of treatment, the doses of immunosuppressive therapy were gradually lowered, but occasional red blood cell and platelet transfusions were still required. The fasciitis remained in remission.

Comment: This patient presented with the characteristic features of eosinophilic fasciitis: limb pain and swelling, normal strength (although strength testing is often difficult to perform if patients have pain); and laboratory findings of elevated ESR, hypergammaglobulinemia, and anemia. Eosinophilia, present in this patient, may be absent, but tissue eosinophilic infiltration is always present. The response to corticosteroids is typical. The association with hematologic disorders is well described, especially aplastic anemia. More selective, persistent thrombocytopenia, as observed in this patient, is more unusual. The response to immunosuppressive therapy, including faciitis and hematologic features, suggests an immune-mediated pathogenesis for both conditions. In fact, antiplatelet antibodies have been described in this condition.[231]

Eosinophilia-Myalgia Syndrome Associated with Tryptophan

The eosinophilia-myalgia syndrome associated with ingestion of tryptophan is a newly recognized disorder related to a chemical contaminant of the manufacturing process.[17,68,93,191,209] Careful epidemiologic case surveillance methods conducted by regional (The New Mexico State Health Department) and national (Center for Disease Control) health agencies led to recognition of this syndrome in 1989.[68]

CLINICAL FEATURES

All patients with the eosinophilia-myalgia syndrome have muscle pain and tenderness, with a subacute onset, evolving over several weeks. The myalgia may be incapacitating and accompanied by varying degrees of muscle weakness and fatigue. Other manifestations, which may be more fleeting, include an erythematous rash (maculopapular, vesicular, or urticarial), mucocutaneous ulcers, abdominal pain, and dyspnea on exertion. A peripheral neuropathy occurs in some patients and may be the presenting symptom.[209] Distal weakness, loss of muscle stretch reflexes, and a "stocking-glove" sensory loss alert the clinician to peripheral nerve involvement. A generalized polyneuropathy, simulating Guillain-Barré syndrome, can lead to respiratory insufficiency.[209]

LABORATORY FEATURES

The majority of patients have an absolute eosinophil count exceeding 2000/mm^3. The CK level may be elevated. The ESR is usually normal, and autoantibodies are absent, providing evidence against an underlying connective tissue disease.

Electrodiagnostic studies can be confusing. Needle EMG examination may show membrane irritability and myopathic motor unit potentials, but large, long-duration motor unit potentials typical of neurogenic disease may also be present. Normal or mildly reduced nerve conduction velocities with low-amplitude evoked potentials accompany the peripheral neuropathy and favor axonal rather than demyelinating disease.[209]

Biopsies of affected tissues show eosinophilic infiltration accompanied by other mononuclear cells in muscle, nerve, and other organ systems. In muscle specimens, inflammation remains predominantly in the fascia and perimysial connective tissue and is similar to that seen in diffuse fasciitis with eosinophilia (see Fig. 5-17).

TREATMENT

High doses of corticosteroids have been used to treat most patients. The regimen outlined for polymyositis and dermatomyositis is usually effective (see Table 5-4), but relapses often occur after steroid withdrawal. Some fatal cases have been unresponsive to all treatment. No long-term follow-up studies are available.

PATHOGENESIS

Use of tryptophan as an over-the-counter dietary supplement became popular for insomnia, premenstrual syndrome, and depression. Case surveillance studies demonstrated that the eosinophilia-myalgia syndrome occurring in 1989 was the result of tryptophan manufactured by a single company (Showa Denko K.K.).[17] High-pressure liquid chromatography analysis of tryptophan samples from patients with eosinophilia-myalgia syndrome revealed that a chemical contaminant, identified as peak E, was strongly associated with the outbreak.[17] Further testing identified the chemical structure of peak E as a compound synthesized from L-tryptophan and acetaldehyde.[191]

The mechanism of tissue damage remains unclear. Unexplained features of the outbreak include the long latency reported by some patients following the ingestion of tryptophan (weeks to years) and the persistence of symptoms long after the drug has been stopped. The nature of the inflammatory infiltrate suggests an allergic or autoimmune phenomenon. Both eosinophil-granule major basic protein and eosinophil-derived neurotoxin have been identified in tissue samples, serum, and urine of affected patients,[93] but their precise role is still obscure.

Toxic-Oil Syndrome

Toxic-oil syndrome has remarkable similarities to the eosinophilia-myalgia syndrome associated with tryptophan.[112,227] This condition was related to the ingestion of denatured rapeseed oil used as a substitute for olive oil. The toxic-oil syndrome reached epidemic proportions, affecting approximately 20,000 people and causing more than 300 deaths. The outbreak was restricted to Spain, particularly around Madrid, and has not recurred since 1981. Nevertheless, because both this syndrome and the similar eosinophilia-myalgia syndrome were reported within less than a decade, we will review the clinical data because other, similar syndromes may occur in the future.

CLINICAL FEATURES

The clinical picture of toxic-oil syndrome involved several well-defined phases of evolution. Myalgia, muscle weakness, and anorexia were seen throughout the course of the illness. During the first week, patients developed fever, headache, skin exanthems, cough, and dyspnea. Chest radiographs showed pulmonary infiltrates and in some cases effusion. During the second week, patients developed gastrointestinal symptoms: abdominal pain, nausea, vomiting, and diarrhea, with hepatomegaly in some patients. Peripheral blood eosinophilia developed during this second phase. After 2 months, and especially in the third month, a more profound neuromuscular syndrome developed, in which myalgias intensified and distal muscle weakness became generalized, including the respiratory muscles of some patients. Patients developed paresthesias, loss of muscle stretch reflexes, and joint contractures. Pulmonary hypertension contributed to

morbidity and mortality, as did a susceptibility to thromboembolic disease to many organs, including the brain. About 10% of patients were left with residual skin lesions similar to progressive systemic sclerosis, Raynaud's phenomenon, sicca syndrome, and dysphagia.

In some cases the disorder was self-limiting, but severe early manifestations were predictive of a worse outcome. More females were seriously affected than males.

LABORATORY FEATURES

The CK level was normal but liver enzyme, bilirubin, alkaline phosphatase, ANA, IgE levels, and ESR were all elevated. Peripheral blood eosinophilia occurred in nearly all patients after the second week, and many also developed thrombocytopenia.

The EMG was often normal early in the course of the illness but later showed fibrillation potentials, positive sharp waves, and reduced recruitment of enlarged motor unit potentials. Small sensory and motor evoked potentials, along with normal or mildly reduced nerve conduction velocities, all suggested an axonal neuropathy. The muscle biopsy contained mononuclear cell inflammation in the fascia, perimysial connective tissue, and the perivascular space, with occasional fibers undergoing necrosis.[137] Sural nerve biopsy showed mononuclear infiltration in the epineurial and perineurial connective tissue, associated with nerve fiber loss. Samples of tissues taken at biopsy or autopsy from many organ systems showed a nonnecrotizing vasculitis involving the intima and affecting blood vessels of every type and size.[137]

TREATMENT

No specific treatment was found for the toxic-oil syndrome. Fortunately the epidemic resolved spontaneously and no subsequent cases have appeared.

PATHOGENESIS

The association with the ingestion of illegally marketed cooking oil containing a high proportion of rapeseed oil was well documented.[112,227] Nevertheless, the exact contaminant was never uncovered, and an association between the extent of exposure and the outcome was never established. The lack of a clear dose-response relationship is also true for the eosinophilia-myalgia syndrome associated with tryptophan.

MYOSITIS AND MYOPATHIES CAUSED BY INFECTIOUS AGENTS

Viral Infections

HIV-1

An inflammatory myopathy occurs in patients with HIV-1 infection,[9,54,150,161] and the histologic and other laboratory features suggest that three or more different types of myopathy may be present (Table 5–10). Because the histology of all three forms often overlaps, it is not certain that they are distinct disorders. In addition, patients with HIV-1 infection are subject to other neurologic disorders that may be present simultaneously with myopathy or closely resemble it (Table 5–11).[47,128] Particu-

Table 5–10 MYOPATHY IN PATIENTS WITH HIV-1 INFECTION

Cachexia from Inanition, Malignancy, Immobility
Opportunistic Infections
  Mycobacteria
  Pyomyositis
  Other (parasitic, etc.)
Inflammatory Myopathy
Nemaline Myopathy
Necrotizing Myopathy
Mixed Forms
Toxic
  Zidovudine toxicity
  Vinca alkaloids
  Ranitidine

Table 5–11 NEUROLOGIC MANIFESTATIONS OF HIV-1 INFECTION

Central Nervous System
  Opportunistic infections
  Lymphomas and other malignancies
  Acute HIV-1 meningoencephalitis
  AIDS dementia (HIV-1 encephalitis)
  Subacute combined degeneration (B_{12} deficiency)
  Vacuolar myelopathy
Neuromuscular Disease
  Neuropathy
    Chronic inflammatory demyelinating polyneuropathy
  Mononeuropathy multiplex
    Distal symmetric sensorimotor neuropathy
    Polyradiculopathy — infectious (e.g., cytomegalovirus)
            — neoplastic
Myopathy (see Table 5–10)

larly important in differential diagnosis are the peripheral neuropathies, especially chronic inflammatory demyelinating polyradiculoneuropathy, which may present with proximal weakness suggesting a myopathy.[47,151]

Clinical Features. The most characteristic HIV-1-related myopathy is an inflammatory myopathy that on biopsy is often associated with nemaline rods.[9,53,54,80,161] Typically the patient is in the early stage of HIV-1 infection, and indeed, this condition can be the earliest manifestation of HIV disease. Patients develop progressive, painless, proximal weakness with a predilection for shoulder-girdle musculature. Respiratory muscles are typically spared, and dysphagia is infrequent.[205] There is no rash or any other evidence for dermatomyositis. Hyporeflexia is usual unless there is accompanying central nervous system (CNS) disease. Sensory symptoms such as pain, cramps, or paresthesias point to an additional central or peripheral nervous system abnormality.

The clinical picture of HIV-1 myopathy is indistinguishable from that of zidovudine myotoxicity (see p. 373), except that myalgia is often present in the latter patients. Zidovudine myopathy, which usually occurs after 9 months or longer of full-dose therapy,[38,52] is much more common than HIV-1 myopathy. Some improvement follows complete cessation of the drug for 8 to 12 weeks.[38,52]

Laboratory Studies. The CK level is elevated in most patients.[38] Myoglobinuria has been observed but may reflect coincidental disease.[238] EMG reveals active myopathy with fibrillations, positive waves, complex repetitive discharges, and brief, polyphasic motor unit potentials. Even weak muscles show early recruitment of motor units and a full interference pattern. Muscle biopsy shows inflammatory cell infiltrates, particularly in the interstitium and perimysial tissues.[80] Widespread muscle fiber necrosis and invasion of fibers by macrophages are usual, and in about half the cases of this HIV-1-related inflammatory myopathy, nemaline rods and the selective loss of thick (myosin) filaments are noted.[80] The presence of numerous rods is the sole feature distinguishing HIV-1 myopathy from polymyositis.

Pathogenesis. The spectrum of HIV-1-related myopathies has not yet been fully characterized. Direct viral invasion of muscle fibers has been sought, but studies thus far are negative. On the other hand, HIV-1 antigen has been identified within macrophages in muscle cellular infiltrates.[37,127] The improvement of many patients during treatment with prednisone (see below) suggests an autoimmune basis for many cases. However, the problem is complicated by the finding that the serum CK level may be elevated, and myopathic changes, including muscle inflammation, may both be present in patients without clinical signs or symptoms of myopathy.[124b]

Severe muscle wasting with preserved muscle strength and endurance[149] is a relatively early and characteristic sign of the development of acquired immunodeficiency syndrome (AIDS) in HIV-1-infected patients. The specific causes of this cachexia have not

been defined, but they are likely to include a combination of generalized systemic infection, diminished activity, and poor nutrition.[206]

Treatment. In uncontrolled studies, prednisone treatment has been associated with improvement in a high proportion of patients with an inflammatory myopathy and HIV-1 infection.[9,52,54,80,150,161,205] Patients have responded to prednisone, relapsed with its withdrawal, and responded again with its reintroduction.[38,52] The regimen is similar to that used for dermatomyositis (see Table 5–4), but the decision to use prednisone in HIV-infected patients with weakness is often difficult, because many patients already have a compromised immune status. Two other strategies are potentially safer and have been effective in anecdotal reports: plasma exchange[38] and high doses of intravenous immunoglobulin.[114]

The HIV-infected patient who appears to have an HIV-related myopathy must be evaluated for other treatable causes of myopathy and neuropathy. Subacute combined degeneration of the peripheral nerves and spinal cord, for example, may respond to vitamin B_{12}. Other important neuropathic disorders include chronic inflammatory demyelinating polyradiculoneuropathy and cytomegalovirus polyradiculopathy.[152] Myopathies from zidovudine, vincristine, rifampin, and other drugs, as well as infection from myocobacteria or other pathogens,[77,177] must be excluded. A dilemma is often posed when HIV-1-infected patients receiving zidovudine experience progressive weakness. If myalgias are a prominent complaint, and if the patient has received zidovudine for 9 months or more, it should be discontinued if possible and an alternative agent used. Myalgia should improve within 4 to 6 weeks, but weakness may take 1 to 3 months to improve.[38] Patients with progressive, painless weakness should be evaluated with electrodiagnostic studies and muscle biopsy; if evidence suggests active inflammatory myopathy, a trial of corticosteroids should be considered. Because both a toxic and an inflammatory myopathy may be present concurrently, it is occasionally necessary to both treat with corticosteroids and stop zidovudine treatment.

Case History

A 29-year-old bisexual man had progressive muscle weakness for 6 months. He first noticed pain in the shoulder-girdle muscles while lifting weights. He attributed this to muscle strain, and the pain resolved over 6 weeks with no exercise. He then developed difficulty running· but denied dysphagia, arthralgia, or symptoms of Raynaud's phenomenon. Over the ensuing 4 months, he noticed painless, progressive weakness and wasting of the deltoid, biceps brachii, pectoral, and scapular muscles bilaterally. In addition, he developed an exaggerated lumbar lordosis. His medical history included surgical repair of an anal fistula and cutaneous herpes zoster 1 year before the onset of muscle weakness. There was no history of opportunistic infection, unexplained fever, lymphadenopathy, drug abuse, or cognitive difficulties.

The general physical examination was normal. There was marked wasting bilaterally in the deltoid, scapular, biceps brachii, triceps, and pectoral muscles. Strength was 2/5 (MRC) in the deltoids, 3/5 in other shoulder-girdle muscles, and 4/5 in biceps brachii, triceps, gluteal, and iliopsoas muscles bilaterally. Strength was nearly normal in the hamstring, quadriceps, and intrinsic hand muscles. The patient could not support himself in a "sit-up" position, and had an exaggerated lumbar lordosis. Muscle stretch reflexes, mental status, cranial nerve, and sensory examinations were normal. The CK level was 900 U/L, the test for HIV-1 antibody was positive, and there was a polyclonal increase in serum immunoglobulin by immunoelectrophoresis. The T-cell ratio was normal. Needle EMG revealed rare fibrillations and positive waves in proximal muscles, with early recruitment of brief, small motor unit potentials. Nerve conduction studies were normal.

Histopathologic studies of a deltoid muscle showed numerous small, predominantly type I fibers containing basophilic and fuchsinophilic granules (see p. 62). Myosin adenosine triphosphatase (ATPase) staining was reduced in intensity. Scattered aggregates of mononuclear cells and several foci of macrophages were seen. Vacuolated fibers and an occasional regenerating fiber with basophilic cytoplasm could be identified.

Electron microscopy revealed widespread rod bodies ($< 1\mu m$) with selective loss of thick filaments. The rods were randomly distributed in affected fibers, and thin filaments were continuous with their margins. In situ hybridization and cultures were negative for HIV-1. Direct and indirect immunofluorescence showed no evidence of immunoglobulin or complement deposition.

Following plasmapheresis (20 treatments over 8 weeks), muscle strength improved both subjectively and on manual muscle testing (one half to a full grade [MRC]); but substantial weakness persisted. Subsequently, the patient improved to almost normal on high doses of prednisone. After tapering to lower doses of alternate-day prednisone, weakness recurred, but then responded again to high doses. Eventually the patient stabilized and his condition is currently stable with only mild weakness on prednisone 10 mg every other day.

Comment: Polymyositis was the presenting manifestation of this patient's HIV infection. This further confirms the need to consider retroviral infection in patients with autoimmune disorders who are at risk for HIV infection. Plasma exchange was tried in an attempt to avoid corticosteroids, with only limited improvement. More marked improvement followed prednisone treatment.

HTLV-1

Although human T-cell leukemia virus type I (HTLV-1) retrovirus has been much more commonly implicated as the cause of a myelopathy, infected patients may suffer from myositis[69] and may present with a clinical picture of polymyositis.[155] HTLV-1 infection is endemic in the tropics, and most cases of inflammatory myopathy have come from Africa and Jamaica. Cases have occurred in patients who have received blood transfusions, as well as in patients with HIV-1 infection.[235] In patients with both HIV-1 infection and HTLV-1 infection, it is difficult to attribute myopathy to either virus alone. HTLV-1 myositis should be considered in patients who live in endemic areas or who have received blood transfusions. The diagnosis is established by serologic studies of blood and virologic study of muscle.

ECHOVIRUS

Patients with acute echovirus infections often experience myalgias, but muscle weakness and laboratory evidence of myositis seldom occur unless the patient is immune-compromised. Several reports document rhabdomyolysis and myoglobinuria in patients with echovirus 9.[103,105] In patients with X-linked hypogammaglobulinemia, a variety of neurologic disorders have been associated with persistent echovirus infections.[141] A dermatomyositis-like disorder with biopsy, EMG, and elevation of CK level typical of dermatomyositis has been observed.[12] The disorder may respond to repeated infusions of immune globulin.[141] A similar disorder in a patient with multiple myeloma also responded to intravenous immune globulin.[211]

INFLUENZA

Acute infection with influenza A and B viruses causes mylagias in most patients.[142] In adults, muscle destruction and myoglobinuria[20,153,156] are common and can lead to renal failure.[156] A severe, acute, painful myopathy, myalgia cruris epidemica,[131] may develop, particularly in children. It is characterized by leg pain that often precludes ambulation. The CK level is elevated to 2 to 20 times normal.[16] The legs, particularly the calf muscles, are often swollen and tender.[16] The disorder is usually self-limited and resolves over a period of 3 days to 3 months. In rare instances, joint contractures develop and a protracted course of limb pain ensues. An isolated case with well-documented persistent influenza virus infection was associated with dermatomyositis.[76]

The syndrome of severe leg pain with a viral illness is not specific for influenza virus. Parainfluenza virus, mumps virus, measles virus, and mycoplasma have all produced the same clinical picture.[16]

OTHER VIRUSES

Numerous other viruses cause an acute myopathy.* In many instances, rhabdomyolysis has been sufficient to cause myoglobinuria and renal failure.[20,153,156] Hepatitis B,[20,174] infectious mononucleosis,[153] and adenovirus[156] have all been implicated. The infrequency of such reports and the relative frequency of viral infections in population studies suggests that some of the viral infections could be coincidental occurrences. The rhabdomyolysis of McArdle's disease (p. 254) is often associated with generalized symptoms that may be the result of a viral infection.

KAWASAKI DISEASE

Kawasaki disease, also termed the mucocutaneous lymph node syndrome, is an acute inflammatory disease characterized by nonsuppurative enlargement of cervical lymph nodes, inflammatory lesions of skin and mucous membranes, and arteritic aneurysms of the coronary arteries.[59] The cause is unknown but the disease has often been considered to be viral in origin. Cardiac myositis occurs in a few cases, and skeletal myositis is seen in occasional patients.[119] Whereas skeletal muscle involvement has usually been overshadowed by the other features of the illness, myositis can be severe and lead to respiratory failure. The CK level is markedly elevated in severely affected patients. Certain manifestations of the disease, particularly coronary arteritis,

---

*References 16,20,107,131,142,153,156,157, 236

respond to treatment with high doses of intravenous gammaglobulin in combination with high doses of aspirin. The same treatment may also improve the myositis. Because gammaglobulin-aspirin treatment is mandatory for the prevention of coronary aneurysms, the natural history of the myositis is not known.

Protozoa

TOXOPLASMOSIS

Systemic infection with *Toxoplasma gondii* produces a multisystemic illness characterized by lymphadenopathy, fever, pharyngitis, headache, malaise, and myalgias. Splenomegaly and hepatomegaly can occur. The illness resembles infectious mononucleosis. Muscle pain and generalized weakness are occasionally dominant features of the illness, and a picture resembling dermatomyositis has occurred.[176] Toxoplasma organisms can be identified on muscle biopsy.[82] A report of serologic evidence for *T gondii* in 10% of patients with idiopathic inflammatory myopathy[106] has prompted others to look for toxoplasmosis in patients with polymyositis, but we have never encountered evidence for toxoplasmosis in such patients. Because the prevalence of clinically inapparent infection with *T gondii* is high, a considerable number of patients with any myopathy are likely to have serologic evidence of infection.[139] Infection with *T gondii* is common in immunocompromised patients, but evidence that myopathy even in these patients is related to *T gondii* myositis is not established.[190]

Helminths

TRICHINOSIS

The nematode *Trichinella spiralis* causes an inflammatory myopathy. Trichinosis occurs when infected, inadequately cooked meat (usually pork) is eaten. With greater awareness of this problem, however, cooks now take more care in preparing foods containing pork, so that an increasing proportion of trichinosis results from ingestion of other meats, including bear, horse, wild boar, and walrus.[35] The disease incidence has recently increased in the United States because of the large refugee population from Southeast Asia who are largely unaware of the need to cook pork.[218] Unlike many other countries, the United States does not test pork for trichinosis.

Clinical Findings. Patients destined to have severe myositis following ingestion of infected meat usually have diarrhea 1 to 7 days after consuming the cyst-containing meat. Myopathic symptoms of myalgia, swelling, and weakness begin up to a week after meat ingestion.[171] Fever and periorbital edema are common. Other findings include a maculopapular rash, splinter hemorrhages, retinal and subconjunctival hemorrhages, hemoptysis, and pulmonary infiltrates. Cardiac involvement can be severe and cause fatal congestive heart failure. Tachycardia is usually present, and arrhythmias, including heart block, can occur.[146] Brain infestation with larvae may cause encephalitis with normal spinal fluid. Both a diffuse encephalopathy and focal signs have been described.[171]

Laboratory Findings. Eosinophilia is present in virtually all patients except for the most severely ill. It appears by the second week of illness and ranges from 5% to 90%. The ESR is usually normal. The CK levels are elevated, the degree of elevation paralleling the severity of disease. EMG shows a picture characteristic of an inflammatory myopathy (see pp. 158–159) without distinguishing findings. Muscle biopsy is the most helpful test for diagnosis. Trichinella larvae can be identified in muscle biopsies from severely ill patients (Fig. 5–18). Occasionally, only a nondiagnostic inflammatory myopathy is evident. *Any patient with an inflammatory myopathy of 3 months' duration or less who also has an eosinophi-*

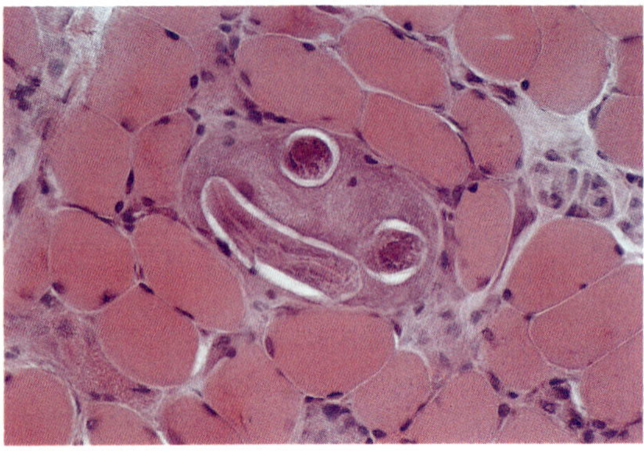

Figure 5–18. Trichinella spiralis in a muscle fiber from a patient with active myositis. The muscle fiber shows a single parasite cut multiple times (H&E).

lia should be suspected of having trichinosis. At times a large muscle biopsy (up to 500–1000 mg) may be needed to find the larvae.[171] The skin test for trichinosis is not reliable, so that serologic tests are important for specific diagnosis. Both the sensitive enzyme-linked immunosorbent assay (ELISA) and the bentonite flocculation test are usually helpful. Serologic tests are usually negative early in the illness (first 1–2 weeks) and become positive later; the rise in titer is particularly valuable in diagnosis.

Pathogenesis. *Trichinella spiralis* is an intraepithelial parasite that inhabits the proximal small intestine of host mammals. When infected meat is ingested, larvae are released in the gut and an *enteric* phase of infection with diarrhea develops. The diarrhea results from increased intestinal motility induced by burrowing of the parasite through the enteric epithelium.[229] The systemic signs and symptoms of trichinosis develop as second-generation larvae migrate into the blood stream and become lodged in the blood vessels of the skeletal muscles, where they provoke an intense local inflammatory reaction. This second phase of infection occurs after the delay necessary for replication of the nematode. The myositis occurs 7 days to 6 weeks after the ingestion of the infected meat. Even the diarrhea may take 2 to 7 days to develop.

Muscle symptoms presumably arise from the intense inflammation that follows the entry of larvae into skeletal muscle. Larvae first coil and then grow in muscle. They become encysted and may eventually become calcified. Both inflammation and muscle destruction usually occur. The extreme eosinophilia (5%–90%) may contribute to tissue damage,[108] but the prompt response of symptoms to prednisone treatment alone, without concomitant antitrichinella agents, suggests that the inflammatory response causes the myopathy, rather than the larvae themselves.

Treatment. Patients with weakness and evidence of active myopathy should receive prednisone (30–80 mg/d). Those with severe disease should receive the higher dose. The necessity of concomitant antitrichinella therapy has not been established, but it is recommended. Albendazole (400 mg three times a day for 2 weeks) kills adult and larval trichinella and appears to be effective. It has few side effects but should not be used in children or pregnant women. Thiabendazole, which does not kill the larvae, has produced improvement in some but not all patients. More than 90% of patients respond promptly to treatment. Those with severe cardiac myositis or with encephalitis, and those who are immunocompromised, may not survive the disease.

Case History: Patient 1

A 68-year-old widow was admitted with a 2-week history of fever, rigor, and muscle weakness. Initial laboratory studies at another hospital indicated eosinophilia (16% of 19,100 cells/mm^3) and findings of nucleated red blood cells on peripheral blood smear. A bone marrow examination showed increased eosinophils and promyelocytes, raising the question of leukemia. There was no history of diarrhea, rash, or muscle pain.

Examination demonstrated proximal

weakness, grade 4 in the arms and grade 2 in the legs. She could not lift her legs off the bed, sit up, or walk. Muscle stretch reflexes were absent in the legs and hypoactive in the arms.

Further laboratory studies included a 10%–13% eosinophilia, hyponatremia, hypoalbuminemia (1.8–2.1 g/dL), abnormal liver function, and mild azotemia. The ESR was normal. Hypergammaglobulinemia (3.7 g/dL) was present. The CK level was elevated fourfold. EMG showed widespread fibrillations and low-amplitude, short-duration, rapidly recruited motor unit potentials. Muscle biopsy showed widespread muscle fiber necrosis and phagocytosis with inflammatory cell infiltrates. Cysts consistent with *T spiralis* were present (see Fig. 5–18). The electrocardiogram (ECG) showed abnormalities of ST-T waves consistent with ischemia. Later, latex flocculation was elevated, and other serologic studies for *T spiralis* were confirmative.

The patient was improving by the time the diagnosis was established and recovered without prednisone or other specific treatment. She denied ingestion of pork.

Case History: Patient 2

One week after Patient 1 was admitted, a 50-year-old housewife (a neighbor of Patient 1) was admitted in a transfer from the same outside hospital. Both had eaten sausage prepared from a garbage-fed, locally slaughtered pig both 6 weeks and then 2 weeks prior to becoming ill. Patient 2 initially had nausea, red eyes, and weak, painful muscles. Her illness was similar to that of Patient 1, and in addition, she had a pleural effusion and congestive heart failure.

Laboratory studies showed a white blood count of 22,300/mm³ with 10% eosinophils; hypoalbuminemia (2.0 g/dL), mild azotemia, and persistent hyperkalemia. The ESR was normal. The ECG showed ventricular ectopy, low QRS voltage and loss of anterior wall forces. The chest radiograph showed pleural effusions, and forced vital capacity was 1.1 L. The CK level was elevated eightfold. Serologic testing for *T spiralis* was positive, and EMG and muscle biopsy were similar to that of Patient 1.

Prednisone (20 mg every 6 hours) was in-

stituted immediately because of suspected myocarditis, and the patient improved rapidly. Prednisone was tapered to 10 mg twice a day after 2 weeks and discontinued over the ensuing month. The patient recovered completely.

Leftover sausage was subsequently located in the patient's freezer and was found to contain cysts consistent with *T spiralis*.

Comment: Both patients had trichinella infection documented by muscle biopsy and serologic tests, but neither had rash or diarrhea. Recent evidence suggests that subspecies of trichinella spiralis may produce markedly different clinical features. For example, gastrointestinal symptoms may be a dominant feature in cases resulting from contaminated walrus meat.

Muscle pain was prominent in only one of the patients. The delay in diagnosis in both cases emphasizes the importance of considering trichinosis when eosinophilia is present in any patient with myopathy. Although one of these patients recovered spontaneously, current treatment recommendations include both prednisone and specific antihelminthic treatment.

CYSTICERCOSIS

A hypertrophic myopathy is a very rare, late complication in patients infected with cysticercosis.[102] Muscle symptoms of pain and generalized fatigue are common in acute infection but are usually overshadowed by involvement of other organs.

ECHINOCOCCOSIS

Echinococcosis is the result of infection with the cestode, *Echinococcus granulosus*. The disease usually occurs in sheep-raising areas of the Middle East, Africa, Australia, Europe, and South America, but can occur in the United States. When ingested, embryo larvae migrate through the intestinal wall to lodge in the liver, lung, brain, and other tissues, including muscle. The larvae then produce cysts and simulate tumors that slowly enlarge over periods ranging from months to decades. In endemic areas the lesions are the commonest cause of a mass lesion in muscle. Eosinophilia is present in less than half the cases, and both diagnosis and treatment are surgical. Patients with multiple lesions and those whose conditions preclude surgery have responded to mebendazole.[198]

Lyme Disease

CLINICAL AND LABORATORY FEATURES

Muscle weakness and pain are common in Lyme disease, the borreliosis caused by *Borrelia burgdorferi*.[217] The pain is often caused by arthritis rather than myositis, and weakness is usually the result of peripheral neuropathy.[90,217] Muscle inflammation has been observed in muscle biopsies from patients with Lyme disease, but it is not yet clear that symptoms are related to involvement of muscle rather than other organ systems.[182,217] Normal CK levels,[8,182] neurogenic findings on EMG,[182] and atrophy rather than cell necrosis on muscle biopsy[8,182] all speak against muscle as the target tissue. Interstitial inflammation in muscle biopsy tissue is inadequate evidence that myositis is a major feature of the disease.

Rarely, a noninflammatory, necrotizing myopathy has been identified in Lyme disease.[195] In patients with muscle weakness, treatment with corticosteroids improved muscle pain, but only antibiotic therapy returned strength to normal.[182,195]

In late-stage Lyme disease, a chronic encephalopathy occurs[168]; it is associated with fatigue, asthenia, sleep disturbances, depression, and abnormal cognition.[168,195] Because many patients at this stage show features of the chronic fatigue syndrome, Lyme disease has been considered as a potential causative agent for that syndrome. Careful study, however, has excluded it as a major cause.[48]

PATHOGENESIS OF MYOPATHY

Direct invasion of muscle by *B. burgdorferi* has been found in only a few patients with Lyme disease who have muscle symptoms.[182,195] An immunologically mediated process in which antibody to the spirochete cross-reacts with myelin (possibly as a result of molecular mimicry) appears to be the triggering process for neuropathy in some patients,[203] but no similar process has been found in muscle. The improvement in muscle pain with corticosteroids could be due to a decrease in the referred pain caused by arthritis. Antibiotic treatment with ceftriaxone has been effective in treating muscle weakness, which could be caused by the organism itself.[182,195]

Bacterial Infections

Bacterial infection of muscle has recently become more frequent in developed countries because of its occurrence in patients with AIDS. Suppurative infection of muscle is common in underdeveloped countries, particularly in the tropics, where it is termed "tropical pyomyositis." Infection is usually caused by *staphylococci* or *streptococci*, but gonococcus, tuberculosis, and other agents are occasionally found.

STAPHYLOCOCCAL PYOMYOSITIS

Pyomyositis caused by *Staphylococcus aureus* presents as a firm, nonfluctuant mass in one or more muscles. Severe pain and tenderness are the usual complaints. Over ensuing days, the illness tends to become generalized, with fever and toxicity. If antibiotic treatment is delayed, the muscle masses suppurate and require surgical drainage. Patients with staphylococcal pyomyositis seldom have signs of generalized myopathy, and the CK level is usually normal.

STREPTOCOCCAL MYOSITIS

This disorder is rare and presents with local muscle pain, tenderness, and swelling, without weakness or signs of generalized myopathy.[181,192] Patients rapidly deteriorate and develop circulatory collapse, which is often associated with disseminated intravascular coagulation. The syndrome often does not respond to antibiotics, and it is not yet known why the relentless, fulminant course can appear in previously healthy individuals.[192] A concomitant viral infection has been implicated in a few instances.[180]

LEPTOSPIROSIS

Severe myalgias are a prominent and early feature of acute leptospirosis.[229b] The disease is typically biphasic. The initial, acute infection, the *leptospiremic phase*, is characterized by headache, chills, fever, and severe pain and tenderness of the thighs and paraspinous muscles. Aseptic meningitis and conjunctivitis are common. Sensory testing often shows hyperpathia. With severe illness, liver and renal failure can develop. Most patients have liver dysfunction, which leads to serum enzyme abnormalities that may obscure the presence of muscle disease. During the acute illness, CK levels are elevated in most patients,[229b] and severe rhabdomyolysis may occur.[94] The late, *immune-mediated phase* of leptospirosis develops 1 to 2 weeks after the leptospiremic phase. Muscle pain is common and the CK level is often elevated.[229b]

In neither phase of leptospirosis is muscle weakness severe enough to suggest a primary disease of skeletal muscle. Diagnosis in the leptospiremic phase is made by blood culture. In the later phase, the diagnosis is usually made by serologic testing, which detects IgM antibody using an ELISA method.[229a]

CLOSTRIDIAL INFECTIONS

Clostridial infection (*C. perfringens*) of traumatic and occasionally of surgical wounds can result in local muscle necrosis. Typically the affected area becomes intensely inflamed, with the cardinal signs of severe pain, swelling, erythema, and heat. Systemic toxicity, with hemolysis, rhabdomyolysis and renal failure, develops rapidly. Emergency surgical and antibiotic treatment are effective in some patients, but mortality is high once the syndrome is fully developed. Other organisms occasionally produce a similar syndrome. Rarely, an unsuspected perforated colonic neoplasm or diverticulum will produce the same picture without a prior history of trauma or surgery.

Tetanus. Infection of wounds with *Clostridium tetani* results in the local production of tetanus toxin, which produces the clinical syndrome of tetanus in nonimmune patients. The disease is most common in underdeveloped countries but continues to be a problem in the United States because of inadequate immunization. Narcotic addiction and minor traumatic wounds lead to most cases in the United States and Europe.

Patients present with focal or generalized muscle spasms and muscle rigidity. Rigidity is the result of the neurotoxic effect of tetanus toxin, which acts to block the release of γ-aminobutyric acid (GABA) and glycine and prevent the normal inhibition of motor activity. Tetanus toxin is transmitted by retrograde transport from muscle to the CNS. The toxin is not directly myotoxic, but the severe muscle spasms invariably elevate the CK level and produce rhabdomyolysis and myoglobinuria. Treatment to prevent myoglobinuria (see Chapter 6) is indicated in most patients.

Fungal Infection

Systemic fungal infections (for example, sporotrichinosis[91]) occasionally cause a focal myositis, usually characterized by granulomas. Biopsy of muscle in patients with overwhelming systemic fungal infections may show asymptomatic granulomas, which occasionally are mistaken for those of sarcoidosis.

GRAFT VERSUS HOST DISEASE

Graft versus host disease (GVHD) occurs in patients receiving bone marrow transplantation. Such transplantation from live, related donors (heterologous transplantation) is increasingly being used to treat leukemia, aplastic anemia, and other hematologic disorders. Patients with chronic GVHD may have an inflammatory myopathy with clinical features resembling polymyositis,[183] and it is likely that the incidence of this disorder will increase along with the number of procedures performed. Other neuromuscular disorders complicating chronic GVHD include myasthenia gravis, mononeuritis multiplex, and a herpes zoster neuritis.[159,210]

The inflammatory myopathy of chronic GVHD usually responds to corticosteroids, but other antiinflammatory agents such as azathioprine are sometimes necessary.[183]

Inflammatory myopathy responsive to prednisone has also been reported in a patient with Hodgkin's disease who received an autologous bone marrow transplant.[194] In this patient, as in cases with heterologous transplantation for malignant disease, the possibility that the malignancy predisposed to polymyositis must be considered.

SUMMARY

The idiopathic inflammatory myopathies can be classified into three major subtypes: dermatomyositis, polymyositis, and inclusion body myositis. Distinctive clinical features and characteristic CK, biopsy, and EMG findings permit separation of the three dis-

orders. There is now considerable understanding of the pathogenesis of each.

Dermatomyositis has a virtually pathognomonic rash that usually establishes the diagnosis on clinical grounds alone. The histologic finding of perifascicular atrophy is also diagnostic, but regional variation in its severity and presence is marked. In dermatomyositis, disturbed humoral immunity is an important early and initiating event. Blood vessel walls appear to be the target of the earliest damage. The inciting factor is not known, but antibody deposition with activation of the complement cascade appears to initiate or perpetuate local vascular damage.

In contrast, polymyositis and inclusion body myositis appear to be cellularly mediated. No unique clinical or laboratory feature allows the specific diagnosis of polymyositis, which must be made on the basis of clinical evidence of weakness and a constellation of abnormal CK, biopsy, and EMG findings. A large number of disorders may produce the same clinical picture, and other inflammatory myopathies resulting from known pathogens (such as HIV-1, other viruses, and *T spiralis*) can produce identical laboratory abnormalities. These diseases and a host of other conditions must be excluded to allow a diagnosis of polymyositis.

Inclusion body myositis often has a distinctive pattern of weakness that suggests the diagnosis: painless proximal weakness accompanied by prominent and characteristic weakness and wasting of wrist flexors, finger flexors, quadriceps, and the ankle dorsiflexors. The distinctive microscopic feature is the presence of rimmed vacuoles, which contain 15- to 18-nm tubulofilaments. Vacuolated muscle fibers show amyloid-positive material, ubiquitin immunoreactivity, and β-amyloid protein. Inclusion body myositis and polymyositis share some pathologic features: partial invasion of nonnecrotic muscle cells by cytotoxic lymphocytes and the presence of class 1 major histocompatibility complex products on the surface of muscle fibers.

Dermatomyositis responds to corticosteroid or cytotoxic treatment. When the disease occurs in childhood, adequate treatment results in remission. Treatment can ultimately be discontinued in most, if not all, children. Adult dermatomyositis also responds to treatment but usually requires lifelong medication. Judicious medical management, begun early, can usually prevent complications of treatment.

In a small number of patients with inflammatory myopathy, the condition is the result of another disorder such as systemic lupus erythematosus, rheumatoid arthritis, or other connective-tissue disorders. In these diseases, neuropathy or central nervous system disease is more often the cause of weakness than is myopathy. Some connective-tissue diseases cause overlap syndromes with features of dermatomyositis or polymyositis.

Finally, in a large number of infectious disorders, an inflammatory myopathy may cause muscle pain and weakness. Trichinosis, HIV-1, Lyme disease, and influenza viruses may produce prominent muscle symptoms. Specific treatment is available for many of these disorders.

REFERENCES

1. Agrawal BL and Giesen PC: Eosinophilic myositis: an unusual cause of pseudotumor and eosinophilia. JAMA 246:70, 1981.
2. Arahata K and Engel AG: Monoclonal antibody analysis of mononuclear cells in myopathies. I: Quantitation of subsets according to diagnosis and sites of accumulation and demonstration and counts of muscle fibers invaded by T cells. Ann Neurol 16: 193, 1984.
3. Arkin CR, Rothschild BM, Florendo NT, and Popoff N: Behçet syndrome with myositis: A case report with pathologic findings. Arthritis Rheum 23:600, 1980.
4. Arnett FC, Hirsch TJ, Bias WB, Nishikai M, and Reichlin M: The Jo-1 antibody system in myositis: relationships to clinical features and HLA. J Rheumatol 8:925, 1981.
5. Ashworth B and Tait GBW: Trigeminal neuropathy in connective tissue disease. Neurology 21:609, 1971.
5a. Askanas V, Serdaroglu P, Engel WK, and Alvarez RB: Immunolocalization of ubiquitin in muscle biopsies of patients with inclusion body myositis and oculopharyngeal muscular dystrophy. Neurosci Lett 130:73, 1991.
5b. Askanas V, Serdaroglu P, Engel WK, and Alvarez RB: Immunocytochemical localization of ubiquitin in inclusion body myositis allows its light-microscopic distinction from polymyositis. Neurology 42:460, 1992
5c. Askanas V, Engel WK, and Alvarez RB: Light and electron microscopic localization of β-amyloid protein in muscle biopsies of patients with inclusion-body myositis. Am J Pathol 141:31, 1992.
6. Askari AD: Cardiac abnormalities. Clinics in Rheumatic Diseases 10: 131, 1984.
7. Askari AD and Huettner TL: Cardiac abnormalities in polymyositis/dermatomyositis. Semin Arthritis Rheum 12:208, 1982.
8. Atlas E, Novak SN, Duray PH, and Steere AC: Lyme myositis: muscle invasion by Borrelia burgdorferi. Ann Intern Med 109:246, 1988.
9. Bailey RO, Turok DI, Jaufmann BP, and Singh JK: Myositis and acquired immunodeficiency syndrome. Hum Pathol 18:749, 1987.
10. Banker BQ: Dermatomyositis of childhood: Ultrastructural alterations of muscle and intramuscular blood vessels. J Neuropathol Exp Neurol 34:46, 1975.
11. Banker BQ and Victor M: Dermatomyositis (systemic angiopathy) of childhood. Medicine 45:261, 1966.
12. Bardelas JA, Winkelstein JA, Seto DSY, Tsai T, and Rogol AD: Fatal ECHO 24 infection in a patient with hypogammaglobulinemia: Relationship to dermatomyositis-like syndrome. J Pediat 90:396, 1977.

13. Barnes BE: Dermatomyositis and malignancy: A review of the literature. Ann Intern Med 84:68, 1976.

14. Neville HE, Baumbach LL, Ringel SP, Russo LS Jr, Sujansky E, and Garcia CA: Familial inclusion body myositis: Evidence for autosomal dominant inheritance. Neurology 42:897–902, 1992.

15. Behan WMH, Behan PO, and Gairns J: Cardiac damage in polymyositis associated with antibodies to tissue ribonucleoproteins. Br Heart J 57:176, 1987.

16. Belardi C, Roberge R, Kelly M, and Serbin S: Myalgia cruris epidemica (benign acute childhood myositis) associated with a mycoplasma pneumonia infection. Ann Emerg Med 16:579, 1987.

17. Belongia EA, Hedberg CW, Gleich GJ, et al: An investigation of the cause of the eosinophilia-myalgia syndrome associated with tryptophan use. N Engl J Med 323:357, 1990.

18. Bennett RM and O'Connell DJ: The arthritis of mixed connective tissue disease. Ann Rheum Dis 37:397, 1978.

19. Bennett RM and O'Connell DJ: Mixed connective tissue disease: A clinicopathologic study of 20 cases. Semin Arthritis Rheum 10:25, 1980.

20. Berlin BS, Simon NM, and Bovner RN: Myoglobinuria precipitated by viral infection. JAMA 227:1414, 1974.

21. Bernstein RM and Mathews MB: Jo-1 and other myositis autoantibodies. In Brooks PM and York JR (eds): Rheumatology-85. Excerpta Medica, Elsevier Science, 1985, pp 273-278.

22. Bidula LP and Myers AR: Eosinophilic fasciitis associated with hematologic disorders: Case reports and review of the literature. Clinical Rheumatology Proceedings 3:117, 1985.

23. Bigger JF, Palmberg PF, and Becker B: Increased cellular sensitivity to glucocorticoids in primary open-angle glaucoma. Invest Ophthalmol Vis Sci 11:832, 1972.

24. Biswas T, Miller FW, Takagaki Y, and Plotz PH: An enzyme-linked immunosorbent assay for the detection and quantitation of anti-Jo-1 antibody in human serum. J Immunol Methods 98:243, 1987.

25. Bitnum S, Daeschner CW, Travis LB, Dodge WF, and Hopps HC: Dermatomyositis. J Pediatr 64:101, 1964.

26. Blumbergs PC, Byrne E, and Kakulas BA: Polymyositis presenting with respiratory failure. J Neurol Sci 65:221, 1984.

27. Bohan A and Peter JB: Polymyositis and dermatomyositis. N Engl J Med 292:344, 1975.

28. Bohan A, Peter JB, Bowman RL, and Pearson CM: A computer-assisted analysis of 153 patients with polymyositis and dermatomyositis. Medicine 56:255, 1977.

29. Bowyer SL, Blane CE, Sullivan DB, and Cassidy JT: Childhood dermatomyositis: factors predicting functional outcome and development of dystrophic calcification. J Pediatr 103:882, 1983.

30. Bunch TW: Prednisone and azathioprine for polymyositis: Long-term followup. Arthritis Rheum 24:45, 1981.

31. Bunch TW, O'Duffy JD, and McLeod RA: Deforming arthritis of the hands in polymyositis. Arthritis Rheum 19:243, 1976.

32. Callen JP: Myositis and malignancy. In Ansell BM (ed): Clinics in Rheumatic Diseases: Inflammatory Disorders of Muscle. London, WB Saunders, 1984, pp 117–130.

33. Carpenter S, Karpati G, Heller I, and Eisen A: Inclusion body myositis: A distinct variety of idiopathic inflammatory myopathy. Neurology 28:8, 1978.

34. Carpenter S, Karpati G, Rothman S, and Watters G: The childhood type of dermatomyositis. Neurology 26:952, 1976.

34a. Cash JM and Klippel JH: Drug therapy: Second-line drug therapy for rheumatoid arthritis. N Engl J Med 330:1368, 1994.

35. Center for Disease Control: Epidemiologic notes and reports. MMWR Morb Mortal Wkly Rep 40:57, 1991.

36. Chad D, Good P, Adelman L, Bradley WG, and Mills J: Inclusion body myositis associated with Sjögren's syndrome. Arch Neurol 39:186, 1982.

37. Chad DA, Smith TW, Blumenfeld A, Fairchild PG, and DeGirolami U: Human immunodeficiency virus (HIV)–associated myopathy: Immunocytochemical identification of an HIV antigen (GP 41) in muscle macrophages. Ann Neurol 28:579, 1990.

38. Chalmers AC, Greco CM, and Miller RG: Prognosis in AZT myopathy. Neurology 41:1181, 1991.

39. Chou SM: Myxovirus-like structures in a case of human chronic polymyositis. Science 158:1453, 1967.

40. Chou SM: Inclusion body myositis: a chronic persistent mumps myositis? Hum Path 17:765, 1986.

41. Clarke JT, Karpati G, and Carpenter S: The effect of vincristine on skeletal muscle in the rat. A correlation histochemical, ultrastructural and chemical study. J Neuropathol Exp Neurol 31:247, 1972.

42. Clements PJ, Furst DE, Campion DS, et al: Muscle disease in progressive systemic sclerosis. Arthritis Rheum 21:62, 1978.

43. Clements PR and Davis J: Cytotoxic drugs: their clinical application to the rheumatic diseases. Sem Arthritis and Rheum 15:231, 1986.

44. Cohen MR, Sulaiman AR, Garancis JC, and Wortmann RL: Clinical heterogeneity and treatment response in inclusion body myositis. Arth Rheum 32:734, 1989.

45. Cole AJ, Kuzniecky R, Karpati G, Carpenter S, Andermann E, and Andermann F: Familial myopathy with changes resembling inclusion body myositis and periventricular leucoencephalopathy. Brain 111:1025, 1988.

46. Conn HO and Blitzer BL: Nonassociation of adrenocorticosteroid therapy and peptic ulcer. N Engl J Med 294:473, 1976.

47. Cornblath DR, McArthur JC, Kennedy PGE, Witte AS, and Griffin JW: Inflammatory demyelinating peripheral neuropathies associated with human T-cell lymphotropic virus type III infection. Ann Neurol 21:32, 1987.

48. Coyle PK and Krupp L: Borrelia burgdorferi infection in the chronic fatigue syndrome [abstract]. Ann Neurol 28:243, 1990.

49. Cram RL, Barmada R, Geho WB, and Ray RD: Diphosphonate treatment of calcinosis universalis. N Engl J Med 285:1012, 1971.

50. Crowe WE, Bove KE, Levinson JE, and Hilton PK: Clinical and pathogenetic implications of histopathology in childhood polydermatomyositis. Arthritis Rheum 25:126, 1982.

51. Cunningham PH, Andrews BS, and Davis JS: Immune complexes in progressive systemic sclerosis and mixed connective tissue disease. J Rheumatol 7:301, 1980.

51a. Dalakas MC, Illa I, Dambrosia JM, et al: A controlled trial of high-dose intravenous immunoglobulin infusions as treatment for dermatomyositis. N Engl J Med 329:1993, 1993.

52. Dalakas MC, Illa I, Pezeshkpour GH, Laukaitis JP, Cohen B, and Griffin JL: Mitochondrial myopathy caused by long-term zidovudine therapy. N Engl J Med 322:1098, 1990.

53. Dalakas MC, Pezeshkpour GH, and Flaherty M. Progressive nemaline (rod) myopathy associated with HIV infection. N Engl J Med 317:1602, 1987.

54. Dalakas MC, Pezeshkpour GH, Gravell M, and Sever JL: Polymyositis associated with AIDS retrovirus. JAMA 256:2381, 1986.

55. De Merieux P, Verity MA, Clements PJ, and Paulus HE: Esophageal abnormalities and dysphagia in polymyositis and dermatomyositis: Clinical, radiographic, and pathologic features. Arthritis Rheum 26:961, 1983.

56. Derderian SS, Tellis CJ, Abbrecht PH, Welton RC, and Rajagopal KR: Pulmonary involvement in mixed connective tissue disease. Chest 88:45, 1985.

57. DeVere R and Bradley WG: Polymyo-

sitis: its presentation, morbidity and mortality. Brain 98:637, 1975.

58. DeVisser M, Emslie-Smith AM, and Engel AG: Early ultrastructural alterations in dermatomyositis. J Neurol Sci 94:181, 1989.

59. Diagnostic guidelines for Kawasaki disease. American Heart Association Committee on Rheumatic Fever, Endocarditis, and Kawasaki Disease. Am J Dis Child 144:1218, 1990.

60. Dickey BF and Myers AR: Pulmonary disease in polymyositis/dermatomyositis. Semin Arthritis Rheum 14:60, 1984.

61. Diez-Jouanen E, Salazar JF, Abud-Mendoza C, and Alarsen-Segovia D: Immune complexes in autoimmune diseases: Differences in immune complexes detected by cellular receptor for complement and for Fc domains of IgG. Revista de Investigacion Clinica 32:153, 1980.

62. Dubowitz V: Treatment of dermatomyositis in childhood. Arch Dis Child 51:494, 1976.

63. Dyck PJ, Conn DL, and Okazaki H: Necrotizing angiopathic neuropathy: Three-dimensional morphology of fiber degeneration related to sites of occluded vessels. Mayo Clin Proc 47:461, 1972.

64. Emslie-Smith AM, Arahata K, and Engel AG: Major histocompatibility complex Class I antigen expression, immunolocalization of interferon subtypes, and T cell-mediated cytotoxicity in myopathies. Hum Pathol 20:224, 1989.

65. Engel AG: Acid maltase deficiency in adults: Studies in four cases of a syndrome which may mimic muscular dystrophy or other myopathies. Brain 93:599, 1970.

66. Engel AG and Hirschhorn R: Acid maltase deficiency. In Engel AG and Franzini-Armstrong C (eds): Myology. New York, McGraw-Hill, 1994, p 1533.

67. Engel AG and Arahata K: Monoclonal antibody analysis of mononuclear cells in myopathies, II. Phenotypes of autoinvasive cells in polymyositis and inclusion body myositis. Ann Neurol 16:209, 1984.

68. Eosinophilia-myalgia syndrome and L-tryptophan-containing products — New Mexico, Minnesota, Oregon, and New York, 1989. MMWR 38:785, 1989.

69. Evans BK, Gore I, Harrell LE, Arnold T, and Oh SJ: HTLV-1-associated myelopathy and polymyositis in a US native. Neurol 39:1572, 1989.

70. Fauci AS: Alternate-day corticosteroid therapy. Am J Med 64:729, 1978.

71. Fauci AS, Harley JB, Roberts WC, Ferrans VJ, and Gralnick HR, and Bjornson BH: The idiopathic hypereosinophilic syndrome. Ann Intern Med 97:78, 1982.

72. Ferreiro JE, Saldana MJ, and Azevedo SJ: Polyarteritis manifesting as calf myositis and fever. Am J Med 80:312, 1986.

73. Florence JM, Fox PT, Planer GJ, and Brook MH: Activity, creatine kinase, and myoglobin in Duchenne muscular dystrophy: A clue to etiology? Neurology 35:758, 1985.

74. Foote RA, Kimbrough SM, and Stevens JC: Lupus myositis. Muscle Nerve 5:65, 1982.

75. Fu TS, Soltani K, Sorensen LB, Levinson D, and Lorincz AL: Eosinophilic fasciitis. JAMA 240:451, 1978.

76. Gamboa ET, Eastwood AB, Hays AP, Maxwell J, and Penn AS: Isolation of influenza virus from muscle in myoglobinuric polymyositis. Neurology 29:1323, 1979.

77. Gaut P, Wong PK, and Meyer RD: Pyomyositis in a patient with the acquired immunodeficiency syndrome. Arch Intern Med 148:1608, 1988.

78. Gilliam JH III, Challa VR, Agudelo CA, Albertson DA, and Huntley CC: Vasculitis involving muscle associated with Crohn's colitis. Gastroenterology 81:787, 1981.

79. Gleich GJ and Adolphson CR: The eosinophilic leukocyte: Structure and function. Adv Immunol 39:177, 1986.

80. Gonzales MF, Olney RK, So YT, Greco CM, McQuinn BA, Miller RG, and DeArmond SJ: Subacute structural

myopathy associated with human immunodeficiency virus infection. Arch Neurol 45:585, 1988.

81. Gordon RM and Silverstein A: Neurologic manifestations in progressive systemic sclerosis. Arch Neurol 22:126, 1970.

82. Greenlee JE, Johnson WD, Campa JF, Adelman LS, and Sande MA: Adult toxoplasmosis presenting as polymyositis and cerebellar ataxia. Ann Intern Med 82:367, 1975.

82a. Griffin JW, Cornblath DR, Alexander E, et al: Ataxic sensory neuropathy and dorsal root ganglionitis associated with Sjögren's syndrome. Ann Neurol 27:304, 1990.

83. Griggs RC: Hypertrophy and cardiomyopathy in the neuromuscular diseases. Circ Res (Suppl) 34:II-145, 1974.

84. Griggs RC and Karpati G: The pathogenesis of dermatomyositis. Arch Neurol 48:21, 1991.

85. Greenstein AJ, Janowitz HD, and Sachar DB: The extra-intestinal complications of Crohn's disease and ulcerative colitis: A study of 700 patients. Medicine 55:401, 1976.

86. Haas DC and Arnason BGW: Cell-mediated immunity in polymyositis. Creatine phosphokinase release from muscle cultures. Arch Neurol 31:192, 1974.

87. Hahn TJ and Hahn BH: Osteopenia in patients with rheumatic diseases: Principles of diagnosis and therapy. Semin Arthritis Rheum 6:165, 1976.

88. Halla JT and Hardin JG: Clinical features of the arthritis of mixed connective tissue disease. Arthritis Rheum 21:497, 1978.

89. Halla JT, Volanakis JE, Schrohenloher RE: Circulating immune complexes in mixed connective tissue disease. Arthritis Rheum 22:484, 1979.

90. Halperin JJ, Little BW, Coyle PK, and Dattwyler RJ: Lyme disease: Cause of a treatable peripheral neuropathy. Neurology 37:1700, 1987.

91. Halverson PB, Lahiri S, Wojno WC, and Sulaiman AR: Sporotrichal arthritis presenting as granulomatous myositis. Arthritis Rheum 28:1425, 1985.

92. Hardin JA: The molecular biology of autoantibodies. In Schumacher HR (ed): Primer on Rheumatic Diseases ed 9. Arthritis Foundation, Georgia, 1988, pp 32–36.

93. Hertzman PA, Blevins WL, Mayer J, Greenfield B, Ting M, and Gleich GJ: Association of the eosinophilia-myalgia syndrome with the ingestion of tryptophan. N Engl J Med 322:869, 1990.

94. Ho KJ and Scully KT: Acute rhabdomyolysis and renal failure in Weil's disease. Alabama Journal of Medical Sciences 17:133, 1980.

95. Hochberg MC, Feldman D, and Stevens MB: Adult onset polymyositis/dermatomyositis: An analysis of clinical and laboratory features and survival in 76 patients with a review of the literature. Semin Arthritis Rheum 15:168, 1986.

96. Hoffman R, Dainiak N, Sibrack L, Pober JS, and Waldron JA Jr: Antibody-mediated aplastic anemia and diffuse fasciitis. N Engl J Med 300:718, 1979.

97. Hoffman R, Young N, Ershler WB, Mazur E, and Gewirtz A: Diffuse fasciitis and aplastic anemia: A report of four cases revealing an unusual association between rheumatologic and hematologic disorders. Medicine 61:373, 1982.

97a. Hohlfeld R, Engel AG, Ii K, and Harper MC: Polymyositis mediated by T lymphocytes that express the γ/δ receptor. N Engl J Med 324:877, 1991.

98. Horowitz M, McNeil JD, Maddern GJ, Collins PJ, and Shearman DJC: Abnormalities of gastric and esophageal emptying in polymyositis and dermatomyositis. Gastroenterology 90:434, 1986.

99. Isenberg D: Myositis in other connective tissue disorders. Clinics in Rheumatic Diseases 10:151, 1984.

100. Isenberg DA and Snaith ML: Muscle disease in systemic lupus erythematosus: a study of its nature. J Rheumatol 8:917, 1981.

101. Itoh J, Akiguchi I, Midorikawa R, and

Kameyama M: Sarcoid myopathy with typical rash of dermatomyositis. Neurology 30:1118, 1980.

102. Jacob JC and Mathew NT: Pseudohypertrophic myopathy in cysticercosis. Neurology 18:767, 1968.

103. Jehn UW and Fink MK: Myositis, myoglobinemia, and myoglobinuria associated with enterovirus echo 9 infection. Arch Neurol 37:457, 1980.

104. Jerusalem F, Rakusa M, Engel AG, and MacDonald RD: Morphometric analysis of skeletal muscle capillary ultrastructure in inflammatory myopathies. J Neurol Sci 23:391, 1974.

105. Josselson J, Pula T, and Sadler JH: Acute rhabdomyolysis associated with an echovirus 9 infection. Arch Intern Med 140:1671, 1980.

105a. Kagen LJ, Hochman RB, and Strong EW: Cricopharyngeal obstruction in inflammatory myopathy (polymyositis/dermatomyositis). Report of three cases and review of the literature. Arthritis Rheum 28:630, 1985.

106. Kagen LJ, Kimball AC, and Christian CL: Serologic evidence of toxoplasmosis among patients with polymyositis. Am J Med 56:185, 1974.

107. Kantor RJ, Norden CW, and Wein TP: Infectious mononucleosis associated with rhabdomyolysis and renal failure. South Med J 71:346, 1978.

108. Kazura JW and Aikawa M: Host defense mechanisms against trichinella spiralis infection in the mouse: Eosinophil-mediated destruction of newborn larvae in vitro. J Immunol 124:355, 1980.

109. Kehoe RF, Bauernfeind R, Tommaso C, Wyndham C, and Rosen KM: Cardiac conduction defects in polymyositis: Electrophysiologic studies in four patients. Ann Intern Med 94:41, 1981.

110. Kelly JJ, Madoc-Jones H, Adelman LS, Andres PL, and Munsat TL: Total body irradiation not effective in inclusion body myositis. Neurology 36:1264, 1986.

111. Kent LT, Cramer SF, and Moskowitz RW: Eosinophilic fasciitis. Clinical, laboratory and microscopic considerations. Arthritis Rheum 24:677, 1981.

112. Kilbourne EM, Rigau-Perez JG, Heath CW Jr, et al: Clinical epidemiology of toxic-oil syndrome. N Engl J Med 309:1408, 1983.

113. Kim RC and Collins GH: The neuropathology of rheumatoid disease. Hum Pathol 12:5, 1981.

114. Kiprov D, Conant MA, Lippert R, Pfaeffl W, Miller R, and Abrams D: Therapeutic apheresis as a treatment modality in AIDS and AIDS-related conditions. In: Carless IB and Pittman-Lindeman M (eds): AIDS: Principles, Practices, and Politics. Harper & Row, New York, 1988.

115. Kissel JT, Halterman RK, Rammohan KW, and Mendell JR: The relationship of complement-mediated microvasculopathy to the histologic features and clinical duration of disease in dermatomyositis. Arch Neurol 48:26, 1991.

116. Kissel JT, Levy RJ, Mendell JR, and Griggs RC: Azathioprine toxicity in neuromuscular disease. Neurology 36:35, 1986.

117. Kissel JT, Mendell JR, and Rammohan KW: Microvascular deposition of complement membrane attack complex in dermatomyositis. N Engl J Med 314:329, 1986.

117a. Kissel JT, Riethman JL, Omerza J, et al: Peripheral nerve vasculitis: Immune characterization of the vascular lesions. Ann Neurol 25:291, 1989.

118. Klinefelter HF, Winkenwerder WL, and Bledsoe T: Single daily dose prednisone therapy. JAMA 241:2721, 1979.

119. Koutras A: Myositis with Kawasaki's disease. Am J Dis Child 136:78, 1982.

120. Lakhanpal S, Bunch TW, Ilstrup DM, and Melton LJ: Polymyositis-dermatomyositis and malignant lesions: Does an association exist? Mayo Clin Proc 61:645, 1986.

121. Lakhanpal S, Duffy J, and Engel AG: Eosinophilia associated with perimyositis and pneumonitis. Mayo Clin Proc 63:37, 1988.

122. Lakhanpal S, Ginsburg WW, Michet CJ, Doyle JA, and Moore SB: Eosinophilic fasciitis: Clinical spectrum and

therapeutic response in 52 cases. Semin Arthritis Rheum 17:221, 1988.

123. Lakhanpal S, Lie JT, Conn DL, and Martin WJ: Pulmonary disease in polymyositis/dermatomyositis: A clinicopathological analysis of 65 autopsy cases. Ann Rheum Dis 46:23, 1987.

124. Laloux P, Brucher JM, Guerit JM, Sindic CJM, and Laterre EC: Subacute sensory neuropathy associated with Sjögren's sicca syndrome. J Neurol 235:352, 1988.

124a. Lang BA, Laxer RM, Thorner P, Greenberg M, and Silverman ED: Pediatric onset of Behçet syndrome with myositis: case report and literature review illustrating unusual features. Arthritis Rheum 33:418, 1990.

124b. Lange DJ: Neuromuscular diseases associated with HIV-1 infection. Muscle Nerve 17:16, 1994.

125. Layzer RB, Shearn MA, and Satya-Murti S: Eosinophilic polymyositis. Ann Neurol 1:65, 1977.

126. Leon-Monzon M and Dalakas MC: Absence of persistent infection with enteroviruses in muscles of patients with inflammatory myopathies. Ann Neurol 32:219, 1992.

127. Levy JA: Human immunodeficiency viruses and the pathogenesis of AIDS. JAMA 261:2997, 1989.

128. Lipkin WI, Parry G, Kiprov D, and Abrams D: Inflammatory neuropathy in homosexual men with lymphadenopathy. Neurology 35:1479, 1985.

129. Lipton JH, McLeod BD, and Brownell AKW: Dermatomyositis and granulomatous myopathy associated with sarcoidosis. Can J Neurol Sci 15:426, 1988.

130. Lotz BP, Engel AG, Nishino H, Stevens JC, and Litchy WJ: Inclusion body myositis: observations in 40 patients. Brain 112:727, 1989.

131. Lundberg A: Myalgia cruris epidemica. Acta Paediatr 46:18, 1957.

132. MacDonald RD and Engel AG: Experimental chloroquine myopathy. J Neuropathol Exp Neurol 29:479, 1970.

133. Manchul LA, Jin A, Pritchard KI, et al: The frequency of malignant neoplasms in patients with polymyositis-dermatomyositis: A controlled study. Arch Intern Med 145:1835, 1985.

134. Maricq HR, LeRoy EC, D'Angelo WA, et al: Diagnostic potential of in vivo capillary microscopy in scleroderma and related disorders. Arthritis Rheum 23:183, 1980.

135. Maricq HR, Spencer-Green G, and LeRoy EC: Skin capillary abnormalities as indicators of organ involvement in scleroderma (systemic sclerosis), Raynaud's syndrome and dermatomyositis. Am J Med 61:862, 1976.

136. Markand ON and D'Agostino AN: Ultrastructural changes in skeletal muscle induced by colchicine. Arch Neurol 24:72, 1971.

137. Martinez-Tello FJ, Navas-Palacios JJ, Ricoy JR, et al: Pathology of a new toxic syndrome caused by ingestion of adulterated oil in Spain. Virchows Arch A Pathol Anat Histopathol 397:261, 1982.

138. Matteson EL and Michet CJ: Sarcoid myositis with pseudohypertrophy. Am J Med 87:240, 1989.

139. McCabe RE, Brooks RG, Dorfman RF, and Remington JS: Clinical spectrum in 107 cases of toxoplasmic lymphadenopathy. Reviews of Infectious Diseases 9:754, 1987.

140. McFarlin DE and Griggs RC: Treatment of inflammatory myopathies with azathioprine. Transactions of the American Neurological Association 93:244, 1968.

141. Mease PJ, Ochs HD, and Wedgwood RJ: Successful treatment of echovirus meningoencephalitis and myositis-fasciitis with intravenous immune globulin therapy in a patient with X-linked agammaglobulinemia. N Engl J Med 304:1278, 1981.

142. Mejlszenkier JD, Safran AP, Healy JJ, Embree L, and Ouellette EM: The myositis of influenza. Arch Neurol 29:441, 1973.

143. Mellgren SI, Conn DL, Stevens JC, and Dyck PJ: Peripheral neuropathy in primary Sjögren's syndrome. Neurology 39:390, 1989.

144. Ménard DB, Haddad H, Blain JG, Beaudry R, Devroede G, and Massé S: Granulomatous myositis and myopathy associated with Crohn's colitis. N Engl J Med 295:818, 1976.

144a. Mendell JR, Kissel JT, Stevens R, et al: Prospective, controlled trial of six monthly myoblast transfers in Duchenne dystrophy. Neurology 44 (suppl 2):A268, 1994.

144b. Mendell JR, Sahenk Z, Gales T, and Paul L: Amyloid filaments in inclusion body myositis. Novel findings provide insight into nature of filaments. Arch Neurol 48:1229, 1991.

145. Metzger AL, Bohan A, Goldberg LS, Bluestone R, and Pearson CM: Polymyositis and dermatomyositis: Combined methotrexate and corticosteroid therapy. Ann Intern Med 81:182, 1974.

146. Metzler MH, Sahgal KK, and Wolff GS: Second degree atrioventricular block in acute trichinosis. Am J Dis Child 124:598, 1972.

147. Michaels RM: Eosinophilic fasciitis complicated by Hodgkin's disease. J Rheumatol 9:473, 1982.

148. Michet CJ Jr, Doyle JA, and Ginsburg WW: Eosinophilic fasciitis. Report of 15 cases. Mayo Clin Proc 56:27, 1981.

149. Miller RG, Carson PJ, Moussavi RS, Green AT, Baker AJ, and Weiner MW: Fatigue and myalgia in AIDS patients. Neurology 41:1603, 1991.

150. Miller RG, Kiprov DD, Parry G, and Bredesen DE: Peripheral nervous system dysfunction in acquired immunodeficiency syndrome. In Rosenblum ML, Levy RM, and Bredesen DE (eds): AIDS and the Nervous System. Raven Press, New York, 1988, p 65.

151. Miller RG, Parry GJ, Pfaeffl W, Lang W, Lippert R, and Kiprov D: The spectrum of peripheral neuropathy associated with ARC and AIDS. Muscle Nerve 11:857, 1988.

152. Miller RG, Storey JR, and Greco CM: Ganciclovir in the treatment of progressive AIDS-related polyradiculopathy. Neurology 40:569, 1990.

153. Minow RA, Gorbach S, Johnson BL Jr, and Dornfeld L: Myoglobinuria associated with influenza A injection. Ann Intern Med 80:359, 1974.

154. Morgan GJ Jr, McGuire JL, and Ochoa J: Penicillamine-induced myositis in rheumatoid arthritis. Muscle Nerve 4:137, 1981.

155. Morgan OS, Rodgers-Johnson P, Mora C, and Char G: HTLV-1 and polymyositis in Jamaica. Lancet 2:1184, 1989.

156. Morgensen JL: Myoglobinuria and renal failure associated with influenza. Ann Intern Med 80:362, 1974.

156a. Moutsopoulos HM, Webber BL, Pavlidis NA, Fostiropoulos G, Goules D, and Shulman LE: Diffuse fasciitis with eosinophilia: A clinicopathologic study. Am J Med 68:701, 1980.

157. Mustafa MM, Scarvey L, Rollins N, and Siegel JD: Primary suppurative myositis associated with haemophilus influenzae type B septicemia. Pediatr Infect Dis J 7:815, 1988.

158. Namba T, Brunner NG, and Grob D: Idiopathic giant cell polymyositis. Report of a case and review of the syndrome. Arch Neurol 31:27, 1974.

159. Nelson KR and McQuillen MP: Neurologic complications of graft-versus-host disease. Neurol Clin 6:389, 1988.

160. Nishino H, Engel AG, and Rima BK: Inclusion body myositis: The mumps virus hypothesis. Ann Neurol 25:260, 1989.

161. Nordstrom DM, Petropolis AA, Giorno R, Gates RH, and Reddy VB: Inflammatory myopathy and acquired immunodeficiency syndrome. Arthritis Rheum 32:475, 1989.

162. Norton WL, Velayos E, and Robison L: Endothelial inclusions in dermatomyositis. Ann Rheum Dis 29:67, 1970.

163. Nussbaum AI, Silver RM, and Maricq HR: Serial changes in nailfold capillary morphology in childhood dermatomyositis. Arthritis Rheum 26:1169, 1983.

164. O'Connell DJ and Bennett RM: Mixed connective tissue disease—clinical and radiological aspects of 20 cases. Br J Radiol 50:620, 1977.

165. Oxenhandler R, Hart MN, Bickel J, Scearce D, Durham J, and Irvin W: Pathologic features of muscle in systemic lupus erythematosus: A biopsy series with comparative clinical and immunopathologic observations. Hum Pathol 13:745, 1982.

166. Oxenhandler R, Hart M, Corman L, Sharp G, and Adelstein E: Pathology of skeletal muscle in mixed connective tissue disease. Arthritis Rheum 20:985, 1977.

167. Pachman LN and Maryjowski MC: Juvenile dermatomyositis and polymyositis. Clinics in Rheumatic Diseases 10:95, 1984.

168. Pachner AR, Duray P, and Steere AC: Central nervous system manifestations of Lyme disease. Arch Neurol 46:790, 1989.

169. Parrillo JE, Fauci AS, and Wolff SM: Therapy of the hypereosinophilic syndrome. Ann Intern Med 89:167, 1978.

170. Pavlidis NA, Karsh J, and Moutsopoulos HM: The clinical picture of primary Sjögren's syndrome: A retrospective study. J Rheumatol 9:685, 1982.

171. Pawlowski ZS: Clinical aspects in man. In Campbell WC (ed): Trichinella and Trichinosis. Plenum Press, New York, 1983, p. 367.

172. Pettersson I, Wang G, Smith EI, et al: The use of immunoblotting and immunoprecipitation of (U) small nuclear ribonucleoproteins in the analysis of sera of patients with mixed connective tissue disease and systemic lupus erythematosus. A cross-sectional, longitudinal study. Arthritis Rheum 29:986, 1986.

173. Peura DA and Johnson LF: Cimetidine for prevention and treatment of gastroduodenal mucosal lesions in patients in an intensive care unit. Ann Intern Med 103:173, 1985.

174. Pittsley RA, Shearn MA, and Kaufman L: Acute hepatitis B simulating dermatomyositis. JAMA 239:959, 1978.

175. Plotz PH, Dalakas M, Leff RL, et al: Current concepts in the idiopathic inflammatory myopathies: Polymyositis, dermatomyositis, and related disorders. Ann Intern Med 111:143, 1989.

176. Pollock JL: Toxoplasmosis: Appearing to be dermatomyositis. Arch Dermatol 115:736, 1979.

177. Pouchot J, Vinceneux P, Barge J, Laparre F, Boussougant Y, and Michon C: Tuberculous polymyositis in HIV infection. Am J Med 89:250, 1990.

178. Prystowsky SD: Mixed connective tissue disease. West J Med 132:288, 1980.

179. Rammohan KW, Wolinsky J, Omerza J, Gales T, Kissel J, and Mendell J: Mumps virus in IBM: Studies implicating cross-reactivity accounting for antigen localization [abstract]. Neurology 38:151, 1988.

180. Raphael SA, Longenecker SC, Wolfson BJ, and Fisher MC: Post-varicella streptococcal pyomyositis. Pediatric Infect Dis J 8:187, 1989.

181. Raphael SA, Wolfson BJ, Parker P, Lischner HW, and Faerber EN: Pyomyositis in a child with acquired immunodeficiency syndrome. Patient report and brief review. Am J Dis Child 143:779, 1989.

182. Reimers CD, Pongratz DE, Neubert U, Pilz A, Hübner G, Naegele M, Wilske B, Duray PH, and Koning J: Myositis cause by Borrelia burgdorferi: report of four cases. J Neurol Sci 91:215, 1989.

183. Reyes MG, Noronha P, Thomas W Jr, and Heredia R: Myositis of chronic graft versus host disease. Neurology 33:1222, 1983.

184. Riggs JE, Schochet SS Jr, Gutmann L, and Lerfald SC: Childhood onset inclusion body myositis mimicking limb-girdle muscular dystrophy. J Child Neurol 4:283, 1989.

185. Ringel SP, Forstot JZ, Tan EM, Wehling C, Griggs RC, and Butcher D: Sjögren's syndrome and polymyositis or dermatomyositis. Arch Neurol 39:157, 1982.

186. Ringel SP, Kenny CE, Neville HE, Giorno R, and Carry MR: Spectrum of inclusion body myositis. Arch Neurol 44:1154, 1987.

187. Ringel SP, Thorne EG, Phanuphak P,

Lava NS, and Kohler PS: Immune complex vasculitis, polymyositis, and hyperglobulinemic purpura. Neurology 29:682, 1979.

188. Rosenberg NL, Rotbart HA, Abzug MJ, et al: Evidence for a novel picornavirus in human dermatomyositis. Ann Neurol 26:204, 1989.

189. Rosenthal J and Benson MD: Diffuse fasciitis and eosinophilia with symmetric polyarthritis. Ann Intern Med 92:507, 1980.

190. Ruskin J and Remington JS: Toxoplasmosis in the compromised host. Ann Intern Med 84:193, 1976.

191. Sakimoto K: The cause of the eosinophilia-myalgia syndrome associated with tryptophan use. N Engl J Med 323:992, 1990.

191a. Sambrook P, Birningham J, Kelly P, et al: Prevention of corticosteroid osteoporosis. N Engl J Med 328:1747, 1993.

192. Schattner A, Hay E, Lifschitz-Mercer B, Gorbacz S, and Bentwich Z: Fulminant streptococcal myositis. Ann Emerg Med 18:320, 1989.

193. Schaumburg HH, Neilsen SL, and Yurchak PM: Heart block in polymyositis. N Engl J Med 284:480, 1971.

194. Schmidley JW and Galloway P: Polymyositis following autologous bone marrow transplantation in Hodgkin's disease. Neurology 40:1003, 1990.

195. Schoenen J, Sianard-Gainko J, Carpentier M, and Reznik M: Myositis during Borrelia burgdorferi infection (Lyme disease). J Neurol Neurosurg Psychiatry 52:1002, 1989.

196. Schwarz MI, Matthay RA, Sahn SA, et al: Interstitial lung disease in polymyositis and dermatomyositis: Analysis of six cases and review of the literature. Medicine 55:89, 1976.

197. Serratrice G, Pellissier JF, Cros D, Gastaut JL, and Brindisi G: Relapsing eosinophilic perimyositis. J Rheumatol 7:199, 1980.

198. Shantz PM: Effective medical treatment for hydatid disease? JAMA 253:2095, 1985.

199. Sharp GC, Irvin WS, Tan EM, Gould RG, and Holman HR: Mixed connective tissue disease: An apparently distinct rheumatic disease syndrome associated with a specific antibody to extractable nuclear antigen (ENA). Am J Med 52:148, 1972.

200. Shevell M, Rosenblatt B, Silver K, Carpenter S, and Karpati G: Congenital inflammatory myopathy. Neurology 40:1111, 1990.

201. Shulman LE: Diffuse fasciitis with eosinophilia: a new syndrome. Arthritis Rheum 20:S205, 1977. Abstract.

202. Shulman LE, Hoffman R, Dainiak N, et al: Antibody-mediated aplastic anemia and thrombocytopenic purpura in diffuse eosinophilic fasciitis [abstract]. Arthritis Rheum 22:659, 1979.

203. Sigal LH and Tatum AH: Lyme disease patients' serum contains IgM antibodies to Borrelia burgdorferi that cross-react with neuronal antigens. Neurology 38:1439, 1988.

204. Silverstein A and Siltzbach LE: Muscle involvement in sarcoidosis. Arch Neurol 21:235, 1969.

205. Simpson DM and Bender AN: Human immunodeficiency virus–associated myopathy: Analysis of 11 patients. Ann Neurol 24:79, 1988.

206. Simpson DM, Bender AN, Farraye J, Mendelson SG, and Wolfe DE: Human immunodeficiency virus wasting syndrome may represent a treatable myopathy. Neurology 40:535, 1990.

207. Singsen BH, Swanson VL, Bernstein BH, Heuser ET, Hanson V, and Landing BH: A histologic evaluation of mixed connective tissue disease in childhood. Am J Med 68:710, 1980.

208. Sladek GD, Vasey FB, Sieger B, Behnke DA, Germain BF, and Espinoza LR: Relapsing eosinophilic myositis. J Rheumatol 10:467, 1983.

209. Smith BE and Dyck PJ: Peripheral neuropathy in the eosinophilia-myalgia syndrome associated with L-tryptophan ingestion. Neurology 40:1035, 1990.

210. Smith CIE, Aarli JA, Biberfeld P, et al: Myasthenia gravis after bone-marrow transplantation: Evidence for a

donor origin. N Engl J Med 309:1565, 1983.

211. Smith JK, Chi DS, Guarderas J, Brown P, Verghese A, and Berk SL: Disseminated echovirus infection in a patient with multiple myeloma and a functional defect in complement. Arch Intern Med 149:1455, 1989.

212. Sokoloff MC, Goldberg LS, and Pearson CM: Treatment of corticosteroid-resistant polymyositis with methotrexate. Lancet:14, 1971.

213. Soueidan SA and Dalakas MC: Treatment of inclusion-body myositis with high-dose intravenous immunoglobulin. Neurology 43:876, 1993.

214. Spencer CH, Hanson V, Singsen BH, Bernstein BH, Kornreich HK, and King KK: Course of treated juvenile dermatomyositis. J Pediatr 105:399, 1984.

215. Spencer-Green G, Crowe WE, and Levinson JE: Nailfold capillary abnormalities and clinical outcome in childhood dermatomyositis. Arthritis Rheum 25:954, 1982.

216. Stark RJ: Eosinophilic polymyositis. Arch Neurol 36:721, 1979.

217. Steere AC: Lyme disease. N Engl J Med 321:586, 1989.

218. Stehr-Green JK and Schantz PM: Trichinosis in Southeast Asian refugees in the United States. Am J Public Health 76:1238, 1986.

219. Stern R, Godbold JH, Chess Q, and Kagen LJ: ECG abnormalities in polymyositis. Arch Intern Med 144:2185, 1984.

220. Stjernberg N, Cajander S, Truedsson H, and Uddenfeldt P: Muscle involvement in sarcoidosis. Acta Medica Scandinavica 209:213, 1981.

221. Sullivan DB, Cassidy JT, and Petty RE: Dermatomyositis in pediatric patient. Arthritis Rheum 20:327, 1977.

222. Taborn J, Bole GG, and Thompson GR: Colchicine suppression of local and systemic inflammation due to calcinosis universalis in chronic dermatomyositis. Ann Intern Med 89:648, 1978.

223. Tan EM: Autoantibodies to nuclear antigens (ANA): their immunobiology and medicine. Adv Immunol 33:167, 1982.

224. Thompson CE: Infantile myositis. Dev Med Child Neurol 24:307, 1982.

224a. Thornton CA and Griggs RC: Plasma exchange and intravenous immunoglobulin treatment of neuromuscular disease. Ann Neurol 35:260, 1994.

225. Tomé FMS and Fardeau M: Nuclear inclusions in oculopharyngeal dystrophy. Acta Neuropathol Berl 49:85, 1980.

226. Torch WC: Computerized tomography of muscle: A useful technique in the differential diagnosis and study of infantile hypotonia and a variety of neuromuscular disorders in children and adults. Ann Neurol 8:233, 1980.

227. Toxic Epidemic Study Group. Toxic epidemic syndrome, Spain, 1981. Lancet 2:697, 1982.

228. Tsokos GC, Moutsopoulos HM, and Steinberg AD: Muscle involvement in systemic lupus erythematosus. JAMA 246:766, 1981.

229. Vermillion DL and Collins SM: Increased responsiveness of jejunal longitudinal muscle in trichinella-infected rats. Am J Physiol 254:G124, 1988.

229a. Watt G, Alquiza LM, Padre LP, Tuazon ML, and Laughlin LW: The rapid diagnosis of leptospirosis: A prospective comparison of the dot enzyme-linked immunosorbent assay and the genus-specific microscopic agglutination test at different stages of illness. J Infect Dis 157:840, 1988.

229b. Watt G, Padre LP, Tuazon M, and Calubaquib C: Skeletal and cardiac muscle involvement in severe, late leptospirosis. J Infect Dis 162:266, 1990.

230. Webb DR and Currie GD: Pulmonary fibrosis masking polymyositis: Remission with corticosteroid therapy. JAMA 222:1146, 1972.

231. Weltz M, Salvado A, Rosse W, and Berenberg J: Humoral suppression of hematopoiesis in eosinophilic fasciitis [abstract]. Blood 52 (Suppl):218, 1978.

232. West SG, Killian PJ, and Lawless OJ: Association of myositis and myocar-

ditis in progressive systemic sclerosis. Arthritis Rheum 24:662, 1981.

233. Whitaker JN and Engel WK: Vascular deposits of immunoglobulin and complement in idiopathic inflammatory myopathy. N Engl J Med 286:332, 1972.

234. Wiener-Kronish JP, Solinger AM, Warnock ML, Churg A, Ordonez N, and Golden JA: Severe pulmonary involvement in mixed connective tissue disease. Am Rev Respir Dis 124:499, 1981.

235. Wiley CA, Nerenberg M, Cros D, and Soto-Aguilar MC: HTLV-1 polymyositis in a patient also infected with the human immunodeficiency virus. N Engl J Med 320:992, 1989.

236. Wright J, Couchonnal G, and Hodges GR: Adenovirus type 21 infection: Occurrence with pneumonia, rhabdomyolysis, and myoglobinuria in an adult. JAMA 241:2420, 1979.

237. Yonker RA and Panush RS: Idiopathic eosinophilic myositis with preexisting fibromyalgia. J Rheumatol 12:165, 1985.

238. Younger DS, Hays AP, Uncini A, Lange DJ, Lovelace RE, and DiMauro S: Recurrent myoglobinuria and HIV seropositivity: incidental or pathogenic association? Muscle Nerve 12:842, 1989.

239. Yunis EJ and Samaha FJ: Inclusion body myositis. Lab Invest 25:240, 1971.

Chapter 6

CONGENITAL MYOPATHIES

DEFINITION OF CONGENITAL MYOPATHY
PRESENTATION OF A PATIENT WITH CONGENITAL MYOPATHY
COMMON TYPES OF CONGENITAL MYOPATHIES
UNCOMMON TYPES OF CONGENITAL MYOPATHIES
DUBIOUS TYPES OF CONGENITAL MYOPATHIES

DEFINITION OF CONGENITAL MYOPATHY

The term "congenital myopathy" was introduced by Shy and Magee in 1956.[154] In their description of central core disease, congenital myopathy was meant to imply a *nonprogressive muscle disease, existing at birth* but very different from muscular dystrophy. This point of view was clearly indicated by the title of the report "A New Congenital Non-Progressive Myopathy."[154] Unfortunately, subsequent additions to the list of congenital myopathies, especially nemaline (rod)[153] and centronuclear myopathies,[136] have destroyed the notion that "congenital myopathy" can be equated with a benign disorder. Many patients with nemaline and centronuclear myopathies have progressed and even died, clearly blurring distinctions from the muscular dystrophies.

By tradition, the term congenital myopathy also implies the presence of a specific morphologic feature on muscle biopsy, for example, the cores in central core disease and rods in nemaline myopathy. Unfortunately, as the list of congenital myopathies has grown, the specificity of the distinguishing morphologic features has not always stood the test of time. This raises the issue of how many of the conditions reported as congenital myopathies actually warrant a separate nosologic designation. We have grouped the congenital myopathies under three subheadings — the common, the uncommon, and those of dubious nature (Table 6–1) — to reflect the consistency of clinical and muscle histology features.

PRESENTATION OF A PATIENT WITH CONGENITAL MYOPATHY

Differential Diagnosis of Floppy Infant

A congenital myopathy should be considered in the evaluation of any floppy infant, although hypotonia in infants will usually have central nervous system rather than a neuromuscular cause. As shown in Table 6–2, of disorders affecting the motor unit, the spinal muscular atrophies account for most floppy infants, followed by (in order of frequency) the congenital myopathies, the muscular dystrophies (especially congenital muscular dystrophy and congenital myotonic dystrophy; see Chapter 4), congenital myasthenic syndromes,[50,51] metabolic disorders of muscle (see Chapter 7), and least commonly, the congenital peripheral neuropathies (amyelinating and hypomyelinating varieties).[27] Bedside differentiation of these disorders can be difficult in the neonatal period. In most

Table 6–1 CONGENITAL MYOPATHIES

COMMON TYPES
Central core disease
Nemaline (rod) myopathy
Centronuclear myopathies
  Neonatal type
  Late infantile–early childhood type
  Late childhood–adult type

UNCOMMON TYPES
Multicore disease
Fingerprint body myopathy
Sarcotubular myopathy
Hyaline body myopathy (familial myopathy
  with probable lysis of myofibrils)

**DUBIOUS TYPES (variable course or
pathology; or inadequate characterization)**
Congenital fiber-type disproportion
Congenital hypotonia with type 1 fiber
  predominance
Reducing body myopathy
Cytoplasmic body myopathy
Myopathy with tubular aggregates
Zebra body myopathy
Trilaminar myopathy

cases, hypotonia and weakness are the major manifestations; some distinguishing features of the congenital myopathies, like ophthalmoplegia or skeletal abnormalities (scoliosis or pes cavus), may not be apparent at birth. In addition, muscle stretch reflexes, which would help identify a central nervous system disease, may not be exagger-

**Table 6–2 NEUROMUSCULAR
DISEASES CAUSING A FLOPPY INFANT**

Spinal muscular atrophy
Congenital myopathy (see Table 6–1)
Congenital muscular dystrophies
Congenital myotonic dystrophy
Congenital myasthenic syndrome(s)
Acid maltase deficiency (Pompe's disease)
Debranching enzyme deficiency (type 3 glycogen
  storage disease)
Branching enzyme deficiency (type 4 glycogen
  storage disease)
Carnitine deficiency
Mitochondrial myopathies
Congenital peripheral neuropathies

ated, and the Babinski sign is not necessarily a sign of central disease.

Clinical and Laboratory Features of Congenital Myopathies

Most congenital myopathies present to the physician for diagnosis in late infancy or early childhood. A history of infantile hypotonia can often be elicited, but more commonly patients present because of delayed motor milestones or varying degrees of weakness noticed in activities such as arising from the floor, climbing stairs, or running. Skeletal abnormalities and dysmorphic features, common accompaniments of congenital myopathies, can be recognized at this later period of childhood; and central nervous system disorders are more easily differentiated because at this later age patients will usually demonstrate upper motor neuron signs (hyperreflexia, increased muscle tone, Babinski sign) or the ataxia typical of some disorders.

The diagnosis of a congenital myopathy rests unequivocally on the muscle biopsy features for which the disorder has usually been named (see Table 6–1). Other laboratory features, including a normal or only minimally elevated creatine kinase (CK) level, will help to differentiate a congenital myopathy from the muscular dystrophies. The CK level is markedly elevated in the latter (see Chapter 4). In the congenital myopathies, the electromyographic (EMG) findings may be normal or show small, polyphasic, and abundant motor unit potentials. These findings, in the absence of abnormal spontaneous activity, point away from the spinal muscular atrophies. Normal results from repetitive nerve stimulation studies exclude the congenital myasthenic syndromes,[50,51] and normal findings in nerve conduction studies exclude the congenital hypomyelinating peripheral neuropathies.[27]

Table 6–3 CENTRAL CORE DISEASE

CLINICAL FEATURES
Hypotonia
Delayed motor milestones
Proximal weakness, especially legs
Skeletal abnormalities, include congenital hip
  dislocation, scoliosis, pes cavus, pes
  planus, clubfeet
Predisposition to malignant hyperthermia
Mild or nonprogressive course

GENETICS
Usually autosomal dominant; sporadic cases

MUSCLE BIOPSY
See Figs. 6–1 and 6–2.

COMMON TYPES OF CONGENITAL MYOPATHIES

Central Core Disease

The first description of central core disease (Table 6–3) represented an important landmark in myology, demonstrating the value of careful histologic examination of muscle.[154]

CLINICAL FEATURES

Patients with central core disease may have decreased fetal movements, breech presentation,[73,154] or congenital hip dislocation,[1,4,73] but a normal birth history is not unusual. Motor milestones, particularly walking, are delayed. Later in childhood, patients develop problems with stair-climbing, running, and getting up from the floor. The course is usually nonprogressive, but exceptions have been documented.[130] Muscle cramps following exercise can be the only clinical symptom.[10]

Clinical examination shows the proximal lower-extremity muscles to be the most affected. Patients may use their arms to push off from chairs or to climb up their legs in getting up from the floor (Gowers' sign; see Fig. 2–1). Upper-extremity proximal muscles are affected to a lesser degree. Mild weakness of the facial muscles and neck flexors may be

present, but sparing of cranial nerve musculature distinguishes central core disease from the other common congenital myopathies (nemaline and centronuclear). Skeletal abnormalities are frequent and include congenital hip dislocation,[1,4,73] scoliosis,[154] pes cavus,[43] pes planus,[57,154] and clubfeet (talipes). Pes cavus may be the only manifestation of the disorder.[162] Muscle stretch reflexes may be normal or depressed.

LABORATORY FEATURES

The CK level is usually normal. Electrophysiologic studies show normal motor and sensory nerve conduction. Needle EMG examination of clinically affected muscles demonstrates an underlying myopathy, with either absent or sparse spontaneous activity and brief, small, abundant, polyphasic motor unit potentials. Some patients show a second population of long-duration, high-amplitude motor unit potentials. Single-fiber EMG studies show an increase in motor unit fiber density that is consistent with an increased terminal innervation ratio.[35]

The muscle biopsy findings are the most important diagnostic feature of central core disease (Figs. 6–1 and

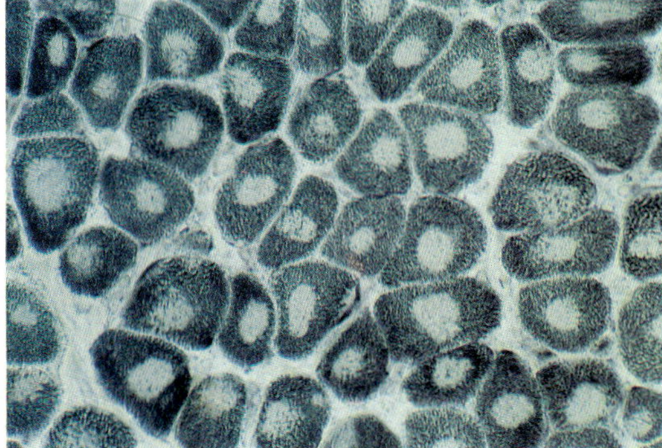

Figure 6–1. Central core disease. Central cores appear as central or eccentric areas of muscle fibers devoid of oxidative enzyme activity. Cores occur predominantly in type 1 fibers, as shown here. NADH-tetrazolium reductase.

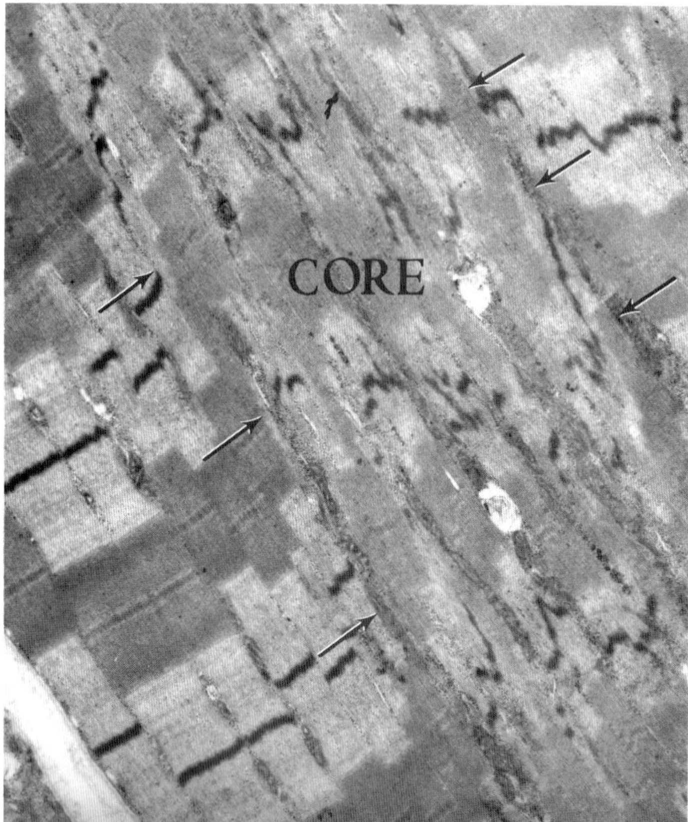

Figure 6–2. Central core disease. Electron micrograph showing poorly aligned sarcomeres and Z disk streaming in region of core (*outlined by arrows*).

6–2). Abnormalities can be recognized in paraffin sections, as originally observed,[76,154] but histochemical alterations are the most distinctive features.[57] Oxidative enzyme staining is likely to reveal one or more central or eccentric cores showing reduced activity. The cores also have decreased glycogen, causing pale staining in phosphorylase and periodic acid–Schiff (PAS) stains. The most common cores have decreased adenosine triphosphatase (ATPase) activity and have been referred to as unstructured cores.[124] In some cases, so-called structured cores have preserved ATPase activity. A smudgy appearance distinguishes the core from the surrounding normal margins of the muscle fiber. Type 1 fibers contain central cores more commonly than do type 2 fibers, and predominance of type 1 fibers is frequent. On electron microscopy, cores appear as poorly aligned sarcomeres associated with Z disc streaming, decreased numbers of mitochondria, and reduced amounts of glycogen (see Fig. 6–2). Unstructured cores show marked disruption of the A, I, and Z bands, accompanied by disorientation of the triads and elongation of the T tubules.

GENETICS

Autosomal dominant inheritance is the usual mode of genetic transmission for central core disease, although sporadic cases also occur.[11,121] An identical twin of an affected central core patient was said to be normal, but because appropriate muscle biopsy findings were not provided, the reliability of this report is questionable.[32] The gene for central core disease has been localized to chromosome 19q.[93] The gene for the ryanodine receptor maps to the same region of chromosome 19q.[104,109] This colocalization appears to account for the frequent occurrence of malignant hyperthermia in central core disease. In fact, at least three distinct mutations of the human ryanodine receptor gene have now been associated with central core disease.[136a,174]

PATHOGENESIS

Central core disease is most likely an inherited primary defect of muscle, but its cause has not been determined, and the mechanism of core formation remains unknown. The obvious similarities in appearance between target fibers and central cores[62] (see Chapter 2), and the results of muscle biopsy[31] and single-fiber EMG[35] studies that demonstrate collateral sprouting at the nerve terminals raise the possibility of an abnormal neural innervation. Cores extend the entire length of the muscle fiber, a feature not typical for targets. Although changes appearing similar to central cores can be produced experimentally by tenotomy,[91] close inspection reveals that tenotomy-induced cores consist of the products of myofibrillar lysis with a central area of granular debris different from a central core.[91]

TREATMENT

Patients with central core disease usually have a mild, nonprogressive condition with few physical limitations. Proximal weakness may cause trouble in stair-climbing and in exercise participation. Patients rarely may require orthotic devices for foot deformities. Recognition of central core disease, however, remains of the utmost importance because patients have a well-established predisposition for malignant hyperthermia during general anesthesia.[41,48,81,120] Because central core disease has associated skeletal abnormalities that may require surgical intervention, appropriate precautions must be taken (see Chapter 7, pp. 279–283). The life-threatening nature of malig-

nant hyperthermia emphasizes the need to diagnose underlying conditions causing congenital hip dislocation. Patients with central core disease must be encouraged to wear a medic-alert bracelet or necklace that indicates their predisposition to anesthesia-related complications.

Nemaline Myopathy

The second congenital myopathy to be recognized was nemaline (or rod) myopathy (Table 6–4).* The term "nemaline" was chosen[153] because the distinctive feature was the presence of rods or coils of threadlike structures (G. *nema*, thread). Others who reported cases concurrently[33] referred to the rodlike structures as "myogranules."

CLINICAL FEATURES

Nemaline myopathy presents as severe neonatal hypotonia with decreased fetal movements and early respiratory distress, resulting in death days to months after birth.† More typically, nemaline patients appear hypotonic dur-

Table 6–4 NEMALINE MYOPATHY

CLINICAL FEATURES
Hypotonia
Delayed milestones
Proximal and distal muscle weakness
Skeletal abnormalities including long thin face, high-arched palate, short jaw, pectus excavatum, kyphoscoliosis, pes cavus, clubfeet
Mild to severely progressive course with possible fatal outcome

GENETICS
Autosomal dominant; sporadic cases

MUSCLE BIOPSY
See Figs. 6–3 and 2–47.

---

*References 33,49,59–61,68,78,89,90,97, 110,123,142,150,153.
†References 68,90,97,110,123,142,150.

ing the neonatal period but do not have catastrophic respiratory distress. Delayed motor milestones, especially walking, are common, as in the originally reported cases.[33,153] Children escaping diagnosis in infancy present with varying degrees of proximal weakness that are noticed because of difficulty in running or arising from the floor.

The physical appearance of children may be striking because of the long, narrow facies or head (dolichocephalic), high-arched palate, and open-mouthed appearance due to an abnormally short or prognathous jaw. In addition, patients often exhibit pectus excavatum, kyphoscoliosis, pes cavus, and clubfoot (talipes) deformities. Nemaline myopathy patients exhibit a slender appearance (dolichomorphic) out of proportion to the degree of weakness. Mild facial weakness can be present, but sparing of extraocular muscle movements helps distinguish nemaline myopathy from centronuclear myopathy (see p. 218). In nemaline myopathy, patients have generalized muscle weakness, which is most apparent in the pelvic girdle and anterior compartment muscles and is commonly associated with absent tendon reflexes. Sensation is normal.

The course of congenital nemaline myopathy may be static and non-progressive,[33,153] mildly progressive,[61] or fatal in infancy or childhood.[90] Intranuclear nemaline rods (see below) serve to identify the most severe form.[140]

An adult-onset form of nemaline myopathy has also been observed.[20,49,59,60,89] Despite the presence of rods in muscle biopsies of these cases, evidence indicates that this is a different entity from the congenital form of the disease. These adult patients lack the skeletal and dysmorphic features characteristic of the childhood cases, and no familial cases have been reported. The presence of typical nemaline rods in adult patients with human immunodeficiency virus (HIV) infection (see Chapter 5) raises the possibility that adult cases are acquired as the result of an infectious or other exogenous process.

Myocardial involvement is an unusual manifestation of nemaline myopathy.[112,113,158] A 29-year-old woman presented with congestive heart failure secondary to a dilated cardiomyopathy but lacked other clinical features of nemaline myopathy.[113] Nevertheless, rods were found at autopsy in the tongue and several skeletal muscles, as well as in the heart muscle and cardiac conduction system. Her mother and one of her sisters also died suddenly at ages 47 and 37 years, respectively. The sister's myocardium demonstrated rods. In one other case with typical features of congenital myopathy, death at age 46 was attributed to congestive heart failure, but rods were not seen in the heart at autopsy.[158]

LABORATORY FEATURES

The CK level is usually normal in nemaline myopathy. Electrophysiologic studies show normal nerve conduction. The EMG of clinically weak muscles, particularly tibialis anterior, usually shows rare fibrillations and a myopathic pattern with early recruitment of small-amplitude, short-duration, polyphasic motor unit potentials. Sequential studies in patients with progressive disease have demonstrated that motor unit potentials of increased duration and polyphasia become more conspicuous, while fiber density increases.[171] As muscles become very weak, the routine EMG may appear "neurogenic," with reduced recruitment and long-duration, polyphasic motor units.

In the muscle biopsy stained with modified trichrome, rods appear as subsarcolemmal and perinuclear clusters of red-staining bodies, measuring 1 to 7 μm in length and 0.3 to 3 μm in width (see Fig. 2–47). The distribution of rods does not correlate with the degree of muscle weakness. Rods have been described in virtually every muscle of the body, including the tongue and diaphragm. Rods occur preferentially but not exclusively in type 1 fibers, and muscle biopsies often show a predominance of type 1 muscle fibers. Rods may be found in both intrafusal and extrafusal muscle fibers.[74,123,150]

Rods originate from the Z disk of skeletal muscle. Ultrastructural examination (Fig. 6–3) reveals distinct features: a tetragonal filamentous array when the rods are cut transversely, structural continuity with thin filaments, and periodic lines perpendicular to the long axis.[103] In addition to the usual location of rods in the cytoplasm, intranuclear rods have been described in both adult[49] and congenital cases. Congenital cases with intranuclear rods have a more severe form of the disease.[140]

GENETICS

The first reports were of sporadic cases,[33,153] but overwhelming evidence favors autosomal dominant inheritance with a reduced penetrance.[98,155] In two families, an autosomal recessive pattern was suggested on the basis that small numbers of fibers with rods were identified in both parents of index cases.[5] The lack of male-to-male transmission, with the exception of one documented case,[74] has raised considerations of X-linked recessive inheritance. The recent localization of autosomal dominant nemaline myopathy to chromosome 1q should clarify the pattern of inheritance and address the issue of whether there is more than one form of the disease.

PATHOGENESIS

The cause of nemaline myopathy remains obscure. Experimentally, rods can be induced following tenotomy[91,137] and ischemic muscle damage.[157] Rods may also be seen in muscle biopsies associated with diverse clinical conditions, including polymyositis,[145] HIV-related myopathy,[39] hypothyroid myopathy,[70] and in muscle biopsies from schizophrenic patients.[114] Evidence suggests that alpha-actinin represents the major protein component of both Z discs and rods.[84] Additional work has demonstrated a twofold to threefold enrichment of alpha-actinin in the skeletal muscle of nemaline myopathy pa-

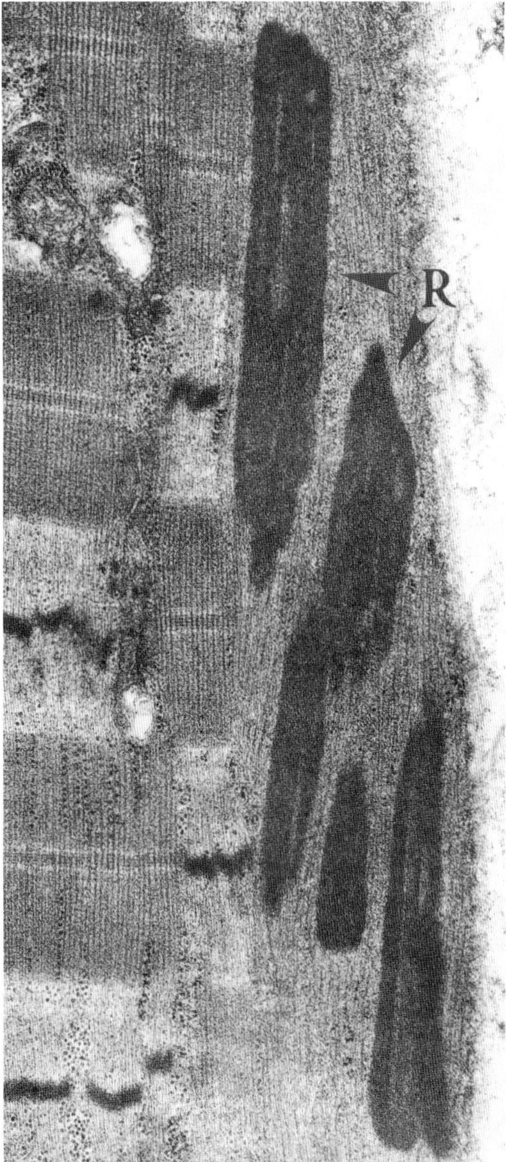

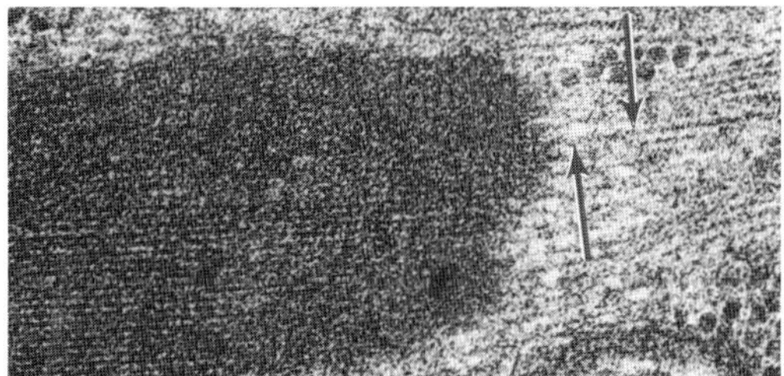

Figure 6–3. Nemaline myopathy. (*Top*) Electron micrograph of muscle fiber showing rods (R) in subsarcolemmal location. Rods appear as dense, osmiophilic bodies. (*Bottom*) At high magnification rods show periodicity and insertion of thin filaments (*arrows*).

tients as compared with muscle from normal controls.[159] Collectively these observations still provide very few clues into the pathogenesis of nemaline myopathy.

TREATMENT

As with other congenital myopathies, patients benefit from supportive treatment. No specific treatment exists for nemaline myopathy. Some patients may require bracing or surgery for the scoliosis, as well as ankle-foot orthoses for foot drop.

Centronuclear Myopathy

The term "myotubular myopathy," originally introduced by Spiro and coworkers,[156] was chosen to describe a distinct morphologic alteration of the muscle fiber that closely resembled the myotubular stage of development. The authors of this first report believed that they had defined a distinct congenital myopathy. Subsequent events have revealed at least three different clinical presentations that exhibit different modes of inheritance, despite overlapping muscle biopsy features (Table 6–5). The most common variety of the disease, depicted in the first reported case,[156] has its onset in infancy or early childhood and has a slowly progressive course. The other forms include a severe neonatal type with a usually fatal outcome,[167] and a late childhood–adult type.[111]

Myotubes, prominent at 10 weeks of gestation, develop by fusion of myoblasts, and form syncytial cells with centrally placed nuclei.[65,122] The myofilaments organize into myofibrils at the periphery, while the central area contains the large, oval nuclei, which are arranged in chains and surrounded by a perinuclear region enriched with ribosomes and other cytoplasmic elements. Between 10 and 14 weeks of gestation, the cytoplasm becomes filled with myofibrils, and the nuclei migrate to the periphery. This transition of myotubes to

Table 6–5 CENTRONUCLEAR MYOPATHIES

CLINICAL FEATURES
  Neonatal type
    Severe hypotonia and weakness
    Respiratory insufficiency
    Ptosis and ophthalmoplegia
    Fatal outcome common
  Late infantile–early childhood type
    Hypotonia
    Delayed motor milestones
    Ptosis and opthalmoplegia
    Skeletal abnormalities include long thin
      face, high-arched palate, scoliosis, clubfeet
    Mild to severely progressive course
  Late childhood–adult type
    Mild limb-girdle muscle weakness

GENETICS
  Neonatal type: X-linked recessive
  Late infantile–early childhood type:
    autosomal recessive
  Late childhood–adult type: autosomal
    dominant

MUSCLE BIOPSY
  See Figs. 6–4, 6–5, and 6–6.

mature muscle fibers concludes by 20 weeks (5 months) of gestation.

The histologic changes observed by Spiro and colleagues[156] suggest an arrest of maturation, but others[7] criticize the term based on features that contradict myotubular arrest, including muscle fibers with a more normal-appearing nuclear-cytoplasmic ratio and larger muscle fibers compared to myotubes, indicating a growth of the fiber with the addition of myofilaments. Sequential studies of a single patient have shown that the central nucleation appears after infancy.[166] The evidence against maturational arrest is therefore convincing, and the name "centronuclear myopathy" is now the accepted term. Another descriptive term, less often used, is "type 1 fiber hypotrophy and central nuclei," emphasizing the appearance of developmentally small type 1 fibers.[58]

CLINICAL FEATURES

Children with *late infantile–early childhood form of centronuclear myop-*

athy are usually products of a normal pregnancy and delivery. Attainment of motor milestones is typically delayed, especially walking.[156] Later, difficulty with running and stair-climbing become apparent. Ptosis and varying degrees of ophthalmoplegia distinguish this condition from other congenital myopathies. The eye muscle findings, in association with generalized weakness, hypotonia, and areflexia, are hallmarks of this disease. Some patients have facial weakness as well. A marfanoid appearance with typical slender body habitus, long narrow face, and high-arched palate may be present. Skeletal abnormalities include an accentuated lordosis, scoliosis, and clubfeet.[12,82,133,149] Focal or generalized seizures[7,169] and involvement of the heart or great vessels[149,169] have been reported but do not consistently occur. The course of this form of centronuclear myopathy varies from nonprogression, to degrees of weakness requiring ambulatory aids, including wheelchair assistance.

The *neonatal form of centronuclear myopathy* presents with severe hypotonia and weakness at birth.* Respiratory assistance may be required, and swallowing difficulties may necessitate a feeding tube to prevent aspiration. Ptosis and ophthalmoplegia are found less often than in the late infantile–childhood cases but may become more apparent after the newborn period. The neonatal form carries a poor prognosis, and the condition is often fatal.[8,136] If patients survive through infancy, they usually remain severely impaired.

A third variant, the *late childhood–adult type of centronuclear myopathy*, has an onset in the second or third decade.[92,111] This least common form, first described by Karpati and associates in 1970,[92] differs markedly from the other types. Patients have full extraocular muscle movements and only rarely exhibit ptosis.[111] Mild, usually nonprogressive limb weakness is manifest as clumsiness in activities like running or

bicycle riding. The dysmorphic features and skeletal abnormalities characteristic of the late infantile–early childhood type usually do not appear. In fact, this late childhood–adult form of centronuclear myopathy resembles a limb-girdle syndrome without notable features other than mild proximal weakness.

LABORATORY FEATURES

Normal or slightly elevated CK levels occur in any of the forms of centronuclear myopathy.[133,152,156,169]

Electrophysiologic studies sometimes appear more distinctive in this disorder than in other congenital myopathies. Positive sharp waves and fibrillation potentials, complex repetitive discharges, and myotonic discharges have all been observed, in addition to the usual myopathic pattern.[101,122,131] In the appropriate clinical setting, abundant spontaneous activity on needle EMG examination should suggest the possibility of centronuclear myopathy.

Muscle biopsy findings provide an unequivocal diagnosis of centronuclear myopathy (Figs. 6–4, 6–5, and 6–6). Longitudinal sections demonstrate the rows of central nuclei, often surrounded by a halo. In transverse sections, the number of muscle fibers with central nuclei varies from as few as 25%, to more than 80%. Some fibers have both normal and centrally placed nuclei. The late childhood–adult cases usually have increased numbers of nuclei more randomly located throughout the fiber, in addition to rows of central nuclei (see Fig. 6–6). Histochemical staining often reveals a predilection for greater involvement of type 1 fibers, and type 1 fiber predominance, especially in the late infantile–early childhood cases (see Fig. 6–5c). The central area of the muscle fibers may show increased oxidative enzyme activity and glycogen staining, with reduced amounts of ATPase activity. By ultrastructural examination, corresponding changes include a reduction in myofilaments, but an excess of mitochondria, Golgi apparatus, and glycogen. Motor nerve ter-

---

*References 2,6,8,101,117,136,146,167.

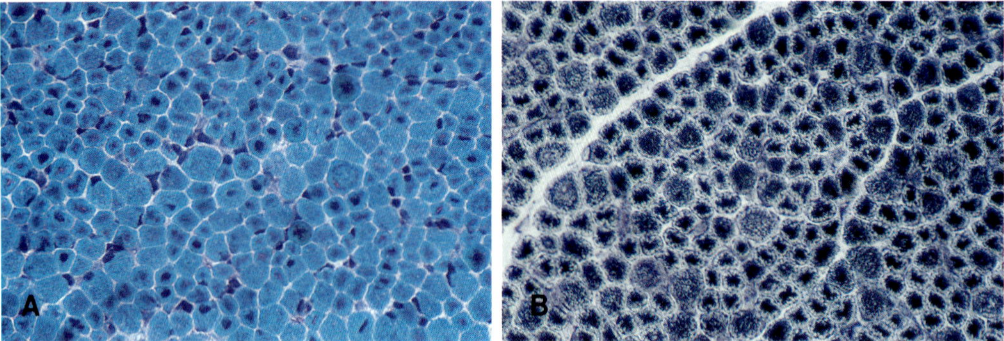

Figure 6–4. Neonatal centronuclear myopathy. (*A*) Central nuclei seen in many muscle fibers (modified trichrome). (*B*) Oxidative enzyme stain shows central region of fibers to be dark in appearance (NADH-tetrazolium reductase).

minal and postsynaptic structures appear normal.[9]

GENETICS

Indisputable evidence for X-linked recessive inheritance exists in the neonatal form of centronuclear myopathy.[2,6,8,117,136,146,167] The gene for the X-linked form has been localized to Xq28, so that linkage analysis can now identify carriers.[100,163] The histologic changes reported in some carriers raise the issue of whether the muscle biopsy can be used for genetic counseling and carrier detection. One report that four of five obligate carriers demonstrated some fibers with central nuclei pro-

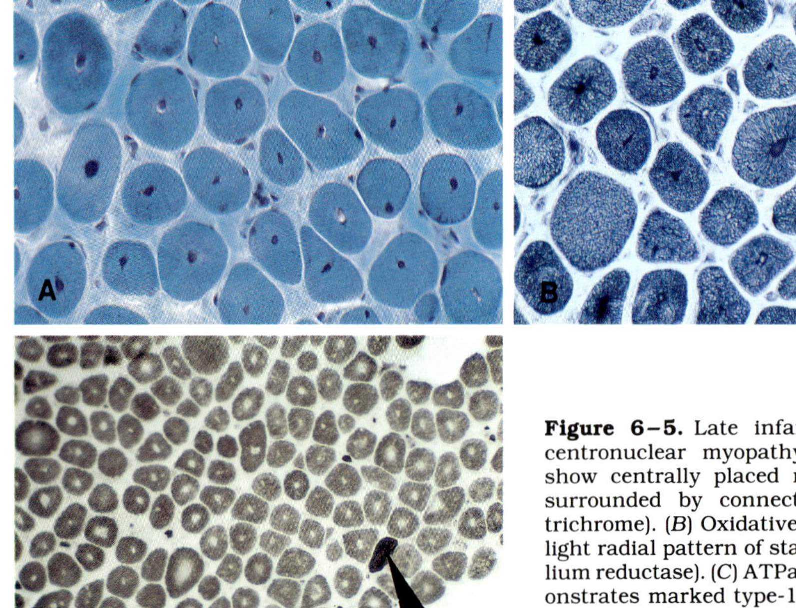

Figure 6–5. Late infantile-early childhood centronuclear myopathy. (*A*) Muscle fibers show centrally placed nuclei. Each fiber is surrounded by connective tissue (modified trichrome). (*B*) Oxidative enzyme stains highlight radial pattern of staining (NADH-tetrazolium reductase). (*C*) ATPase stain (pH 9.4) demonstrates marked type-1 predominance. Only one type-2 fiber is seen (*arrowhead*). The centronuclear region of muscle fibers remains unstained.

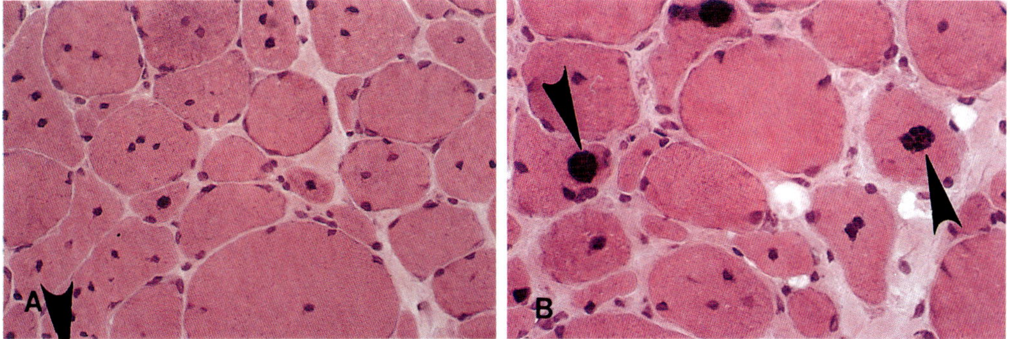

Figure 6–6. Late childhood-adult variety of centronuclear myopathy. (*A*) Variability in fiber size and increased number of internal nuclei scattered throughout the fibers is apparent. Fewer nuclei are restricted to the center of the fiber than in other forms of centronuclear myopathy (H&E). (*B*) Another area of the same biopsy emphasizes variability in fiber size and shows clusters of centrally placed nuclei in some muscle fibers (*arrowheads*) (H&E).

moted this idea,[8] but in other cases, muscle biopsy analysis for carrier detection has been disappointing.[136]

In the late infantile–early childhood disorder, the existence of families with multiple affected sibs and no prior family history favors autosomal recessive inheritance.[122,127,149,152,169] Consanguinity has also been reported.[127,131] There are reports that muscle biopsy has shown evidence of increased central nuclei in asymptomatic mothers of affected patients with this form of centronuclear myopathy,[122,152] but histologic examination of muscle for carrier detection has a low yield for positive results and is not helpful.

In the late childhood–adult form of centronuclear myopathy, there is convincing evidence of autosomal dominant inheritance.[92,167] In one pedigree, 16 family members were affected over five generations.[167]

PATHOGENESIS

The cause of the centronuclear change has been repeatedly addressed. Opposition to the idea of maturational arrest was discussed earlier. The possibility of an altered trophic influence from the neuron has been suggested by experimental denervation studies.[58] In cats, sciatic neurectomy causes persis-

tence of the myotube stage beyond the usual 10-day postnatal period.[58] The applicability of this model has been challenged, however, because extensive autopsy studies have not demonstrated abnormalities of the brain, spinal cord, or peripheral nerve in humans.[8,47,117,136,167]

A more viable explanation for the centronuclear change is an abnormality in nuclear migration from an inherited defect of a cytoskeletal protein of muscle.[23,166]

TREATMENT

No specific treatment is available. Patients with the neonatal form of centronuclear myopathy may require respiratory support and gastric feeding. These life-support systems are often introduced at birth or shortly thereafter, prior to an established diagnosis. Some improvement can be expected with developmental maturation, but neonatal patients usually remain totally dependent on life-support systems.

For patients with the late infantile–early childhood disorder, ambulatory aids and orthotic devices (and less often, wheelchairs) may be necessary. Specific indications depend on the severity of involvement. Occasional patients may benefit from scoliosis surgery.

UNCOMMON TYPES OF CONGENITAL MYOPATHIES

The three common congenital myopathies described earlier have long been recognized as distinct entities. Patients with central core disease, nemaline myopathy, and the different forms of centronuclear myopathy each present a clinically and morphologically consistent picture; thus, they represent distinct nosologic entities. The conditions discussed in this next group of congenital myopathies are rare and have less well-defined inheritance patterns. Whether they represent distinct nosologic entities has not been unequivocally established.

Multicore Disease

Multicore disease,[53] also referred to as minicore disease or myopathy with multiple minicores,[139] has histologic features that resemble central core disease but are sufficiently different to warrant a separate designation. Following the first report of two sporadic cases by A. G. Engel and colleagues in 1971,[53] additional reports have attested to a reasonably homogeneous phenotype.[19,77,160,168]

CLINICAL FEATURES

Typically, patients with multicore disease have an uneventful neonatal period, although hypotonia and poor head control have been described.[77,139] Motor milestones are delayed, with proximal muscle weakness and depressed tendon reflexes (Table 6–6).[19,53,77,139,160,168] Ptosis was observed in one individual,[53] and another was described with more extensive ophthalmoplegia.[160] Skeletal abnormalities, including a slender body habitus, high-arched palate, and scoliosis, are shared with more common congenital myopathies.[53,77,160] The condition either progresses slowly or remains static.

In one distinctive case, the onset of

Table 6–6 MULTICORE DISEASE

CLINICAL FEATURES
  Delayed motor milestones
  Proximal muscle weakness
  Rarely, ptosis and ophthalmoplegia
  Skeletal abnormalities including slender body
    habitus, high-arched palate, scoliosis,
    clubfeet
  Predisposition to malignant hyperthermia
  Stable, or nonprogressive course

GENETICS
  Autosomal dominant

MUSCLE BIOPSY
  See Figs. 6–7 and 6–8.

symptoms occurred in adult life, with a 12-year history of progressive proximal weakness.[13] The skeletal and dysmorphic features of younger cases were absent. This disparity of phenotype, in which adult cases lack the skeletal and dysmorphic features of the childhood congenital myopathy, also occurs in nemaline and centronuclear myopathies.

LABORATORY FEATURES

The CK level is typically normal, and the EMG confirms myopathic changes. The muscle biopsy shows fibers with focal zones of diminished oxidative enzyme activity (Fig. 6–7). These changes are similar to those of central core dis-

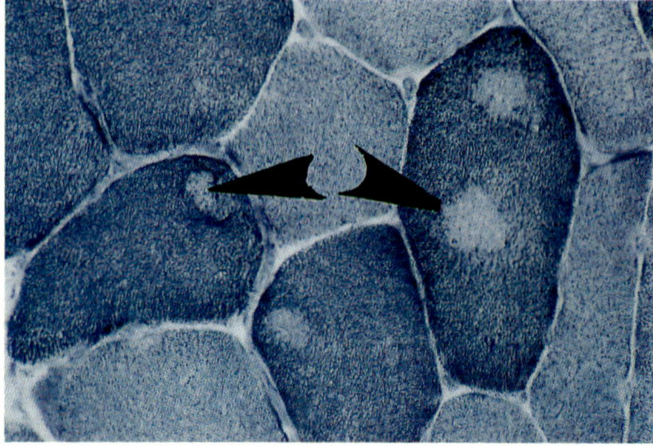

Figure 6–7. Multicore disease. Three fibers show one or more focal regions of loss of oxidative enzymes (*arrowheads*) (NADH-tetrazolium reductase).

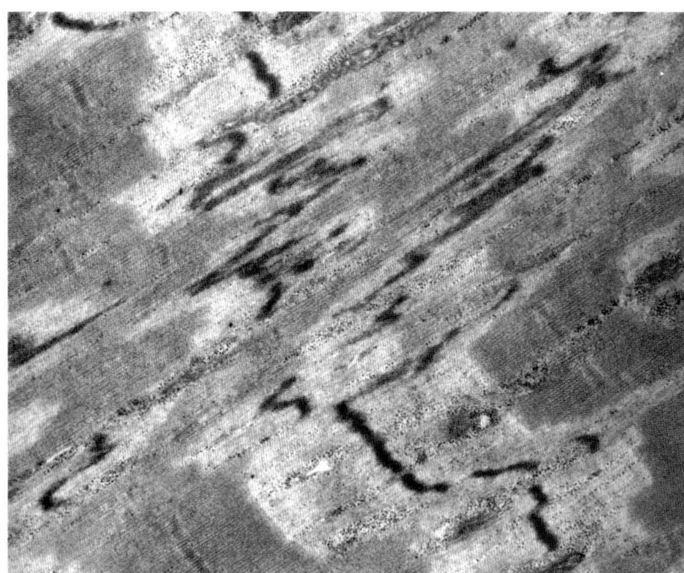

Figure 6-8. Multicore disease. Myofibrillar disarray and Z disk streaming seen in focal area of muscle fiber. In multicore disease these changes do not extend the length of the fiber.

ease. Multicores are composed of Z disk streaming and myofibrillar disarray extending for up to 75 μm along the length of the fiber (Fig. 6-8). In comparison to central cores, the lesions of multicore disease appear smaller and more numerous and do not extend the length of the fiber. Both type 1 and type 2 fibers have multicores, often in association with a predominance of type 1 muscle fibers.

GENETICS

In certain cases, the involvement of multiple generations indicates autosomal dominant inheritance.[19,53,168] Identical twins have been reported to be affected,[77] and sporadic cases also occur.

PATHOGENESIS

Z disk streaming, the hallmark of multicore disease, is a nonspecific finding in muscle pathology. These focal abnormalities occur in greater numbers in multicore disease, but are common in muscle biopsies from patients with various types of neuromuscular disorders, including muscular dystrophy and inflammatory myopathies.[53] In addition, target fibers, typical of denervation at-

rophy, demonstrate Z disk streaming.[115] The first report of multicore disease pointed out that the focal myofibrillar abnormalities correspond to areas of mitochondrial loss.[53] The importance of reduced oxidative enzyme activity remains unknown, as does the cause of multicore disease.

TREATMENT

Patients with multicore disease usually do not require ambulatory aids. The skeletal abnormalities, however, especially the scoliosis, may necessitate surgical intervention. As in central core disease, malignant hyperthermia may be associated with multicore disease.[134] The incidence of malignant hyperthermia with multicore disease has not been defined, but patients should be advised to avoid general anesthesia whenever possible and to wear a medic-alert bracelet or necklace in case of emergency surgery (see Chapter 7).

Fingerprint Body Myopathy

Following the initial report of fingerprint body myopathy in 1972,[52] only a few additional cases have been re-

Table 6–7 FINGERPRINT BODY MYOPATHY

CLINICAL FEATURES
  Hypotonia
  Delayed motor milestones
  Weakness of truncal and extremity muscles
  Skeletal abnormalities include kyphosis,
    pectus excavatum
  Mental retardation
  Mild or nonprogressive course

GENETICS
  Unknown

MUSCLE BIOPSY
  See Fig. 6–9.

ported,[37,63,75,132] but the relative homogeneity of the phenotype justifies regarding fingerprint body myopathy as a separate form of congenital myopathy.

CLINICAL FEATURES

The initial case, diagnosed at age 5, was characterized by hypotonia during infancy, delayed walking, and mild, diffuse truncal and extremity weakness, findings also typical of subsequent cases (Table 6–7).[37,52,63,75,132] Involvement of cranial nerve musculature has not occurred. Skeletal abnormalities have been an inconsistent finding, but a kyphotic posture and pectus excavatum were seen in two families.[132] Muscle stretch reflexes may be depressed. Subnormal intelligence has been observed in several instances.[37,52,63] The clinical course has been nonprogressive.

LABORATORY FEATURES

The CK level is usually normal, and the EMG demonstrates a myopathic pattern. The muscle biopsy shows subsarcolemmal or juxtanuclear inclusions made up of concentric lamellae arranged in a fingerprint pattern (Fig. 6–9). The lamellae contain sawtooth projections. Fingerprint bodies may be seen in as many as 50% of fibers[52] and can be observed, in the light microscope, as small, greenish (modified trichrome) or eosinophilic (H&E) oval structures, 1 to 10 μm in length. Their presence, however, must be confirmed by electron microscopy. Fingerprint bodies show a predilection for type 1 fibers and, as in many of the congenital

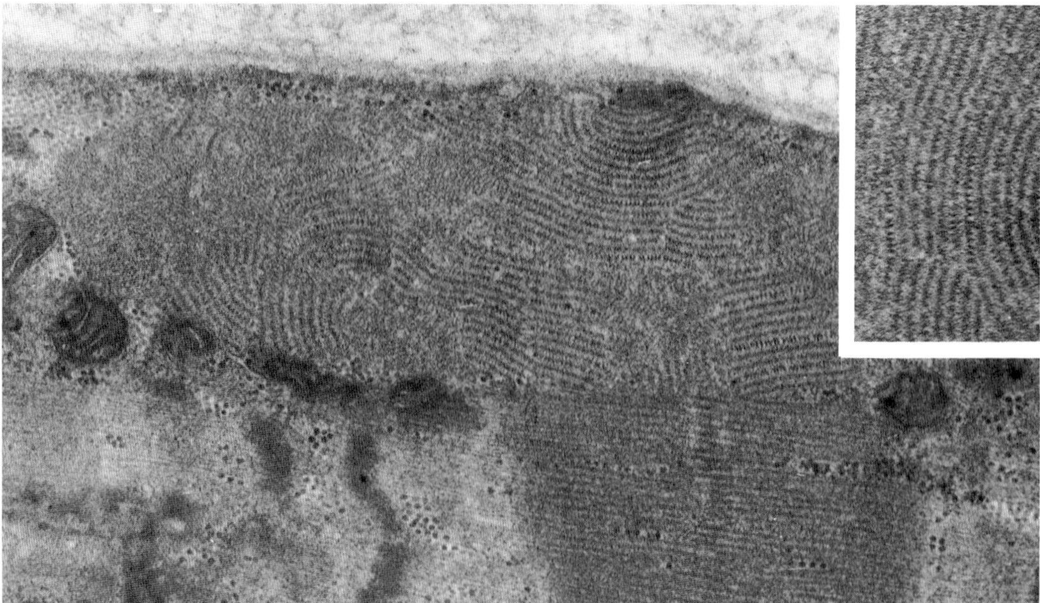

Figure 6–9. Fingerprint body myopathy. Electron micrograph of subsarcolemmal fingerprint body showing the concentric lamellae arranged in fingerprint pattern. Inset shows lamellae at higher magnification.

myopathies, type 1 muscle fibers may predominate. Atrophy of type 1 muscle fibers also occurs.

GENETICS

The genetic pattern has not been well delineated. The condition was reported in a set of male twins[37] and was also seen in a boy and girl with a common mother and different fathers.[63]

PATHOGENESIS

Although it has been suggested that fingerprint bodies originate in degenerating mitochondria,[37] it is more likely that they represent a cytoskeletal protein. They are not a myofibrillar protein, since they resist procedures that remove thick and thin filaments, M-band protein, and Z disk associated material.[52] The stimulus for induction of fingerprint bodies remains completely unknown, but they have been observed in other conditions including dermatomyositis,[24] myotonic dystrophy,[147] oculopharyngeal dystrophy,[88] in muscle from uremic patients,[108] and in nemaline myopathy.

TREATMENT

Fingerprint body myopathy usually does not require specific treatment for the neuromuscular manifestations. Special education may be necessary for those with subnormal intelligence. Febrile seizures, reported in twins, have not been a consistent feature.[37]

Sarcotubular Myopathy

Only two patients, brothers from a consanguineous marriage, have been described with sarcotubular myopathy.[85] Although the clinical features of this rare entity were typical of the overall group of congenital myopathies (Table 6–8), it is difficult to consider this as an established entity because of the lack of further case reports since 1973.

Table 6–8 SARCOTUBULAR MYOPATHY

CLINICAL FEATURES
Hypotonia
Delayed motor milestones
Weakness of neck and proximal muscles
Nonprogressive course

GENETICS
Unknown

MUSCLE BIOPSY
The membrane-bound vacuoles, originating from sarcoplasmic reticulum, are seen preferentially in type 2 muscle fibers. The vacuoles are of variable size and may be empty or contain amorphous material.

CLINICAL FEATURES

The patients with sarcotubular myopathy were affected in infancy. One demonstrated decreased fetal movements and delayed walking. Both brothers had difficulty climbing stairs and awkwardness in running; neither demonstrated progression of weakness. Skeletal abnormalities were not present. Neck flexor and proximal muscle weakness were present in both, whereas only one had weakness in ankle dorsiflexion.

LABORATORY FEATURES

In one brother, the CK level was elevated to four times normal. The EMG showed myopathic motor unit potentials confined to selected muscles. The muscle biopsy features were unique. Approximately 20% to 30% of the type 2 fibers and fewer than 4% of the type 1 fibers showed vacuolar changes. By ultrastructural examination, the vacuoles were membrane bound; they appeared empty or showed traces of amorphous material. Using electron cytochemical markers and peroxidase labeling, the membranes of the vacuoles showed activity for sarcoplasmic-reticulum–associated ATPase and did not communicate with the extracellular space. These findings suggested an origin in the sarcoplasmic reticulum of muscle. In addition to the vacuolated fibers, the muscle demonstrated a slight increase in connective tissue, occasional fiber splitting, and a slight increase in internal nuclei.

GENETICS

On the basis of a single family, it is impossible to establish the pattern of inheritance. The fact that this was a consanguineous marriage and 2 of 10 siblings were affected suggests autosomal recessive inheritance.

PATHOGENESIS

Segmental vacuolization, degeneration, and coalescence of the sarcoplasmic reticulum results in vacuoles of differing size. The stimulus has not been determined. Although a similar reaction can occasionally be seen in nonspecific myopathies, the relatively selective involvement of the type 2 fibers suggests a unique process. The vacuoles in sarcotubular myopathy can be distinguished from those occurring in periodic paralysis, inclusion body myositis, distal myopathies, and various autophagic processes, and from those of lysosomal origin.[85]

TREATMENT

There is no treatment for sarcotubular myopathy.[85]

Hyaline Body Myopathy (Familial Myopathy with Probable Lysis of Myofibrils)

Familial myopathy with probable lysis of myofibrils in type 1 fibers deserves mention because of the uniqueness of the muscle fiber change and its onset in infancy or early childhood.[7a,22,144] Although the name of this condition suggests a degenerative process, the clinical features indicate a nonprogressive course more consistent with a congenital myopathy (Table 6–9).

Table 6–9 HYALINE BODY MYOPATHY (FAMILIAL MYOPATHY WITH LYSIS OF MYOFIBRILS)

CLINICAL FEATURES
 Hypotonia
 Delayed motor milestones
 Weakness of proximal and distal muscles
 Mild or nonprogressive course

GENETICS
 Unknown

MUSCLE BIOPSY
 See Figs. 6–10 and 6–11.

CLINICAL FEATURES

Familial myopathy with probable lysis of myofibrils in type 1 fibers has been reported only rarely.[7a,22,144] The brother and sister described by Cancilla and colleagues[22] had a history typical of congenital myopathy. The birth of one of the siblings was breech. Both children demonstrated hypotonia and had delayed motor milestones. Mild proximal and distal weakness was apparent. In a third case, symptoms were first recognized in early childhood following a normal developmental history.[144] The clinical course was nonprogressive. A recently described case also demonstrated hypotonia and delayed milestones from infancy.[7a] She has slight nonprogressive proximal weakness, preserved muscle stretch reflexes, and high-arched feet.

LABORATORY FEATURES

The CK level is normal, and the EMG is myopathic. The unusual muscle biopsy features are characterized by a prominent hyaline appearance (Fig. 6–10), lacking oxidative enzyme activity. Increased oxidative enzyme activity surrounds the hyaline bodies, which are characteristically present at the periphery of muscle fibers. ATPase reactivity may be retained or reduced, depending on pH. With regard to ultrastructure, the hyaline body is devoid of myofibrils and demonstrates a matrix of granular and filamentous material measuring 6 to 8 nm in diameter (Fig. 6–11). Muscle nuclei can be seen scat-

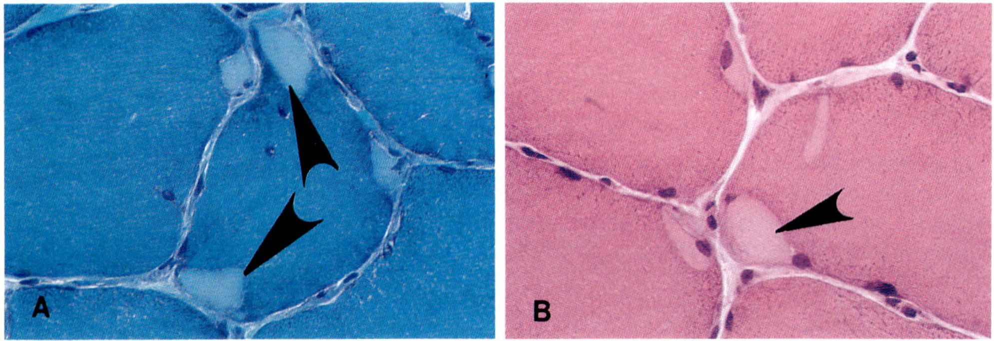

Figure 6–10. Hyaline body myopathy. (A) Muscle fibers show subsarcolemmal hyaline bodies (*arrowheads*) (modified trichrome). (B) Hyaline bodies seen in H&E stain (*arrowhead*).

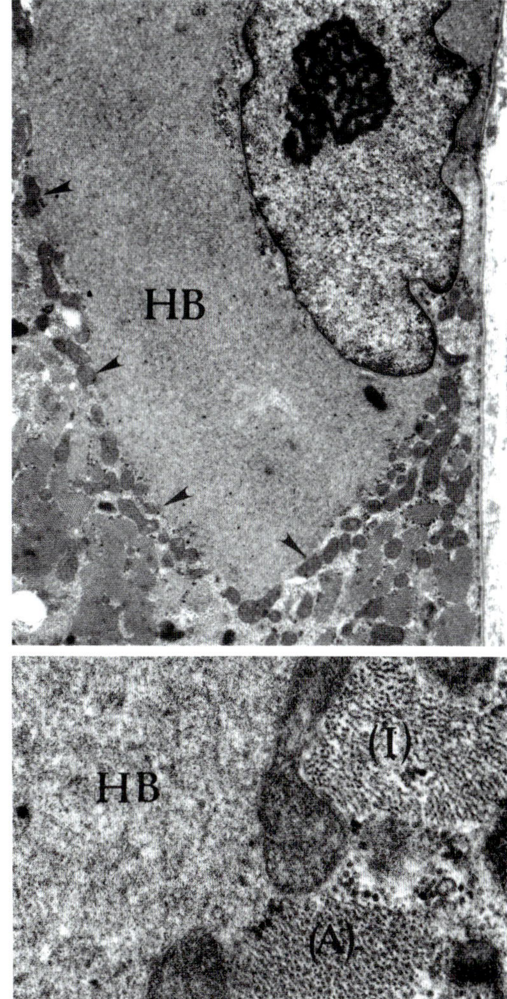

Figure 6–11. Hyaline body myopathy. (*Top*) Electron micrograph of hyaline body (HB) composed of granular matrix and bordered by mitochondria (*arrowheads*). (*Bottom*) Higher magnification shows fine granular matrix of HB compared with filaments of normal muscle in A band and I band.

tered within or closely associated with the granular matrix.

GENETICS

The report involving two of six siblings without additional family history gives no clue to the genetic basis for this disease.[22] The other reported cases[7a,144] were sporadic.

PATHOGENESIS

Composition of the granular and filamentous material has not been identified and in view of the rather abrupt transition to these peripheral hyaline zones it seems unlikely that this material results from lysis of myofibrils. The course of the illness does not suggest a degenerative process. We agree with A. G. Engel that these peripheral zones are better referred to as hyaline bodies.[52a] Others suggest that the condition is due to a maturational arrest because of the associated histologic findings, including nuclei with prominent nucleoli and the dispersion of chromatin, Golgi apparatus, and rough endoplasmic reticulum.[144] The cause, however, remains obscure.

TREATMENT

No treatment exists for this rare congenital myopathy.

DUBIOUS TYPES OF CONGENITAL MYOPATHIES

Congenital Fiber-Type Disproportion

In an extensive study of childhood muscle biopsies, Brooke and Engel[17] observed that a group of patients with hypotonia and weakness in infancy demonstrated uniform smallness of the type 1 fibers, which was not accounted for by known disorders (e.g., myotonic dystrophy). Brooke[14] later introduced the term "congenital fiber-type disproportion" to refer to this condition.[14] The

Table 6–10 CONGENITAL FIBER-TYPE DISPROPORTION

CLINICAL FEATURES
Hypotonia
Delayed motor milestones
Weakness of proximal and distal muscles
Skeletal abnormalities including short stature, high-arched palate, kyphoscoliosis, congenital hip dislocation, clubfeet
Mild or nonprogressive course

GENETICS
Unknown

MUSCLE BIOPSY
See Fig. 6–12.

muscle biopsy features were believed to be important in establishing a favorable prognosis for hypotonic infants. Unfortunately, these muscle biopsy changes have not been consistent in predicting the clinical course and prognosis.

CLINICAL FEATURES

Typical cases of congenital fiber-type disproportion show hypotonia and weakness at birth or in the neonatal period (Table 6–10). Delay in attainment of motor milestones is common. Small stature and contractures of hands and feet may be seen, as well as skeletal abnormalities including a high-arched palate, clubfeet, kyphoscoliosis, and congenital hip dislocation. These children have normal intelligence. As originally described, a diagnosis of congenital fiber-type disproportion implied a static course or one associated with improvement. Patients with a progressive and even fatal course were subsequently reported, and the same biopsy findings are seen in other neuromuscular diseases.*

LABORATORY FEATURES

The CK level is normal. The EMG may be normal or myopathic. By definition, the muscle biopsy shows small type 1

---

*References 3,16,26,29,46,69,80,170.

fibers, whose mean diameter is at least 12% smaller than that of type 2 fibers.[14,17] The number of type 1 fibers is usually excessive, and the type 2 fibers, especially type 2B, are normal or have an increased fiber diameter for age. Therefore, a typical muscle biopsy shows type 1 fiber smallness, type 1 fiber predominance, and type 2 fiber hypertrophy (Fig. 6–12). Unfortunately, the specificity of these changes has not been borne out by experience.† Patients with more serious disorders, including congenital muscular dystrophy,[26] centronuclear myopathy,[101] spinal muscular atrophy,[80] and central nervous system disorders.[29,69] have shown muscle biopsy features typical of congenital fiber-type disproportion.

---

†References 3,15,16,26,29,46,69,80,170

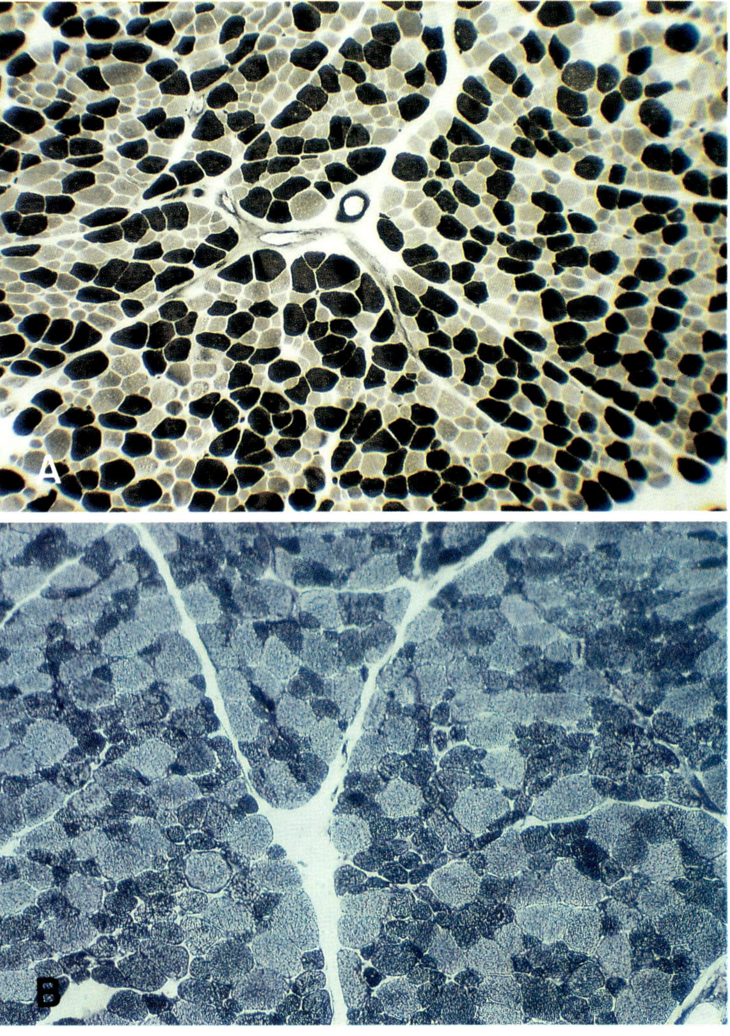

Figure 6–12. Congenital fiber-type disproportion. (A) Muscle biopsy shows many more type 1 muscle fibers (predominance), which have a significantly smaller mean fiber diameter than the darker type 2 muscle fibers. ATPase pH 9.4. (B) Oxidative enzyme stain shows type 1 fibers to be smaller and more numerous than type 2 fibers (NADH-tetrazolium reductase).

Congenital fiber-type disportion differs from *congenital hypotonia with type 1 fiber predominance*, in which the muscle biopsy does not show a decrease in the size of type 1 fibers, but only an increase in their number, so that they comprise more than 60% of the total.[16] This muscle biopsy picture showing only an alteration in fiber-type ratio does not justify recognition as a distinct congenital myopathy.

GENETICS

Because congenital fiber-type disproportion does not represent a specific disease entity, no inheritance pattern can be determined. Nevertheless, muscle biopsies fulfilling the criteria for this condition have been described in identical twins,[36] in multiple sibs within a single generation,[26] and in successive generations.[94]

PATHOGENESIS

The nonspecificity of muscle biopsies demonstrating small type 1 fibers or predominance of type 1 fibers has already been emphasized. In fact, a substantial number of muscle biopsies from normal children show a reduced size of type 1 fibers compared to type 2 fibers.[170] These changes appear to represent an alteration in muscle fiber maturation and development. This interpretation may be relevant to families with one or more affected children, as inherited influences on muscle fiber maturation and development may also cause hypotonia.

TREATMENT

Despite all the debates regarding the specificity of congenital fiber-type disproportion, most clinicians will be faced with hypotonic infants exhibiting type 1 fiber smallness, type 1 fiber predominance, and type 2 fiber hypertrophy on muscle biopsy. Although the findings are not exclusive to a static (or improving) condition, many children will have a favorable outcome. For this reason,

Table 6–11 REDUCING BODY MYOPATHY

CLINICAL FEATURES
Presentations include
1. Severe weakness and hypotonia with fatal infantile outcome
2. Delayed motor milestones and nonprogressive course
3. Focal onset with asymmetric weakness leading to death

GENETICS
Unknown

MUSCLE BIOPSY
Reducing bodies appear in variable numbers, autofluoresce, reduce nitroblue tetrazolium when mediated by menadione, and have no oxidative enzyme activity. Electron microscopy shows osmophilic densities composed of tubular filaments.

these patients deserve supportive measures. Skeletal abnormalities may need attention, including congenital hip dislocation and foot deformities. Physical therapy for contractures of hands and feet also may be required.

Reducing Body Myopathy

Evidence that reducing body myopathy is an inherited congenital myopathy has been inconclusive. The clinical picture has been inconsistent (Table 6–11), and even the number of reducing bodies considered to be diagnostic has varied greatly.[18,25,44,79,126,165]

CLINICAL FEATURES

In the initial report, two unrelated patients with severe weakness and hypotonia at birth developed respiratory failure at 9 months and 2 years, respectively.[18] One patient had ptosis and facial weakness. Subsequent reports included a 14-year-old boy who had delayed milestones but a nonprogressive course[165] and cases with focal upper-extremity onset, asymmetric weakness, and variable outcome, including death.[18,44] No consistent clinical pattern has emerged from these case histories.

LABORATORY FEATURES

Serum CK levels have been normal or slightly increased,[165] and the EMG changes are usually described as myopathic. Reducing bodies are the distinctive pathologic feature for which the disorder was named. In some cases, however, fewer than 0.5% of fibers exhibited reducing bodies, whereas in others reducing bodies have been abundant and easy to identify.[18,25,44,79,126,165] The name "reducing body" is derived from the presence of sulfhydryl groups that reduce nitroblue tetrazolium when mediated by menadione.[18] The reducing bodies stain purple with modified trichrome and pink with H&E and show autofluorescence.[25] They may be subsarcolemmal or occupy a large portion of the cross-sectional area of the muscle fiber. Reducing bodies do not exhibit oxidative enzyme activity and do not show a predilection for fiber type. On ultrastructural examination, reducing bodies appear electron-dense and consist of tubular filaments varying from 12 to 17 nm in diameter,[25] associated with a granular matrix. Lucent islands, containing typical glycogen particles, give the reducing bodies a porous appearance. Reducing bodies have no limiting membrane.

GENETICS

A total of seven cases have been reported.[18,25,44,79,126,165] Because all reports have been sporadic cases except for one family involving two sisters,[79] no conclusion can be reached regarding a possible genetic basis.

PATHOGENESIS

The origin of reducing bodies remains unclear. Biochemical studies have shown the presence of two unidentified proteins of 62,000 kd and 53,000 kd in muscle homogenates.[25] The smaller of these proteins showed reducing activity when isolated by sucrose density gradient fractionation. The presence of tubular filaments on electron microscopy accounts for speculation of a possible viral cause.[25] Others have suggested that the granular material arises from an undefined myofibrillary component.[165]

TREATMENT

No effective treatment has been found for patients diagnosed with reducing-body myopathy.

Cytoplasmic (Spheroid) Body Myopathy

Cytoplasmic bodies are a nonspecific abnormality consisting of aggregates of filaments of Z disk origin and are found in muscle in diverse conditions.* W. K. Engel[54] chose the name "cytoplasmic body" for these small, round or elongated structures measuring 2 to 5 μm in diameter. They are usually present in the subsarcolemmal region of the muscle fiber (Fig. 6–13). These structures have also been referred to as spheroid bodies,[71] inclusion bodies,[30] myofibrillar aggregates,[95] and sarcoplasmic bodies.[45] Attempts to define specific congenital myopathies by the presence of cytoplasmic bodies has not been justified by consistency of phenotype or inheritance patterns.

CLINICAL FEATURES

Three clinical pictures emerge from the heterogeneity of reports of myopathies with cytoplasmic bodies (Table 6–12). One group of patients, with onset in childhood, have severe limb-girdle and respiratory muscle weakness leading to death in early adult life.[86,95,129] One of these cases, exhibiting hypertrophied calf muscles, may have had a form of muscular dystrophy.[129] In contrast, a second clinical picture associated with cytoplasmic bodies displays mild limb-girdle muscle

---

*References 30, 38, 45, 54, 66, 67, 71, 86, 95, 102, 129, 148, 151.

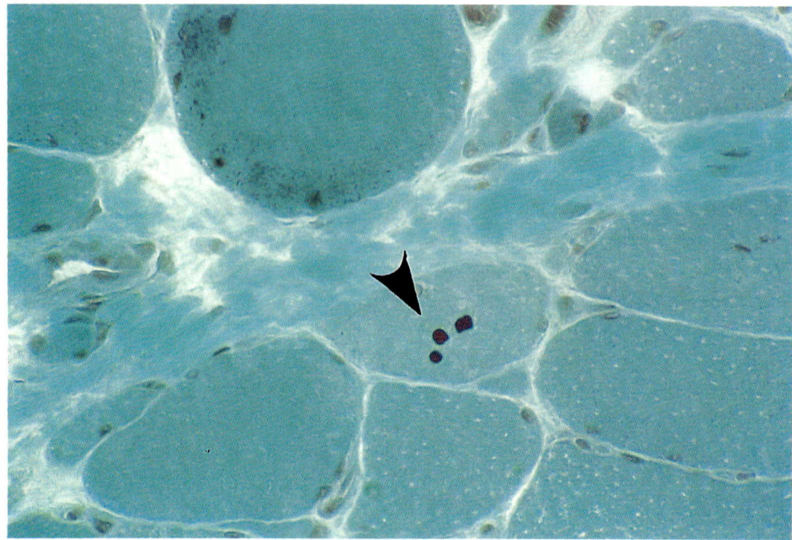

Figure 6–13. Cytoplasmic bodies. Muscle fiber shows three cytoplasmic bodies (*arrowhead*) (modified trichrome).

weakness without dysmorphic features or skeletal abnormalities.[38,71] A third clinical picture consists of a late-onset distal myopathy, beginning in the hand muscles and resulting in severe generalized weakness and respiratory muscle compromise.[45]

LABORATORY FEATURES

A normal or mildly elevated CK level occurred in these myopathies. The EMG changes have been myopathic,[30,95] neurogenic,[45,86] or mixed.[172] The histologic features in all cases included the presence of cytoplasmic bodies, but their number and other muscle pathology features varied greatly. In some cases, cytoplasmic bodies were the only change present in scattered fibers,[71] but severe changes in others included marked variability in muscle fiber size, fiber splitting, increased central nuclei, and prominent connective tissue proliferation, suggesting a form of muscular dystrophy.[45]

GENETICS

In families with the mild limb-girdle syndrome, the inheritance pattern was autosomal dominant,[30,71] although sporadic cases also appeared.[72] Patients with clinical features of the late-onset distal myopathy with cytoplasmic bodies also exhibit an autosomal dominant inheritance pattern,[45] but in the severely affected childhood cases less insight could be gained into the genetic pattern. These cases were sporadic,[86,95] except in one family where two of four offspring of first-cousin parents were afflicted, suggesting autosomal recessive inheritance.[129]

Table 6–12 CYTOPLASMIC BODY MYOPATHY

CLINICAL FEATURES
Presentations include
1. Childhood-onset, severely progressive limb-girdle syndrome with fatal outcome
2. Mild or nonprogressive limb-girdle syndrome
3. Late-onset, severely progressive, distal myopathy beginning in hands

GENETICS
Childhood-onset disorder: unknown
Mild limb-girdle syndrome: autosomal dominant
Late-onset distal myopathy: autosomal dominant

MUSCLE BIOPSY
See Figs. 6–13 and 6–14.

PATHOGENESIS

Cytoplasmic bodies appear in response to the muscle injury associated with many conditions, including denervation atrophy,[66,105] inflammatory myopathies,[102,151] and muscular dystrophies of various types.[54,102,105] Careful studies have demonstrated that cystoplasmic bodies originate in the Z disk and provide a matrix composed of a tangle of filaments intermixed with amorphous osmiophilic material (Fig. 6–14).[102] Surrounding the central dense matrix appears a zone of decreased lucency composed of haphazardly oriented filaments; at the periphery, radially oriented thick and thin filaments can be seen, contiguous with nearby disrupted myofibrils.

TREATMENT

Patients with early-childhood limb-girdle syndrome and late-onset distal myopathy with cytoplasmic bodies have respiratory insufficiency requiring special attention. These severely affected patients also require braces and wheelchairs, as do patients with muscular dystrophies (see Chapter 4). The mild limb-girdle syndrome with cytoplasmic bodies does not require treatment.

Myopathy with Tubular Aggregates

Tubular aggregates, first described in hypokalemic periodic paralysis and myotonia congenita,[55] accumulate in the subsarcolemmal regions or in more interior regions of muscle fibers. They appear as masses of blue (H&E), red (modified trichrome) or dark (NADH-tetrazolium reductase) staining material derived from sarcoplasmic reticulum (see Fig. 2–49). Tubular aggregates in muscle do not define a specific congenital myopathy, but they have occurred in association with three different clinical pictures (Table 6–13).*

---

*References 21,23,40,42,87,118,119,143.

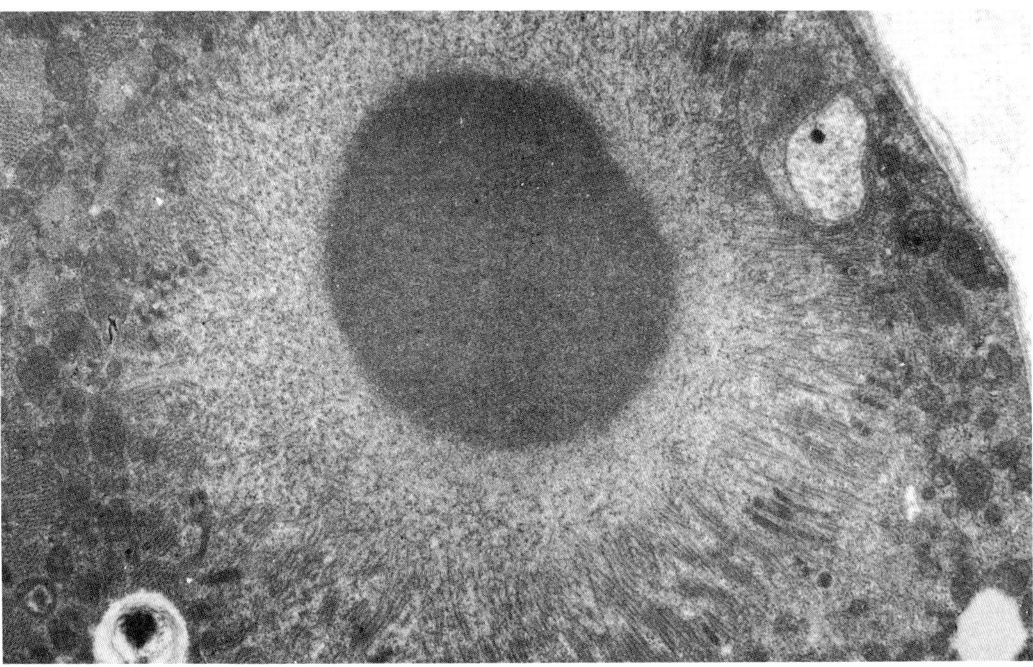

Figure 6–14. Cytoplasmic body. Electron micrograph of muscle fiber shows typical cytoplasmic body with dense osmiophilic core surrounded by a zone of loosely packed filaments and an outer zone of radially oriented filaments.

Table 6–13 MYOPATHY WITH TUBULAR AGGREGATES

CLINICAL FEATURES
Presentations include
1. Slowly progressive limb-girdle syndrome
2. Myasthenic syndrome with childhood onset, proximal weakness, and easy fatigability
3. Syndrome of exercise-induced muscle pain and stiffness

GENETICS
Limb girdle syndrome: autosomal dominant or autosomal recessive
Myasthenic syndrome: autosomal recessive
Muscle pain syndrome: unknown

MUSCLE BIOPSY
See Figs. 6–15 and 2–49.

CLINICAL FEATURES

A limb-girdle syndrome that shows tubular aggregates on muscle biopsy has been associated with slowly progressive, mild weakness in childhood[40] or early adult life.[143] A second condition with myopathy and tubular aggregates represents a myasthenic syndrome.[42,87,118] These patients have a childhood onset of proximal weakness, easy fatigability with moderate exercise, and a nonprogressive course. Some of these patients exhibit dysphagia, dysphonia, and fluctuating eyelid ptosis. Despite the presence of a decremental response with repetitive nerve stimulation, the features of these cases have not been sufficiently characterized to permit a comparison with other congenital myasthenic syndromes.[50,51]

The third clinical syndrome of myopathy with tubular aggregates consists of exercise-induced muscle pain and stiffness with little or no weakness.[21,23,119] The discomfort occurs in both upper and lower extremities with moderate activity, and disappears with rest (see Chapter 9).

LABORATORY FEATURES

The CK level was found to be normal or slightly elevated in patients with all three clinical pictures. EMG findings consistent with myopathy were seen in the limb-girdle[40,143] and myasthenic[42] syndromes. The decremental response to repetitive nerve stimulation in patients with the myasthenic syndrome was improved by pyridostigmine,[42,87,118] and acetylcholine-receptor antibody titers were normal in these patients.

In one family with the myasthenic syndrome, three affected sisters showed consistent electrocardiogram abnormalities with a vertical axis; inverted T waves in leads I, aVL, and V_3 to V_6; and an occasional wandering atrial pacemaker.[42]

Muscle biopsies from patients with these clinical syndromes showed tubular aggregates (see Fig. 2–49) in a large percentage of muscle fibers, usually type 2.[56,64,116] Other muscle biopsy abnormalities were usually meager, without evidence of muscle fiber degeneration. Variation in fiber size and atrophy of type 2 fibers accompanied tubular aggregates in the limb-girdle syndrome.[40,143]

GENETICS

The limb-girdle syndrome may show either an autosomal recessive[40] or a dominant[143] pattern of inheritance. Evidence favoring autosomal recessive inheritance occurs in the myasthenic syndrome with tubular aggregates.[42,87] The condition of exercise-induced muscle pain and stiffness and tubular aggregates occurs sporadically.

PATHOGENESIS

Tubular aggregates were originally thought to represent accumulations of mitochondria because of their strong affinity for NADH-tetrazolium reductase.[55] Later observations, however, demonstrated a lack of histochemical staining by succinic dehydrogenase, and electron microscopy showed parallel aggregates of inner and outer tubules arranged in bundles (Fig. 6–15).[56] Studies also demonstrated continuity with the sarcoplasmic reticulum of muscle.[56] The stimulus for proliferation of these tubules has not been determined, but

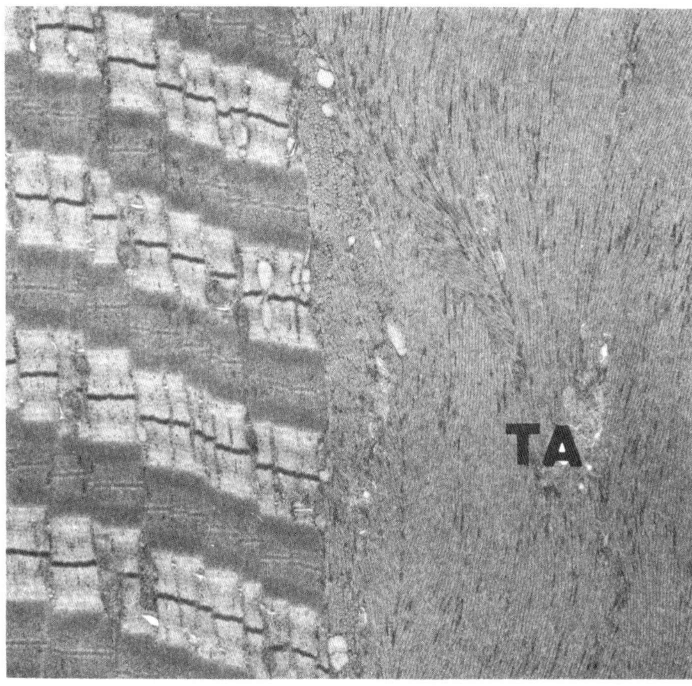

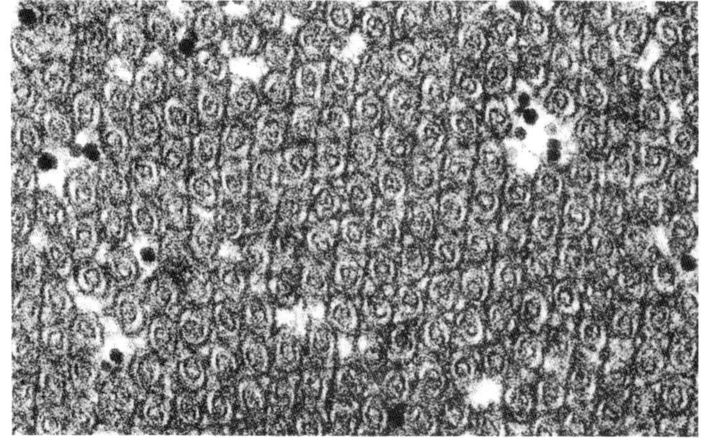

Figure 6–15. Tubular aggregates. (*Top*) Electron micrograph of tubular aggregate (TA) shows parallel rows of tubules adjacent to normal muscle. (*Bottom*) Higher magnification of cross section of tubular aggregates shows inner and outer tubules.

they occur in all types of periodic paralysis[56,116] and in the muscle of patients with a history of ingestion of drugs and alcohol.[28,64] Tubular aggregates werc observed following an episode of rhabdomyolysis in a patient with phosphoglycerate mutase deficiency,[96] an observation of interest in relation to the exercise-induced muscle pain and stiffness syndrome.

TREATMENT

The symptoms of patients suffering from the limb-girdle syndrome with tubular aggregates have been mild and require no specific treatment. In the myasthenic syndrome, patients have benefited from anticholinesterase inhibitors, particularly pyridostigmine. Dantrolene has been reported to yield marked improvement for some but not all patients experiencing exercise-induced muscle pain and stiffness associated with tubular aggregates.

Zebra Body Myopathy

Zebra bodies, also called leptomeres or microladders, occur normally at the myotendinous junctions,[106] in intrafusal fibers,[128] in extraocular muscle,[107] and in cardiac muscle.[164] The function of zebra bodies has remained unknown. In two cases with congenital weakness, zebra bodies were reported to be the distinguishing feature,[99,138] other prominent histologic changes could also account for muscle weakness.

CLINICAL FEATURES

Zebra body myopathy was characterized by hypotonia and delayed motor milestones for sitting and walking (Table 6–14). Running, hopping, and climbing were also impaired. Mild facial weakness occurred,[99] but neck and proximal limb muscles were more affected. Body habitus appeared slender. The condition was mildly progressive. Other organ systems were unaffected.

LABORATORY FEATURES

The CK level was two to three times normal, and the EMG showed a myo-

Table 6–14 ZEBRA BODY MYOPATHY

CLINICAL FEATURES
Hypotonia
Delayed motor milestones
Weakness of facial, neck, and pelvic-girdle
  muscles
Mild or nonprogressive course

GENETICS
Unknown

MUSCLE BIOPSY
See Fig. 6–16.

pathic pattern. Zebra bodies cannot be seen by light microscopy and must be examined with an electron microscope. They measure up to 2 nm in length, with osmiophilic stria resembling Z disks spaced at 0.15- to 0.27-nm intervals and connecting fine filaments of unknown composition (Fig. 6–16).

In the reported cases, abnormalities included marked variation in muscle fiber size, fiber splitting, and fibers with increased central nuclei and vacuoles. The amount of connective tissue was excessive in one patient.[99] Rods were also present in the muscle of both cases.[99,138]

GENETICS

The two reported cases of zebra body myopathy have been sporadic.[99,164]

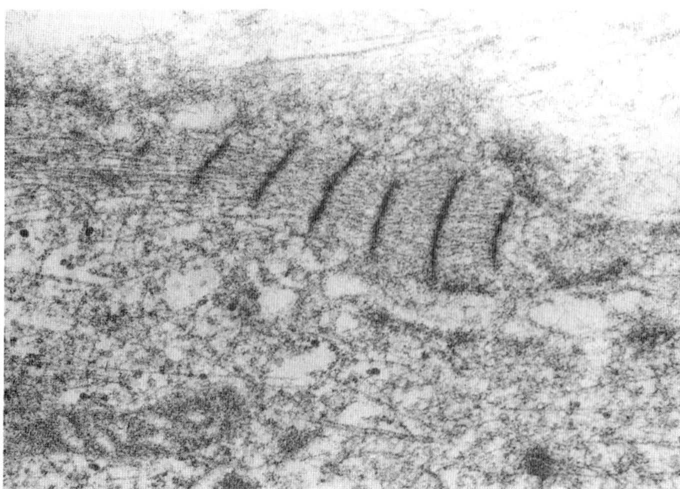

Figure 6–16. Zebra body. Ultrastructure of zebra body showing dense osmiophilic stria connected by fine filaments.

PATHOGENESIS

Zebra bodies are a normal component of skeletal and cardiac muscle.[106,107,128,164] They have also been observed in the late-distal myopathy associated with cytoplasmic bodies.[45] The stimulus for their proliferation in damaged muscle has not been identified.

TREATMENT

No specific treatment can be offered. Bracing or ambulatory aids were not required in the reported cases.[99,138]

Trilaminar Myopathy

The report of a single patient with trilaminar myopathy[141] does not justify its designation as a specific congenital myopathy.

CLINICAL FEATURES
(Table 6–15)

A newborn girl demonstrated marked rigidity of trunk and limbs following a precipitous delivery at 37 week's gestation. There were no abnormal spontaneous muscle movements. Increased muscle tone persisted during sleep. Muscle stretch reflexes and sensation were normal. Follow-up, at 10 months, demonstrated clinical improvement with reduction in muscle tone and decreased spontaneous movements. The patient later learned to walk with difficulty.

Table 6–15 TRILAMINAR MYOPATHY

CLINICAL FEATURES
  Severe muscle rigidity in newborn period
  No spontaneous movements
  Increased muscle tone persists during sleep

GENETICS
  Unknown

MUSCLE BIOPSY
  Muscle fibers show three concentric zones: innermost with densely packed mitochondria, glycogen, electron-dense material, and filaments; middle with Z disc streaming; outer with loosely packed cytoplasm

LABORATORY FEATURES

The CK level was markedly elevated (in the range of 40 times normal) at birth and was 7 times normal at 10 months. The EMG of resting muscles was electrically silent, without spontaneous activity. Motor unit potentials observed during spontaneous movement were normal. Motor conduction velocities were normal.

The muscle biopsy showed fibers composed of three concentric zones, accounting for the term "trilaminar." The innermost zone contained densely packed sarcoplasm composed of mitochondria, glycogen, osmiophilic electron-dense material, and single filaments. The middle zone consisted of myofibrils with Z disk streaming, and the outer zone contained loosely packed sarcoplasm completely encircling the other zones. Using labelled α-bungarotoxin, a band of extrajunctional acetylcholine receptors was demonstrated between the middle and outer zones.

GENETICS

This single reported case was a sporadic occurrence.

PATHOGENESIS

The cause for this condition could not be determined. The authors speculated that the extrajunctional acetylcholine receptors in the trilaminar fibers suggested an altered neural influence, but no other features of abnormal nerve input were found by electrophysiologic or muscle biopsy studies.

TREATMENT

There is no known treatment for this poorly understood condition.

Other Rare, Morphologically Distinct Myopathies

Unique structural abnormalities have been noted in other single cases of muscular weakness or have been found in at most two or three individuals or families. In many patients, symptoms have been lifelong, raising the notion of a "congenital myopathy." The identity or similarity of the biopsy findings in these cases to many other conditions, however, and the lack of evidence that the morphologic features correlate with a clinical entity, have lead us to omit them from this chapter. Examples include cylindrical spirals,[161] rings,[34] and accumulations or degeneration of contractile or structural proteins.[173,135] Similarly, some morphologically striking abnormalities of mitochondria have been described in patients or families with myopathy (e.g., megaconial myopathy), but recent molecular studies have shown these mitochondrial myopathies to result from defects of mitochondrial DNA (see Chapter 8).

SUMMARY

Congenital myopathies are heterogeneous in clinical features, natural history, and histopathology. Nonetheless, most patients have onset of signs and symptoms in infancy, or very early in life, with symmetric and often more proximal than distal limb weakness. Depressed muscle stretch reflexes, normal or only modestly elevated CK levels, and, in most instances, a distinctive histopathologic picture on muscle biopsy are all common features. Some have distinctive clinical features such as the ptosis of centronuclear myopathy and the dysmorphic facial and skeletal features of nemaline myopathy. The natural history of these disorders is also variable, but the majority are either static or only very slowly progressive.

Histopathology has provided the key for specific diagnosis. Central cores, nemaline rods, and the appearance of many central nuclei suggesting a defect in nuclear migration (centronuclear myopathy) are three of the typical, distinctive morphologic features of the most common congenital myopathies. It is presumed that most of these disorders will prove to have a genetic basis, and precise localization of the genetic defect is either emerging or under investigation. Thus far, central core disease has been localized to chromosome 19, nemaline myopathy to chromosome 1q, and the neonatal form of centronuclear myopathy to chromosome Xq28.

REFERENCES

1. Afifi AK, Smith JW, and Zellweger H: Congenital non-progressive myopathy: Central core disease and nemaline myopathy in one family. Neurology 15:371, 1965.
2. Ambler MW, Neave C, Tutschka BG, Pueschel SM, Orson JM, and Singer DB: X-linked recessive myotubular myopathy: I. Clinical and pathologic findings in a family. Hum Pathol 15:566, 1984.
3. Argov Z, Gardner-Medwin D, Johnson MA, and Mastaglia FL: Patterns of muscle fiber-type disproportion in hypotonic infants. Arch Neurol 41:53, 1984.
4. Armstrong RM, Koenigsberger R, Mellinger J, and Lovelace RE: Central core disease with congenital hip dislocation: Study of two families. Neurology 21:369, 1971.
5. Arts WF, Bethlem J, Dingemans KP, and Eriksson AW: Investigations on the inheritance of nemaline myopathy. Arch Neurol 35:72, 1978.
6. Askanas V, Engel WK, Reddy NB, et al: X-linked recessive congenital muscle fiber hypotrophy with central nuclei: Abnormalities of growth and adenylate cyclase in muscle tissue cultures. Arch Neurol 36:604, 1979.
7. Banker BQ: Discussion of the presentation by Sher JH, Rimalovski AB, Athanassiades TJ, and Aronson SM: Familial myotubular myopathy: A clinical, pathological, histochemical and ultrastructural study. J Neuropath Exp Neurol 26:132, 1967.
7a. Barohn RJ, Mendell JR, and Brumback RA: Hyaline body myopathy. Neuromuscul Disord, in press.
8. Barth PG, van Wijngaarden GK, and Bethlem J: X-linked myotubular my-

opathy with fatal neonatal asphyxia. Neurology 25:531, 1975.

9. Bergen BJ, Carry MP, Wilson WB, Barden MT, and Ringel SP: Centronuclear myopathy: Extraocular- and limb-muscle findings in an adult. Muscle Nerve 3:165, 1980.

10. Bethlem J, Van Gool J, Hülsmann WC, and Meijer AE: Familial non-progressive myopathy with muscle cramps after exercise: A new disease associated with cores in the muscle fibres. Brain 89:569, 1966.

11. Bethlem J and Posthumus Meyjes FEP: Congenital, non-progressive central core disease of Shy and Magee. Psychiatr Neurol Neurochir 63:246, 1960.

12. Bill PLA, Cole G, and Proctor NSF: Centronuclear myopathy. J Neurol Neurosurg Psychiatry 42:548, 1979.

13. Bonnette H, Roelofs R, and Olson WH: Multicore disease: report of a case with onset in middle age. Neurology 24:1039, 1974.

14. Brooke MH: Congenital fiber type dysproportion. In Kakulas BA (ed): Clinical Studies in Myology. Proceedings of the Second International Congress on Muscle Diseases, Perth, Australia, pt 2. Excerpta Medica, Amsterdam, 1973, p 147.

15. Brooke MH: A Clinician's View of Neuromuscular Diseases, ed 2. Williams & Wilkins, Baltimore, 1986.

16. Brooke MH, Carroll JE, and Ringel SP: Congenital hypotonia revisited. Muscle Nerve 2:84, 1979.

17. Brooke MH and Engel WK: The histographic analysis of human muscle biopsies with regard to fiber types. 4: Children's biopsies. Neurology 19:591, 1969.

18. Brooke MH and Neville HE: Reducing body myopathy. Neurology 22:829, 1972.

19. Brownell AKW: Familial multicore disease. Ann Neurol 6:155, 1979.

20. Brownell AKW, Gilbert JJ, Shaw DT, Garcia B, Wenkebach GF, and Lam AKS: Adult onset nemaline myopathy. Neurology 28:1306, 1978.

21. Brumback RA, Staton RD, and Susag ME: Exercise-induced pain, stiffness, and tubular aggregation in skeletal muscle. J Neurol Neurosurg Psychiatry 44:250, 1981.

22. Cancilla PA, Kalyanaraman K, Verity MA, Munsat T, and Pearson CM: Familial myopathy with probable lysis of myofibrils in type 1 fibers. Neurology 21:579, 1971.

23. Carpenter S and Karpati G: Pathology of Skeletal Muscle. Churchill Livingstone, New York, 1984.

24. Carpenter S, Karpati G, Eisen A, Andermann F, and Watters G: Childhood dermatomyositis and familial collagen disease. Neurology 22:425, 1972. Abstract.

25. Carpenter S, Karpati G, and Holland P: New observations in reducing body myopathy. Neurology 35:818, 1985.

26. Cavanagh NPC, Lake BD, and McMeniman P: Congenital fibre type disproportion myopathy: A histological diagnosis with an uncertain clinical outlook. Arch Dis Child 54:735, 1979.

27. Charnas L, Trapp B, and Griffin J: Congenital absence of peripheral myelin: Abnormal Schwann cell development causes lethal athrogryposis multiplex congenita. Neurology 38:966, 1988.

28. Chui LA, Neustein H, and Munsat TL: Tubular aggregates in subclinical alcoholic myopathy. Neurology 25:405, 1975.

29. Clancy RR, Kelts KA, and Oehlert JW: Clinical variability in congenital fiber type disproportion. J Neurol Sci 46:257, 1980.

30. Clark JR, D'Agostino AN, Wilson J, Brooks RR, and Cole GC: Autosomal dominant myofibrillar inclusion body myopathy: Clinical, histologic, histochemical, and ultrastructural characteristics. Neurology 28:399, 1978. Abstract.

31. Coers C, Telerman-Toppet N, Gerard JM, Szliwowski H, Bethlem J, and van Wijngaarden GK: Changes in motor innervation and histochemical pattern of muscle fibers in some congenital myopathies. Neurology 26:1046, 1976.

32. Cohen ME, Duffner PK, and Heffner

R: Central core disease in one of identical twins. J Neurol Neurosurg Psychiatry 41:659, 1978.

33. Conen PE, Murphy EG, and Donohue WL: Light and electron microscopic studies of "myogranules" in a child with hypotonia and muscle weakness. Can Med Assoc J 89:983, 1963.

34. Coulter CL, Marks WA, Bodensteiner JB, et al: An adult-onset myopathy characterized by a double ring appearance of muscle fibers. Neuromuscular Disorders 1:205, 1991.

35. Cruz Martinez A, Ferrer MT, López-Terradas JM, Pascual-Castroviejo I, and Mingo P: Single fibre electromyography in central core disease. J Neurol Neurosurg Psychiatry 42:662, 1979.

36. Curless RG and Nelson MB: Congenital fiber type disproportion in identical twins. Ann Neurol 2:455, 1977.

37. Curless RG, Payne CM, and Brinner FM: Fingerprint body myopathy: A report of twins. Dev Med Child Neurol 20:793, 1978.

38. D'Agostino AN, Ziter FA, Rallison ML, and Bray PF: Familial myopathy with abnormal muscle mitochondria. Arch Neurol 18:388, 1968.

39. Dalakas MC, Pezeshkpour GH, and Flaherty M: Progressive nemaline (rod) myopathy associated with HIV infection. N Engl J Med 317:1602, 1987.

40. de Groot JG and Arts WF: Familial myopathy with tubular aggregates. J Neurol 227:35, 1982.

41. Denborough MA, Dennett X, and Anderson RM: Central-core disease and malignant hyperpyrexia. Br Med J 1:272, 1973.

42. Dobkin BH and Verity MA: Familial neuromuscular disease with type 1 fiber hypoplasia, tubular aggregates, cardiomyopathy, and myasthenic features. Neurology 28:1135, 1978.

43. Dubowitz V: The "new" myopathies. Neuropäediatrie 1:137, 1969.

44. Dubowitz V and Brooke MH: Muscle Biopsy: A Modern Approach. WB Saunders, Philadelphia, 1973.

45. Edström L, Thornell LE, and Eriksson A: A new type of hereditary distal myopathy with characteristic sarcoplasmic bodies and intermediate (skeletin) filaments. J Neurol Sci 47:171, 1980.

46. Eisler T and Wilson JH: Muscle fiber-type disproportion: Report of a family with symptomatic and asymptomatic members. Arch Neurol 35:823, 1978.

47. Elder GB, Dean D, McComas AJ, Paes B, and DeSa D: Infantile centronuclear myopathy: Evidence suggesting incomplete innervation. J Neurol Sci 60:79, 1983.

48. Eng GD, Epstein BS, Engel WK, McKay DW, and McKay R: Malignant hyperthermia and central core disease in a child with congenital dislocating hips. Arch Neurol 35:189, 1978.

49. Engel AG: Late-onset rod myopathy (a new syndrome?): Light and electron microscopic observations in two cases. Mayo Clin Proc 41:713, 1966.

50. Engel AG: Myasthenia gravis and myasthenic syndromes. Ann Neurol 16:519, 1984.

51. Engel AG: Congenital disorders of neuromuscular transmission. Semin Neurol 10:12, 1990.

52. Engel AG, Angelini C, and Gomez MR: Fingerprint body myopathy: A newly recognized congenital muscle disease. Mayo Clin Proc 47:377, 1972.

52a. Engel AG and Banker BQ: Ultrastructural changes in diseased muscle. In Engel AG and Banker BQ (eds): Myology. McGraw-Hill, 1986, p 961.

53. Engel AG, Gomez MR, and Groover RV: Multicore disease: A recently recognized congenital myopathy associated with multifocal degeneration of muscle fibers. Mayo Clin Proc 46:666, 1971.

54. Engel WK: The essentiality of histo- and cytochemical studies of skeletal muscle in the investigation of neuromuscular disease. Neurology 12:778, 1962.

55. Engel WK: Mitochondrial aggregates in muscle disease. J Histochem Cytochem 12:46, 1964.

56. Engel WK, Bishop DW, and Cunningham GG: Tubular aggregates in

type II muscle fibers: Ultrastructural and histochemical correlation. J Ultrastruct Res 31:507, 1970.

57. Engel WK, Foster JB, Hughes BP, Huxley HE, and Mahler R: Central core disease—an investigation of a rare muscle cell abnormality. Brain 84:167, 1961.

58. Engel WK, Gold GN, and Karpati G: Type I fiber hypotrophy and central nuclei: A rare congenital muscle abnormality with a possible experimental model. Arch Neurol 18:435, 1968.

59. Engel WK and Oberc MA: Abundant nuclear rods in adult-onset rod disease. J Neuropathol Exp Neurol 34:119, 1975.

60. Engel WK and Resnick JS: Late-onset rod myopathy: A newly recognized, acquired, and progressive disease. Neurology 16:308, 1966.

61. Engel WK, Wanko T, and Fenichel GM: Nemaline myopathy. A second case. Arch Neurol 11:22, 1964.

62. Engel WK and Warmolts JR: The motor unit: Diseases affecting it in toto or in portio. In Desmedt JE (ed): New Developments in Electromyography and Clinical Neurophysiology, vol 1, 1973, p 141.

63. Fardeau M, Tomé FMS, and Derambure S: Familial fingerprint body myopathy. Arch Neurol 33:724, 1976.

64. Fardeau M, Tomé FMS, and Simon P: Muscle and nerve changes induced by perhexiline maleate in man and mice. Muscle Nerve 2:24, 1979.

65. Fischman DA: Development of striated muscle. In Bourne GH (ed): The Structure and Function of Muscle, ed 2, vol 1. Academic Press, New York, 1972, p 75.

66. Fukuhara N, Hoshi M, and Mori S: Core/targetoid fibres and multiple cytoplasmic bodies in organophosphate neuropathy. Acta Neuropathol 40: 137, 1977.

67. Ghatak NR, Hirano A, Poon TP, and French JH: Trichopoliodystrophy. II. Pathological changes in skeletal muscle and nervous system. Arch Neurol 26:60, 1972.

68. Gillies C, Raye J, Vasan U, Hart WE, and Goldblatt PJ: Nemaline (rod) myopathy: A possible cause of rapidly fatal infantile hypotonia. Arch Pathol Lab Med 103:1, 1979.

69. Glick B, Shapira Y, Stern A, Blank A, and Rosenmann E: Congenital muscle fiber-type disproportion myopathy: a follow up study of twenty cases. Ann Neurol 16:405, 1984. Abstract.

70. Godet-Guillain J and Fardeau M: Hypothyroid myopathy: Histological and ultrastructural study of an atrophic form. In Walton JN, Canal N, and Scarlato G (eds): Muscle Diseases. Proceedings of an International Congress. Excerpta Medica, Amsterdam, 1970, p 512.

71. Goebel HH, Muller J, Gillen HW, and Merritt AD: Autosomal dominant "spheroid body myopathy." Muscle Nerve 1:14, 1978.

72. Goebel HH, Schloon H, and Lenard HG: Congenital myopathy with cytoplasmic bodies. Neuropediatrics 12: 166, 1981.

73. Gonatas NK, Perez MC, Shy GM, and Evangelista I: Central "core" disease of skeletal muscle: Ultrastructural and cytochemical observations in two cases. Am J Pathol 47:503, 1965.

74. Gonatas NK, Shy GM, and Godfrey EH: Nemaline myopathy: The origin of nemaline structures. N Engl J Med 274:535, 1966.

75. Gordon AS, Rewcastle NB, Humphrey JG, and Stewart BM: Chronic benign congenital myopathy: Fingerprint body type. Can J Neurol Sci 1:106, 1974.

76. Greenfield JG, Cornman T, and Shy GM: The prognostic value of the muscle biopsy in the "floppy infant." Brain 81:33, 1958.

77. Heffner R, Cohen M, Duffner P, and Daigler G: Multicore disease in twins. J Neurol Neurosurg Psychiatry 39: 602, 1976.

78. Hopkins IJ, Lindsey JR, and Ford FR: Nemaline myopathy: A long-term clinicopathologic study of affected mother and daughter. Brain 89:299, 1966.

79. Hüber G and Pongratz D: Granularkörpermyopathie (sog. reducing body myopathy): Beitrag zur Feinstruktur

und Klassifizierung. Virchows Archiv A Pathol Anat Histopathol 392:97, 1981.

80. Iannaccone ST, Bove KE, Vogler CA, and Buchino JJ: Type I fiber size disproportion: morphometric data from 37 children with myopathic, neuropathic, or idiopathic hypotonia. Pediatr Pathol 7:395, 1987.

81. Isaacs H and Barlow MB: Central core disease associated with elevated creatine phosphokinase levels: Two members of a family known to be susceptible to malignant hyperpyrexia. S Afr Med J 48:640, 1974.

82. Jadro-Šantel N, Grčević N, Dogan S, Franjić J, and Benc H: Centronuclear myopathy with type I fibre hypotrophy and "fingerprint" inclusions associated with Marfan's syndrome. J Neurol Sci 45:43, 1980.

83. Jenis EH, Lindquist RR, and Lister RC: New congenital myopathy with crystalline intranuclear inclusions. Arch Neurol 20:281, 1969.

84. Jennekens FGI, Roord JJ, Veldman H, Willemse J, and Jockusch BM: Congenital nemaline myopathy, I. Defective organization of α actinin is restricted to muscle. Muscle Nerve 6:61, 1983.

85. Jerusalem F, Engel AG, and Gomez MR: Sarcotubular myopathy: A newly recognized, benign, congenital, familial muscle disease. Neurology 23:897, 1973.

86. Jerusalem F, Ludin H, Bischoff A, and Hartmann G: Cytoplasmic body neuromyopathy presenting as respiratory failure and weight loss. J Neurol Sci 41:1, 1979.

87. Johns TR, Campa JF, and Adelman LS: Familial myasthenia with "tubular aggregates" treated with prednisone [abstract]. Neurology 23:426, 1973.

88. Julien J, Vital CL, Vallat JM, Vallat M, and LeBlanc M: Oculopharyngeal muscular dystrophy—a case with abnormal mitochondria and "fingerprint" inclusions. J Neurol Sci 21:165, 1974.

89. Kamieniecka Z: Late onset myopathy with rod-like particles. Acta Neurol Scand 49:547, 1973.

90. Karpati G, Carpenter S, and Andermann F: A new concept of childhood nemaline myopathy. Arch Neurol 24:291, 1971.

91. Karpati G, Carpenter S, and Eisen AA: Experimental core-like lesions and nemaline rods: A correlative morphological and physiological study. Arch Neurol 27:237, 1972.

92. Karpati G, Carpenter S, and Nelson RF: Type I muscle fibre atrophy and central nuclei: A rare familial neuromuscular disease. J Neurol Sci 10:489, 1970.

93. Kausch K, Lehmann-Horn F, Janka M, Wieringa B, Grimm T, and Müller CR: Evidence for linkage of the central core disease locus to the proximal long arm of human chromosome 19. Genomics 10:765, 1991.

94. Kinoshita M, Satoyoshi E, and Kumagai M: Familial type I fiber atrophy. J Neurol Sci 25:11, 1975.

95. Kinoshita M, Satoyoshi E, and Suzuki Y: Atypical myopathy with myofibrillar aggregates. Arch Neurol 32:417, 1975.

96. Kissel JT, Beam W, Bresolin N, Gibbons G, DiMauro S, and Mendell JR: Physiologic assessment of phosphoglycerate mutase deficiency: Incremental exercise tests. Neurology 35:828, 1985.

97. Kolin IS: Nemaline myopathy. A fatal case. Am J Dis Child 114:95, 1967.

98. Kondo K and Yuasa T: Genetics of congenital nemaline myopathy. Muscle Nerve 3:308, 1980.

99. Lake BD and Wilson J: Zebra body myopathy: Clinical, histochemical and ultrastructural studies. J Neurol Sci 24:437, 1975.

100. Liechti-Gallati S, Müeller B, and Grimm T, et al: X-linked centronuclear myopathy: Mapping the gene to Xq28. Neuromuscular Disorders 1:239, 1991.

101. Lo WD, Barohn RJ, Bobulski RJ, Kean J, and Mendell JR: Centronuclear myopathy and type-I hypotrophy without central nuclei: Distinct nosologic entities? Arch Neurol 47:273, 1990.

102. MacDonald RD and Engel AG: The

cytoplasmic body: Another structural anomaly of the Z disk. Acta Neuropathol 14:99, 1969.

103. MacDonald RD and Engel AG: Observations on organization of Z-disk components and on rod-bodies of Z-disk origin. J Cell Biol 48:431, 1971.

104. MacLennan D, Duff C, Zorzato F, et al: Ryanodine receptor gene is a candidate for predisposition to malignant hyperthermia. Nature 343:559, 1990.

105. Mair WGP and Tomé FMS: Atlas of the Ultrastructure of Diseased Human Muscle. Williams & Wilkins, Baltimore, 1972, p 48.

106. Mair WGP and Tomé FMS: The ultrastructure of the adult and developing human myotendinous junction. Acta Neuropathol (Berl) 21:239, 1972.

107. Martinez AJ, Hay S, and McNeer KW: Extraocular muscles: Light microscopy and ultrastructural features. Acta Neuropathol (Berl) 34:237, 1976.

108. Mastaglia FL and Hudgson P: Ultrastructural studies of diseased muscle. In Walton J (ed): Disorders of Voluntary Muscle. Churchill Livingstone, Edinburgh, 1981, p 296.

109. McCarthy T, Healy J, Heffron J, et al: Localization of the malignant hyperthermia susceptibility locus to human chromosome 19q12. Nature 343:562, 1990.

110. McComb RD, Markesbery WR, and O'Connor WN: Fatal neonatal nemaline myopathy with multiple congenital abnormalities. J Pediatr 94:47, 1979.

111. McLeod JG, Baker WDC, Lethlean AK, and Shorey CD: Centronuclear myopathy with autosomal dominant inheritance. J Neurol Sci 15:375, 1972.

112. Meier C, Gertsch M, Zimmerman A, Voellmy W, and Geissbuhler J: Nemaline myopathy presenting as cardiomyopathy. N Engl J Med 308:1536, 1983.

113. Meier C, Voellmy W, Gertsch M, Zimmerman A, and Geissbühler J: Nemaline myopathy appearing in adults as cardiomyopathy: A clinicopatho-

114. Meltzer HY, McBride E, and Poppei RW: Rod (nemaline) bodies in the skeletal muscle of an acute schizophrenic patient. Neurology 23:769, 1973.

115. Mendell JR and Engel WK: The fine structure of type II fiber atrophy. Neurology 21:358, 1971.

116. Meyers KR, Gilden DH, Rinaldi CF, and Hansen JL: Periodic muscle weakness, normokalemia, and tubular aggregates. Neurology 22:269, 1972.

117. Meyers KR, Golomb HM, Hansen JL, and McKusick VA: Familial neuromuscular disease with "myotubes." Clin Genet 5:327, 1974.

118. Morgan-Hughes JA, Lecky BRF, Landon DN, and Murray NM: Alterations in the number and affinity of junctional acetylcholine receptors in a myopathy with tubular aggregates: A newly recognized receptor defect. Brain 104:279, 1981.

119. Morgan-Hughes JA, Mair WGP, and Lascelles PT: A disorder of skeletal muscle associated with tubular aggregates. Brain 93:873, 1970.

120. Moulds RFW and Denborough MA: Myopathies and malignant hyperpyrexia [abstract]. Br Med J 3:520, 1974.

121. Mrozek K, Strugalska M, and Fidziańska A: A sporadic case of central core disease. J Neurol Sci 10:339, 1970.

122. Munsat TL, Thompson LR, and Coleman RF: Centronuclear ("myotubular") myopathy. Arch Neurol 20:120, 1969.

123. Neustein HB: Nemaline myopathy. A family study with three autopsied cases. Arch Pathol 96:192, 1973.

124. Neville HE and Brooke MH: Central core fibers: structured and unstructured. In Kakulas BA (ed): Basic Research in Myology. Proceedings of the Second International Congress on Muscle Diseases, Perth, Australia, November 22–26, 1971, pt 1. Excerpta Medica, Amsterdam, 1973, p 497, ICS 294.

125. Norton P, Ellison P, Salaiman AR,

and Harb J: Nemaline myopathy in the neonate. Neurology 33:351, 1983.

126. Oh SJ, Meyers GJ, Wilson ER, and Alexander CB: A benign form of reducing body myopathy. Muscle Nerve 6:278, 1983.

127. Oritz de Zarte JC and Maruffo A: The descending ocular myopathy of early childhood myotubular or centronuclear myopathy. Eur Neurol 3:1, 1970.

128. Ovalle WK: Fine structure of rat intrafusal muscle fibers: The equatorial region. J Cell Biol 52:382, 1972.

129. Patel H, Berry K, MacLeod P, and Dunn HG: Cytoplasmic body myopathy: Report on a family and review of the literature. J Neurol Sci 60:281, 1983.

130. Patterson VH, Hill TRG, Fletcher PJH, and Heron JR: Central core disease: Clinical and pathological evidence of progression within a family. Brain 102:581, 1979.

131. Pavone L, Mollica F, Grasso A, and Pero G: Familial centronuclear myopathy. Acta Neurol Scand 62:33, 1980.

132. Payne CM and Curless RG: Fingerprint inclusions: ultrastructural demonstration of muscle fiber type specificity. J Neurol Sci 31:379, 1977.

133. PeBenito R, Sher JH, and Cracco JB: Centronuclear myopathy: Clinical and pathologic features. Clin Pediatr 17:259, 1978.

134. Penn AS: Myoglobin and myoglobinuria. In Vinken PJ and Bruyn GW (eds): Handbook of Clinical Neurology, vol 41. North Holland Publishing, 1979, p 268.

135. Prelle A, Moggio M, Comi GP, et al: Congenital myopathy associated with abnormal accumulation of desmin and dystrophin. Neuromuscular Disorders 2:169, 1992.

136. Raju TNK, Vidyasagar D, Reyes MG, and Chokroverty S: Centronuclear myopathy in the newborn period causing severe respiratory distress. Pediatrics 59:29, 1977.

136a. Quane KA, Healy JMS, Keating KE, et al: Mutations in the ryanodine receptor gene in central core disease and malignant hyperthermia. Nat Genet 5:51, 1993.

137. Resnick JS, Engel WK, and Nelson PG: Changes in the Z disk of skeletal muscle induced by tenotomy. Neurology 18:737, 1968.

138. Reyes MG, Goldbarg H, Fresco K, and Bouffard A: Zebra body myopathy: A second case of ultrastructurally distinct congenital myopathy. J Child Neurol 2:307, 1987.

139. Ricoy JR, Cabello A, and Goizueta G: Myopathy with multiple minicore: Report of two siblings. J Neurol Sci 48:81, 1980.

140. Rifai Z, Kazee AM, Kamp C, and Griggs RC: Intranuclear rods in severe congenital nemaline myopathy. Neurology 43:2372, 1993.

141. Ringel SP, Neville HE, Duster MC, and Carroll JE: A new congenital neuromuscular disease with trilaminar muscle fibers. Neurology 28:282, 1978.

142. Robertson WC Jr, Kawamura Y, and Dyck PJ: Morphometric study of motoneurons in congenital nemaline myopathy and Werdnig-Hoffman disease. Neurology 28:1057, 1978.

143. Rohkamm R, Boxler K, Ricker K, and Jerusalem F: A dominantly inherited myopathy with excessive tubular aggregates. Neurology 33:331, 1983.

144. Sahgal V and Sahgal S: A new congenital myopathy: A morphological, cytochemical and histochemical study. Acta Neuropathol (Berl) 37:225, 1977.

145. Sato T, Walker DL, Peters HA, Reese HH, and Chou SM: Chronic polymyositis and myxovirus-like inclusions: Electron microscopic and viral studies. Arch Neurol 24:409, 1971.

146. Schochet SS Jr, Zellweger H, Ionasescu V, and McCormick WF: Centronuclear myopathy: Disease entity or a syndrome? Light- and electron-microscopic study of two cases and review of the literature. J Neurol Sci 16:215, 1972.

147. Sengel A and Stoebner P: Une inclusion musculaire atypique rare: Les "corps en empreintes digitales" ou

"fingerprint bodies." Acta Neuropathol (Berl) 27:61, 1974.

148. Serratrice G, Roux H, Aquaron R, Gambarelli D, Baret R, and Recordier AM: Myopathy associated with arthropathic psoriasis. In Walton JN, Canal N, and Scarlato G (eds): Muscle diseases: Proceedings of an International Congress. Excerpta Medica, Amsterdam, 1970, p 642.

149. Serratrice G, Pellissier JF, Faugere MC, and Gastaut JL: Centronuclear myopathy: Possible central nervous system origin. Muscle Nerve 1:62, 1978.

150. Shafiq SA, Dubowitz V, Peterson HDC, and Milhorat AT: Nemaline myopathy: Report of a fatal case, with histochemical and electron microscopic studies. Brain 90:817, 1967.

151. Shafiq SA, Milhorat AT, and Gorycki MA: An electron microscope study of muscle degeneration and vascular changes in polymyositis. J Pathol Bacteriol 94:139, 1967.

152. Sher JH, Rimalovski AB, Athanassiades TJ, and Aronson SM: Familial centronuclear myopathy: A clinical and pathological study. Neurology 17:727, 1967.

153. Shy GM, Engel WK, Somers JE, and Wanko T: Nemaline myopathy: A new congenital myopathy. Brain 86:793, 1963.

154. Shy GM and Magee KR: A new congenital non-progressive myopathy. Brain 79:610, 1956.

155. Spiro AJ and Kennedy C: Hereditary occurrence of nemaline myopathy. Arch Neurol 13:155, 1965.

156. Spiro AJ, Shy GM, and Gonatas NK: Myotubular myopathy: Persistence of fetal muscle in an adolescent boy. Arch Neurol 14:1, 1966.

157. Staley NA and Benson ES: Z lines in early anoxic injury to red skeletal muscle [abstract]. J Cell Biol 39:128a, 1968.

158. Stoessl AJ, Hahn AF, Malott D, Jones DT, and Silver MD: Nemaline myopathy within associated cardiomyopathy: Report of clinical and detailed autopsy findings. Arch Neurol 42:1084, 1985.

159. Stuhlfauth I, Jennekens FG, Wilemse J, and Jockusch BM: Congenital nemaline myopathy, II. Quantitative changes in α-actinin and myosin in skeletal muscle. Muscle Nerve 6:69, 1983.

160. Swash M and Schwartz MS: Familial multicore disease with focal loss of cross-striations and ophthalmoplegia. J Neurol Sci 52:1, 1981.

161. Taratuto AL, Matteucci M, Barreiro C, Saccolitti M, and Sevlever G: Autosomal dominant neuromuscular disease with cylindrical spirals. Neuromuscular Disorders 1:433, 1991.

162. Telerman-Toppet N, Gerard JM, and Coers C: Central core disease: A study of clinically unaffected muscle. J Neurol Sci 19:207, 1973.

163. Thomas NST, Williams H, Cole G, et al: X-linked neonatal centronuclear/myotubular myopathy: Evidence for linkage to Xq28 DNA marker loci. J Med Genet 27:284, 1990.

164. Thornell LE, Sjöström MX, and Andersson KE: The relationship between mechanical stress and myofibrillar organization in heart Purkinje fibres. J Mol Cell Cardiol 8:689, 1976.

165. Tomé FMS and Fardeau M: Congenital myopathy with "reducing bodies" in muscle fibres. Acta Neuropathol (Berl) 31:207, 1975.

166. van der Ven PFM, Jap PHK, Wetzels RHW, et al: Postnatal centralization of muscle fibre nuclei in centronuclear myopathy. Neuromuscular Disorders 1:211, 1991.

167. van Wijngaarden GK, Fleury P, Bethlem J, and Meijer AEFH: Familial "myotubular" myopathy. Neurology 19:901, 1969.

168. Vanneste JAL and Stam FC: Autosomal dominant multicore disease. J Neurol Neurosurg Psychiatry 45:360, 1982.

169. Verhiest W, Brucher JM, Goddeeris P, Lauweryns J, and DeGeest H: Familial centronuclear myopathy associated with "cardiomyopathy." Br Heart J 38:504, 1976.

170. Vogler C and Bovek KE: Morphology of skeletal muscle in children: An assessment of normal growth and dif-

ferentiation. Arch Pathol Lab Med 109:238, 1985.

171. Wallgren-Pettersson C, Sainio K, and Salmi T: Electromyography in congenital nemaline myopathy. Muscle Nerve 12:587, 1989.

172. Wolburg H, Schlote W, Langohr HD, Peiffer J, Reiher KH, and Heckl RW: Slowly progressive congenital myopathy with cytoplasmic bodies: Report of two cases and a review of the literature. Clin Neuropathol 1:55, 1982.

173. Yarom R and Shapira Y: Myosin degeneration in a congenital myopathy. Arch Neurol 34:114, 1977.

174. Zhang Y, Chen HS, Khanna VK, et al: A mutation in the human ryanodine receptor gene associated with central core disease. Nature Genet 5:46, 1993.

METABOLIC MYOPATHIES

Recent developments in molecular biology and biochemistry have defined the fundamental biochemical defect in many disorders resulting from an abnormality of muscle metabolism (or suspected of resulting from such disorders). Some of these metabolic myopathies are treatable, and genetic counseling is possible in most of them, so recognition is increasingly important. In the majority of metabolic myopathies, the clinical features are *dynamic* rather than *static*, so that exercise intolerance rather than fixed weakness is the chief complaint (Table 7–1). Nonetheless, progressive muscular weakness, which can mimic limb-girdle muscular dystrophy or an inflammatory myopathy, is characteristic of some metabolic muscle diseases, including acid maltase deficiency, both branching and debranching enzyme deficiencies, and carnitine deficiency. For most patients with a defect in glycogen, lipid, or purine metabolism, however, the major clinical problems are reduced exercise tolerance and intermittent muscle pain or myoglobinuria. Thus, the presence of intermittent, exercise-related symptoms suggests a diagnosis of metabolic muscle disease and a defect in muscle bioenergetics. Patients with persistent pain or with pain or fatigue with minimal activity are less likely to have a metabolic disorder (see Chapter 11).

ENERGY METABOLISM IN EXERCISING MUSCLE

The evaluation of a patient suspected of having a metabolic myopathy requires exercise tests or other biochemical studies to uncover the defect of muscle metabolism. Before considering the evaluation, we will briefly review the normal pathways for the use of muscle fuel during exercise (Fig. 7–1). Muscle contraction depends on the chemical energy of adenosine triphosphate (ATP). Numerous processes within the muscle cell work together to maintain a supply of ATP to support muscle contraction. Four major pathways supply ATP to meet the energy demands of exercising muscle: glycogen metabolism, lipid metabolism, phosphocreatine stores, and the purine nucleotide cycle (see Fig. 7–1).

Glycogen Metabolism

ANAEROBIC EXERCISE

Glycolysis provides energy for high-intensity muscular activity, particularly when blood flow is reduced and the availability of oxygen to the muscle cell is limited (Fig. 7–2). Myophosphorylase is the enzyme responsible for initiating the metabolism of glycogen. The enzyme phosphofructokinase (PFK) catalyzes the rate-limiting step in

Table 7–1 METABOLIC MYOPATHIES CHARACTERIZED BY DYNAMIC SYMPTOMS (EXERCISE INTOLERANCE)

GLYCOGEN METABOLIC DEFECTS
  Myophosphorylase
  Phosphofructokinase
  Phosphoglycerate kinase
  Phosphoglycerate mutase
  Lactate dehydrogenase
  Phosphorylase *b* kinase

LIPID METABOLIC DEFECT
  Carnitine palmitoyl transferase

MITOCHONDRIAL MYOPATHIES

PURINE NUCLEOTIDE CYCLE DEFECT
  Myoadenylate deaminase (rarely clinically
    significant)

the glycolytic pathway, converting fructose-6-phosphate to fructose 1,6-diphosphate. During anaerobic exercise, phosphofructokinase activity, critical to the regulation of the glycolytic pathway, is reduced by lowered intracellular pH, and by elevated adenosine diphosphate (ADP) and high ATP concentrations. Under anaerobic conditions, glycolysis proceeds through the conversion of pyruvate to lactate. It has been known for more than 100 years that lactate builds up in exercising muscle, contributing to increased acidification of the muscle cell, and to the development of fatigue. The accumulation of three other products of ATP

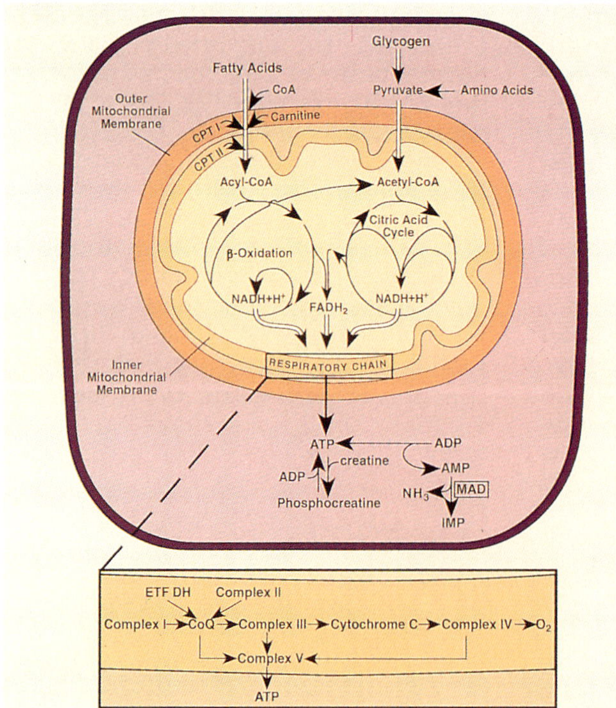

Figure 7–1. Overview of muscle energy metabolism, showing the major pathways supplying ATP. Glycogen is broken down through the steps of glycolysis to form pyruvate, which undergoes oxidative decarboxylation to acetyl-CoA before entering the citric acid cycle. The use of lipids as a source of energy requires release of free fatty acids from cytoplasmic fat stores. Long-chain fatty acids attached to carnitine penetrate the mitochondrial membranes. Acyl-CoA must be converted to acylcarnitine by the enzyme carnitine palmitoyl transferase (CPT 1), present on the outer mitochondrial membrane, followed by reconversion to acyl-CoA by CPT 2, found on the inner mitochondrial membrane. Acyl-CoA then undergoes β-oxidation. The hydrogen carriers NADH + H⁺ and FADH₂ transfer electrons to the respiratory chain on the inner mitochondrial membrane. Progressive oxidation of the hydrogen electrons through the respiratory chain releases energy to synthesize ATP. An alternative reservoir of energy is stored in muscle as phosphocreatine, a high-energy compound found in equilibrium with ATP. ATP in muscle may also be derived from adenosine monophosphate (AMP) produced by adenylate kinase deaminated by the enzyme myoadenylate deaminase (MAD). The resulting ammonia and inosine monophosphate (IMP) may be reconverted to AMP or degraded to hypoxanthine (not shown). Formation of IMP without reconversion to AMP will result in ATP production.

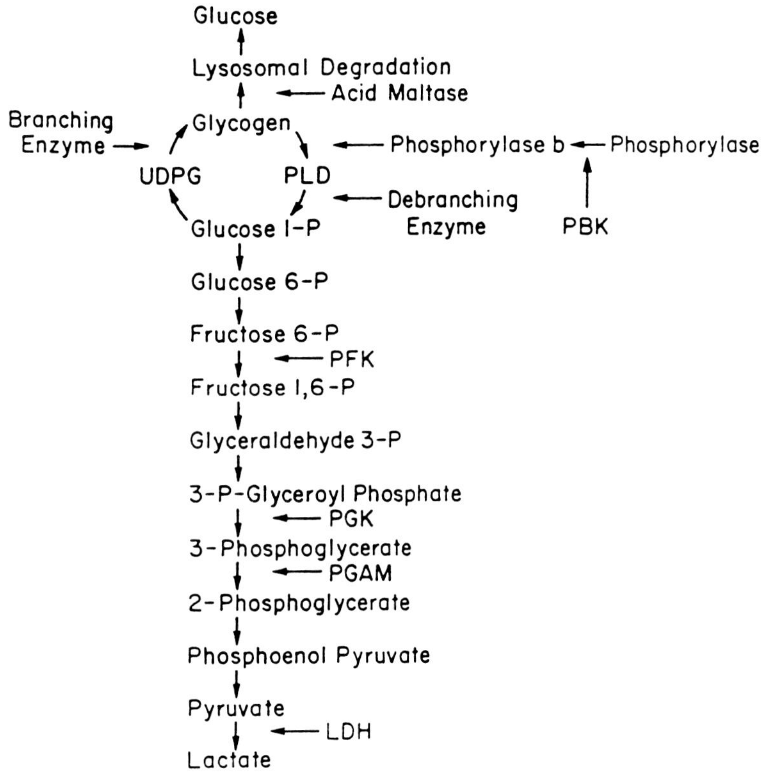

Figure 7–2. Scheme of glycolysis showing the sites of defects causing clinical muscle disorders. These include deficiencies of various enzymes: acid maltase; myophosphorylase (McArdle's disease); phosphorylase *b* kinase (PBK); phosphofructokinase (PFK); phosphoglycerate kinase (PGK); phosphoglycerate mutase (PGAM); and lactic acid dehydrogenase (LDH).

hydrolysis—inorganic phosphate, ADP, and particularly the monovalent form of organic phosphate—appears also to play an important role in fatigue, as discussed below.

AEROBIC EXERCISE

When muscular exercise is intermittent or submaximal (less than approximately 15% of maximum contraction) (see Fig. 11–1) and blood flow to muscle is unimpaired, then oxidative phosphorylation is the major pathway for carbohydrate metabolism. The metabolism of glycogen (and blood glucose) proceeds through the same steps as in anaerobic glycolysis, down to the formation of pyruvate. At that point, oxidative decar-

boxylation of pyruvate through the pyruvate dehydrogenase complex generates acetyl coenzyme A (acetyl-CoA), which then enters the tricarboxylic acid (TCA) cycle and is ultimately converted to carbon dioxide and water (see Fig. 7–1).

ELECTRON TRANSPORT

In the TCA cycle, acetyl-CoA undergoes a series of oxidation-reduction reactions. In three reactions, hydrogen ions are transferred to three molecules of nicotinamide adenine dinucleotide (NAD), and in one, a pair of hydrogen ions is transferred to a molecule of flavin adenine dinucleotide (FAD). The mitochondrion then uses these electron carriers to yield ATP when they are oxidized by oxygen in the electron transport chain. This process occurs within the mitochondrial inner membrane, in the respiratory chain, which consists of a series of enzymes that serve as electron and hydrogen carriers responsible for transferring reducing equivalent derived from the TCA cycle to molecular oxygen. This process, usually referred to as electron transport, releases a large amount of free energy stored as ATP, in a process called oxidative phosphorylation.

The reduced forms of NAD and succinate dehydrogenase (NADH and SDH) formed from the citric acid cycle and the fatty acid oxidation pathway in the mitochondrial matrix are funneled into the respiratory chain found in the inner mitochondrial membrane. The components of the respiratory chain can be separated into four multienzyme complexes (see Fig. 7–1):

Complex I (NADH-ubiquinone oxido-reductase)
Complex II (succinate-ubiquinone oxido-reductase)
Complex III (dihydro-ubiquinone-cytochrome *c* oxido-reductase)
Complex IV (cytochrome *c* oxidase).

Hydrogen from NADH is delivered directly to Complex I, whereas hydrogen from succinate is obtained from Complex II. These electrons are then transferred to coenzyme Q, which in turn donates electrons to Complex III. Cytochrome *c* is located on the outside of the inner membrane and donates the electrons to Complex IV, where they are combined with an oxygen atom and two hydrogen ions to produce water. This flow of electrons releases energy that is used in the synthesis of ATP by Complex V (ATP synthetase), also found in the inner mitochondrial membrane. The oxidation of NADH yields three molecules of ATP, whereas two ATP molecules arise from oxidation of SDH.

It is theorized that the transfer of electrons through the respiratory chain results in the pumping of protons (hydrogen ions) from the mitochondrial matrix to the cytoplasmic side of the inner mitochondrial membrane. The hydrogen ion concentration becomes higher on the cytoplasmic side, and a membrane potential is generated. According to this model, the electron transport chain interacts with the ATP-synthesizing complex only through the membrane potential. ATP synthetase (Complex V) allows some of the protons to flow back into the mitochondrion and uses the released energy to synthesize ATP.

Lipid Metabolism

Saturated, long-chain fatty acids are a major source of energy for sustained submaximal exercise, usually more than 40 to 45 minutes in duration. Fatty acids are derived from circulating very-low-density lipoproteins in the blood via endothelial lipoprotein lipase or from stored triglycerides within muscle fibers, again via a lipase system. These fatty acids in the muscle cytoplasm are activated by acyl-CoA synthetase so that they can be transported across the mitochondrial membrane (see Fig. 7–1), a process that also depends on carnitine palmitoyl transferase (CPT). There are two forms of CPT: CPT 1 is localized to the inner face of the outer membrane of the mitochondria, and CPT 2 is localized on the inner surface of the inner membrane. The fatty-acid-derived acyl group (two-carbon fragment) is linked with carnitine by the enzyme CPT 1 to allow transport into the mitochondria. The carnitine is removed by CPT 2 after passage through the mitochondrial membrane, and the acyl-CoA is then oxidized to carbon dioxide and water, a process termed beta oxidation. This pathway for muscle energy metabolism is used during resting conditions but becomes increasingly important during prolonged aerobic exercise.

Other Sources of Energy

PHOSPHOCREATINE

Two other pathways are significant during muscular exercise: the phosphocreatine pathway and the purine nucleotide cycle. As shown in Figure 7 – 1, the creatine kinase reaction permits the rapid formation of ATP through the reaction of stored phosphocreatine with ADP. This pathway is particularly important during very-high-intensity exercise, but because stores are limited, the duration of this metabolic reaction is very brief. Phosphocreatine levels are restored in muscle when the oxygen supply is again adequate.

THE PURINE NUCLEOTIDE CYCLE

The second pathway that can replace ATP over short periods uses the enzymes adenylate kinase and myoadenylate deaminase. Adenylate kinase converts ADP to ATP plus adenosine monophosphate (AMP). The AMP is then converted to inosine monophosphate (IMP) by myoadenylate deaminase, with simultaneous ammonia production. This pathway is also only used for brief, high-intensity exercise and may be preferentially used by fast (type 2) muscle fibers, because myoadenylate deaminase activity is higher in type 2 than in type 1 fibers.

EVALUATION OF THE PATIENT

Clinical Features

The clinical features of patients suspected of having a metabolic myopathy should be considered in terms of both *dynamic* and *static* symptoms (see Table 7 – 1). *Dynamic* symptoms include fatigue, myalgia, and muscle stiffness that emerge during the exercise. In addition, when the exercise load outstrips the available energy, muscle breakdown or rhabdomyolysis occurs, releasing myoglobin from the muscle cell. Significant muscle breakdown causes the brownish-red color of urine resulting from myoglobinuria; lesser amounts of myoglobin release can be

detected in the serum in the absence of grossly visible urine pigment.

Static symptoms reflect fixed muscle weakness and result from abnormal storage of lipid or glycogen in muscle. The storage product appears to affect not only muscle metabolism (no doubt contributing to dynamic symptoms) but also the normal structure-function relationship of important intracellular muscle components. The clinical result is generalized muscle weakness, more often affecting proximal muscles. Respiratory muscles and other organ systems (especially cardiac muscle, as in patients with acid maltase deficiency) can also be affected. The clinical picture may be indistinguishable from limb-girdle muscular dystrophy.

Any of the metabolic myopathies may have both dynamic and static symptoms to some degree. The juxtaposition of dynamic and static symptoms is particularly apparent in the mitochondrial myopathies (Chapter 8). These patients display dynamic symptoms consisting of marked fatigability during sustained or repeated exercise; cardiovascular hyperreactivity is especially apparent. They also show static features such as progressive external ophthalmoplegia and a variety of abnormalities of the nervous system, including seizures, dementia, strokelike symptoms, ataxia, and peripheral neuropathies.

Laboratory Findings

The laboratory evaluation of a patient suspected of having a metabolic muscle disorder should include the tests listed in Table 7 – 2.

BLOOD TESTING

The creatine kinase (CK) level is often elevated in glycogen storage diseases, carnitine deficiency, and malignant hyperthermia. Serum lactate may be elevated in mitochondrial disorders.

Table 7–2 LABORATORY INVESTIGATION FOR SUSPECTED METABOLIC MYOPATHY

BLOOD TESTS
  CK
  Lactate
  Pyruvate
  Lactic acid dehydrogenase

ELECTROMYOGRAPHY
  Routine
  Quantitative (selected cases)
  Repetitive nerve stimulation (selected cases)

FOREARM EXERCISE TESTING

MUSCLE BIOPSY
  Histology
  Histochemistry
  Electron microscopy (selected cases)
  Biochemical analysis

ELECTROMYOGRAPHY

Electromyography (EMG) can exclude a neurogenic disorder in a patient with static weakness and will reveal a myopathic pattern in carnitine deficiency, acid maltase deficiency, debranching enzyme deficiency (with abundant myotonic discharges), and long-standing myophosphorylase deficiency. Quantitative EMG (see Chapter 2) may be useful in patients with mild weakness. Repetitive nerve stimulation should be used to evaluate neuromuscular transmission in patients with excessive fatigability.

FOREARM EXERCISE TESTING

Exercise testing is a critical part of the evaluation of a patient with exercise intolerance. The exercise test should be carried out *without the blood pressure cuff*, as ischemic exercise may be hazardous to patients with glycolytic defects (see p. 272). Repetitive maximum isometric contractions (using a hand grip dynamometer), consisting of sustained contractions for 1.5 seconds separated by rest periods of 0.5 seconds, are performed for 1 full minute. A resting blood sample for venous lactate and ammonia is obtained prior to exercise, with further sampling at 1, 2, 4, 6, and 10 minutes following the termination of exercise. A threefold rise in lactate level constitutes a normal response and indicates excellent effort (Fig. 7–3). The concentration of venous lactate rises rapidly after exercise, whereas that of ammonia rises more gradually (3 to 4 minutes after starting exercise).

The results of the forearm exercise test help to detect different metabolic errors. Lactate production is absent (e.g., PFK, myophosphorylase) or diminished (e.g., phosphoglycerase mutase [PGAM] deficiency) in defects of glycogenolysis; there is excessive production of lactate at low levels of work in patients with mitochondrial myopathy; and finally, there is an absence of ammonia production in myoadenylate deaminase deficiency.[132]

NUCLEAR MAGNETIC RESONANCE SPECTROSCOPY

Nuclear magnetic resonance (NMR) spectroscopy is a new, noninvasive technique for the study of muscle metabolism. It may elucidate mechanisms of fatigue in normal muscle and in patients with metabolic myopathies.[12,12a,93a,119] Phosphocreatine, inorganic phosphate, intracellular pH, ATP, and lactate levels are continuously monitored during exercise (Fig. 7–4). The role of NMR spectroscopy in the diagnosis of muscle disease is only beginning to emerge.[4a,119] With glycolytic defects (e.g., myophosphorylase deficiency), it can quickly reveal the absence of intracellular acidification during exercise.[8,144] In mitochondrial myopathies, the elevated ratio of inorganic phosphate to phosphocreatine at rest, as well as the delayed resynthesis of phosphocreatine after exercise, both reflect impaired mitochondrial function.[6,113a]

MUSCLE BIOPSY

Muscle biopsy should usually be carried out in a patient suspected of having

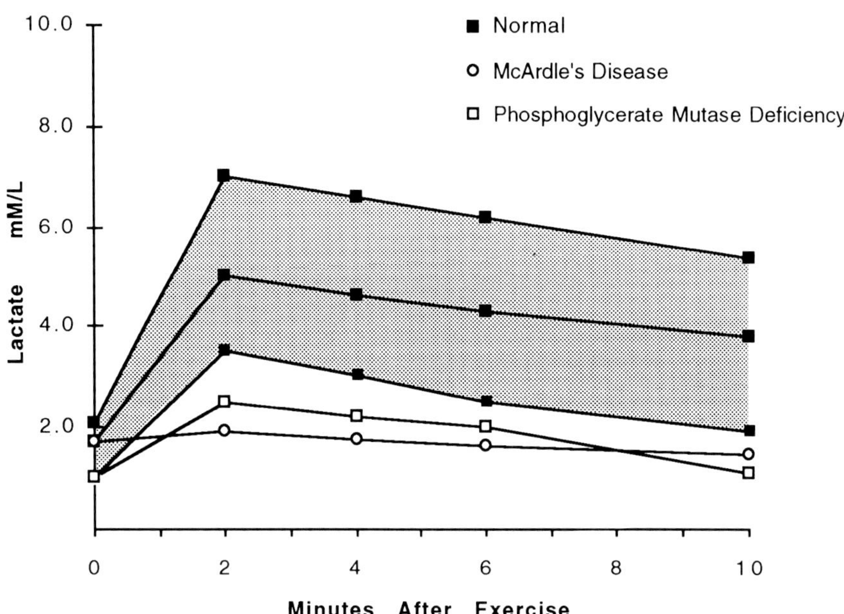

Figure 7–3. The shaded area shows the response of venous lactate in normal controls following 1 minute of forearm exercise. The maximum rise occurs 2 minutes after exercise and gradually falls toward baseline. The open circles (O) demonstrate the failure of lactate to increase following exercise in a patient with McArdle's disease. The open boxes (□) show a partial rise in lactate following exercise in a patient with phosphoglycerate mutase deficiency.

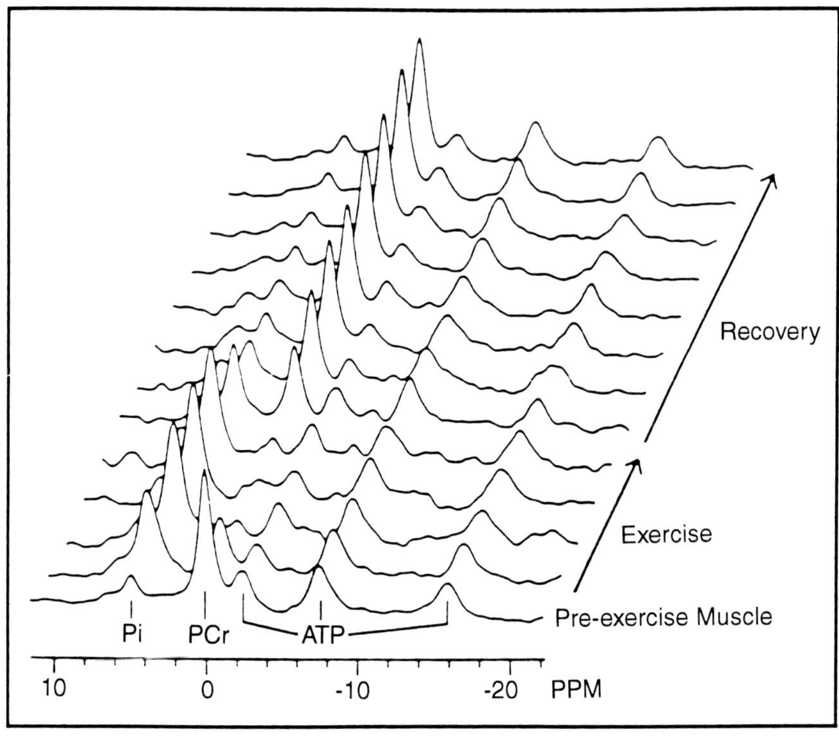

Figure 7–4. Stacked plots of ^{31}P NMR spectra obtained before, during, and after sustained submaximal exercise of the tibialis anterior muscle. Pi = inorganic phosphate; PCr = phosphocreatine.

a metabolic muscle disease only after the rest of the evaluation is complete. One cannot screen biopsy tissue for all metabolic defects, and so the data derived from the clinical evaluation, and CK, lactate, EMG, and exercise testing can usually provide direction. Muscle samples should be taken for microscopic examination, including electron microscopy and histochemistry, as well as for biochemical testing. The microscopic examination can demonstrate glycogen or lipid storage and mitochondrial disorders with ragged red fibers. Histochemical staining for myophosphorylase, PFK, and myoadenylate deaminase may reveal specific defects, which should then be biochemically quantified. Some metabolic defects, such as CPT deficiency or partial carnitine deficiency, may not be apparent by any microscopic studies and must be diagnosed by the biochemical analysis of muscle tissue.

DEFECTS OF GLYCOGEN METABOLISM

Disorders Producing Dynamic Symptoms (Exercise Intolerance)

Patients with these conditions usually complain of easy fatigability with exercise. Muscle stiffness also may be provoked by exercise. These dynamic symptoms are characteristic of many metabolic myopathies.

MYOPHOSPHORYLASE DEFICIENCY (McARDLE'S DISEASE)

Case History

A 38-year-old woman first developed difficulties with exercise tolerance in high school. She noted rigidity and pain in abdominal muscles when attempting sit-ups in a physical education class. A few months later, while learning wrestling, she developed cramping and rigidity of leg muscles, followed by dark, pigmented urine. Two

years later, while maintaining a prolonged crouch position during work in cramped quarters, she developed spasms in the leg muscles and then dark, pigmented urine and vomiting. Renal function was only mildly impaired, and she recovered within 2 weeks. She subsequently learned to modify her physical activity and only one further experience of pigmented urine has been noted, after a prolonged hike. She also learned that when walking for prolonged distances, her endurance was improved by a warm-up period.

Her older brother is more severely affected with the same symptoms, and her mother had similar symptoms.

Physical examination was normal except for mild pelvic-girdle weakness. The serum CK level was twice the normal value. The EMG was abnormal, with occasional fibrillations and trains of positive sharp waves. Motor unit potentials were substantially reduced in duration and amplitude, with early recruitment. On the forearm exercise test, serum lactate did not rise. NMR spectroscopy study of the anterior tibial muscle demonstrated that exercise produced a slight rise in intracellular pH from 7.0 to 7.1 (whereas pH normally falls to 6.7 or less); there was no excessive fall in phosphocreatine (see Fig. 7–4). Repetitive nerve stimulation (20 Hz, 50 seconds) of the first dorsal interosseous muscle disclosed a 28% decrement in muscle action potential amplitude (normal <20%) (Fig. 7–5, shown as "McArdle's 1"). A muscle biopsy of the vastus lateralis disclosed occasional degenerating fibers undergoing phagocytosis, as well as excessive accumulation of periodic acid–Schiff (PAS)-positive material in the subsarcolemmal region. Myophosphorylase was absent by histochemical analysis (Fig. 7–6). Biochemical studies of muscle disclosed no measurable phosphorylase activity and an increased glycogen concentration.

Comment: In this patient, the appearance of symptoms following brief episodes of intense exercise is typical of McArdle's disease. The results of laboratory studies, including the elevated CK level, and the EMG evidence of fibrillations and small early recruited motor units in a patient with long-standing symptoms, are also characteristic.

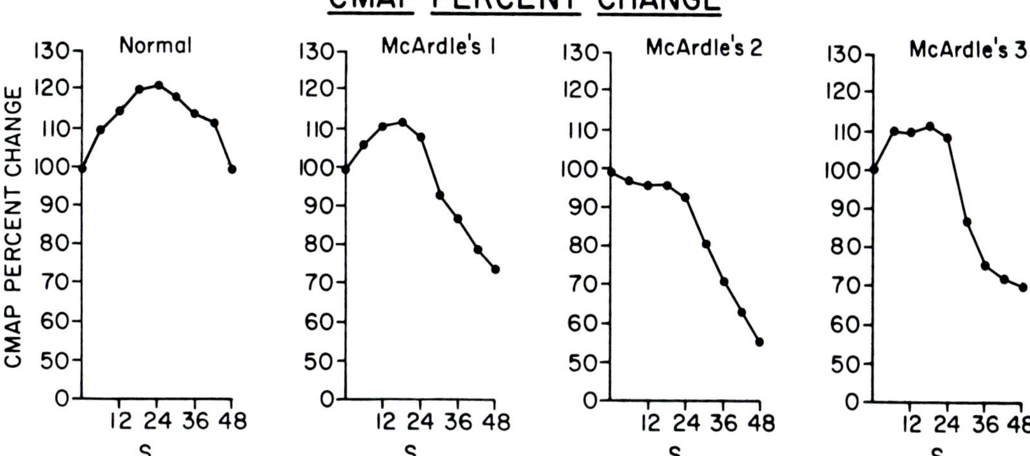

Figure 7–5. Repetitive nerve stimulation (20 Hz, 50 seconds) of the first interosseous muscle decreases the compound muscle action potential (CMAP) amplitudes by 25 to 50% in patients with McArdle's disease but less than 20% in controls.

The family history is most consistent with an autosomal dominant inheritance pattern. McArdle's disease is autosomal dominant in a small proportion of patients; most cases are autosomal recessive (see below).

Clinical Features. Exercise intolerance with myalgia, easy fatigability, and stiffness in exercising muscles are the cardinal manifestations of McArdle's disease (myophosphorylase defi-

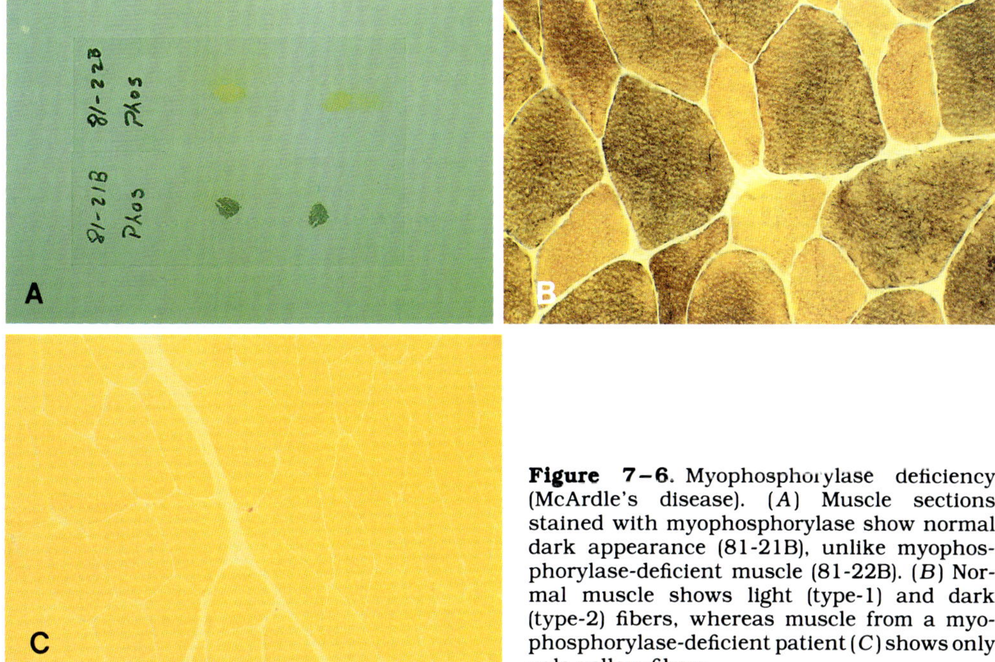

Figure 7–6. Myophosphorylase deficiency (McArdle's disease). (*A*) Muscle sections stained with myophosphorylase show normal dark appearance (81-21B), unlike myophosphorylase-deficient muscle (81-22B). (*B*) Normal muscle shows light (type-1) and dark (type-2) fibers, whereas muscle from a myophosphorylase-deficient patient (*C*) shows only pale yellow fibers.

ciency). Patients with this condition have variable exercise tolerance. Symptoms are often precipitated by brief bursts of high-intensity exercise such as carrying heavy objects, squatting for sustained periods, or sprinting, although sustained low-intensity exercise such as jogging, swimming, or tennis can also produce them. Almost all patients give a history of exercise intolerance, usually since adolescence, and most report episodes of dark-colored urine and cramping of the muscles following vigorous exercise (Table 7–3). Most patients learn to modify their exercise activity and avoid further attacks. Myalgia and muscle stiffness usually precede the intensely painful muscle contracture (defined in Chapter 2) and myoglobinuria, and patients learn to recognize these warning signs. Approximately 25% of patients experience an episode of renal failure complicating myoglobinuria.[50] Fixed proximal weakness develops in nearly one third of patients and tends to become more conspicuous as patients get older. The "second wind" phenomenon, in which exercise tolerance improves following a brief rest after the initial appearance of myalgia and muscle stiffness, is common in McArdle's disease.[20]

Although most patients with McArdle's disease conform to the above description, at least four other clinical syndromes deserve mention:

1. Some patients have no definite history of cramps or myoglobinuria but simply report slight fatigability. This lack of typical dynamic symptoms may add considerable difficulty to establishing a diagnosis.[50]

2. Some patients with no clear history of myoglobinuria or cramps have gradually progressive weakness which usually becomes obvious by the sixth or seventh decade.[61]

3. A few patients have been described with a mild congenital weakness.[39]

4. Rare cases have developed rapidly progressive weakness shortly after birth, with respiratory failure and death before the age of 4 months.[53]

This dramatic clinical heterogeneity is independent of the severity of the enzyme defect or the amount of glycogen accumulation in muscle.[157] Most patients have no detectable myophosphorylase, but the presence or absence of enzyme is not clearly correlated with the clinical presentation or with the concentration of muscle glycogen.

Laboratory Findings. The serum CK level is elevated in the absence of symptoms in more than 90% of patients and is a useful indicator of an underlying muscle disease. As discussed earlier, p. 252, in this syndrome fatiguing exercise of the forearm produces no significant rise in venous lactate concentration; however, this test requires standardization and care to avoid false positives and false negatives. It is now clear that the forearm *ischemic* exercise test may be hazardous, producing a compartment syndrome with ulnar nerve damage or myoglobinuria and a risk of renal failure in some patients.[117]

Cardiac and pulmonary function may be assessed in specialized laboratories using a motorized treadmill or cycle ergometry with analysis of expired ventilation.[58] With increasing exercise, the heart rate, systolic blood pressure, and oxygen consumption all steadily rise to a plateau at peak exertion. In normal subjects, aerobic metabolism is suffi-

---

Table 7–3 MYOPHOSPHORYLASE DEFICIENCY

CLINICAL FEATURES
Exercise intolerance
Myoglobinuria
Muscle weakness in 30% of cases

LABORATORY FINDINGS
CK level elevated
Forearm exercise test — no lactate rise
Decremental response (>20%) to repetitive
　nerve stimulation (20 Hz, 50 s)
Absent or reduced myophophorylase in muscle

GENETICS
Autosomal recessive (in rare cases, autosomal
　dominant) — chromosome 11
Male predominance

TREATMENT
None

cient to meet energy needs initially. With more demanding exercise, glycolysis begins and serum lactate rises. Ventilation rates begin to rise more steeply, in response to increased carbon dioxide production, and muscle glycogen and blood glucose become the main source of fuel. Blood lactate and the respiratory exchange ratio (CO_2 production/O_2 consumption) can be used to monitor anaerobic metabolism. Patients with defects of glycolysis (especially myophosphorylase and PFK deficiency) have the greatest difficulty during short bursts of intense exercise. They show an exaggerated cardiovascular response, with a premature increase in cardiac output, which is up to 300% greater than that seen in normal subjects for a given rise in oxygen uptake.[179]

Electrodiagnostic Studies. The EMG may be abnormal at rest, with fibrillations and positive waves. Motor unit potential duration is usually shortened and polyphasic wave activity increased, with early recruitment, especially as the disease becomes more advanced.[135] The exercise-induced painful contractures are electrically silent, unlike cramps. As shown on Figure 7-5, repetitive nerve stimulation produces a marked decremental response. The high-frequency (20 Hz) repetitive stimulation used for these patients is more uncomfortable than the low-frequency stimulation used to evaluate myasthenia gravis, and it requires complete immobilization of the hand with an armboard. Nonetheless, the test is usually well tolerated and is a safe method of supporting the diagnosis.[21] The ulnar nerve is stimulated at the wrist, with recording from the abductor digiti minimi; no ischemia is necessary. Although a slight contracture may be triggered, there have been no serious ill effects.

Muscle Biopsy. The muscle biopsy is usually abnormal, with subsarcolemmal vacuoles that are PAS-positive. Both degenerating and regenerating fibers are present, and the variability of fiber size is increased (see Fig. 7-6).

The histochemical reaction for phosphorylase is absent in muscle fibers, but this absence is not invariably diagnostic of McArdle's disease. A marked reduction of phosphorylase reactivity may be seen in any muscle biopsy depleted of glycogen. This "phosphorylase deficiency" may occur in severe malnutrition, in severely denervated muscles, with ischemia of muscle, or in biopsy specimens held for several hours before freezing (e.g., in those transported to regional laboratories). The apparent absence of phosphorylase activity is an artifact of staining, as the histochemical reaction requires preformed glycogen in the tissue for demonstration.[62] Biochemical assay of phosphorylase usually discloses markedly reduced activity in patients with McArdle's disease; as much as 10% of normal activity may be found in some patients.

Genetics. At least 50% of patients have a positive family history.[50] Most have autosomal recessive inheritance, but some families with autosomal dominant transmission have been described.[33] A gene that encodes muscle phosphorylase has been localized to the long arm of chromosome 11.[101] The gene was recently sequenced and DNA analysis from patient's leukocytes can now be used for diagnosis.[172] For unexplained reasons, the condition more commonly affects men. Preliminary results of muscle messenger RNA (mRNA) analysis indicate substantial heterogeneity of the gene defect in McArdle's disease. Some patients have normal mRNA and others have none, with no clear correlation between clinical severity and mRNA content.[157] In patients who have normal mRNA but no phosphorylase protein, either a point mutation or a small deletion may prevent mRNA translation or may produce an unstable, readily degraded protein. It has been proposed that patients with no mRNA may have either a gene deletion or a regulatory mutation, but no deletions have yet been identified. At least five different mutations have been postulated to account for variations observed in mRNA levels.[157]

Pathophysiology of Fatigue. The physiologic basis of excessive fatigability and contracture in patients with McArdle's disease remains unclear. Myophosphorylase catalyzes the cleavage of the 1-4 glycoside linkage of glycogen, the last step in glycogen breakdown prior to entering the glycolytic chain (see Fig. 7 – 2). In normal muscle, periods of brief, high-intensity exercise require that intramuscular high-energy phosphates be replenished through glycolysis. Recent studies of normal human muscle have demonstrated that the accumulation of ATP hydrolysis products, including both total inorganic phosphate[29,37] and the monovalent form of inorganic phosphate, $H_2PO_4^-$, may be linked to decreased muscle force.[19,42,118,125] Clearly, impaired glycogenolysis in patients with phosphorylase deficiency is important in limiting exercise tolerance. NMR spectroscopy studies following exercise-induced fatigue, however, have shown neither a buildup of hydrogen ions nor excessive changes in the concentration of ATP, inorganic phosphate, diprotonated phosphate, or phosphocreatine.[8,29,144] The accumulation of ADP, however, may be increased in patients with McArdle's disease; this might limit oxidative phosphorylation and reduce energy availability during exercise.[16] Other studies have demonstrated an abnormally large decrement on repetitive nerve stimulation, suggesting that the fatigue in such patients may result at least in part from impaired muscle activation rather than from energy deficiency per se within the muscle. Increased extracellular potassium has also been documented in these patients[131]; this could cause the reduced membrane excitability that accompanied excessive fatigue in many (but not all) circumstances.[38,103] Finally, although exercise increases water accumulation in the extracellular space in normal muscle, magnetic resonance imaging (MRI) studies revealed an absence of water buildup in McArdle's patients.[65] This finding could be due to either reduced activation or absent lactate accumulation. Thus, identification of the precise mechanisms of fatigue in McArdle's disease still requires further study.

The second-wind phenomenon, common to both normal subjects and to myophosphorylase-deficient patients during vigorous athletic activity, follows only brief exercise in McArdle's disease. After an initial period of adjustment due to their inability to use muscle glycogen, a transition toward using blood-borne glucose and free fatty acids for muscle fuel allows the myophosphorylase-deficient patient to experience a second wind. The excessive cardiovascular response to exercise in these patients appears to be centrally mediated,[179] and produces an early and excessive intramuscular blood flow that permits increased delivery of blood-borne glucose and free fatty acids. Uptake of free fatty acid increases during the first 5 to 15 minutes of exercise.[20,102] Infusing free fatty acids, both during this adaptation period and during sustained exercise, improves exercise tolerance in patients with McArdle's disease, suggesting that fat may be the major substrate during the second-wind period. Similarly, infusion of glucose can induce a second wind, suggesting that increased uptake of glucose also plays a role.[78]

Treatment. Some patients with myophosphorylase deficiency benefit from a graduated exercise program with emphasis on aerobic activity. Training, dietary modification, or intermittent rest could be important factors in modifying the second-wind phenomenon and may have potential treatment applications. Therapeutic attempts to raise blood glucose or increase peripheral use of glucose have had no demonstrable effect, however, and dietary manipulation has not proved beneficial.[87,98]

PHOSPHOFRUCTOKINASE DEFICIENCY

Clinical Features. Phosphofructokinase (PFK) deficiency (Tarui's dis-

Table 7–4 PHOSPHOFRUCTOKINASE (PFK) DEFICIENCY

CLINICAL FEATURES
Exercise intolerance
Myoglobinuria
Mild hemolytic anemia
Normal muscle strength

LABORATORY FINDINGS
Hemolytic anemia
CK level elevated
Forearm exercise test — no lactate rise
Decremental response to repetitive nerve
   stimulation
Absent PFK in muscle

GENETICS
Autosomal recessive trait — chromosome 1
Male predominance in Ashkenazi Jews

TREATMENT
None

---

ease) is far less common than McArdle's disease; fewer than 30 cases have been reported.[147] The clinical manifestations closely resemble those of myophosphorylase deficiency (Table 7–4). Impaired exercise tolerance with muscle pain or contracture and myoglobinuria are the usual symptoms. Unlike McArdle's disease, however, progressive weakness does not appear later in life. The partial PFK deficiency in red blood cells leads to episodes of hemolysis and jaundice, which help to distinguish PFK deficiency from other disorders of glycogen metabolism. The mechanism underlying the hemolysis remains uncertain. Anemia is slight or absent despite a diminished erythrocyte survival time.[147] A fatal infantile form with generalized weakness and cardiomyopathy has also been described.[2]

Laboratory Findings. Serum CK levels may be elevated, and a slight anemia with an increased percentage of reticulocytes is common. As in McArdle's disease, venous lactate concentration does not rise during forearm exercise. EMG and repetitive nerve stimulation studies are also similar to those in myophosphorylase deficiency, showing early recruitment of small motor units and abnormal decremental responses

to 20-Hz stimulation for 50 seconds. The muscle biopsy shows subsarcolemmal, PAS-positive vacuoles. A histochemical reaction demonstrates a lack of PFK; biochemical analysis of muscle tissue is usually necessary to confirm the diagnosis.

Genetics and Pathophysiology. PFK deficiency is an autosomal recessive disorder but has an unexplained male predominance (9:1) and an overrepresentation in Ashkenazi Jews.

PFK catalyzes the phosphorylation of fructose-6-phosphate to fructose 1,6-diphosphate. Because this reaction is essential and rate-limiting for the metabolism of glucose, the absence of PFK prevents ATP formation from glycogen or glucose. In affected patients, PFK activity is completely absent in muscle, present at approximately 50% of normal levels in red cells, and normal in platelets and white blood cells. The M subunit, the muscle form of the enzyme, is normally present in both muscle and red blood cells. The M subunit defect accounts for the phenotype of muscle fatigue and hemolysis.[41] The abnormality of the M subunit of the PFK protein is localized to a defect on chromosome 1.[138,182]

As in McArdle's disease, the precise mechanism causing the premature fatigue in patients with PFK deficiency is still not entirely clear. Exercise studies, including data obtained by ^{31}P NMR, demonstrate a distinctive rise in phosphorylated sugars, a reduced decline in phosphocreatine, absence of lowered pH, and no excessive fall in ATP.[7,55] These findings do not explain the excessive fatigue, but recent evidence suggests that the accumulation of ADP may be a critical factor in muscular fatigue.[139] Thus the buildup of muscle ADP, which would ordinarily be phosphorylated via glycolysis or oxidative phosphorylation, may play a major role in the development of excessive fatigue in patients with PFK deficiency.[16] Creatine kinase and the adenylate-kinase–AMP-deaminase reactions have limited capacity to remove ADP. The combined data from patients with PFK deficiency and McArdle's disease suggest that ADP accumulation may be the common denominator accounting for premature fatigability. ADP accumulation may well inhibit either sodium-potassium or calcium ATPase, thus interfering with activation of muscle fibers,[38] as well as decreasing force generation by inhibiting myosin ATPase. Impaired activation of muscle fibers would explain the similar decline in force production and compound muscle action potential amplitude during repetitive nerve stimulation in patients with PFK and phosphorylase deficiency.[38]

Treatment. Physical conditioning may improve exercise tolerance and increase the capacity for muscle oxygen extraction and the oxidation of free fatty acids. Thus, in PFK deficiency, as in McArdle's disease, there may be substantial improvement through training, but in contrast to McArdle's disease, the second-wind phenomenon does not occur.[80] Evidence suggests that glucose infusion actually impairs exercise tolerance,[80] probably because the concentrations of free fatty acids in the plasma are lowered by glucose-induced inhibition of lipolysis.[80] The anemia of PFK deficiency is mild and is only of consequence when red cell production is impaired by coincidental disease. No treatment is available for the anemia.

UNCOMMON DEFECTS OF GLYCOLYSIS

Other defects of glycolysis are uncommon. They include deficiency of phosphoglycerate kinase, phosphoglycerate mutase, lactate dehydrogenase, and phosphorylase *b* kinase. Each of these conditions can cause dynamic symptoms such as pain and recurrent myoglobinuria; the first three involve the second stage of glycolysis, distal to the PFK reaction.

Phosphoglycerate Kinase Deficiency. *Clinical Features.* Most patients with phosphoglycerate kinase (PGK) deficiency do not have symptoms

Table 7–5 PHOSPHOGLYCERATE KINASE (PGK) DEFICIENCY

CLINICAL FEATURES
Two presentations
1. Seizures, mental retardation
2. Exercise intolerance and myoglobinuria with slowly progressive weakness

LABORATORY FINDINGS
Hemolytic anemia
CK level elevated
Forearm ischemic test — no rise in lactate level
Electromyography usually normal
Absent or reduced PGK in muscle

GENETICS
X-linked recessive trait

TREATMENT
None

of muscle disease but instead have a central nervous system disorder including seizures and mental retardation in childhood, as well as a severe hemolytic anemia (Table 7–5). However, three patients with a purely myopathic syndrome and recurrent myoglobinuria have been reported.[51,52,142,170] Myalgia and pigmented urine after brief, intense exercise occurred in adolescence, followed by slowly progressive proximal weakness. One patient had retinitis pigmentosa.[170]

Laboratory Findings. Most patients show evidence of hemolysis, including reticulocytosis, anemia, raised serum bilirubin, and reduced serum haptoglobin. The serum CK level is elevated to two to three times normal. Forearm exercise produced no significant rise in venous lactate concentration in two patients.[142,170] EMG is usually normal.

The muscle histology appears normal unless there has been recent rhabdomyolysis. In this circumstance, the biopsy shows muscle fiber degeneration. Electron microscopy usually demonstrates only slight glycogen accumulation. The diagnosis is made by biochemical analysis of PGK activity, either in red blood cells or in muscle.[51] Some patients show evidence of decreased enzyme activity, but in others the enzyme is normal except for abnormal electrophoretic mobility.[170]

Genetics. Phosphoglycerate kinase deficiency has been localized to the short arm of the X chromosome.[170] It is transmitted as an X-linked recessive trait, and decreased enzyme activity has been found in the muscle of mothers and sisters of affected patients. Evidence suggests genetic heterogeneity in this disorder.[69,170]

Therapy. Some patients with hemolytic anemia have benefited from splenectomy. No other therapy is available at this time.

Phosphoglycerate Mutase Deficiency. *Clinical Features.* Patients have dynamic muscle symptoms, including exercise intolerance, beginning in childhood or adolescence (Table 7–6). Muscle cramping and pain follow intense exercise and are often accompanied by myoglobin in the urine.[5,95,173] Patients do not develop proximal weakness.

Laboratory Findings. The serum CK level is usually elevated up to three times normal even when patients are symptom-free. The forearm exercise test produces a subnormal rise in venous lactate level, not reaching the fourfold rise seen in normal subjects (see Fig. 7–3).[95] In contrast, patients with myophosphorylase, PFK, and PGK

Table 7–6 PHOSPHOGLYCERATE MUTASE (PGAM) DEFICIENCY

CLINICAL FEATURES
   Exercise intolerance
   Myoglobinuria
   Muscle strength normal

LABORATORY FINDINGS
   CK level elevated
   Forearm exercise test — reduced (not absent) lactate rise
   Electromyography usually normal
   PGAM reduced in muscle

GENETICS
   Autosomal recessive trait
   Predominantly African-Americans

TREATMENT
   None

deficiencies produce a flat lactate curve. Intracellular pH, measured by NMR spectroscopy, falls to intermediate levels (6.85) during ischemic exercise (compared to 6.6 or less in controls), an observation that documents the partial nature of the glycolytic block.[5] EMG and nerve conduction studies are usually normal.

Muscle biopsies contain increased glycogen, as demonstrated by PAS staining in the subsarcolemmal region. Tubular aggregates in type 2 B fibers have also been seen.[95] Surprisingly, glycogen concentrations in muscle tissue are normal,[95] but phosphoglycerate mutase activity is markedly reduced (less than 10% of normal).

Genetics and Pathogenesis. Phosphogylcerate mutase (PGAM) is a dimeric enzyme that catalyzes the conversion of 3-phosphoglycerate to 2-phosphoglycerate. In normal muscle, PGAM consists predominantly of the slow-migrating muscle (MM) type on starch-gel electrophoresis, with only low concentrations of the brain (BB) and intermediate (MB) forms. The BB band has been preserved in patients with PGAM deficiency, a finding which suggests that the genetic defect primarily involves the M subunit. All but one of the patients described thus far have been African-American.[173] Molecular genetic analysis has confirmed the autosomal recessive pattern of inheritance.[171]

Lactate Dehydrogenase Deficiency. *Clinical Features.* In the first well-documented case of this disorder, the patient developed symptoms at age 16.[90] Both this patient and another recently described[26] had excessive fatigue and exercise intolerance, myalgia, and myoglobinuria (Table 7–7). Both patients also had a generalized, scaling, erythematous rash.

Laboratory Findings. The serum CK level after an episode of myoglobinuria may be elevated to more than 100 times normal, while the serum lactate dehydrogenase (LDH) is normal. The differential increases in these two en-

Table 7–7 LACTATE DEHYDRO-GENASE (LDH) DEFICIENCY

CLINICAL FEATURES
  Excessive fatigue and exercise intolerance,
    especially for maximal exercise
  Myoglobinuria
  Normal muscle strength

LABORATORY FINDINGS
  CK level elevated (*with normal serum LDH*)
  Forearm exercise test — no lactate rise;
    normal pyruvate rise
  Absent or reduced LDH in muscle and red
    blood cells

GENETICS
  Autosomal recessive trait — chromosome 11

TREATMENT
  None

zymes, whose activities normally rise together, is helpful in suggesting a defect in the LDH enzyme. A forearm exercise test produces a minimal elevation in the lactate level, but the serum pyruvate level rises substantially, indicating that the glycolytic defect lies just beyond pyruvate on the metabolic pathway, and involves conversion to lactate. Thus, maximal exercise, which depends on anaerobic glycolysis, is most impaired in these patients. The diagnosis is confirmed by electrophoretic studies of erythrocytes, serum, and muscle tissue, where activity of the skeletal muscle isoform of LDH (LDH-M) is substantially reduced (less than 5% of normal).[119b] DNA analysis of blood is now possible as well.[106a,107]

Genetics. There are five isoforms of LDH. The skeletal muscle isoform (LDH-M) has been localized to chromosome 11. This isoform is absent in LDH deficiency, accounting for the exercise intolerance. The defect is inherited as an autosomal recessive trait.[18] A deficiency of the cardiac isoform (LDH-H) has also been described, but has no associated skeletal muscle symptoms; coding for LDH-H is localized to chromosome 12.[115]

Phosphorylase *b* Kinase Deficiency.
Clinical Features. Nine children and 13 adults have been described with phosphorylase *b* kinase (PBK) deficiency.[1,34,164,176,183a] The clinical picture is heterogeneous (Table 7–8). Children have weakness and liver enlargement. Adult patients have exercise-induced cramps and myoglobinuria; three patients had progressive weakness. Progressive distal or proximal weakness has been noted without associated dynamic symptoms.[183a]

Laboratory Findings. The serum CK level is usually elevated more than twofold, and lactate production with forearm exercise may be impaired, although it was normal in one patient.[34] PBK is important in initiating glycogenolysis by converting the inactive form of myophosphorylase (type b) to the active form (type a).[34] PBK also down-regulates glycogen synthesis by converting the active form of glycogen synthetase (type a) to the inactive form (type b). Muscle biopsy shows slight accumulation of glycogen; necrotic muscle fibers are found in the patient with progressive distal weakness. Muscle PBK activity is usually less than 12% of normal. In adults with only muscle manifestations, PBK activity is found to be normal in red blood cells and liver. In two adult patients, the analysis of Western blots with an anti-PBK antibody revealed a selective deficiency of the beta subunit of PBK.[34]

Table 7–8 PHOSPHORYLASE *b* KINASE (PBK) DEFICIENCY

CLINICAL FEATURES (VARIABLE)
  Exercise intolerance and myoglobinuria
  Distal muscle weakness
  Muscle weakness and liver enlargement in
    children

LABORATORY FINDINGS
  CK level elevated
  Forearm exercise test normal
  Repetitive nerve stimulation normal
  PBK reduced to <12% in muscle

GENETICS
  Inheritance pattern autosomal recessive
    — chromosome 16

  None

Genetics. The inheritance pattern of muscle PBK deficiency appears to be autosomal recessive.[183a] The condition appears to result from a selective defect in the beta-gamma subunits of PBK[183a] the beta subunit has recently been mapped to chromosome 16.[67] In contrast, PBK deficiency of liver is X-linked,[40] while the childhood disorder involving the liver, muscle, red blood cells, and leukocytes is inherited as an autosomal recessive trait.[34,67]

Disorders Producing Static Symptoms (Fixed Weakness)

In contrast to the foregoing disorders, which are characterized by *dynamic* symptoms of exercise intolerance, the following diseases produce the *static* symptom of progressive muscular weakness. These conditions include deficiencies of acid maltase, debranching enzyme, and branching enzyme.

ACID MALTASE DEFICIENCY

Case History

A 28-year-old woman described a 12-year history of progressive proximal weakness. Her early development was normal, but she was never able to climb a rope or perform chin-ups. At age 15, she was able to do 15 sit-ups and climb steps without difficulty. By age 18 she required a railing to climb stairs. By age 26 she had difficulty lifting objects, and falling became frequent. She had no dysphagia, dyspnea, cramps, or dark urine. Her sister had a similar condition.

On examination, the weakest muscles were the hip flexors and extensors (MRC grade 2) and other pelvic-girdle muscles (grade 3). Shoulder-girdle muscles were grade 4. She was unable to perform a sit-up and could not rise from the floor without assistance. She had a waddling gait and an exaggerated lumbar lordosis, and she could not walk on her heels. Muscle stretch reflexes were absent at the knees but normal elsewhere. The results of cardiac examination were normal, and the liver was not enlarged. The forced vital capacity was 2.4 L (63% predicted).

The serum CK level was three times normal. The EMG showed trains of myotonic discharges, fibrillations, and positive waves (Fig. 7–7) in the lumbosacral paraspinal muscles. In the vastus lateralis, no abnormal spontaneous activity was observed, but motor unit potentials were reduced in duration (mean 9.9 milliseconds, normal > 10.6 milliseconds). The recruitment was abnormal and early, with 25% polyphasia. Forearm exercise produced a 13-fold increase in serum lactate concentration. Alpha glucosidase (acid maltase) levels in leukocytes were markedly depressed (0.8 nmol/h per mg protein compared to a normal value of > 25 nmol/h).

Muscle biopsy of the vastus lateralis disclosed extensive vacuolar change in 50% of fibers; vacuoles contained PAS-positive material. Many also showed prominent acid phosphatase-positive granular material indicative of lysosomal activity (Fig. 7–8). Electron microscopy demonstrated vacuoles containing free and membrane-bound glycogen and autophagic material (Fig. 7–9). A high-protein diet was rigorously followed for 1 year with no improvement in manual muscle testing or forced vital capacity.

Comment: As this patient's history illus-

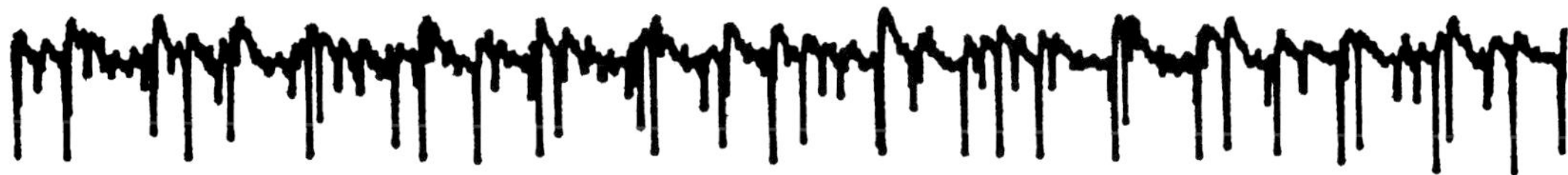

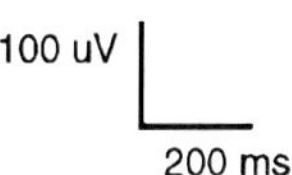

Figure 7–7. Trains of positive waves in the lumbosacral paraspinal muscles of a 26-year-old woman with acid maltase deficiency.

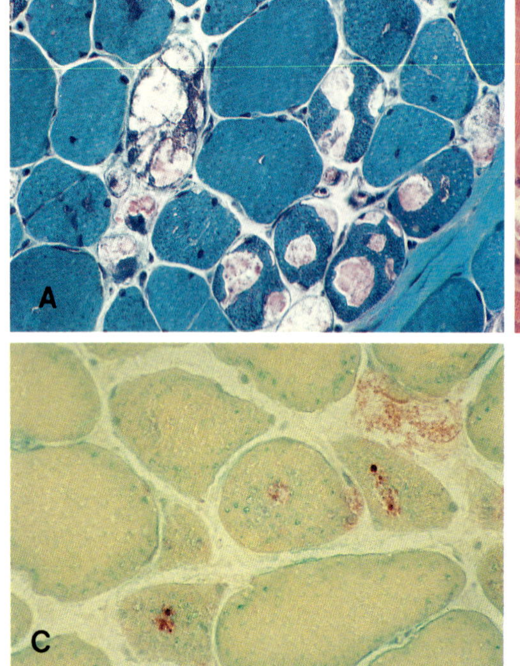
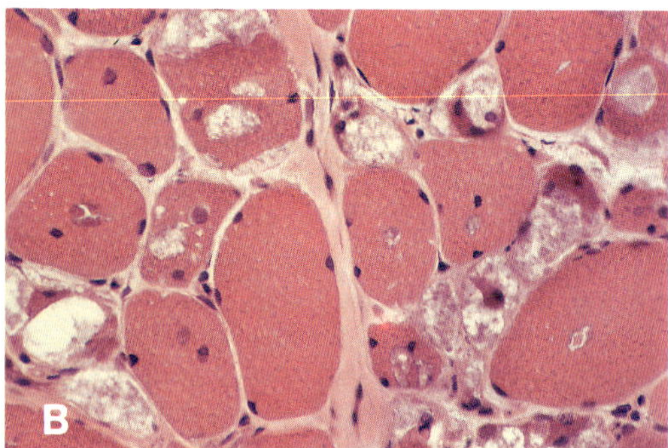

Figure 7–8. Acid maltase deficiency. Muscle fibers in (*A*) modified trichrome stain and (*B*) H&E stain show marked variability in fiber size and many vacuolated muscle fibers. Some vacuoles contain amorphous material. (*C*) Acid-phosphatase–positive granular material (red granules) can be seen within the muscle fibers.

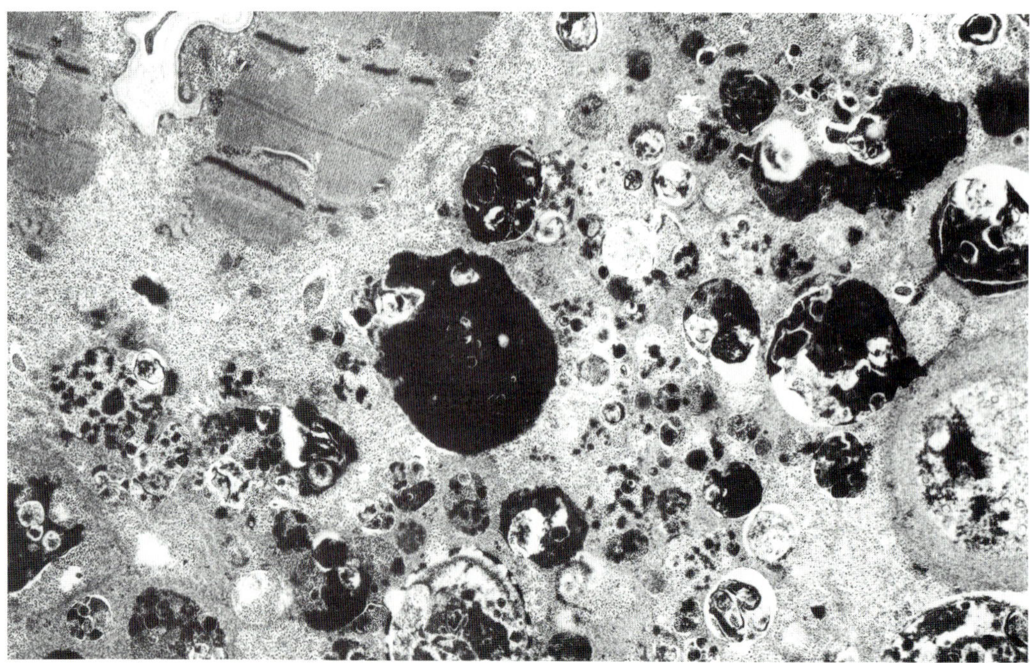

Figure 7–9. Acid maltase deficiency. Electron micrograph of muscle fibers shows autophagic vacuoles containing degradative material and glycogen.

trates, acid maltase deficiency (AMD) may begin in the second or third decade with slowly progressive proximal weakness. Excessive fatigue and myoglobinuria are generally not present. Respiratory failure is noted at onset in approximately one third of adult cases, and the diaphragm appears to be selectively involved.[119c] Some patients develop pulmonary hypertension, but heart and liver involvement are otherwise absent. Dietary treatment has not proven successful, as will be discussed below.

Clinical Features. Acid maltase (also termed alpha glucosidase) deficiency is a glycogen storage disease that causes progressive proximal weakness. It can present at any age, and has three major forms (Table 7–9):

Infantile. Infantile AMD, the most common form, produces a floppy-infant syndrome with onset of symptoms in the first 3 months of life. It is characterized by progressive weakness and enlargement of the heart, tongue, and liver, as well as respiratory insufficiency and feeding difficulty.[59] Death from cardiorespiratory failure usually occurs before age 2.

Childhood. This is the least common of the three forms. Weakness begins in infancy or early childhood and is accompanied by delayed motor milestones and progressive proximal weak-

ness with involvement of respiratory muscles.[113] Unlike the infantile-onset cases, these patients usually have few if any clinical signs that the heart, liver, or nervous system are involved.

Adult. This disorder presents in adolescence or early adulthood with progressive proximal weakness. Diaphragmatic involvement is frequent and may be the earliest manifestation of the disease.[143] The clinical picture is not specific, so that adult AMD often resembles limb-girdle muscular dystrophy, but a scapuloperoneal form has also been described.[13a]

Laboratory Findings. The serum CK level is usually moderately elevated (2–10 times normal). The EMG examination is especially helpful in AMD, because in addition to the usual changes of motor unit potentials seen in myopathy, there are abundant myotonic discharges, trains of fibrillations and positive waves, and complex repetitive discharges (see Fig. 7–7). The abnormal spontaneous activity is particularly prominent in the lumbosacral paraspinal muscles. Lactic acid production is normal (more than a fourfold elevation) on forearm exercise testing. The electrocardiogram (ECG) often shows left ventricular hypertrophy in infantile

Table 7–9 ACID MALTASE DEFICIENCY

CLINICAL FEATURES

Infancy:	floppy infant with generalized weakness; cardiac and liver involvement; early death
Childhood:	progressive proximal weakness; respiratory muscle insufficiency; occasional cardiac abnormalities
Adult:	progressive proximal weakness; respiratory muscle insufficiency; no heart or liver abnormalities

LABORATORY FINDINGS
CK level elevated
Forearm ischemic test — normal
EMG — myotonic and complex repetitive discharges
Muscle biopsy — vacuolar myopathy with glycogen storage and autophagic features
Acid maltase reduced in muscle to <10% of normal
Enzyme deficiency demonstrable in white blood cells and urine

GENETICS
Autosomal recessive trait — multiple mutations chromosome 17

TREATMENT
None (bone marrow transplant under investigation)

patients, whereas in adults the ECG is usually normal until respiratory failure occurs. Because respiratory failure results in pulmonary hypertension, the ECG shows peaked P waves and other signs of cor pulmonale. The P-R interval is often abnormally short in infantile AMD.[59]

The muscle biopsy is often distinctive, but care must be taken to avoid very weak muscles (less than MRC grade 4), which may be so fibrotic that the diagnosis is obscured. Abundant vacuoles are usually present, and a high glycogen content can be demonstrated within the vacuoles. Vacuoles contain both glycogen and lysosomes. These autophagic vacuoles accumulate material as a result of incomplete digestion. The glycogen accumulation can be membrane-bound or free within the sarcoplasm. A specific diagnosis depends on the demonstration of acid maltase deficiency in cultured fibroblasts or in lymphocytes, urine, or muscle. The enzyme assay of urine and of lymphocytes is rapid, noninvasive, and adequate for all three forms of the deficiency.[104]

Genetics. All forms of AMD are transmitted by an autosomal recessive pattern of inheritance. The gene has been localized to chromosome 17 (17q21–23).[109] There appear to be at least six different mutations, based on the heterogeneity of size and amount of mRNA, enzyme activity, and protein cross-reactivity to antibody.[110] The molecular basis of AMD is becoming clearer.[85] Prenatal diagnosis has been accomplished using chorionic villus biopsy in the 10th week of gestation,[76] using antibodies for human liver acid (alpha) glucosidase.

Pathophysiology. The enzyme is a lysosomal glucosidase, which releases glucose from glycogen, maltose, and oligosaccharides. The metabolic role of acid maltase is still not established. The mechanism of progressive muscular weakness is presumed to relate to the deposition of excessive glycogen, indiscriminate organelle digestion, or the ill effect of releasing lysosomal enzymes

when secondary lysosomes rupture. The use of glycogen and glucose for muscular fuel is normal in AMD, so there is no exercise intolerance or myoglobinuria. Enzyme activity is diminished in liver, heart, and brain, but abnormal glycogen storage in these organs is usually seen only in the infantile form.[59] It is not clear why glycogen storage is not usually found in organs other than muscle.[175]

The clinical diversity of the three forms of acid maltase deficiency remains incompletely understood. In general, early-onset patients have a more profound deficiency, suggesting a relationship to clinical course and severity, but other factors must also be important, since some adult patients have very low activity of acid maltase.[141]

Treatment. No satisfactory treatment exists. A high-protein diet has been advocated, but efficacy has not been documented.[120,130] Parenteral administration of exogenous, donor acid maltase enzyme has produced no therapeutic benefit.[47,165] The use of bone marrow transplantation to treat lysosomal storage disorders is currently under investigation.[177]

DEBRANCHING ENZYME DEFICIENCY

Debranching enzyme deficiency results in incomplete glycogen degradation within liver and skeletal muscle. Both debranching enzyme transferase activity and the debranching enzyme glucosidase are needed to release glucose from glycogen, and either or both may be deficient in this disorder.[35] In approximately 85% of patients, debranching enzyme is deficient in both liver and muscle, and a progressive myopathy and possibly cardiomyopathy develop in the third or fourth decade of life. In a few patients the deficiency occurs only in the liver and such patients appear to have no risk of myopathy or cardiomyopathy.[35]

Clinical Features. Patients with debranching enzyme deficiency may present in childhood or as adults; the presentations differ depending upon age of onset. Infants and young children usually present with hepatomegaly, failure to thrive, hypoglycemia, and abnormal liver enzymes. Weakness and hypotonia with delayed motor development are also common, and cardiomyopathy may occur.[145]

Adult patients present with gradually progressive proximal muscle weakness. Some patients have also had marked distal weakness and wasting,[35,154] and cardiomyopathy. They usually do not have cramping, myoglobinuria, or severe exercise intolerance, though they frequently report a history of diminished physical activity in childhood and a protuberant abdomen in infancy. These patients comprise approximately 25% of those with glycogen storage disease.[25]

Laboratory Findings. The serum CK level is usually elevated (2 to 20 times normal). Venous lactate does not rise during forearm exercise testing, but ammonia rises excessively.[35] The electrocardiogram often shows left ventric-

ular hypertrophy. On EMG, abundant spontaneous activity (fibrillations, complex repetitive discharges, and myotonic discharges) is often seen in proximal muscles. Weak muscles show early recruitment and brief, small, polyphasic motor unit potentials.[154] The results of nerve conduction studies are usually normal, but a mild neuropathy has been observed.[35] Muscle biopsy (Figs. 7–10 and 7–11) demonstrates excessive glycogen between and within the myofibrils, and beneath the sarcolemma.[123] Biochemical assay of muscle biopsy tissue, fibroblasts, or lymphoblasts, for the debranching enzyme is needed to establish the diagnosis.[25,35] Distinctive morphologic findings in the skin biopsy tissue of five patients were recently reported.[154] Large amounts of free glycogen in secretory cells of eccrine sweat glands and in smooth muscle fibers appear to occur only in this disorder and may also be helpful in diagnosis.

Genetics. The disorder is transmitted in an autosomal recessive pattern; the very large gene has been cloned and localized to chromosome 1.[185,186]

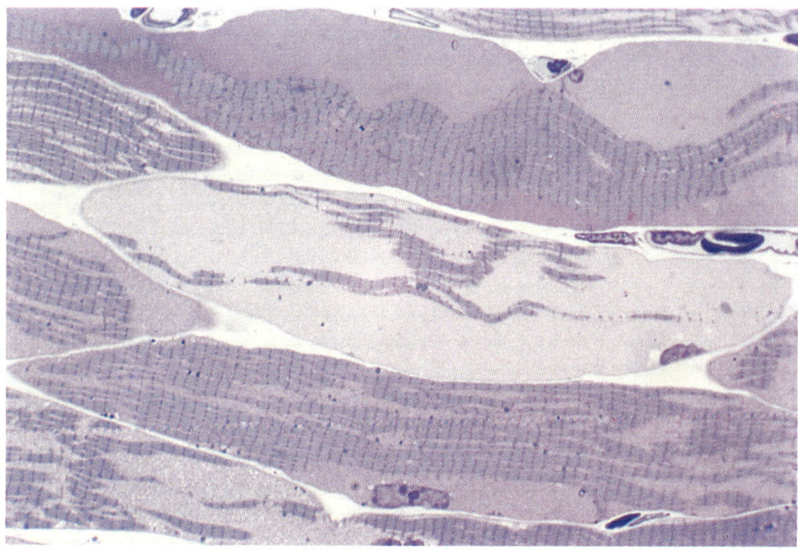

Figure 7–10. Debranching enzyme deficiency. Plastic sections (1 μ thick) show glycogen accumulation (pale blue regions) in subsarcolemmal and intermyofibrillar regions of muscle fibers. Toluidine blue.

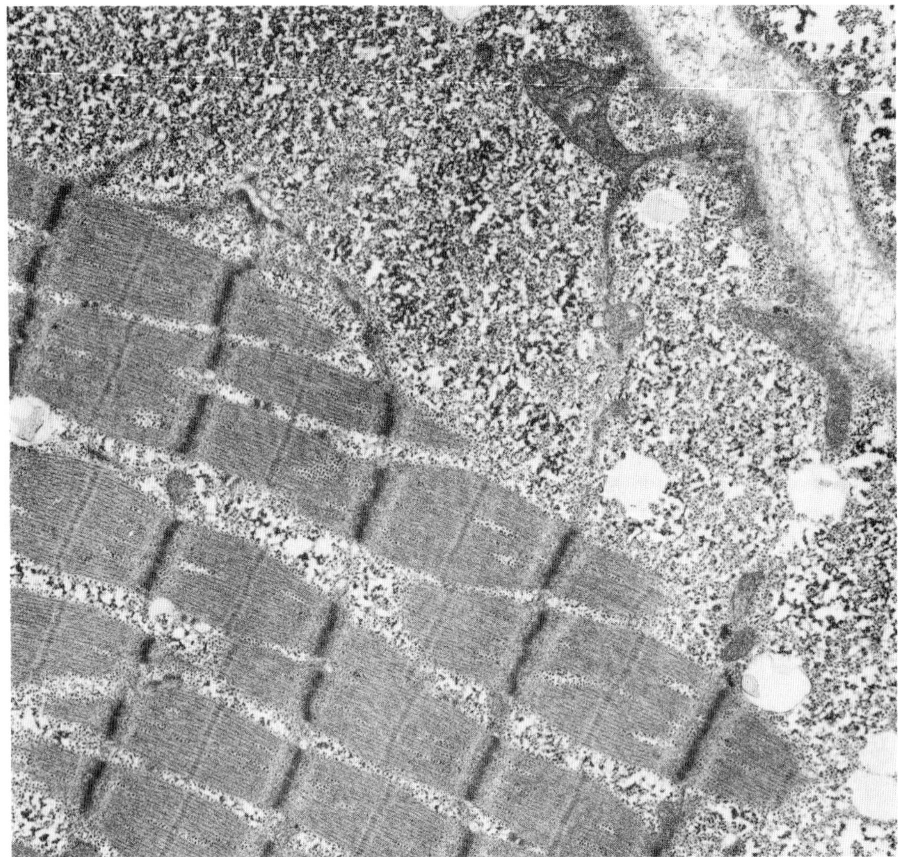

Figure 7–11. Debranching enzyme deficiency. Electron micrograph of muscle fiber shows intermyofibrillar and subsarcolemmal glycogen accumulation.

Treatment. Frequent small meals are necessary to avoid hypoglycemia, particularly during episodes of infection, because of the failure to degrade glycogen. Patients with cardiomyopathy may require treatment for congestive heart failure. No treatment improves muscle weakness.

BRANCHING ENZYME DEFICIENCY

Branching enzyme deficiency is a rare and uniformly fatal congenital disorder characterized by the accumulation of polysaccharide in liver, heart, skeletal muscle, and the central nervous system.[116]

Clinical Features. Patients usually present with failure to thrive and liver failure. Muscle weakness is usually not conspicuous. Death generally occurs in the second year of life, by which time all patients have hepatomegaly as well as weakness and hypotonia.

Laboratory Findings. The diagnosis may be established by demonstrating branching enzyme deficiency in skin fibroblasts.[116]

Genetics. This condition is transmitted by an autosomal recessive mode of inheritance, but the gene has not yet been identified.

Treatment. Liver transplantation has produced normal growth and development (after an average follow-up of 42 months).[156] Glycogen accumulation in both heart and skeletal muscle has also been reduced; the mechanism for these beneficial effects is unclear, but the discovery of cells containing the donor HLA phenotypes in the heart and skin suggests that migration of cells from the allograft may alleviate the enzyme deficiencies.[163]

DEFECTS OF LIPID METABOLISM

Carnitine Deficiency and Related Disorders

Carnitine deficiency is the most common form of lipid storage myopathy (Table 7–10). Insufficient free carnitine within the muscle cell prevents the transport of long-chain fatty acids into mitochondria, and interferes with the modulation of coenzyme A (see Fig. 7–1).[3] Thus, abnormal amounts of lipid accumulate, particularly in type 1 fibers, with less accumulation in type 2A fibers, and the least accumulation in type 2B fibers. Carnitine deficiency occurs as a *myopathic* form and a *systemic* form; a secondary form of carnitine deficiency may result from a heterogeneous group of conditions (Table 7–11).

Table 7–10 MYOPATHIC CARNITINE DEFICIENCY

CLINICAL FEATURES
   Myopathic form: progressive muscle
      weakness, childhood or young adults
   Systemic form: episodes resembling Reye's
      syndrome in children, progressive weakness

LABORATORY FINDINGS
   CK level elevated
   Forearm exercise test normal
   EMG myopathic
   Muscle biopsy: lipid storage and reduced carnitine
   Low levels of carnitine in blood, muscle, liver, kidneys (systemic form)

GENETICS
   Autosomal recessive trait

TREATMENT
   Low-fat diet (<20% of calories)
   L-Carnitine administration, 2 to 4 g/day
      (children 100 mg/kg per day)

Table 7–11 CAUSES OF SECONDARY CARNITINE DEFICIENCY

Renal failure
Organic aciduria
Mitochondrial disorders
Reye's syndrome
Liver failure
Muscular dystrophy
Endocrinopathies
Chronic myopathies
Valproate therapy
Total parenteral nutrition
Malnutrition
Pregnancy

CLINICAL FEATURES

Myopathic Form. In the myopathic form, the deficiency in carnitine usually is confined to muscle. Patients develop progressive, painless proximal muscle weakness in childhood or early adult life. An infantile form has also been described.[158] Exercise intolerance is uncommon. Rare patients have experienced myoglobinuria. Severe cardiomyopathy with congestive heart failure can occur. Most patients have wasting of proximal muscles, with diminished tendon reflexes and preserved sensory function. Three patients have worsened substantially during pregnancy.[60] The cause of this deterioration is uncertain, but may involve increased fetal demand for carnitine.

Systemic Form. Systemic carnitine deficiency usually presents in early childhood with progressive cardiomyopathy and attacks of hypoglycemia resembling Reye's syndrome.[162] During acute episodes, all patients have evidence of hepatic dysfunction and hepatomegaly. Proximal weakness may be prominent but often it is overshadowed by the cardiomyopathy or the acute episodes. Carnitine levels are reduced in muscle, liver, kidney, and heart, often because of a carnitine uptake defect that particularly affects cardiac and skeletal muscle.[162] The rate of uptake is also reduced in cultured skin fibroblasts.[168a] The serum carnitine level is usually reduced as well. Death may occur during the acute attacks, most often between the ages of 7 and 28.[60]

Secondary Form. A decrease in muscle carnitine levels occurs in a variety of other metabolic disorders during treatment with certain drugs,[32,60,155a] as well as in many other chronic myopathies (see Table 7–11). Carnitine deficiency syndromes should be considered as secondary until all other known causes of this deficiency have been excluded.[56] The clinical consequences of the moderate decreases in muscle carnitine levels seen in most of these disorders is unclear. Treatment strategies directed at the carnitine deficiency per se have a salutary effect only for glutaric aciduria.[141a]

LABORATORY FINDINGS

The serum CK level has been normal in 50% of reported cases of the myopathic form, but has been elevated up to 15 times in others. EMG studies show occasional fibrillations and positive waves with reduced motor unit potential duration and amplitude as well as increased polyphasic wave activity. The recruitment pattern is increased in weak muscles. Patients may develop a hypertrophic cardiomyopathy; left axis deviation with high voltage in precordial T waves may be present in the ECG.[14]

Muscle biopsy shows an excess of lipid droplets, which are demonstrated by oil red O staining (Fig. 7–12). The lipid droplets frequently distend the intermyofibrillar space (Fig. 7–13).[60] Atrophic and angular fibers may be present. The amount of lipid in normal muscle may vary considerably, however, making the biochemical assay for carnitine an absolute requirement to establish the diagnosis of carnitine-deficiency myopathy. Muscle carnitine levels can be reduced in other neuromuscular diseases, particularly in Duchenne dystrophy.[32] Patients with symptomatic carnitine deficiency usually have a reduction in muscle carnitine to below 25% of control levels, but

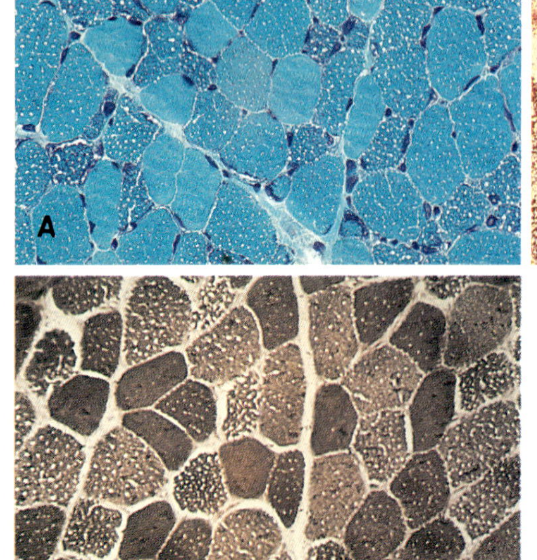

Figure 7–12. Carnitine deficiency. Sequential sections of muscle show the appearance of lipid accumulation in (A) (modified trichrome). (B) Oil red O. (C) ATPase pH 9.4. The lipid accumulates predominantly in type 1 muscle fibers.

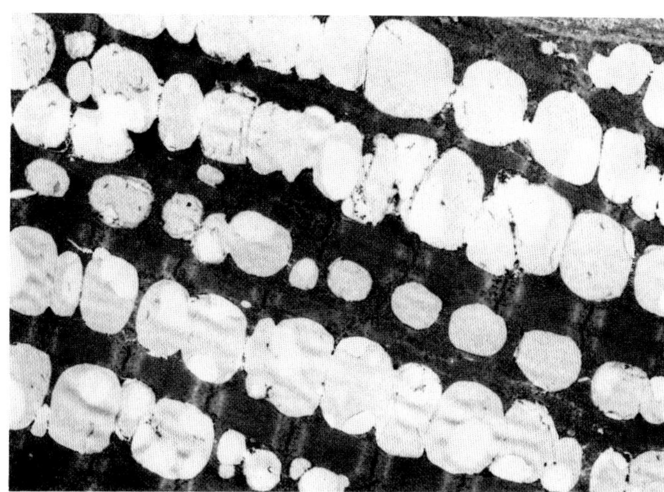

Figure 7–13. Carnitine deficiency. Electron micrograph shows rows of lipid accumulation.

the precise level that defines clinically significant carnitine deficiency is still not clear. Some recent evidence suggests that carnitine does not limit fatty-acid oxidation in muscle until it falls to below 5% of normal.[162] In other disorders of muscle, like the dystrophies, in which secondary carnitine deficiency occurs, excess lipid in muscle fibers is usually not observed.

GENETICS

Autosomal recessive inheritance is likely,[178] although most cases have been sporadic. A recent report described a family with autosomal dominant transmission of hypertrophic cardiomyopathy responsive to carnitine replacement; the condition was associated with asymptomatic muscle carnitine deficiency (muscle carnitine levels 0.9 to 1.4 μmol/g, compared to a normal value of > 3.0 μmol/g).[14]

PATHOPHYSIOLOGY

The cause of myopathic carnitine deficiency is still not entirely clear. Defective transport of carnitine into muscle was proposed,[140] and more recent studies have shown that the rate of carnitine entry into muscle in these patients is in fact reduced.[60] Some patients have excessive renal excretion, but this is

clearly not the primary cause of the disorder. The role of carnitine in the transport of long-chain fatty acids into mitochondria appears not to be critical, since these patients do not experience dynamic symptoms such as exercise intolerance.

TREATMENT

Systemic. Treatment of systemic carnitine deficiency consists of reduced dietary fat intake (less than 20% of daily caloric ingestion) and administration of divided doses of supplemental L-carnitine (available in health food stores or from Sigma-tau, Costa Mesa, CA), as shown in Table 7–10. This regimen has improved the organic acid profile in the urine, restored serum levels of free carnitine to normal in patients with the systemic disease, reduced hepatomegaly, and prevented hypoglycemic attacks.[49,108] Both cardiomyopathy and strength have improved in many, but not all, patients.[162] Patients should avoid fasting and take frequent meals of high carbohydrate content. L-Carnitine is generally well tolerated except for modest gastric upset, and no serious side effects have been reported.[30] In some patients with an apparent clinical response to carnitine, low muscle levels of carnitine have persisted.

Myopathic. The same doses of supplemental L-carnitine are usually helpful in treating patients with the myopathic form.[158] Some patients unresponsive to carnitine replacement have improved with prednisone.[178] Propranolol,[111] a medium-chain triglyceride diet,[10] and riboflavin[43] have each been reported to be effective in a small number of patients.

Carnitine Palmitoyl Transferase Deficiency

Case History

A 30-year-old woman complained of myalgia and cramps with two episodes of pigmented urine after prolonged vigorous exercise. The patient had normal early development and gave no history of limitation in athletic activity. Her problem emerged during a period of training for bicycle racing. On two occasions after bicycling for 40 to 60 minutes she developed myalgia in the thighs with stiffness that was followed within 2 hours by darkly pigmented urine. The second episode was more severe and occurred during a period of fasting. The pigmented urine did not clear for several days, and the myalgia persisted for nearly 48 hours. She was admitted to hospital, where myoglobin was found in the urine, and a 20-fold elevation in serum CK level was documented.

No other family members were affected, and the neuromuscular examination, several months after the last episode, was entirely normal. The serum CK level was within normal limits, and forearm exercise testing disclosed a ninefold rise in serum lactate level. Quantitative EMG gave normal results. A muscle biopsy disclosed no histologic abnormality, but there was a substantial reduction in carnitine palmitoyltransferase activity (0.12 μmol substrate utilized per mg per minute, less than 5% of normal values).

Comment: This patient presents a typical history of the dynamic symptoms of patients with carnitine palmitoyl transferase (CPT) deficiency, but is atypical in that the majority of patients are men. Her history illustrates the importance of fasting as one predisposing factor and the characteristic onset of symptoms after prolonged exercise. The clinical presentation of CPT deficiency is heterogeneous, and the onset of muscle pain and tightness may be more subtle than in patients with defects of glycogenolysis or glycolysis.[70]

CLINICAL FEATURES

CPT deficiency is the most common currently recognized cause of recurrent myoglobinuria (Table 7–12).[54] Prolonged exercise and prolonged fasting are antecedent precipitating factors. Patients do not develop true muscular cramps or contracture and do not experience the second-wind phenomenon,[32] but pain, stiffness, and tightness of the muscles are common. Other predisposing factors include infection; cold exposure; general anesthesia; emotional stress; a low-carbohydrate, high-fat diet; and lack of sleep.[70,91] In a few patients, no precipitating cause of myoglobinuria can be found. The first attacks tend to appear during adolescence. Most patients have a normal neuromuscular examination except during an attack of muscle destruction. Fixed weakness has only been described in one patient, a 60-year-old woman with partial CPT deficiency (50% reduction), whose son

Table 7–12 CARNITINE PALMITOYL TRANSFERASE (CPT) DEFICIENCY

CLINICAL FEATURES
Myalgia, stiffness, and myoglobinuria triggered by prolonged exercise, fasting, infection, cold, stress, or low-carbohydrate, high-fat diet
Normal strength between attacks

LABORATORY FINDINGS
CK level normal
Forearm exercise test normal
EMG normal
Muscle biopsy normal except for reduced CPT activity (7% to 21% of normal)

GENETICS
Autosomal recessive trait—chromosome 1 (other loci possible)
Male predominance

TREATMENT
Avoid prolonged exercise without carbohydrate loading or during infection

had nearly complete absence of CPT (95% reduction) but normal strength.[94] An infantile form characterized by hypoketotic hypoglycemia, high serum CK level, and sudden death, has also been observed.[44]

LABORATORY FINDINGS

The serum CK level and the EMG are usually normal between episodes. The venous lactate level rises normally during forearm exercise.[54] Prolonged fasting (24–72 hours) has been used to screen for the disorder and may cause increased serum CK or a delayed rise of ketone bodies in the blood.[54] EMG studies, including quantitative studies of motor units, usually give normal results, as does the muscle biopsy. Biochemical analysis of muscle tissue for CPT activity (which varies between 7% and 21% of normal) is necessary for diagnosis. The procedure of choice is an isotope exchange assay on biopsied muscle,[187] although some workers advocate an enzyme-linked immunosorbent assay as well.[181] This latter method detects primarily CPT 2, the enzyme form that appears to be more important than CPT 1 in skeletal muscle function. No clear-cut relationship exists between the degree of residual activity and the number or severity of attacks.[169] Reduced CPT activity in both liver and leukocytes has been documented in a few patients.[54]

GENETICS

The condition is much more common in men (5.5:1), but all other evidence points to transmission as an autosomal recessive trait; the reason for the male preponderance is not known. The recent cloning of the gene for CPT localizes the disorder, at least in some cases, to chromosome 1.[63] Further studies of individual cases should clarify whether genetic heterogeneity is the explanation for the disparity between the incidence in males and females. Alternatively, overall differences may place greater demands on muscle metabolism in males.[54] Better definition of the localization of CPT 1 and CPT 2 may also shed light on clinical heterogeneity.[121] Recently, the molecular basis for the disorder has been identified,[167] and diagnostic DNA analysis is now possible.[166] In all cases thus far found to have a genetic defect, the mutation was observed in the gene for CPT 2.[166,167]

PATHOPHYSIOLOGY

As discussed earlier in the chapter, lipid metabolism becomes important during prolonged exercise of moderate intensity, as the source of energy shifts after about 40 minutes from glycogen and glucose to lipid. A similar shift to lipid occurs after prolonged fasting. In patients with CPT deficiency, muscle glycogen content and metabolism are normal, and patients can tolerate intense exercise for short periods, as long as carbohydrate availability is adequate. With prolonged exercise, however, a fuel shortage occurs because of the absence of CPT. Prolonged fasting also can seriously compromise exercise performance, presumably because muscle glycogen is depleted. CPT acts as a translocation enzyme that normally enables long-chain fatty acids to pass through the inner mitochondrial membrane to become oxidized to CO_2 and water. Fasting reduces both the amount of muscle glycogen and the availability of blood glucose, aggravating the dependence of muscle on CPT. In spite of our general understanding of these events, it is not clear which factors are critical in causing myoglobinuria.[169]

It is still uncertain whether CPT deficiency involves only muscle. Some, but not all, patients with CPT deficiency exhibit ketone body formation during fasting.[32] The development of ketosis implies adequate hepatic CPT activity.

TREATMENT

Treatment consists of frequent meals and a low-fat, high-carbohydrate diet. Prolonged exertion, particularly following fasting or in the setting of infection, must be avoided. Patients with CPT deficiency should receive intravenous glucose prior to and during general anesthesia because prolonged fasting may provoke an attack.[91]

OTHER DISORDERS OF MUSCLE METABOLISM

Myoadenylate Deaminase Deficiency

Myoadenylate deaminase (MAD) is deficient in skeletal muscle in 1% to 2% of patients undergoing muscle biopsy.[64,93,160] The enzyme is normally present in very high concentration in skeletal muscle, and its absence has been noted in a number of patients who have exercise intolerance and myalgia.[13b,184] The deficiency is an incidental finding, however, in patients with a variety of possibly coincidental neuromuscular diseases. MAD is an enzyme of the purine nucleotide cycle and has the potentially important role of supplying ATP during periods of intense muscular exercise (see Fig. 7–1). The clinical importance of MAD is controversial. Its deficiency is benign in virtually all instances.[151] Although some cases of a stereotypic syndrome of exercise intolerance have been well documented, this pattern has not emerged in many others. More information is needed before this condition can be placed in clear clinical perspective.

CLINICAL FEATURES

Patients with exertional myalgia who are deficient in this enzyme have been reported to develop muscular pain and fatigue that worsens steadily during intensive exercise (Table 7–13). They do not develop a second wind. Symptoms usually do not appear until the second to fourth decade. They most often involve the legs, especially during running, and the hands during continuous use. Rarely, back and chest muscles appear to be affected, but not bulbar or ocular muscles. Some patients subsequently found to be MAD-deficient have a history of benign congenital hypotonia.

Table 7–13 MYOADENYLATE DEAMINASE (MAD) DEFICIENCY

CLINICAL FEATURES
Exercise intolerance with myoglobinuria in some patients
Myalgia and muscle fatigue syndrome
Often asymptomatic

LABORATORY FINDINGS
CK level variable (normal or slightly elevated)
EMG normal
Forearm exercise test—normal lactate rise, but reduced ammonia rise

GENETICS
Autosomal recessive—chromosome 1

TREATMENT
None

A cause-and-effect relationship between the enzyme deficiency and the clinical symptoms of exertional myalgia and fatigability is yet to be proven.[149] In one series, a fivefold higher incidence of the enzyme deficiency was found in patients with exertional myalgia,[93] including 14 members of four families with a hereditary syndrome of exercise-related myalgia and MAD deficiency. Two family members with myalgia had normal enzyme levels, however, and a patient with a sporadic case of the enzyme deficiency swam competitively without myalgia. In another report, two brothers with exercise-exacerbated myalgia had marked differences in enzyme activity; one was completely deficient and the other had 60% of normal activity (which should permit normal muscle function).[82] Some authorities have suggested that MAD deficiency may have no clinical correlate[159,160]; others consider it a cause of myoglobinuria.[169] In a review of 250 muscle biopsies, only 2 patients with exercise-induced myalgia were completely deficient in the enzyme, whereas many who had no enzyme activity suffered no exercise-induced symptoms, but had other neuromuscular disease such as motor neuron disease, myasthenia gravis, and facioscapulohumeral dystrophy.[23] Thus, the role of this enzyme and its link to exertional myalgia remain controversial.

LABORATORY FEATURES

The serum CK level is slightly elevated in half the reported cases. Nonspecific EMG abnormalities have been reported, although the findings have not been analyzed in a quantitative fashion. Measurements of MAD in the blood are not helpful. Elevated serum uric acid levels and clinical gout have been described in association with the enzyme deficiency.[64]

The forearm exercise test appears to be an effective screening test since ammonia is normally liberated in this type of exercise. It is not necessary to produce ischemia in exercising muscle to demonstrate the reduced rise in ammonia in enzyme-deficient patients.[64] The ammonia increase (in mM) is approximately 1.5% of the lactate rise (in mM) in normal subjects. All patients with MAD deficiency mount less than a 0.4% increase in ammonia with respect to lactate. No false positives, but some false negatives, have been described.[64]

Analysis of muscle biopsy tissue remains the only definitive way to establish MAD deficiency. The histochemical stain for myadenylate deaminase is easily performed; all deficient patients have a complete absence of staining (Fig. 7–14). The biochemical assay is recommended to confirm the enzyme deficiency.[64]

GENETICS

Exercise-induced myoglobinuria was described in two brothers with MAD deficiency.[82] Males and females are equally affected and the trait appears to conform to an autosomal recessive pattern of inheritance. The gene has been localized to chromosome 1, in the region p13–p21,[152] and recently the gene has been cloned and sequenced.[151,184]

PATHOPHYSIOLOGY

MAD appears to have two major roles during muscular exercise. First, MAD converts AMP to inosine monophosphate (IMP) and ammonia, thus preventing levels of ADP and reducing the fatigue-exacerbating effect of ADP accumulation (see Fig. 7–1). Second, by stimulating the purine nucleotide cycle, MAD increases fumarate production and makes intermediates of the citric acid cycle more available as an energy source during exercise. Both of these functions would suggest that the enzyme may be important in increasing the efficiency of both oxidative phosphorylation and glycolysis during very demanding exercise.

Systematic studies of patients with MAD deficiency are few. During bicycle exercise, reduced work and endurance time was found in MAD-deficient patients compared to others who had myalgia without enzyme deficiency or

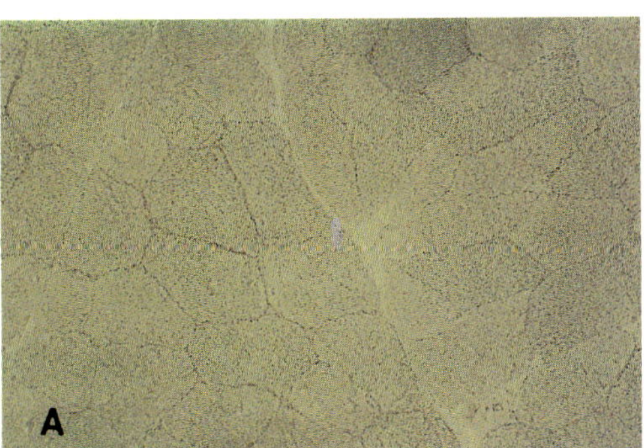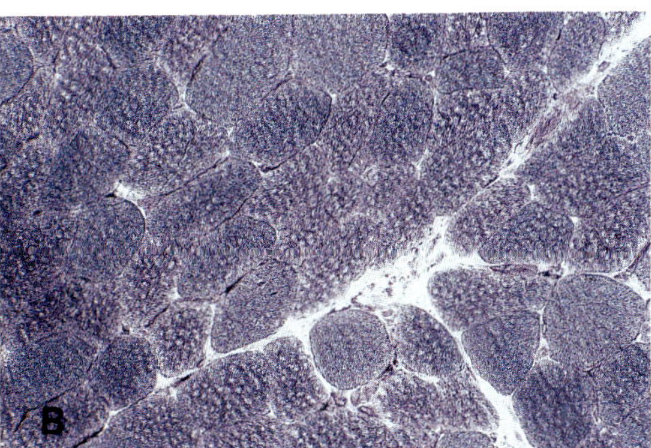

Figure 7–14. MAD deficiency. (*A*) Muscle deficient for MAD enzyme demonstrates pale fibers. (*B*) Control muscle for myoadenylate shows normal purple-blue staining of muscle fibers.

other neuromuscular disease. Enzyme-deficient patients had a significantly greater reduction in phosphocreatine and ADP levels than did controls, a finding which suggests a reduced capacity for aerobic energy metabolism.[153] A study of sustained, isometric muscular contraction during ischemia, however, found no difference in endurance time between MAD-deficient patients and healthy controls. The levels of resting phosphocreatine and lactate elevation after exercise also were similar in the two groups. These results suggest that patients with the enzyme deficiency have normal anaerobic exercise capacity. Finally, oxygen utilization during exercise in patients with MAD deficiency was normal.[179]

Thus, while it appears that myoadenylate deaminase may be important in expanding energy metabolism during extreme aerobic exercise, and its absence could contribute to exercise-induced myalgia and fatigue, more studies are needed to clarify this point.

TREATMENT

No treatment has yet been described to alleviate the symptoms ascribed to MAD deficiency. Moderate degrees of exercise, however, appear not to be harmful and may improve exercise tolerance through training.[64]

Myoglobinuria

Many of the metabolic disorders detailed in this chapter cause myoglobinuria (Table 7–14). Myoglobinuria may also occur in normal individuals following unaccustomed, demanding exercise, particularly in hot weather. For example, during military training, the appearance of myoglobinuria in otherwise healthy individuals is well documented.[45] In addition, many viral or bacterial disorders (Chapter 5) as well as numerous drugs (Chapter 10) cause myoglobinuria.

Table 7–14 DIFFERENTIAL DIAGNOSIS OF MYOGLOBINURIA

1. Vigorous exercise
2. Metabolic disturbances: deficiencies of
   a. Carnitine palmitoyl transferase
   b. Glycogenolytic/glycolytic defects
      1. Myophosphorylase
      2. Phosphofructokinase
      3. Phosphoglycerate kinase
      4. Phosphoglycerate mutase
      5. Lactate dehydrogenase
      6. Phosphorylase *b* kinase
   c. Myoadenylate deaminase
3. Ischemia
4. Mechanical injury or burn
5. Infection
   a. Viral (esp. influenza and Coxsackie)
   b. Gram negative sepsis
6. Drugs
   a. Alcohol, barbiturates
   b. Cocaine, heroin, amphetamines
   c. Neuroleptics
   d. Succinylcholine, halothane (MH-susceptible)
7. Electrolyte disturbance
   a. Hypokalemia
   b. Hypophosphatemia

CLINICAL FEATURES

Regardless of cause, myoglobinuria results from the necrosis of muscle tissue (rhabdomyolysis) and is usually associated with weakness, pain, tenderness, and swelling of affected muscles. Ecchymosis may be visible in the overlying skin. Occasionally, however, myoglobinuria may occur in the absence of pain, swelling, or weakness.[133] Myoglobinuria during exercise is associated with fatigue and myalgia, which becomes increasingly severe as exercise continues. If exercise is not terminated (as in military training situations) progressive weakness develops and constitutional symptoms including nausea, vomiting, and headache ensue. Fasting and high ambient air temperatures are major contributory factors. Pigment in the urine may appear immediately or may be delayed for up to 24 hours. Muscles contained within a closed compartment, such as the forearm or the anterior compartment of the leg, are vulnerable to increased pressure and ischemia and may require a therapeutic fasciotomy to prevent total occlusion of blood flow and subsequent gangrene. Renal failure with acute tubular necrosis is the other frequent serious complication of myoglobinuria.

DIFFERENTIAL DIAGNOSIS

Various infections predispose to myoglobinuria. Influenza virus (A_2) infection is the most common, but other viruses have been implicated, including Coxsackie, herpes simplex, Epstein-Barr, adenoviruses, and echoviruses.[155] Particularly with influenza and Coxsackie viruses, evidence indicates that direct muscle infection and injury lead to myoglobinuria.[9] Mechanical injury of muscle, due either to compression during prolonged coma or to increased pressure within fixed compartments following trauma, may lead to myoglobinuria. Pressures measured in fixed compartments may exceed 200 mm Hg; such pressures may produce severe focal ischemia[129] and contribute to massive muscle necrosis and myoglobinuria.

A number of drugs are associated with myoglobinuria, especially alcohol, heroin, cocaine, barbiturates, and the combination of lovastatin and gemfibrozil (see Chapter 10).[77,134,150,174] Moreover, patients with polymyositis or dermatomyositis may develop rhabdomyolysis with myoglobinuria, although this is a most uncommon presentation of these inflammatory myopathies.[27] Cramps and myoglobinuria may be the presenting features of Becker muscular dystrophy.[54a,119a] Patients with genetically determined metabolic errors in muscle, as well as some mitochondrial disorders,[126] are much more prone to develop myoglobinuria; these disorders are discussed earlier in this chapter and in Chapter 8.

LABORATORY FINDINGS

Pigment in the urine from myoglobin must be distinguished from hemoglobinuria, hematuria, and porphyria (see Chapter 2). The urine dip stick test (benzidine) is negative in porphyria and positive if myoglobin, hemoglobin, or hematuria are present. The identification of red blood cells in the urine establishes hematuria. With recent hemoglobinuria, there may be staining of the serum since the hemoglobin molecule does not pass through the glomerulus as rapidly as the smaller myoglobin molecule. In practice, however, it is essential to do direct determinations for urinary myoglobin. A fresh urine sample, which has been neutralized to prevent myoglobin breakdown, should be employed for a specific myoglobin radioimmunoassay. When myoglobinuria is visible to the naked eye, it implies destruction of more than 200 g of muscle and a serum concentration of myoglobin exceeding 1 mg/mL.[146] Normally, serum myoglobin is less than 80 ng/mL, and in urine, levels are less than 12 μg/mL. The serum CK level is always elevated in the presence of myoglobinuria; the elevation in CK level persists for 3 to 7 days, whereas the myoglobin in the serum usually falls to normal levels within 24 to 48 hours. Renal function may be impaired in the absence of overt renal failure, and abnormal creatinine clearance and increased levels of serum creatinine and urea nitrogen may persist for 1 to 2 months. Elevated serum potassium is common in myoglobinuria, and may in itself be life-threatening because of cardiac arrhythmia. The release of potassium from damaged muscle, particularly when complicated by impaired renal function, may require urgent intervention to lower potassium levels.

Analysis of muscle tissue may be necessary to establish the cause of myoglobinuria when there is no obvious predisposing cause (see Table 7–14). The most common cause of recurrent myoglobinuria is carnitine palmitoyl transferase deficiency.[169] As already discussed, a number of inherited defects of glycogen metabolism may also produce recurrent myoglobinuria. Recurrent myoglobinuria is distinctly unusual in mitochondrial myopathy, carnitine deficiency, and acid maltase deficiency. Other defects in energy metabolism may yet be uncovered, since nearly half of the cases of familial, recurrent myoglobinuria cannot be assigned to a specific diagnostic category.[133]

The muscle biopsy from patients with myoglobinuria characteristically shows extensive necrosis, regeneration, or inflammation, depending upon the timing of the biopsy in relation to the episode. A biopsy done while myoglobinuria is present invariably shows necrotic fibers. A biopsy done 2 to 7 days later shows regenerating fibers. Later biopsies may show little change, although internally placed nuclei are usually present for weeks.

PATHOPHYSIOLOGY

The precise mechanism of muscular injury leading to rhabdomyolysis during heavy exertion, whether in normal individuals or those with inborn errors of metabolism, is still not clear. Depletion of ATP is presumed to predispose to muscle breakdown, but this has not been substantiated, even in patients with known enzyme defects such as phosphorylase deficiency.[179] Moreover, studies of normal individuals using ^{31}P NMR spectroscopy have shown very little depression of ATP even during exhaustive exercise. Possibly a critical compartment of ATP, not detected by current methods, is depleted selectively. Recent studies of muscle injury during heavy exercise have demonstrated a particular susceptibility to damage following eccentric contractions (Fig. 7–15); marked elevation of CK levels (2 to 20 times normal), the development of muscle pain, and histologic evidence of injury have been observed,[124] but the mechanism of tissue injury has yet to be clarified.

Training appears important in protecting against muscle injury. Untrained individuals are much more susceptible to developing myoglobinuria, a phenomenon that often appears very early in military basic training.[148] Individuals who become deconditioned and attempt to resume a previous level of athletic performance are also more susceptible to myoglobinuria.[81] Training increases capillary density, mitochondrial density and size, myoglobin concentration, and mitochondrial enzymes.[57] Thus, training reduces susceptibility to myoglobinuria; however, trained individuals may still develop myoglobinemia and myoglobin-

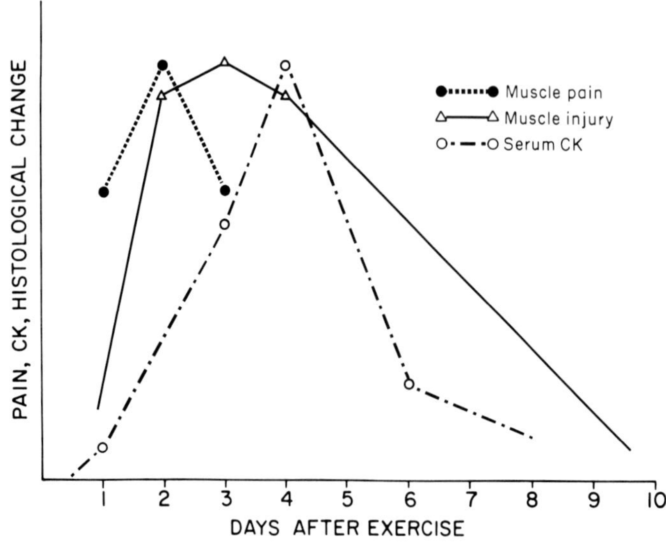

Figure 7–15. Time course of muscle pain, histologically detectable muscle fiber damage, and elevated serum CK after vigorous eccentric muscle exercise.

uria.[114] Elevated ambient air temperature increases susceptibility to myoglobinuria, although acclimatization can alleviate the effect of this factor. Patients have also developed myoglobinuria during periods of prolonged involuntary muscle contraction, as occurs in status epilepticus and tetanus.[48]

TREATMENT

Respiratory support may be necessary during episodes of rhabdomyolysis associated with severe generalized weakness. Acute tubular necrosis can often be prevented by administering sodium bicarbonate, mannitol, furosemide, and large volumes of intravenous fluid (Table 7-15).[146] Hyperkalemia ($K^+ > 5.5$ mEq/L) may warrant urgent intervention and may be worsened by mannitol infusion.[96] Infusion of isotonic sodium bicarbonate may prevent or treat hyperkalemia and is useful in preventing renal tubular damage from myoglobin and uric acid.[28] Hypocalcemia may lead to symptomatic tetany. Vascular collapse with severe hypotension may occur because of the depletion of intravascular volume as fluid diffuses into necrotic muscle. Finally, disseminated intravascular coagulation may appear and require aggressive treatment.

Table 7-15 TREATMENT OF MYOGLOBINURIA

A. Maintain airway and circulation
B. Prevent acute tubular necrosis
  1. Infusion of physiologic saline: 10-15 mL/kg immediately; maintain high rates of infusion if urine output adequate
  2. Infusion of isotonic sodium bicarbonate
  3. Mannitol (0.3-0.5 g/kg IV). *Caution:* may worsen hyperkalemia
  4. Furosemide (40-80 mg IV immediately, up to 200 mg total)
C. Reverse hyperkalemia
D. Treat disseminated intravascular coagulopathy, if present

IV = intravenous.

Malignant Hyperthermia

Malignant hyperthermia is a rare but potentially lethal disorder. It usually appears in patients without a recognized muscle disorder but may occur in association with other muscle diseases.[183] Malignant hyperthermia is both preventable and treatable and therefore diagnosis is of great importance to clinicians.

CLINICAL FEATURES

Patients destined to develop malignant hyperthermia rarely complain of dynamic or static symptoms such as fatigability, cramp, myoglobinuria, or weakness. The disorder presents as a dramatic syndrome usually triggered by a general anesthetic. This state of hypermetabolism within skeletal muscle is most frequently provoked by halogenated inhalational anesthetics and the depolarizing muscle relaxant, succinylcholine. Very rarely, patients have developed this syndrome as a result of physical or emotional stress while awake.[122] Recently, a subset of patients with malignant hyperthermia was also found to have CPT deficiency, which might explain some cases of "awake" malignant hyperthermia.[180] Occasionally the attack has occurred during recovery from general anesthesia, or the patient has recovered and then relapsed during the next few days.[112] Local anesthetics, in conventional doses, appear to be safe,[15] but intravenous lidocaine may trigger an attack.[168] Both exercise and coffee, which may cause muscle cramps in susceptible patients, have triggered episodes of malignant hyperthermia in rare instances.[75]

The incidence of malignant hyperthermia is approximately 1 in 1200 anesthetic administrations in children and 1 in 50,000 in adults. The reason for the higher incidence in children is unknown. At least 50% of patients developing malignant hyperthermia have had prior anesthesia without a recognized episode.

The clinical features of evolving malignant hyperthermia include tachypnea, sinus tachycardia, rising blood pressure, and masseter spasm, particularly during induction of anesthesia using succinylcholine for intubation. Areas of bright red flushing of the skin are seen near mottled areas that appear cyanotic. Generalized rigidity usually develops in skeletal muscles, and body temperature rises as a result of the excessive muscular activity. The rise in temperature may not occur until late in the evolution of the syndrome, often after 15 to 60 minutes. The temperature increase is approximately 0.2°C per minute, but in severe cases, shock and ventricular fibrillation with acidosis may all develop before the temperature elevation.

A marked metabolic and respiratory acidosis with increased oxygen consumption and hypopoxemia are all indicative of the profound increase in oxygen uptake, lactate release, and heat production by skeletal muscle.[72] Increased levels of circulating catecholamines produce vasoconstriction, increased cardiac output, and reduced peripheral blood flow. Serum potassium values may rise dramatically. Myoglobinuria, with elevation in the serum CK level to over 100 times normal and disseminated intravascular coagulation, may complicate the attack. Myoglobinemia may be detectable immediately, while the elevation in CK level may take several hours to appear. Significant danger of relapse exists during the first few days after an episode, even with no further exposure to anesthetic agents.

Association with Other Conditions. A susceptibility to malignant hyperthermia should be considered in patients with other muscle diseases. Attacks have been documented in patients with central core disease[68] and in Duchenne muscular dystrophy.[100] The possibility of an increased susceptibility also has been raised in myotonic disorders. Denborough and King[46] described a rare syndrome in four children with malignant hyperthermia and short stature, mild nonprogressive myopathy, delayed motor development, and congenital anomalies (webbed neck, pectus carinatum).

The increased incidence of malignant hyperthermia is particularly significant in Duchenne muscular dystrophy.[100] In one recent report, two of five Duchenne patients and one of two Becker patients had positive contracture tests (abnormal sensitivity of muscle biopsy tissue to caffeine).[84] It is not clear whether such results are related to the skeletal muscle abnormalities resulting from the dystrophy, or whether these are primary cases of malignant hyperthermia.[73] In porcine malignant hyperthermia, cell injury enhances halothane sensitivity, so the muscle damage that is part of the dystrophic process could increase the sensitivity to contracture testing. The possibility remains, however, that X-linked muscular dystrophies and malignant hyperthermia susceptibility share common pathophysiologic abnormalities.

Neuroleptic Malignant Syndrome. The neuroleptic malignant syndrome (NMS) is a condition that has some features in common with malignant hyperthermia.[31,83] NMS occurs most often in young men, and usually complicates neuroleptic drug treatment. Approximately 1% of patients receiving any neuroleptic, especially haloperidol or fluphenazine, develop NMS. The disorder has a mortality rate of 9% to 25%.[92] NMS may also occur in patients with Parkinson's disease who are being withdrawn from medication.[128] The features of NMS include fever, rigidity, confusion, tachycardia, labile blood pressure, rhabdomyolysis, and myoglobinuria. Central dopamine blockade appears to be important in the pathogenesis of this disorder. Although some reports have proposed a causal link between NMS and malignant hyperthermia,[4] recent evidence suggests that they are not related.[86]

Differential Diagnosis of Malignant Hyperthermia. Other syndromes can produce clinical features similar to malignant hyperthermia and may occasionally be mistaken for it. The neuroleptic malignant syndrome (see above) closely resembles malignant hyperthermia, but does not occur in the setting of general anesthesia. Also, it is seen only in patients receiving treatment with neuroleptics such as the phenothiazines.

Patients with myotonia congenita, myotonic dystrophy, and other myotonic disorders often develop generalized rigidity when given depolarizing muscle relaxants such as succinylcholine, but actual malignant hyperthermia seldom, if ever, occurs (see Chapter 9). Similarly, patients with generalized denervating disorders such as amyotrophic lateral sclerosis and spinal muscular atrophy develop generalized fasciculations and cramps after receiving depolarizing muscle relaxants.[75] Hyperthermia does not usually complicate this reaction, but hyperkalemia may occur and can be life-threatening.[168]

Patients who have received antidepressant monoamine oxidase inhibitors are vulnerable to the administration of opiates. Agents such as meperidine and morphine may precipitate severe hyperthermia in such patients.[75] Because this drug-induced syndrome often occurs in the perioperative period, it may suggest malignant hyperthermia. Patients are usually not rigid, however, and CK does not reach the very high levels seen in malignant hyperthermia. Treatment with prompt and aggressive cooling measures is life-saving.[71]

Another neuroleptic-induced disorder, acute dystonia, produces muscle rigidity. Phenothiazines, butyrophenones, and other agents such as metoclopramide and antihistamines can induce a picture of trismus, opisthotonus, or a generalized increase in muscle tone. Choreiform movements may occur, either generalized or isolated to cranial or limb muscles. The CK level is often elevated if the movements or dystonia are severe. This acute, medication-induced disorder occasionally simulates tetanus. Tetanus itself (see Chapter 5) can be confused with malignant hyperthermia.

LABORATORY FINDINGS

Apart from a family history of anesthetic complications, usually nothing in the clinical history or examination of the susceptible patient suggests the diagnosis of malignant hyperthermia. The serum CK level is often elevated interictally, but not reliably so. In one study, the mean value in patients who had an attack was 152 IU; in first-degree relatives it was 93 IU, and in normal controls it was 43 IU. In children less than 10 and in older patients (over 50) who are susceptible, the serum CK level is often normal.[22]

Attempts to develop a reliable and noninvasive diagnostic test for malignant hyperthermia have had significant problems. Compared with controls, patients with malignant hyperthermia susceptibility display significantly shorter contraction time and half-relaxation time, as well as electromechanical delay of contraction, in response to a train of 20-Hz stimulation of the adductor pollicis; however, the overlap with controls is too great to render this finding diagnostically useful.[11] Analysis of tibialis anterior contractile characteristics demonstrate a high degree of overlap between the ranges of all mechanical parameters in susceptible patients, their relatives, and normal controls.[136,137] In recent controlled studies, NMR spectroscopy disclosed higher ratios of inorganic phosphate to phosphocreatine in resting muscle and a significantly slower recovery rate after exercise for patients susceptible to malignant hyperthermia.[127] The bioenergetic changes that accompanied exercise were not significantly different in patients as compared with controls. Unfortunately, these findings are not specific.[89] Nonetheless, in the same way that the serum CK level is useful in detecting the presence of some muscle disorders, ^{31}P NMR, in conjunction with the clinical history, may ultimately become helpful in screening patients who might be at risk.

The diagnostic test for conventional malignant hyperthermia is the *in vitro* contracture test of muscle biopsy tissue. The muscle biopsy is best carried out under local anesthesia or at the time of an elective surgical procedure for other purposes. The test is based on the observation that skeletal muscle from patients with malignant hyperthermia undergoes a contracture in response to caffeine, and that this effect is potentiated by halothane.[75,88] Contracture studies are performed at only a few regional diagnostic centers and require extensive standardization to avoid false positives.[99] In patients with malignant hyperthermia susceptibility, contracture occurs at lower doses of caffeine (1–2 mM) than in normal muscle (>4mM). Similarly, low concentrations of halothane produce a large abnormal contraction response in muscle from susceptible patients, compared with controls.[75] In a patient with abnormal sensitivity to both caffeine and halothane, the diagnosis of malignant hyperthermia is secure.

A new method, using calcium uptake in thin, frozen muscle slices, has been advocated to screen patients for malignant hyperthermia, but it requires further investigation.[36]

The potential advantages of a DNA-based blood test are obvious, but currently only a small percentage of the total number of individuals susceptible to malignant hyperthermia can be recognized by DNA analysis.[105]

GENETICS

The genetic basis for malignant hyperthermia is incompletely understood. The ryanodine receptor is the calcium release channel of the sarcoplasmic reticulum of skeletal muscle. The ryanodine receptor gene of skeletal muscle is located on chromosome 19q13.1,[105] and mutations of this gene have been linked to malignant hyperthermia.[13] The most common point mutation of the human ryanodine receptor gene of skeletal muscle accounts for 2% to 5% of the malignant hyperthermia throughout the world and corresponds to the identical alteration in amino acid sequence found in a highly conserved region of the calcium channel gene of swine.[105] The susceptibility of patients with central core disease to develop malignant hyperthermia is explained by linkage of central core disease to chromosome 19q13.1.[105,135a] Three point mutations of the ryanodine receptor gene appear to cause central core disease.[135a,186a] The potential use of a DNA-based blood test for malignant hyperthermia may be limited by the genetic heterogeneity of the disorder; evidence supports a second locus for malignant hyperthermia susceptibility mapping to chromosome 17q11.2-24.[13]

PATHOPHYSIOLOGY

Insight into the mechanisms of malignant hyperthermia has been obtained from the porcine model. This genetic strain of pigs has a disorder similar to the human condition, although it is more severe and more easily induced.[11,106] The biochemical changes during an attack result almost exclusively from skeletal muscle overactivity. Porcine malignant hyperthermia results from a consistent DNA mutation of the skeletal muscle ryanodine receptor.

The pathophysiology of the skeletal muscle hypermetabolism that characterizes an attack involves a complex series of biochemical changes. During exposure to succinylcholine or halothane, phospholipase A2 activity is enhanced and increases the mitochondrial content of free fatty acids. The elevated concentration of free fatty acids induces calcium release from the sarcoplasmic reticulum and also inhibits calcium reuptake. The high calcium concentration allows continued interaction of the actin and myosin fibers, which demands further energy and, in turn, stimulates glycolysis. The increases in lactate concentration, PCO_2, and temperature are produced by the increased glycolytic activity in contracted muscles.[74]

TREATMENT

Prevention in Previously Diagnosed Patients. Patients who are susceptible to malignant hyperthermia should wear a medic-alert bracelet indicating the diagnosis and the need to avoid succinylcholine and halogenated inhalational anesthetics. Susceptible patients may safely undergo anesthesia with narcotics, barbiturates, diazepam, nitrous oxide, droperidol, and local anesthetics of both amide and ester classes in conventional doses.[75] Earlier concerns about local anesthetics have, for the most part, been dispelled.[75] If skeletal muscle paralysis is necessary, then the nondepolarizing agent pancuronium is recommended. Patients may appreciate a referral to the Malignant Hyperthermia Association of the United States (Box 3231, Darien, CT 06820), to receive a monthly bulletin and additional information.

Treatment of the Acute Episode. Treatment of malignant hyperthermia includes discontinuing triggering drugs, hyperventilation with 100% oxygen, cooling to reduce body temperature, and rapid intravenous administration of dantrolene (2.5 mg/kg), with an additional dose of 7.5 mg/kg if all symptoms have not resolved within 45 minutes. Monitoring arterial blood gases, serum CK level, and myoglobin in serum and urine helps to determine the magnitude of the attack and the potential for renal failure.

Dantrolene sodium is a specific therapy for malignant hyperthermia. The drug is available in a lyophilized form and is easily administered intravenously. Intravenous doses up to 10 mg/kg of body weight may be needed, and occasionally even higher doses have been required[17]; however, a large multicenter prospective study established the efficacy of doses of 2.5 mg/kg in most cases.[97] The dose of dantrolene can be titrated by monitoring maximal muscle relaxation.[66] Oral loading with dantrolene preoperatively at a dose of 4 to 8 mg/kg per day for 1 to 2 days has been practiced in some centers, but most authorities no longer consider oral loading to be necessary.[71,75]

Newer diagnostic methods, as well as rapid recognition and appropriate treatment of acute episodes, have all helped to reduce the earlier mortality rate of 65% to almost zero. Dantrolene sodium appears to act directly upon the sarcoplasmic reticulum, raising the threshold voltage for activation in susceptible muscle and preventing the depolarization of susceptible muscle by halothane. The drug has a primary antiarrhythmic effect on cardiac tissue. It may be safely used in pregnancy. Although liver toxicity may occur with prolonged oral use, it has not been reported during the acute treatment of malignant hyperthermia.

Counseling Families with Malignant Hyperthermia. A complete family history of anesthetic exposure and complications is needed. The serum CK level, obtained in a resting and fasting state, is elevated in 70% of affected people; elevation should be considered diagnostic in a close relative to known susceptible patients.[22] Family members at risk for malignant hyperthermia who have a normal or equivocal CK level should consider undergoing a muscle biopsy for the contracture test. Fresh muscle tissue is needed for this analysis (see reference 75), which should be carried out in a standardized fashion in a specialized center.

Treatment of Disorders That Resemble Malignant Hyperthermia. Treatment of neuroleptic malignant syndrome includes stopping neuroleptics, and ensuring adequate hydration and ventilation. Spontaneous recovery is common.[161] Bromocriptine (7.5–30 mg daily) with dantrolene (100–300 mg daily), both in divided doses for 3 days, provide reversal of dopamine blockade and muscular relaxation, respectively.[128]

SUMMARY

Most metabolic disorders of muscle result from the lack of one of the enzymes necessary for energy metabolism. Defects in the pathways for carbohydrate metabolism (both aerobic and anaerobic), in lipid transport and metabolism, and in the purine nucleotide cycle may each lead to dynamic, exercise-related symptoms or to the static symptoms of weakness. A full understanding of metabolic pathways helps in understanding the clinical features of these various metabolic defects and also in evaluating patients who require exercise testing for clarification of the diagnosis. An appropriate combination of exercise testing for lactate and ammonia production, histologic and biochemical assays of muscle, and NMR spectroscopy can establish the diagnosis and explain symptoms in most patients. The genetic defects responsible for the metabolic disorders are being characterized; specific molecular diagnosis will soon be practical.

Dynamic symptoms, including fatigability, exercise-induced cramp, and myoglobinuria, result from defects of carbohydrate metabolism, including deficiencies of myophosphorylase, phosphofructokinase, phosphoglycerate kinase, phosphoglycerate mutase, and lactate dehydrogenase, as well as phosphorylase *b* kinase. Patients with carnitine palmitoyl transferase deficiency, an important and common cause of recurrent myoglobinuria, also have dynamic symptoms, but only after prolonged exercise. Final conclusions concerning the significance of the controversial category of myoadenylate deaminase deficiency cannot yet be drawn.

Static symptoms of gradually progressive, proximal muscle weakness are typical of patients with acid maltase, debranching enzyme, branching enzyme, and carnitine deficiencies. The clinical picture can mimic limb-girdle muscular dystrophy. The precise explanation for the progressive, fixed deficits is not entirely clear.

Treatment is effective for many patients with carnitine deficiency, and many patients with dynamic symptoms from other metabolic disorders are helped by various strategies of exercise modification. Nearly all patients with metabolic myopathies can be provided with helpful genetic counseling.

A large number of disorders produce the clinical picture of myoglobinuria. This complication of rhabdomyolysis can produce renal failure and severe metabolic abnormalities such as hyperkalemia and hyperuricemia. All of these severe complications can be prevented by early recognition and treatment. For malignant hyperthermia, a life-threatening condition, the important considerations are identifying the susceptible patient, using safe anesthetic agents, and instituting early treatment with intravenous dantrolene. Mortality for this disease was once more than 50% but is now largely preventable.

Skeletal muscle is a complex metabolic machine that is increasingly well understood. The diagnosis and treatment of the various defects of muscle metabolism warrant a full investigation because an increasing number of these disorders are treatable.

REFERENCES

1. Abarbanel JM, Bashan N, Potashnik R, et al: Adult muscle phosphorylase "b" kinase deficiency. Neurology 36:560, 1986.
2. Amit R, Bashan N, Abarbanel JM, Shapira Y, Sofer S, and Moses S: Fatal familial infantile glycogen storage disease: Multisystem phosphofructokinase deficiency. Muscle Nerve 15:455, 1992.
3. Angelini C, Vergani L, and Martinuzzi A: Clinical and biochemical aspects of carnitine deficiency and insufficiency: Transport defects and inborn errors of β-oxidation. Crit Rev Clin Lab Sci 29:217, 1992.
4. Araki M, Takagi A, Higuchi I, et al: Neuroleptic malignant syndrome: Caffeine contracture of single muscle fibers and muscle pathology. Neurology 38:297, 1988.
4a. Argov Z and Bank WJ: Phosphorus magnetic resonance spectroscopy (^{31}P MRS) in neuromuscular disorders. Ann Neurol 30:90, 1991.
5. Argov Z, Bank WJ, Boden B, et al: Phosphorus magnetic resonance spectroscopy of partially blocked muscle glycolysis: An in vivo study of phosphoglycerate mutase deficiency. Arch Neurol 44:614, 1987.
6. Argov Z, Bank WJ, Maris J, et al: Bioenergetic heterogeneity of human mitochondrial myopathies: Phosphorus magnetic resonance spectroscopy study. Neurology 37:257, 1987.
7. Argov Z, Bank WJ, Maris J, et al: Muscle energy metabolism in human phosphofructokinase deficiency as recorded by ^{31}P nuclear magnetic res-

onance spectroscopy. Ann Neurol 22:46, 1987.

8. Argov Z, Bank WJ, Maris J, et al: Muscle energy metabolism in McArdle's syndrome by in vivo phosphorus magnetic resonance spectroscopy. Neurology 37:1720, 1987.

9. Armstrong CL, Miranda AF, Hsu KC, et al: Susceptibility of human skeletal muscle culture to influenza virus infection. J Neurol Sci 35:43, 1978.

10. Avigan J, Askansas V, and Engel WK: Muscle carnitine deficiency: Fatty acid metabolism in cultured fibroblasts and muscle cells. Neurology 33:1021, 1983.

11. Bäckman E, Lennmarken C, Rutberg H, et al: Skeletal muscle contraction characteristics in vivo in malignant hyperthermia susceptible subjects. Acta Neurol Scand 77:278, 1988.

12. Baker AJ, Carson PJ, Miller RG, et al: Investigations of muscle bioenergetics with ^{31}P NMR. Invest Radiol 24:1001, 1989.

12a. Baker AJ, Kostov RG, Miller RG, and Weiner MW: Slow force recovery after long-duration exercise: Metabolic and activation factors in muscle fatigue. Am J Physiol 74:2294, 1993.

13. Ball SP and Johnson KJ: The genetics of malignant hyperthermia. J Med Genet 30:89, 1993.

13a. Barohn RJ, McVey AL, and DiMauro S: Adult acid maltase deficiency. Muscle Nerve 16:672, 1993.

13b. Baumeister FA, Gross M, Wagner DR, Pongratz D, and Eife R: Myoadenylate deaminase deficiency with severe rhabdomyolysis. Eur J Pediatr 152:513, 1993.

14. Bautista J, Rafel E, Martinez A, et al: Familial hypertrophic cardiomyopathy and muscle carnitine deficiency. Muscle Nerve 13:192, 1990.

15. Berkowitz A and Rosenberg H: Femoral block with mepivacaine for muscle biopsy in malignant hyperthermia patients. Anesthesiology 62:651, 1985.

16. Bertocci LA, Haller RG, Lewis SF, Fleckenstein JL, and Nunnally RL: Abnormal high-energy phosphate metabolism in human muscle phosphofructokinase deficiency. J Appl Physiol 70:1201, 1991.

17. Blank JW and Boggs SD: Successful treatment of an episode of malignant hyperthermia using a large dose of dantrolene. J Clin Anesth 5:69, 1993.

18. Boone C, Chen TR, and Ruddle FH: Assignment of three human genes to chromosomes (LDH-A to 11, TK to 17, and 10H to 20) and evidence for translocation between human and mouse chromosomes in somatic cell hybrids. Proc Natl Acad Sci USA 69:510, 1972.

19. Boska MD, Moussavi RS, Carson PJ, et al: The metabolic basis of recovery after fatiguing exercise of human muscle. Neurology 40:240, 1990.

20. Braakhekke JP, De Bruin MI, Stegeman, et al: The second wind phenomenon in McArdle's disease. Brain 109:1087, 1986.

21. Brandt NJ, Buchthal F, Ebbesen F, et al: Post-tetanic mechanical tension and evoked action potentials in McArdle's disease. J Neurol Neurosurg Psychiatry 40:920, 1977.

22. Britt BA, Endreny L, Peters PL, et al: Screening of malignant hyperthermia susceptible families by creatine phosphokinase measurement and other clinical investigations. Can Anaesth Soc J 23:263, 1976.

23. Brooke MH (ed): A Clinician's View of Neuromuscular Diseases, ed 2. Williams & Wilkins, Baltimore, 1977, p 313.

24. Brooke MH, Patterson VH, and Kaiser KK: Hypoxanthine and McArdle's disease: a clue to metabolic stress in the working forearm. Muscle Nerve 6:204, 1983.

25. Brown BI: Debranching and branching enzyme deficiencies. In Engel AG and Banker BQ (eds): Myology: Basic and Clinical. McGraw-Hill, New York, 1986, p 1653.

26. Bryan W, Lewis SF, Bertocci L, et al: Muscle lactate dehydrogenase deficiency: A disorder of anaerobic glycogenolysis associated with exertional myoglobinuria. Neurology 40 (Suppl 1):203, 1990.

27. Caccamo DV, Keene CY, Durham J, and Peven D: Fulminant rhabdomyolysis in a patient with dermatomyositis. Neurology 43:844, 1993.

28. Cadnapaphornchai P, Taher S, and McDonald FD: Acute drug-associated rhabdomyolysis: An examination of its diverse renal manifestations and complications. Am J Med Sci 280:66, 1980.

29. Cady EB, Jones DA, Lynn J, et al: Changes in force and intracellular metabolites during fatigue of human skeletal muscle. J Physiol 418:311, 1989.

30. Campos Y, Huertas R, Lorenzo G, et al: Plasma carnitine insufficiency and effectiveness of L-carnitine therapy in patients with mitochondrial myopathy. Muscle Nerve 16:150, 1993.

31. Caroff SN and Mann SC: Neuroleptic malignant syndrome. Med Clin North Am 77:185, 1993.

32. Carroll JE: Myopathies caused by disorders of lipid metabolism. Neurol Clin 6:563, 1988.

33. Chui LA and Munsat TL: Dominant inheritance of McArdle syndrome. Arch Neurol 33:636, 1976.

34. Clemens PR, Yamamoto M, and Engel AG: Adult phosphorylase *b* kinase deficiency. Ann Neurol 28:529, 1990.

35. Coleman RA, Winter HS, Wolf B, Gilchrist JM, and Chen YT: Glycogen storage disease type III (glycogen debranching enzyme deficiency): correlation of biochemical defects with myopathy and cardiomyopathy. Ann Intern Med 116:896, 1992.

36. Condrescu M, López JR, Medina P, et al: Deficient function of the sarcoplasmic reticulum in patients susceptible to malignant hyperthermia. Muscle Nerve 10:238, 1987.

37. Cooke R, Franks K, Luciani GB, et al: Inhibition of rabbit skeletal muscle contraction by hydrogen ions and phosphate. J Physiol 395:77, 1988.

38. Cooper RG, Stokes MJ, and Edwards RHT: Myofibrillar activation failure in McArdle's disease. J Neurol Sci 93:1, 1989.

39. Cornelio F, Bresolin N, DiMauro S, et al: Congenital myopathy due to phosphorylase deficiency. Neurology 33:1383, 1983.

40. Davidson JJ, Özcelik T, Hamacher C, Willems PJ, Francke U, and Kilimann MW: cDNA cloning of a liver isoform of the phosphorylase kinase α subunit and mapping of the gene to Xp22.2-p22.1, the region of human X-linked liver glycogenosis. Proc Natl Acad Sci USA 89:2096, 1992.

41. Davidson M, Miranda AF, Bender AN, et al: Muscle phosphofructokinase deficiency: Biochemical and immunological studies of phosphofructokinase isoenzymes in muscle culture. J Clin Invest 72:545, 1983.

42. Dawson JM: The relation between muscle contraction and metabolism: Studies by ^{31}P nuclear magnetic resonance spectroscopy. In Sugi H and Pollack GH (eds): Molecular Mechanisms of Muscle Contraction. Plenum, New York, 1988, p 433.

43. de Visser M, Scholte HR, Schutgens RBH, et al: Riboflavin-responsive lipid-storage myopathy and glutaric aciduria type II of early adult onset. Neurology 36:367, 1986.

44. Demaugre F, Bonnefont JP, Colonna M, Cepanec C, Leroux JP, and Sandubray JM: Infantile form of carnitine palmitoyltransferase II deficiency with hepatomuscular symptoms and sudden death. Physiopathological approach to carnitine palmitoyltransferase II deficiencies. J Clin Invest 87:859, 1991.

45. Demos MA and Gitin EL: Acute exertional rhabdomyolysis. Arch Intern Med 133:233, 1974.

46. Denborough MA, Ebeling P, King JO, et al: Myopathy and malignant hyperpyrexia. Lancet 1:1138, 1970.

47. Desnick RJ (ed): Enzyme Therapy in Genetic Diseases, ed 2. Alan R Liss, New York, 1980.

48. Diamond I and Aquino TI: Myoglobinuria following unilateral status epilepticus and ipsilateral rhabdomyolysis. N Engl J Med 272:834, 1965.

49. Di Donato S, Pelucchetti D, Rimoldi M, et al: Systemic carnitine defi-

ciency: Clinical, biochemical, and morphological cure with L-carnitine. Neurology 34:157, 1984.

50. Di Mauro S and Bresolin N: Phosphorylase deficiency. In Engel AG and Banker BQ (eds): Myology: Basic and Clinical. McGraw-Hill, New York, 1986, p 1585.

51. DiMauro S and Bresolin N: Newly recognized defects in distal glycolysis. In Engel AG and Banker BQ (eds): Myology: Basic and Clinical. McGraw-Hill, New York, 1986, p 1619.

52. DiMauro S, Dalakas M, and Miranda AF: Phosphoglycerate kinase deficiency: another cause of recurrent myoglobinuria. Ann Neurol 13:11, 1983.

53. DiMauro S and Hartlage PL: Fatal infantile form of muscle phosphorylase deficiency. Neurology 28:1124, 1978.

54. DiMauro S and Papadimitriou A: Carnitine palmitoyltransferase deficiency. In Engel AG and Banker BQ (eds): Myology: Basic and Clinical. McGraw-Hill, New York, 1986, p 1697.

54a. Doriguzzi C, Palmucci L, Mongini T, et al: Exercise intolerance and recurrent myoglobinuria as the only expression of Xp21 Becker type muscular dystrophy. J Neurol 240:269, 1993.

55. Duboc D, Jehenson P, Dinh ST, et al: Phosphorus NMR spectroscopy study of muscular enzyme deficiencies involving glycolgenolysis and glycolysis. Neurology 37:663, 1987.

56. Editorial: Carnitine deficiency. Lancet 335:631, 1990.

57. Edström L and Grimby L: Effect of exercise on the motor unit. Muscle Nerve 9:104, 1986.

58. Elliot DL, Buist NRM, Goldberg L, et al: Metabolic myopathies: Evaluation by graded exercise testing. Medicine 68:163, 1989.

59. Engel AG: Acid maltase deficiency. In Engel AG and Banker BQ (eds): Myology: Basic and Clinical. McGraw-Hill, New York, 1986, p 1629.

60. Engel AG: Carnitine deficiency syndromes and lipid storage myopathies.

In Engel AG and Banker BQ (eds): Myology: Basic and Clinical. McGraw-Hill, New York, 1986, p 1663.

61. Engel WK, Eyerman EL, and Williams HE: Late-onset type of skeletal-muscle phosphorylase deficiency: A new familial variety with completely and partially affected subjects. N Engl J Med 268:135, 1963.

62. Feit H and Brooke MH: Myophosphorylase deficiency: Two different molecular etiologies. Neurology 26:963, 1976.

63. Finocchiaro G, Taroni F, Rocchi M, et al: cDNA cloning, sequence analysis, and chromosomal localization of the gene for human carnitine palmitoyl transferase. Proc Natl Acad Sci USA 88:661, 1991.

64. Fishbein WN: Myoadenylate deaminase deficiency. In Engel AG and Banker BQ (eds): Myology: Basic and Clinical. McGraw-Hill, New York, 1986, p 1745.

65. Fleckenstein JL, Haller RG, Lewis SF, et al: Absence of exercise-induced MRI enhancement of skeletal muscle in McArdle's disease. J Appl Physiol 71:961, 1991.

66. Flewellen EH and Nelson TE: Dantrolene dose response in malignant hyperthermia-susceptible (MHS) swine: Method to obtain prophylaxis and therapeusis. Anesthesiology 52:303, 1980.

67. Francke U, Darras BT, Zander NF, et al: Assignment of human genes for phosphorylase kinase subunits α (PHKA) to Xq12-q13 and β (PHKB) to 16q12-q13. Am J Hum Genet 45:276, 1989.

68. Frank JP, Harati Y, Butler IJ, et al: Central core disease and malignant hyperthermia syndrome. Ann Neurol 7:11, 1980.

69. Fujii H, Kanno H, Hirono A, Shiomura T, and Miwa S: A single amino acid substitution (157 Gly$\rightarrow$Val) in a phosphoglycerate kinase variant (PGK Shizuoka) associated with chronic hemolysis and myoglobinuria. Blood 79:1582, 1992.

70. Galdi AP and Clark JB: An unusual

case of carnitine palmitoyl transferase deficiency. Arch Neurol 46:819, 1989.

71. Gronert GA: Malignant hyperthermia. In Engel AG and Banker BQ (eds): Myology: Basic and Clinical. McGraw-Hill, New York, 1986, p 1763.

72. Gronert GA, Ahern CP, and Milde JH: Treatment of porcine malignant hyperthermia: Lactate gradient from muscle to blood. Can Anaesth Soc J 33:729, 1986.

73. Gronert GA, Fowler W, Cardinet GH III, Grix A, Ellis WG, and Schwartz MZ: Absence of malignant hyperthermia contractures in Becker-Duchenne dystrophy at age 2. Muscle Nerve 15:52, 1992.

74. Gronert GA, Mott J, and Lee J: Aetiology of malignant hyperthermia. Br J Anaesth 60:253, 1988.

75. Gronert GA, Schulman SR, and Mott J: Malignant hyperthermia. In Miller RD (ed): Anesthesia. Churchill-Livingstone, New York, 1990, p 935.

76. Grubisic A, Shin YS, Meyer M, et al: First trimester diagnosis of Pompe's disease (glycogenosis type II) with normal outcome: Assay of acid α-glucosidase in chorionic villous biopsy using antibodies. Clin Genet 30:298, 1986.

77. Haller RG and Drachman DB: Alcoholic rhabdomyolysis: An experimental model in the rat. Science 208:412, 1980.

78. Haller RG and Lewis SF: Abnormal ventilation during exercise in McArdle's syndrome: Modulation by substrate availability. Neurology 36:716, 1986.

79. Haller RG and Lewis SF: Physical conditioning: A rational treatment of muscle phosphofructokinase deficiency [abstract]. Neurology 38:341, 1988.

80. Haller RG and Lewis SF: Glucose-induced exertional fatigue in muscle phosphofructokinase deficiency. N Engl J Med 324:364, 1991.

81. Hamilton RW, Gardner LB, Penn AS, et al: Acute tubular necrosis caused by exercise-induced myoglobinuria. Ann Intern Med 77:77, 1972.

82. Hayes DJ, Summers BA, and Morgan-Hughes JA: Myoadenylate deaminase deficiency or not? Observations on two brothers with exercise-induced muscle pain. J Neurol Sci 53:125, 1982.

83. Heiman-Patterson TD: Neuroleptic malignant syndrome and malignant hyperthermia: Important issues for the medical consultant. Med Clin North Am 77:477, 1993.

84. Heiman-Patterson TD, Natter HM, Rosenberg HR, et al: Malignant hyperthermia susceptibility in X-linked muscle dystrophies. Pediatr Neurol 2:356, 1986.

85. Hermans MM, deGraaff E, Kroos MA, et al: The conservative substitution Asp-645$\rightarrow$Glu in lysosomal α-glucosidase affects transport and phosphorylation of the enzyme in an adult patient with glycogen-storage disease type II. Biochem J 289:687, 1993.

86. Hermesh H, Aizenberg D, Lapidot M, et al: Risk of malignant hyperthermia among patients with neuroleptic malignant syndrome and their families. Am J Psychiatry 145:1431, 1988.

87. Hopewell R, Yeater R, and Ullrich I: The effect of three test meals on exercise tolerance of an individual with McArdle's disease. J Am Coll Nutr 7:485, 1988.

88. Iaizzo PA, Wedel DJ, and Gallagher WJ: In vitro contracture testing for determination of susceptibility to malignant hyperthermia: A methodologic update. Mayo Clin Proc 66:998, 1991.

89. Kalow W, Britt BA, Terreau ME, et al: Metabolic error of muscle metabolism after recovery from malignant hyperthermia. Lancet 2:895, 1970.

90. Kanno T, Sudo K, Takeuchi I, et al: Hereditary deficiency of lactate dehydrogenase M-subunit. Clin Chim Acta 108:267, 1980.

91. Katsuya H, Misumi M, Ohtani Y, et al: Postanesthetic acute renal failure due to carnitine palmityl transferase deficiency. Anesthesiology 68: 945, 1988.

92. Keck PE Jr, Pope HG Jr, and McElroy

SL: Frequency and presentation of neuroleptic malignant syndrome: a prospective study. Am J Psychiatry 144:1344, 1987.

93. Keleman J, Rice DR, Bradley DM, et al: Familial myoadenylate deaminase deficiency and exertional myalgia. Neurology 32:857, 1982.

93a. Kent-Braun JA, Miller RG, and Weiner MW: Phases of metabolism during progressive exercise to fatigue in human skeletal muscle. Am J Physiol 75:573, 1993.

94. Kieval RI, Sotrel A, and Weinblatt ME: Chronic myopathy with a partial deficiency of the carnitine palmityl transferase enzyme. Arch Neurol 46:575, 1989.

95. Kissel JT, Beam W, Bresolin N, et al: Physiologic assessment of phosphoglycerate mutase deficiency: Incremental exercise tests. Neurology 35:828, 1985.

96. Knochel JP: Rhabdomyolysis and myoglobinuria. Annu Rev Med 33:435, 1982.

97. Kolb ME, Horne ML, and Martz R: Dantrolene in human malignant hyperthermia: A multicenter study. Anesthesiology 56:254, 1982.

98. Kushner RF and Berman SA: Are high-protein diets effective in McArdle's disease? Arch Neurol 47:383, 1990.

99. Larach MG, Landis JR, Bunn JS, and Diaz M: Prediction of malignant hyperthermia susceptibility in low-risk subjects: An epidemiologic investigation of caffeine halothane contracture responses. Anesthesiology 76:16, 1992.

100. Larsen UT, Juhl B, Hein-Sørensen O, et al: Complications during anaesthesia in patients with Duchenne's muscular dystrophy (a retrospective study). Can J Anaesth 36:418, 1989.

101. Lebo RV, Gorin F, Fletterick RJ, et al: High-resolution chromosome sorting and DNA spot-blot analysis assign McArdle's syndrome to chromosome 11. Science 225:57, 1984.

102. Lewis SF and Haller RG: The pathophysiology of McArdle's disease: Clues to regulation in exercise and fatigue. J Appl Physiol 61:391, 1986.

103. Linssen WHJD, Jacobs M, Stegeman DF, Joosten EMG, and Moleman J: Muscle fatigue in McArdle's disease: Muscle fibre conduction velocity and surface EMG frequency spectrum during ischaemic exercise. Brain 113:1779, 1990.

104. Loonen MCB, Busch HFM, Koster JF, et al: A family with different clinical forms of acid maltase deficiency (glycogenosis type II): biochemical and genetic studies. Neurology 31:1209, 1981.

105. MacLennan DH, Otsu K, Fujii J, et al: The role of the skeletal muscle ryanodine receptor gene in malignant hyperthermia. Symp Soc Exp Biol 46:189, 1992.

106. MacLennan DH and Phillips MS: Malignant hyperthermia. Science 256:789, 1992.

106a. Maekawa M, Sudo K, Kitajima M, et al: Detection and characterization of new genetic mutations in individuals heterozygous for lactate dehydrogenase-B (H) deficiency using DNA conformation polymorphism analysis and silver staining. Hum Genet 91:163, 1993.

107. Maekawa M, Sudo K, Li SSL, and Kanno T: Genotypic analysis of families with lactate dehydrogenase A (M) deficiency by selective DNA amplification. Human Genet 88:34, 1991.

108. Mandel H, Africk D, Blitzer M, et al: The importance of recognizing secondary carnitine deficiency in organic acidaemias: Case report in glutaric acidaemia type II. J Inher Metab Dis 11:397, 1988.

109. Martiniuk F, Bodkin M, Tzall S, et al: Identification of the base-pair substitution responsible for a human acid alpha glucosidase allele with lower "affinity" for glycogen (GAA 2) and transient gene expression in deficient cells. Am J Hum Genet 47:440, 1990.

110. Martiniuk F, Mehler M, Tzall S, et al: Extensive genetic heterogeneity in patients with acid alpha glucosidase deficiency as detected by abnormali-

ties of DNA and mRNA. Am J Hum Genet 47:73, 1990.

111. Martyn C, Jellinek EH, Webb JN: Lipid storage myopathy: Successful treatment with propranolol. BMJ 282:1997, 1981.

112. Mathieu A, Bogosian AJ, Ryan JF, et al: Recrudescence after survival of an initial episode of malignant hyperthermia. Anesthesiology 51:454, 1979.

113. Matsuishi T, Yoshino M, Terasawa K, et al: Childhood acid maltase deficiency: A clinical, biochemical, and morphologic study of three patients. Arch Neurol 41:47, 1984.

113a. Matthews PM, Allaire C, Shoubridge EA, et al: In vivo muscle magnetic resonance spectroscopy in the clinical investigation of mitochondrial disease. Neurology 41:114, 1991.

114. Maxwell JH and Bloor CM: Effects of conditioning on exertional rhabdomyolysis and serum creatine kinase after severe exercise. Enzyme 26:177, 1981.

115. Mayeda K, Weiss L, Lindahl R, et al: Localization of the human lactate dehydrogenase B gene on the short arm of chromosome 12. Am J Hum Genet 26:59, 1974.

116. McMaster KR, Powers JM, Hennigar GR Jr, et al: Nervous system involvement in type IV glycogenosis. Arch Pathol Lab Med 103:105, 1979.

117. Meinck HM, Goebel HH, Rumpf KW, et al: The forearm ischaemic work test: Hazardous to McArdle patients? J Neurol Neurosurg Psychiatry 45:1144, 1982.

118. Miller RG, Boska MD, Moussavi RS, et al: ^{31}P nuclear magnetic resonance studies of high energy phosphates and pH in human muscle fatigue: Comparison of aerobic and anaerobic exercise. J Clin Invest 81:1190, 1988.

119. Miller RG, Carson PJ, Moussavi RS, et al: The use of magnetic resonance spectroscopy to evaluate muscular fatigue and human muscle disease. Applied Radiology 18:33, 1989.

119a. Minetti C, Tnaji K, Chang HW, et al: Dystrophinopathy in two young boys with exercise-induced cramps and myoglobinuria. Eur J Pediatr 152:848, 1993.

119b. Miyajima H, Takahashi Y, Suzuki M, Shimizu T, and Kaneko E: Molecular characterization of gene expression in human lactate dehydrogenase-A deficiency. Neurology 43:1414, 1993.

119c. Moufarrej NA and Bertorini TE: Respiratory insufficiency in adult-type acid maltase deficiency. South Med J 86:560, 1993.

120. Mumpleby A, Trend PSJ, Chubb D, et al: The effect of a high protein diet on leucine and alanine turnover in acid maltase deficiency. J Neurol Neurosurg Psychiatry 52:954, 1989.

121. Murthy MSR and Pande SV: Malonyl-CoA binding site and the overt carnitine palmitoyltransferase activity reside on the opposite sides of the outer mitochondrial membrane. Proc Natl Acad Sci USA 84:378, 1987.

122. Nelson TE and Flewellen EH: Current concepts: The malignant hyperthermia syndrome. N Engl J Med 309:416, 1983.

123. Neustein HB: Fine structure of skeletal muscle in type III glycogenosis. Arch Pathol 88:130, 1969.

124. Newham DJ, Jones DA, Ghosh G, et al: Muscle fatigue and pain after eccentric contractions at long and short length. Clin Sci 74:553, 1988.

125. Nosek TM, Fender KY, and Godt RE: It is diprotonated inorganic phosphate that depresses force in skinned skeletal muscle fibers. Science 236:191, 1987.

126. Ohno K, Tanaka M, Sahashi K, et al: Mitochondrial DNA deletions in inherited recurrent myoglobinuria. Ann Neurol 29:364, 1991.

127. Olgin J, Argoz VZ, Rosenberg H, et al: Non-invasive evaluation of malignant hyperthermia susceptibility with phosphorus nuclear magnetic resonance spectroscopy. Anesthesiology 68:507, 1988.

128. Olmsted TR: Neuroleptic malignant syndrome: Guidelines for treatment and reinstitution of neuroleptics. South Med J 81:888, 1988.

129. Owen CA, Mubarak SJ, Hargens AR, et al: Intramuscular pressures with

limb compression. Clarification of the pathogenesis of the drug-induced muscle-compartment syndrome. N Engl J Med 300:1169, 1979.

130. Padberg GW, Wintzen AR, Giesberts AH, et al: Effects of a high-protein diet in acid maltase deficiency. J Neurol Sci 90:111, 1989.

131. Paterson DJ, Friedland JS, Bascom DA, et al: Changes in arterial K$^+$ and ventilation during exercise in normal subjects and subjects with McArdle's syndrome. J Physiol (Lond) 429:339, 1990.

132. Patterson VH, Kaiser KK, and Brooke MH: Exercising muscle does not produce hypoxanthine in adenylate deaminase deficiency. Neurology 33:784, 1983.

133. Penn AS: Myoglobinuria. In Engel AG and Banker BQ (eds): Myology: Basic and Clinical. McGraw-Hill, New York, 1986, p 1785.

134. Pierce LR, Wysowski DK, and Gross TP: Myopathy and rhabdomyolysis associated with lovastatin-gemfibrozil combination therapy. JAMA 264:71, 1990.

135. Pourmand R, Sanders DB, and Corwin HM: Late-onset McArdle's disease with unusual electromyographic findings. Arch Neurol 40:374, 1983.

135a. Quane KR, Healy JM, Keating KE, et al: Mutations in the ryanodine receptor gene in central core disease and maligant hyperthermia. Nat Genet 5:51, 1993.

136. Quinlan JG, Wedel DJ, and Iaizzo PA: Multiple-pulse stimulation and dantrolene in malignant hyperthermia. Muscle Nerve 13:904, 1990.

137. Quinlan JG, Iaizzo PA, Lambert EH, et al: Ankle dorsiflexor twitch properties in malignant hyperthermia. Muscle Nerve 12:119, 1989.

138. Raben N, Sherman J, Miller F, Mena H, and Plotz P: A 5' splice junction mutation leading to exon deletion in an Ashkenazic Jewish family with phosphofructokinase deficiency (Tarui disease). J Biol Chem 268:4963, 1993.

139. Radda GK: Control of bioenergetics: from cells to man by phosphorus nuclear-magnetic-resonance spectroscopy. Biochem Soc Trans 14:517, 1986.

140. Rebouche CJ and Engel AG: Kinetic compartmental analysis of carnitine metabolism in the human carnitine deficiency syndromes: Evidence for alterations in tissue carnitine transport. J Clin Invest 73:857, 1984.

141. Reuser AJJ, Kroos M, Willemsen R, et al: Clinical diversity in glycogenosis type II: Biosynthesis and in situ localization of acid q-glucosidase in mutant fibroblasts. J Clin Invest 79:1689, 1987.

141a. Rinaldo P, Schmidt-Sommerfield E, Posca AP, et al: Effect of treatment with glycine and L-carnitine in medium-chain acyl-coenzyme A dehydrogenase deficiency. J Pediatr 122:580, 1993.

142. Rosa R, George C, Fardeau M, et al: A new case of phosphoglycerate kinase deficiency: PGK creteil associated with rhabdomyolysis and lacking hemolytic anemia. Blood 60:84, 1982.

143. Rosenow EC and Engel AG: Acid maltase deficiency in adults presenting as respiratory failure. Am J Med 64:485, 1978.

144. Ross BD, Radda GK, Gadian DG, et al: Examination of a case of suspected McArdle's syndrome by ^{31}P nuclear magnetic resonance. N Engl J Med 304:1338, 1981.

145. Rossignol AM, Meyer M, Rossignol B, et al: La myocardiopathie de la glycogénose type III. Arch Fr Pediatr 36:303, 1979.

146. Rowland LP: Myoglobinuria, 1984. Can J Neurol Sci 11:1, 1984.

147. Rowland LP, DiMauro D, and Layzer RB: Phosphofructokinase deficiency. In Engel AG and Banker BQ (eds): Myology: Basic and Clinical. McGraw-Hill, New York, 1986, p 1603.

148. Rowland LP, Fahn S, Hirschberg E, and Harter DH: Myoglobinuria. Arch Neurol 10: 537, 1964.

149. Rowland LP, Layzer RB, and DiMauro S: Pathophysiology of metabolic muscle disorders. In Asbury AK, McKhann GM, and McDonald WI (eds): Diseases of the Nervous Sys-

tem. WB Saunders, Philadelphia, 1986, p 197.

150. Rubin E: Alcoholic myopathy in heart and skeletal muscle. N Engl J Med 301:28, 1979.

151. Sabina RL, Fishbein WN, Pezeshkpour G, Clarke PRH, and Holmes EW: Molecular analysis of the myoadenylate deaminase deficiencies. Neurology 42:170, 1992.

152. Sabina RL, Morisaki T, Clarke P, et al: Characterization of the human and rat myoadenylate deaminase genes. J Biol Chem 265:9423, 1990.

153. Sabina RL, Swain JL, Olanow W, et al: Myoadenylate deaminase deficiency: Functional and metabolic abnormalities associated with disruption of the perineal nucleotide cycle. J Clin Invest 73:720, 1984.

154. Sancho S, Navarro C, Fernández JM, et al: Skin biopsy findings in glycogenosis III: Clinical, biochemical and electrophysiological correlations. Ann Neurol 27:480, 1990.

155. Schlesinger JJ, Gandara D, and Bensch KG: Myoglobinuria associated with herpes-group viral infections. Arch Intern Med 138:422, 1978.

155a. Sekas G and Harbhajan SP: Hyperammonemia and carnitine deficiency in a patient receiving sulfadiazine and pyrimethamine. Am J Med 95:112, 1993.

156. Selby R, Starzl TE, Yunis E, et al: Liver transplantation for type IV glycogen storage disease. N Engl J Med 324:39, 1991.

157. Servidei S, Shanske S, Zeviani M, et al: McArdle's disease: Biochemical and molecular genetic studies. Ann Neurol 24:774, 1988.

158. Shapira Y, Glick B, Harel S, Vattin JJ, and Gutman A: Infantile idiopathic myopathic carnitine deficiency: Treatment with L-carnitine. Pediatr Neurol 9:35, 1993.

159. Shumate JB, Kaizer KK, Carroll JE, et al: Adenylate deaminase deficiency in a hypotonic infant. J Pediatr 96:885, 1980.

160. Shumate JB, Katnik R, Ruiz M, et al: Myoadenylate deaminase deficiency. Muscle Nerve 2:213, 1979.

161. Srinivasan AV, Murugappan SG, Krishnamurthy SG, et al: Neuroleptic malignant syndrome. J Neurol Neurosurg Psychiatry 53:514, 1990.

162. Stanley CA, DeLeeuw S, Coates PM, et al: Chronic cardiomyopathy and weakness or acute coma in children with a defect in carnitine uptake. Ann Neurol 30:709, 1991.

163. Starzl TE, Demetris AJ, Trucco M, et al: Chimerism after liver transplantation for type IV glycogen storage disease and type 1 Gaucher's disease. N Engl J Med 328:745, 1993.

164. Strugalska-Cynowska M: Disturbances in the activity of phosphorylase-b-kinase in a case of McArdle myopathy. Folia Histochemica et Cytochemica 5:151, 1967.

165. Tager JM, Hooghwinkel GJM, and Daems WTH (eds): Enzyme Therapy in Lysosomal Storage Diseases. North-Holland, Amsterdam, 1974.

166. Taroni F, Verderio E, Dworzak F, et al: Identification of a common mutation in the carnitine palmitoyltransferase II gene in familial recurrent myoglobinuria patients. Nat Genet 4:314,1993.

167. Taroni F, Verderio E, Fiorucci S, et al: Molecular characterization of inherited carnitine palmitoyltransferase II deficiency. Proc Nat Acad Sci USA 89:8429, 1992.

168. Tatsukawa H, Okuda J, Kondoh M, et al: Malignant hyperthermia caused by intravenous lidocaine for ventricular arrhythmia. Internal Medicine 31:1069, 1992.

168a. Tein I, De Vico OC, Ranucci D, and DiMauro S: Skin fibroblast carnitine uptake in secondary carnitine deficiency. J Inherit Metab Dis 16:135, 1993.

169. Tonin P, Lewis P, Servidei S, et al: Metabolic causes of myoglobinuria. Ann Neurol 27:181, 1990.

170. Tonin P, Shanske S, Miranda AF, et al: Phosphoglycerate kinase (PGK) deficiency: Biochemical and molecular genetic studies in a new myopathic variant (PGK Alberta). Neurology 3:387, 1993. Abstract.

171. Toscano A, Messina I, Tsujino S, et al: Molecular basis of muscle phosphog-

lycerate mutase (PGAM-M) deficiency in an Italian kindred. Neurology 43: A279, 1993. Abstract.

172. Tsujino S, Shanske S, and DiMauro S: Molecular genetic heterogeneity of myophosphorylase deficiency (McArdle's disease). N Engl J Med 329:241, 1993.

173. Tsujino S, Shanske S, Sakoda S, Fenichel G, and DiMauro S: The molecular genetic basis of muscle phosphoglycerate mutase (PGAM) deficiency. Am J Hum Genet 52:472, 1993.

174. Urbano-Marquez A, Estruch R, Navarro-Lopez F, et al: The effects of alcoholism on skeletal and cardiac muscle. N Engl J Med 320:409, 1989.

175. Usuki F, Higuchi I, Soejima Y, et al: Human acid maltase-deficient myogenic cell transformation with origin-defective SV40: characterization of a cloned line. Muscle Nerve 14:245, 1991.

176. Van den Berg IET and Berger R: Phosphorylase *b* kinase deficiency in man: A review. J Inherit Metab Dis 13:442, 1990.

177. Van Der Ploeg AT, Loonen MCB, Bolhuis PA, et al: Receptor-mediated uptake of acid a-glucosidase corrects lysosomal glycogen storage in cultured skeletal muscle. Pediatr Res 24:90, 1988.

178. Vandyke DH, Griggs RC, Markesbery W, et al: Hereditary carnitine deficiency of muscle. Neurology 25:154, 1975.

179. Vissing J, Lewis SF, Galbo H, and Haller RG: Effect of deficient muscular glycogenolysis on extramuscular fuel production in exercise. J Appl Physiol 72:1773, 1992.

180. Vladutiu GD, Hogan K, Saponara I, Tassini L, and Conroy J: Carnitine palmitoyl transferase deficiency in malignant hyperthermia. Muscle Nerve 16:485, 1993.

181. Vladutiu GD, Saponara I, Conroy JM, Grier RE, Brady L, and Brady P: Immunoquantitation of carnitine palmitoyl transferase in skeletal muscle of 31 patients. Neuromuscular Disorders 2:249, 1992.

182. Vora S, Durham S, de Martinville B, et al: Assignment of the human gene for muscle-type phosphofructokinase (PFKM) to chromosome 1 (region cen→q 32) using somatic cell hybrids and monoclonal anti-M antibody. Somat Cell Genet 8:95, 1982.

183. Wedel DJ: Malignant hyperthermia and neuromuscular disease. Neuromuscular Disorders 2:157, 1992.

183a. Wilkinson DA, Tonin P, Shanshe S, Lomkes A, Carlson GM, and DiMauro S: Clinical and biochemical features of 10 adult patients with muscle phophorylase kinase deficiency. Neurology 44:461, 1994.

184. Wortmann RL: Metabolic myopathies. Curr Opin Rheumatol 3:925, 1991.

185. Yang BZ, Ding JH, Enghild JJ, Bao Y, and Chen YT: Molecular cloning and nucleotide sequence of cDNA encoding human muscle glycogen debranching enzyme. J Biol Chem 267:9294, 1992.

186. Yang-Feng TL, Zheng K, Yu J, Yang BZ, Chen YT, and Kao FT: Assignment of the human glycogen debrancher gene to chromosome 1p21. Genomics 13:931, 1992.

186a. Zhang Y, Chen HS, Hanna VK, et al: A mutation of the human ryanodine receptor gene associated with central core disease. Nature Genet 5:46, 1993.

187. Zierz S and Engel AG: Are there two forms of carnitine palmitoyltransferase in muscle? Neurology 37:1785, 1987.

Chapter 8

MITOCHONDRIAL MYOPATHIES

The mitochondrial myopathies have only been recognized in the past 30 years. They were first identified when electron microscopic study of muscle found mitochondria of abnormal appearance or in abnormal numbers.[30] The subsequent recognition of a light-microscopic marker for mitochondrial disease, the "ragged red fiber," led to the identification of a number of clinically and biochemically heterogeneous disorders of muscle and other systems.[35]

Mitochondrial replication takes place by the interaction of nonchromosomal, mitochondrial DNA and nuclear, autosomal DNA. The entire mitochondrial genome has been sequenced, and the nuclear genes encoding mitochondrial proteins have also been established. The correlation of clinical syndromes and findings with the molecular biology of mitochondria is rapidly clarifying the extremely confusing literature on mitochondrial myopathies.

This chapter first reviews the structure, biochemistry, and genetics of mitochondria and then describes the generally accepted clinical syndromes related to generalized or specific genetic lesions of mitochondria. The chapter concludes with a review of the still unclear role of mitochondria in other disorders in which muscle mitochondria is abnormal and muscle biopsy may be of diagnostic help, but in which myopathy and muscle weakness are either absent or unimpressive.

MITOCHONDRIAL STRUCTURE

The mitochondrion is an intracellular organelle that is compartmentalized by the outer and inner membranes; the inner membrane is intricately folded into cristae (see Figs. 7–1 and 8–1). The outer membrane is highly permeable and permits access to the intermembrane space. In contrast, the inner membrane serves as an impermeable barrier regulating access of ions and metabolites to the mitochondrial matrix (the space confined by the inner membrane). The respiratory chain enzymes are found within the folded inner membrane.

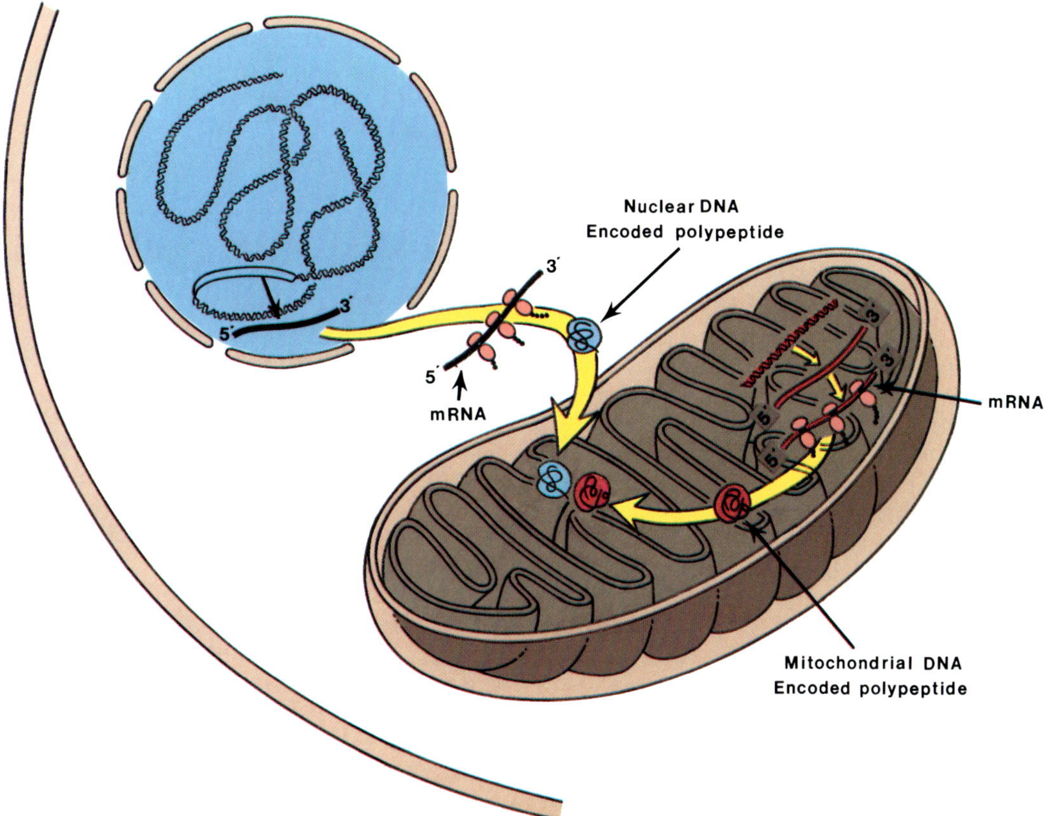

Figure 8–1. Proteins of four respiratory chain enzymes (complexes I, III, IV, V) are encoded by both nuclear and mitochondrial DNA. The polypeptides encoded by nuclear DNA are translated in the cell cytoplasm, transported into the mitochondrion, and assembled with polypeptides translated in the mitochondrion. The diagram shows the mRNA translation in ribosomes in both cytoplasm and mitochondrion.

MITOCHONDRIAL BIOCHEMISTRY

The mitochondria are important in the generation of muscle energy from cellular substrates. The substrates derived from lipids, carbohydrates, and amino acids are oxidized aerobically in mitochondria (see Fig. 7–1). Lipids are first metabolized by the liver and other tissues to form fatty acids; carbohydrates are converted by glycolysis to pyruvate; and protein is first hydrolyzed to amino acids. Fatty acids, pyruvate, and amino acids are then actively transported into the mitochondria.

Long-chain fatty acids, attached to carnitine, enter the mitochondrial ma-trix through the inner mitochondrial membrane (see Chapter 7, p. 250) prior to their degradation through beta-oxidation. Pyruvate must be converted to acetyl coenzyme A (acetyl-CoA) before entry into the citric acid cycle. Amino acids provide a source of energy by conversion to pyruvate or by direct conversion to intermediates of the citric acid cycle. The reduced forms of nicotinamide adenine dinucleotide (NADH) and flavin adenine dinucleotide ($FADH_2$) formed in glycolysis, fatty acid oxidation, and the citric acid cycle each contain a pair of electrons that can be transferred to molecular oxygen; in this process energy is liberated and used to generate adenosine triphosphate (ATP).

Transferring electrons from NADH and FADH$_2$ to oxygen by electron carriers coupled to ATP synthesis is called oxidative phosphorylation. This process takes place in the respiratory chain within the inner membrane of the mitochondria (see Fig. 7–1).

MITOCHONDRIAL GENETICS

The molecular genetics of mitochondria[1,56] differs from that of chromosomally derived organelles. The unique features of mitochondrial reproduction account for the inheritance pattern and the clinical heterogeneity of mitochondrial myopathies (Table 8–1). Each mitochondrion possesses DNA genomes that have been sequestered away from nuclear DNA. Because mitochondrial genes are located on nonchromosomal DNA, the genetics of many mitochondrial diseases are non-Mendelian. Mitochondrial DNA and nuclear DNA combine to direct synthesis of certain proteins; others are encoded by mitochondria alone. Mitochondrial DNA (mtDNA) consists of a double-stranded, circular DNA molecule composed of 16,569 base pairs. It encodes for 22 transfer RNAs, two ribosomal RNAs,

Table 8–1 PROPERTIES OF MITOCHONDRIAL DNA (mtDNA)

Maternally inherited
Genome consists of circular, double-stranded
  DNA with 16,569 base pairs
Mitochondrial genes encode for:
  22 transfer RNA
   2 ribosomal RNA
 13 polypeptide subunits of
  respiratory chain enzymes*

Complex I	7 subunits
Complex III	1 subunit
Complex IV	3 subunits
Complex V	2 subunits

High incidence of mutations
Poor repair of mtDNA
Multiple mtDNA genes in each cell

*Mitochondrial Complex II and other mitochondrial proteins, including subunits of other complexes, are encoded by nuclear DNA. (See pp. 296–297 and Fig. 8–1).

and 13 polypeptide subunits of the five multienzyme complexes that constitute respiratory chain enzymes. Complex I, made up of 25 polypeptides, has 7 of these encoded by mtDNA; Complex III has 1 of 11 from mtDNA; Complex IV includes 13 polypeptides, 3 derived from mtDNA; and 2 of the 12 polypeptides of Complex V arise from mtDNA. Only polypeptides of Complex II have no mtDNA contribution. Components of the respiratory chain enzymes that arise from nuclear (rather than mitochondrial) DNA must be transcribed in the nucleus of the cell and then translated in the ribosomes of the cell cytoplasm (see Fig. 8–1). Following translation, these polypeptides must be transported into the mitochondrion and assembled in conjunction with the translated products of mitochondrial DNA to form the respiratory chain enzymes. The complexity of assembly of the respiratory chain enzymes exposes the system to potential sources of error.

Mitochondrial DNA has unique features that are important in genetics; these include maternal inheritance,[13a] frequent spontaneous mutations, and a large number of copies of mtDNA per cell (versus only two alleles for nuclear DNA). In general, patients with a single mtDNA deletion constitute sporadic cases of mitochondrial disorders, which suggests that deletions arise as fresh mutational events.[5a] The mitochondrial genomes are found within the cytoplasm of germline cells (oocytes and sperm), and inheritance occurs through direct cytoplasmic continuity, independent of nuclear DNA. The minute sperm and the very large egg contribute unequal numbers of mitochondrial genomes to their offspring at the time of fertilization. The cytoplasm of the oocyte accounts for nearly all of the mitochondria contributed to the zygote. Thus, *many mitochondrial genes are derived through maternal inheritance.* The large number of mtDNAs per cell are randomly distributed in ova, so that different offspring receiving mutant mtDNA receive differing numbers of mutant mtDNA as opposed to wild-type (normal) mtDNA. Moreover, in subsequent cell development in the zygote, different populations of mtDNA will give rise to different tissues. Recent work suggests that the proportion of mutant mtDNA is determined during oogenesis or early embryonic development, while random replicative (mitotic) segregation after germ layer establishment accounts for variations between tissues.[30a] This difference in mitochondrial populations, termed *heteroplasmy*, accounts for the marked differences within a kindred in the clinical manifestations of a mutation in mtDNA, both in severity and specific organ involvement.

The nature of the molecular defects in a number of mitochondrial myopathies are now known. In other myopathies, biochemical characterization is possible but the genetic mechanism is uncertain. In still others, histologic evidence for mitochondrial disease has been found, but neither a specific genetic nor biochemical basis has been defined.

THE DIAGNOSIS OF MITOCHONDRIAL DISEASE

The neuromuscular symptoms and signs of mitochondrial disease are often overlooked by both the patient and physician. The commonest indication of a mitochondrial neuromuscular disease is progressive external ophthalmoplegia (PEO), which is insidious in both onset and progression. *Diplopia seldom if ever occurs*, even in patients who have virtually no eye movement. If ptosis is not present, or if it is symmetrical and of slight extent, the unsuspecting physician may overlook major abnormalities in evaluating the patient. The eye muscles must be examined carefully, with emphasis on testing whether the patient has *full* ocular motility. One must assess the ability of the patient to "fill the outer and inner canthi" (that is, move the eye to the extremes of lateral and medial gaze).

Limb muscle weakness is usually only slight in mitochondrial myopathies; most functional tests can be performed, albeit with difficulty. As in other myopathies, patients often deny limb weakness.

Many nonmuscular symptoms and signs should suggest mitochondrial disease. The family history often provides the important clue and must be combed for the disorders listed on Table 8–2. Multiple symmetric lipomas are usually evident but are often ignored; a scar at the site of removal may be the only indication of their previous existence. As discussed earlier, however, heteroplasmy may lead to extreme variation from patient to patient within a kindred.

PROGRESSIVE EXTERNAL OPHTHALMOPLEGIA SYNDROMES AND RAGGED RED FIBERS

Progressive external ophthalmoplegia (PEO) denotes a clinical syndrome in which ptosis and limitation of extraocular muscle movements develop insidiously and progress at a variable but usually relentless rate (see Chapter 2). Prior to 1972, morphologically abnormal

Table 8–2 NONMUSCULAR MANIFESTATIONS OF MITOCHONDRIAL DISEASE

Site	Abnormality
Skin	Lipomas (especially multiple, symmetric); ichthyosis
Eye	Cataracts; retinitis pigmentosa
Heart	Conduction disturbances; cardiomyopathy
Gastrointestinal system	Intestinal pseudo-obstruction
Endocrine system	Short stature; diabetes; goiter; primary ovarian failure
Nervous system	Deafness; ataxia (often intermittent); neuropathy; seizures; strokes

mitochondria in selected muscle biopsies had been described in a variety of conditions, including muscular dystrophy,[37] pleoconial and megaconial myopathies,[48,49] and hypermetabolism of nonthyroid origin.[30] A definite association, however, between abnormal mitochondria and a consistent phenotype that includes PEO went unrecognized until the description by Olson and colleagues[35] of "oculocraniosomatic neuromuscular disease with ragged red fibers." The cumbersome name was adopted originally since the disorder affected many regions of the neuraxis ("oculocraniosomatic"), had no known cause (thus "neuromuscular disease" was used in place of myopathy), and demonstrated muscle fibers with red-staining material in modified trichrome stains ("ragged red fibers") (Fig. 8–2A). Such cases had been described by Kearns and Sayre,[23] Shy and associates,[50] and Drachman,[12] but the clini-

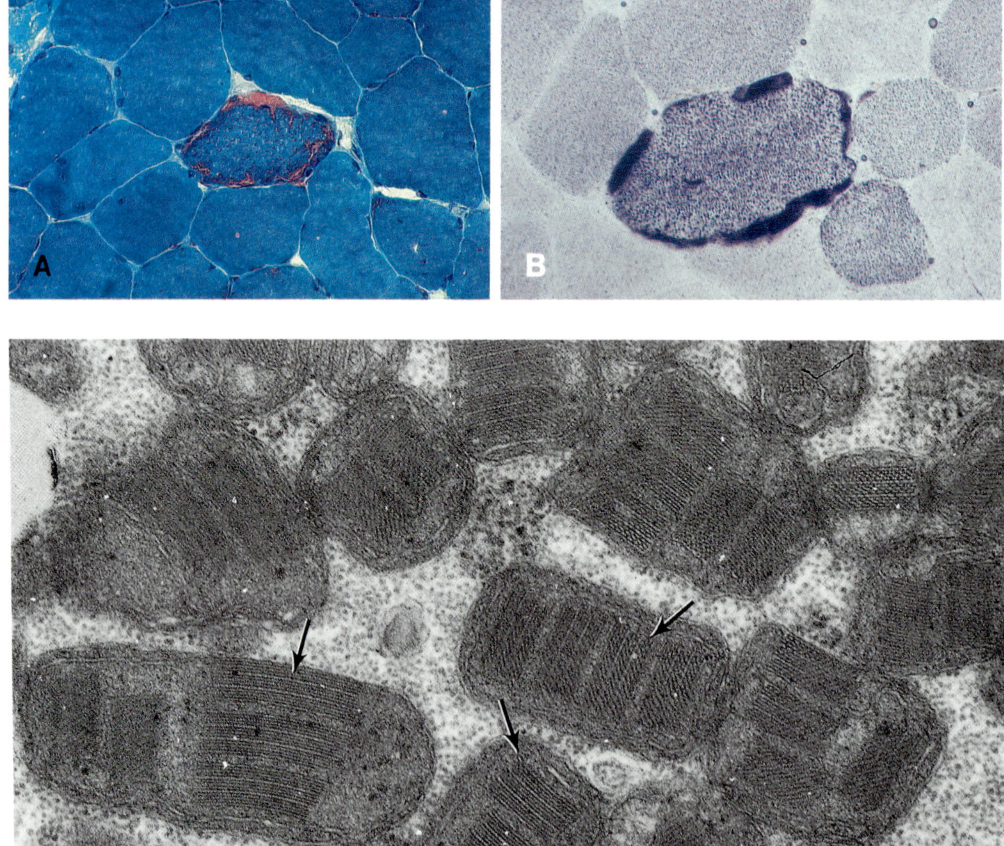

Figure 8–2. (*A*) Typical ragged red fiber showing subsarcolemmal deposits of aggregated mitochondria (red-staining material) (trichrome). (*B*) Subsarcolemmal mitochondrial aggregates positive for succinic dehydrogenase (SDH). (*C*) Boxcar-type intramitochondrial (*arrows*) crystalline inclusions characteristic of ragged red fibers (electron micrograph).

copathologic correlation of mitochondrial myopathy with the PEO syndrome had not been recognized.

Clinical Features

Most patients with fixed, nonfluctuating, insidiously progressive ptosis and ophthalmoplegia have a mitochondrial myopathy. (Less common conditions with similar eye findings include oculopharyngeal muscular dystrophy and centronuclear myopathy, but other features usually differentiate these conditions from mitochondrial PEO disorders; see Chapters 3 and 5.) The degree of eye muscle impairment can vary widely. In some patients, unilateral ptosis may be the only manifestation, but others have severe bilateral ptosis and complete loss of extraocular movements. Patients with PEO and ragged red fibers rarely complain of diplopia; in myasthenia gravis, on the other hand, extraocular muscle weakness fluctuates and diplopia is common.

More recently, the term "oculocraniosomatic neuromuscular disease" has been dropped in favor of dividing the patients into two groups: Kearns-Sayre syndrome (KSS) and familial PEO syndromes (Table 8–3).

KEARNS-SAYRE SYNDROME

The KSS typically has its onset before age 20 and, importantly, has no family history.[43] The characteristic clinical findings are the triad of PEO, pigmentary degeneration of the retina, and

heart block.[5,43] The full-blown expression of KSS also includes other features listed in Table 8–4. These abnormalities emphasize the multisystem nature of this condition. Many patients will have only partial expression of this disorder.

FAMILIAL PEO SYNDROME

A subgroup of PEO with ragged red fibers is clinically distinct from KSS and has an inherited basis. The familial nature was first emphasized in a report by Iannacone and colleagues in 1974.[22]

Table 8–4 FEATURES OF KEARNS-SAYRE SYNDROME

CLINICAL FEATURES
Progressive external ophthalmoplegia*
Mitochondrial myopathy (ragged red fibers)*
Pigmentary degeneration of retina*
Heart block*
Ataxia
Hearing loss
Dementia
Short stature (growth hormone deficiency)
Delayed secondary sexual characteristics
Hypoparathyroidism (basal ganglia calcification)
Hypothyroidism
Peripheral neuropathy
Elevated cerebrospinal fluid protein
Depressed ventilatory drive[3]

GENETIC DEFECT
Single mtDNA deletions causing abnormal protein translation

*Syndrome usually defined by these four features.

Table 8–3 PROGRESSIVE EXTERNAL OPHTHALMOPLEGIA (PEO) SYNDROMES WITH RAGGED RED FIBERS

Disorder	*Mitochondrial (mt) DNA Defect*
Kearns-Sayre syndrome	Single mtDNA deletions
Familial PEO syndromes	
Maternal inheritance	None
Autosomal dominant inheritance	Multiple mtDNA deletions

Two distinct familial syndromes exist: One is maternally inherited via a mitochondrial genetic abnormality,[22] and the other is autosomal dominant.[60,63]

Unlike KSS, the maternally inherited disorder does not have multisystem effects. An important difference is that familial PEO patients do not have the risk of heart block. The major manifestations of familial PEO are varying degrees of muscle weakness of neck and limbs, associated with the ophthalmoplegia. In severe cases, patients may require assisted ambulation (cane or walker or, rarely, a wheelchair) and may have respiratory insufficiency.[3]

In the autosomal dominant variant of PEO with ragged red fibers, the patients exhibit tremor, ataxia, and a sensorimotor peripheral neuropathy, as well as hearing loss. In the absence of a family history, these patients may be difficult to distinguish from those with KSS, but there are distinctions in mtDNA mutations between KSS[33] and the autosomal dominant variant,[60,63] as discussed below (see Table 8–3).

An important feature of PEO syndromes associated with mitochondrial myopathies (both familial cases and KSS) is a depressed ventilatory drive.[3] This feature often goes unrecognized but may predispose patients to life-threatening hypoxia. Central nervous system depressants, high altitude, or respiratory infections may precipitate this complication, which is independent of muscle weakness.[3]

Laboratory Features

In both KSS and familial PEO syndromes, muscle biopsies reveal ragged red fibers in the modified trichrome stain (Fig. 8–2A). The mitochondrial accumulations are highlighted in oxidative enzyme stains (succinate dehydrogenase or nicotinamide adenine dehydrogenase) (Fig. 8–2B). Some ragged red fibers show excess lipid. At the ultrastructural level, increased numbers of mitochondria can be demonstrated, many of which appear enlarged, with altered patterns of mitochondrial cristae (Fig. 8–2C).

The creatine kinase (CK) level is usually normal. Levels of pyruvate, lactate, and alanine may be increased in the blood of these patients.[8]

Electrophysiologic changes vary in limb muscles of patients with mitochondrial myopathies. Many have minimal limb weakness, and the electromyogram (EMG) is normal. In others, a myopathic change will be encountered. In KSS, electrophysiologic abnormalities may show an associated peripheral neuropathy consisting of a mild slowing of motor conduction velocities or small sensory nerve action potentials, reflecting axonal degeneration.[58] These abnormalities are presumably a result of abnormal mitochondria, which have been seen in the Schwann cell cytoplasm.

Cardiac conduction defects are highly characteristic of KSS and range from first-degree to complete atrial-ventricular block.[5,8,43] The electroencephalogram (EEG) may show nonspecific slowing. In KSS patients with hypoparathyroidism, the computed tomography (CT) scan often shows calcification of the basal ganglia.[8,44] Autopsy studies show spongiform changes in the deep white matter of hemispheres, cerebellum, and brain stem.[8] Similar changes are seen in patients with other mitochondrial encephalomyopathies.

Genetics

KEARNS-SAYRE SYNDROME

mtDNA can be isolated and separated from nuclear DNA in any tissue of interest. In patients with KSS, two populations of mtDNA are present: the normal or wild-type, and the abnormal or mutant. Heteroplasmy refers to the presence of both normal and mutant mtDNA in the same cell. In KSS, single mtDNA deletions result in an additional band on Southern blot analysis (Fig. 8–3). The mtDNA deletions vary in size and do not correlate with clinical manifesta-

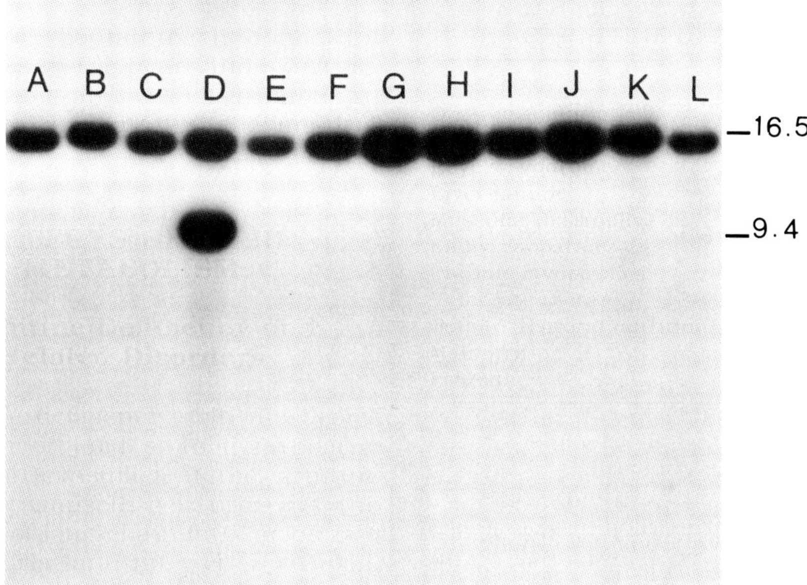

Figure 8–3. Southern blot analysis of mitochondrial DNA in patients with mitochondrial myopathies. Only the patient with Kearns-Sayre syndrome, Lane D, demonstrates heteroplasmy (two populations of mitochondria). The 16.5 kb band is the normal mitochondrial genome; the smaller (9.4 kb) band represents populations of deleted mitochondria. Lanes A to C show mitochondrial DNA from normals. Lanes G to L show mitochondrial DNA from familial PEO patients without deletions. Lane E is from a patient with MERRF syndrome; Lane F is from a MELAS patient.

tions.[21,61] The reported percentage of affected mitochondrial genomes in a muscle biopsy varies widely, from 27% to 85%.[33] Deleted mtDNA can also be seen in other tissues (for example, brain, liver, and fibroblasts), but the percentage is lower than in muscle. The absence of mutant mtDNA from a tissue reflects both mitotic segregation early in embryogenesis and selection against a mutant cell line in a rapidly dividing tissue. The latter explanation accounts for the infrequent number of mtDNA deletions found in peripheral blood leukocytes.

The presence of single mtDNA deletions can be used as a diagnostic test for KSS. Because KSS is a sporadic, nonhereditary disease, it can be determined that other family members are not at risk if a single mtDNA deletion is found. Such analysis is especially helpful for families in which a sporadic case of PEO

and ragged red fibers occurs without the findings of a multisystem disorder. It is now known that KSS with proven mtDNA deletions can occur without full expression of the multisystem features of the disease.[33]

FAMILIAL PEO SYNDROME

Familial PEO with ragged red fibers may be maternally inherited. Deletions of mtDNA have not been found in affected patients with maternal inheritance, an important difference from the laboratory findings with KSS (see Fig. 8–3) or the autosomal dominant variant of PEO.

In the autosomal dominant variant of PEO with ragged red fibers, large-scale multiple mtDNA deletions are found,[60,61,63] in contrast to the single mtDNA deletions found in KSS (see Table 8–3).

Pathogenesis

The lack of correlation of specific respiratory-chain enzyme deficiencies with mtDNA deletions in KSS or the autosomal dominant variant can be explained by the finding that deleted mitochondrial genomes remain transcriptionally active but are not translated. Thus, mitochondrial genomes with deleted mtDNA fail to synthesize polypeptides of the respiratory chain. The extent of clinical expression of the mitochondrial deficit is related to the ratio of wild and mutant mtDNA in the cell as a result of mitotic segregation. The clinical expression increases with age because oxidative capacity falls with age, so that mutant genomes have more profound effects in older patients.[53]

The cause of mtDNA deletions in KSS is unknown. Since KSS cases are sporadic, it has been assumed that the mutation takes place in the zygote (after fertilization). In the autosomal dominant variant associated with multiple deletions, evidence suggests a more complex mechanism, in which there is a mutation of a nuclear gene encoding a protein involved in a nuclear-controlled mechanism of mtDNA replication. A failure or disruption of binding of this nuclear-encoded protein during mtDNA replication results in multiple deletions.[60,63]

Treatment

No specific treatment has emerged for patients with mitochondrial myopathies. Dietary supplementation with artificial electron acceptors such as coenzyme Q has been suggested, but no controlled trials have been done. In some patients with KSS, coenzyme Q was reported to increase exercise tolerance and improve the electrocardiogram.[4a,14,34]

In patients in whom ptosis severely impairs vision, eyelid surgery may be appropriate. Two major approaches are used: lid resection and lid suspension. In lid resection, the highly redundant upper-lid tissue is resected. This plastic surgical procedure yields cosmetically excellent results but needs to be repeated frequently (often within months). Lid suspension employs either autologous fascia or prosthetic materials such as silicone elastomer (Silastic) (Fig. 8–4). This approach permanently corrects ptosis and has the advantage of easy reversibility. Neither procedure should be done if facial weakness interferes with eye closure.

In KSS the risk of progression to complete heart block and sudden death requires monitoring, and consideration of early pacemaker placement. Some patients require special attention for manifestations of endocrinopathies including hypoparathyroidism, hypothyroidism, and growth hormone deficiency. Others may need treatment for seizures. A complicating peripheral neuropathy may cause distal lower-extremity weakness requiring ankle-foot orthoses.

Awareness of depressed ventilatory drive can be extremely important for patients with PEO syndromes associated with mitochondrial myopathies,[3] particularly if surgery or sedation is planned. The following case history illustrates the consequences of reduced ventilatory drive.

Case History

A 31-year-old woman had a familial PEO syndrome with ragged red fibers, associated with neck and proximal limb weakness. She was hospitalized at 39 weeks' gestation in early labor. There was a history of respiratory arrest during a previous delivery after receiving a "sedative." On admission to the labor unit, she had no respiratory symptoms. As spontaneous labor progressed, she became anxious, and 1 mg of butorphanol tartrate was given intravenously. Over the next 5 minutes she became short of breath. An arterial blood gas analysis revealed PO_2 48 mmHg, PCO_2 62 mm Hg, HCO_3^- 28 mEq/L, and pH 7.26. Oxygen was administered by mask, and the patient improved. Within the hour she delivered a baby boy with an Apgar

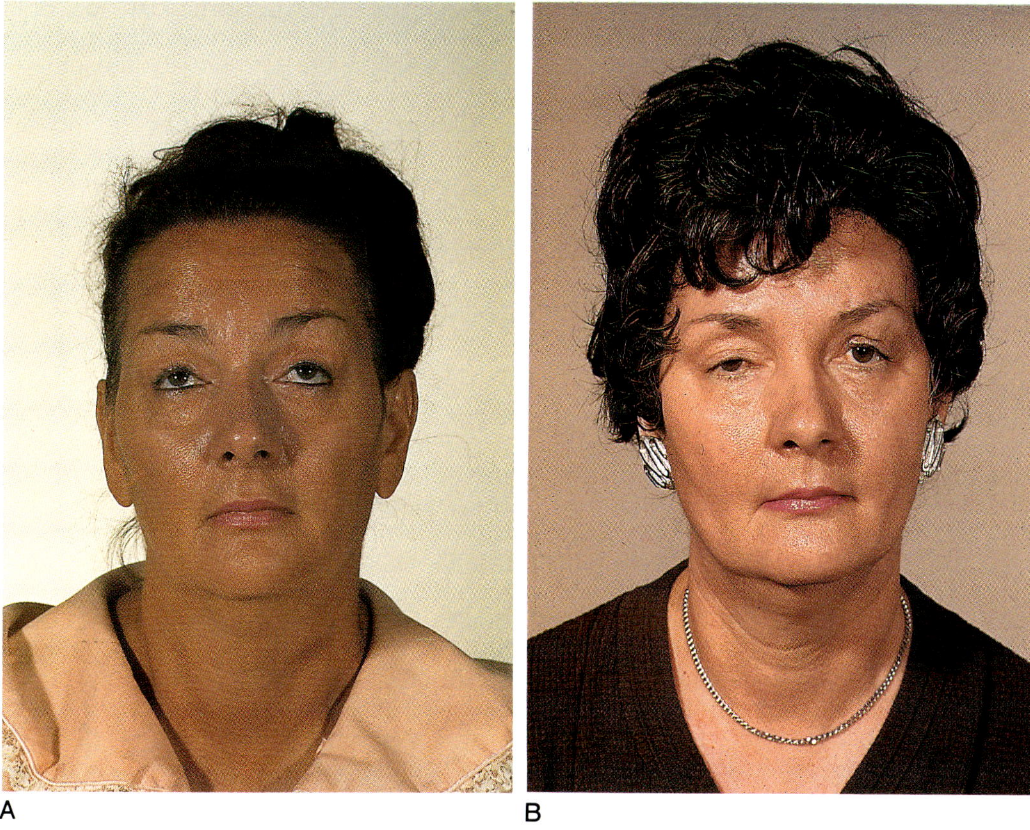

A   B

Figure 8–4. Treatment of ptosis in a woman with progressive external ophthalmoplegia. (*A*) The patient has recurrent, bilateral ptosis that persisted after four previous lid resections. (*B*) Silicone elastomer (Silastic) sling insertion corrected ptosis of the left eye. The cosmetic result is often better if previous lid surgery has not been performed.

score of 5 at 1 minute and 9 at 5 minutes. After the delivery she developed dyspnea, agitation, and cyanosis and required intubation and mechanical ventilation. Attempts to wean her from the ventilator were poorly tolerated initially, but she was extubated after 12 days.

Ventilatory drive studies were performed 4 months after this incident. These studies indicated a markedly depressed response to hypoxia (hypoxic ventilatory response, $+0.03$ L/min per %SaO_2, $n = -0.6$ L/min per %SaO_2) and hypercapnia (hypercapnic ventilatory response, 0.12 L/min per mmHg; $n = < 1.0$ L/min per mmHg).

Comment: The clinical features and ventilatory drive studies in this patient with familial PEO demonstrate that patients with mitochondrial myopathies are extremely sensitive to central nervous system depres-

sants. The ventilatory drive studies demonstrate the lack of response to hypoxia and hypercapnia as a respiratory stimulus. This lack of response, especially to hypoxia, is independent of muscle weakness. Impaired ventilatory drive occurs not only in PEO syndromes but also in other mitochondrial myopathies.[3]

MYOCLONIC EPILEPSY AND RAGGED RED FIBERS

In 1973 Tsairis and colleagues reported a family with the syndrome of myoclonic epilepsy associated with a mitochondrial myopathy.[54] Subsequent reports and molecular genetic studies[13c,16,29,42,57] indicate that this condition, now referred to by the acronym MERRF, is a distinct nosologic entity.

Clinical Features

The full expression of MERRF (Table 8–5) includes a mitochondrial myopathy with limb weakness but no PEO, and myoclonus, generalized seizures, intellectual deterioration, ataxia, and hearing loss. As with most mitochondrial disorders, individual manifestations vary. The original MERRF family, illustrated in Figure 8–5 and further described after 18 years of follow-up,[29] provides an excellent example of the heterogeneity of a mitochondrial disease within a family. The proband developed the full expression of the syndrome by the time of his death at age 36 years. In contrast, his mother was not symptomatic until age 33; she had insidiously progressive weakness in a limb-girdle distribution, indistinguishable from muscular dystrophy. The proband's sisters presented with myoclonus and generalized seizures at ages 10 and 8, respectively, and subsequently developed gait ataxia, hearing loss, and intellectual decline; both died before age 20. Other reported families have exhibited similar heterogeneity.[42,57]

Laboratory Features

The muscle biopsies in MERRF have typical ragged red fibers. Using electron microscopy, accumulations of abnor-

Table 8–5 MYOCLONIC EPILEPSY AND RAGGED RED FIBERS (MERRF)

CLINICAL FEATURES
  Mitochondrial myopathy
  Myoclonus
  Generalized seizures
  Intellectual deterioration
  Ataxia
  Hearing loss

GENETIC DEFECT
  Point mutation of tRNA lysine

mal, large mitochondria can be observed; these often show crystalline inclusions. The CK level may be normal or mildly elevated. Serum lactate is usually increased. The EEG shows diffuse slowing, with bursts of spike and wave discharges. A magnetic resonance imaging (MRI) scan may show cerebral atrophy.

Genetics

A defect in mtDNA has now been identified in MERRF families.[13c,45,47,59] A point mutation, an adenine-to-guanine substitution at nucleotide 8344 in the transfer RNA gene for lysine (tRNA^{Lys}) of mtDNA, causes the disorder (Fig. 8–6). This abnormality can be detected with the polymerase chain reaction of leukocytes or muscle (see Chapter 3 for full discussion of the use of this technique), which can be used for clinical diagnosis. The mtDNA population appears heteroplasmic in the MERRF syndrome, with both wild-type and mutant mtDNA represented. The percentage of residual normal mtDNA correlates with phenotype. The proportion of mutant mtDNA in blood correlates with age of onset and clinical severity.[18a] In rare MERRF cases, this point mutation cannot be found.[59]

Pathogenesis

The mutation of mtDNA correlates with the non-Mendelian maternal inheritance previously observed.[29,42,57] The mutation found in the tRNA gene for lysine in MERRF patients disrupts synthesis of mitochondrial-encoded polypeptides. Each tRNA gene of mitochondria contains approximately 75 nucleotides.[39] Each tRNA for each of the different amino acids has a unique sequence. A point mutation, such as the one found in MERRF (and also for MELAS, as described below) alters the normal structural conformation of the tRNA, impairing translation, probably at the ribosome.

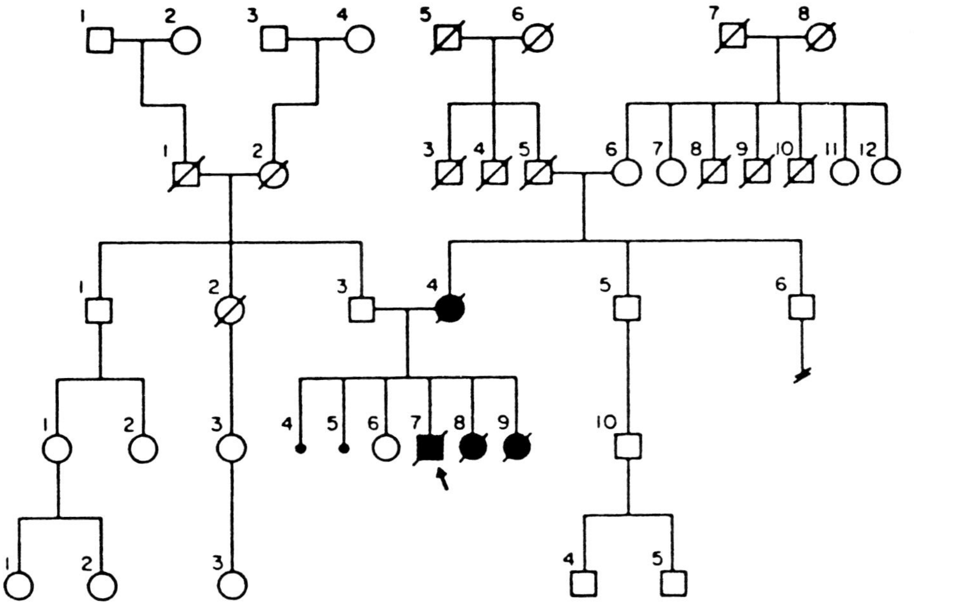

Patient	Age at death (yr)	Mitochondrial Myopathy	Myoclonus	Ataxia	Generalized Seizures	Dementia	Hearing Loss
III-4	47	+ + +	+	+	0	0	0
IV-7	36	+ + +	+ + +	+	+	+	+
IV-8	16	+ + +	+ + +	+ + +	+ +	+	+
IV-9	12	+ + +	+ + +	+ + +	+ +	+	+

Figure 8–5. Pedigree of family with myocionic epilepsy and ragged red fibers (MERRF). O = normal female subjects; □ = normal male subjects, ●,■ = affected members; ∅⊘◐◩ = deceased members; • = miscarriages. The proband is indicated by an arrow. The table shows the heterogeneity of clinical manifestations: 0 = absent; + = mild; ++ = moderate; +++ = severe. (From Lombes, et al.[29] Reprinted with permission from Annals of Neurology 26:20, 1989.)

MERRF Mutation

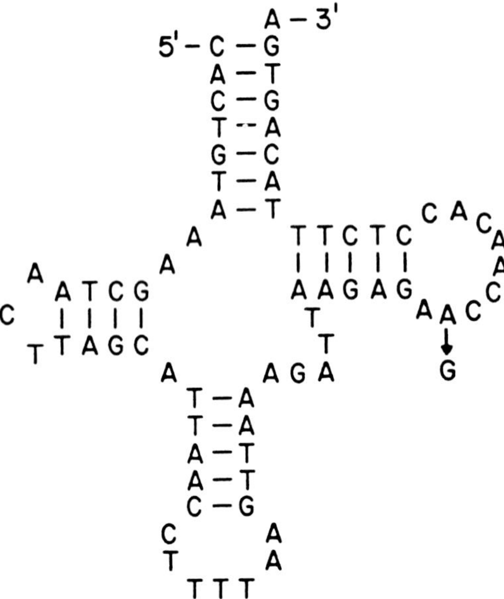

Figure 8–6. The four-arm cloverleaf structure of mitochondrial transfer RNA (mtRNA) for lysine, showing the MERRF point mutation at nucleotide 8344, consisting of an adenine (A) to guanine (G) substitution (*arrow*).

Treatment

No specific treatment has been effective for MERRF patients. Supportive care remains essential and is helpful for aspects of the disease. Myoclonus usually can be controlled effectively with clonazepam; other appropriate anticonvulsants (valproate, carbamazepine, phenytoin, or others) must be used for generalized seizures. Many patients require ambulatory aids for muscle weakness and ataxia.

MITOCHONDRIAL MYOPATHY, ENCEPHALOPATHY, LACTIC ACIDOSIS, AND STROKELIKE EPISODES

This multisystem mitochondrial encephalomyopathy usually is referred to by the acronym MELAS.[36] A specific mutation in mtDNA has been identified as a cause for this condition.[17,24b,51b] Cases of MERRF and MELAS sometimes overlap clinically.[15,20,25]

Clinical Features

Clinical heterogeneity occurs in MELAS, as in all mitochondrial encephalomyopathies (Table 8–6).[2,13,19,36,46,51] The disease begins in childhood after a normal birth and uneventful early development. Patients have stunted growth and recurrent strokelike episodes manifesting as hemiparesis, hemianopsia, or cortical blindness. Episodic vomiting may occur, and some patients have hearing loss. Focal or generalized seizures and occasionally myoclonic epilepsy may be present. Full expression of the disease leads to dementia, a bedridden state, and death, often before 20 years of age.[36]

Although MELAS is usually distinct from other multisystem mitochondrial encephalomyopathies, MERRF patients may have strokelike episodes,[20] and some MELAS patients have a cerebellar syndrome, as well as PEO.[13b,17,32a]

Laboratory Features

A mitochondrial myopathy with typical ragged red fibers occurs in MELAS.

Table 8–6 FEATURES OF MITOCHONDRIAL MYOPATHY, ENCEPHALOPATHY, LACTIC ACIDOSIS, AND STROKELIKE EPISODES (MELAS)

CLINICAL FEATURES
  Mitochondrial myopathy
  Short stature
  Strokelike episodes (hemiparesis, hemianopsia, cortical blindness)
  Episodic vomiting
  Hearing loss
  Seizures
  Intellectual deterioration

GENE DEFECT
  Point mutation of tRNA

Serum CK and lactic acid levels may be elevated. The EMG will be normal in most patients but may be myopathic. In many patients, the CT scan shows focal lucencies and basal ganglia calcifications.[36] Focal areas of encephalomalacia and a spongy state of the brain with microcystic liquefaction may be prominent.[19,46]

Genetics

MELAS may be familial,[19,46] but far less often than MERRF. No large pedigrees of MELAS have been reported. A point mutation of mtDNA causes this disease (Fig. 8–7).[17,24] Like MERRF, the defect occurs in a tRNA gene. An adenine-to-guanine substitution occurs in the tRNA for leucine at nucleotide 3243. This mutation creates a new restriction enzyme site, providing a simple molecular diagnostic test for the disease. The mutant DNA coexists with normal mtDNA (heteroplasmy).

MELAS Mutation

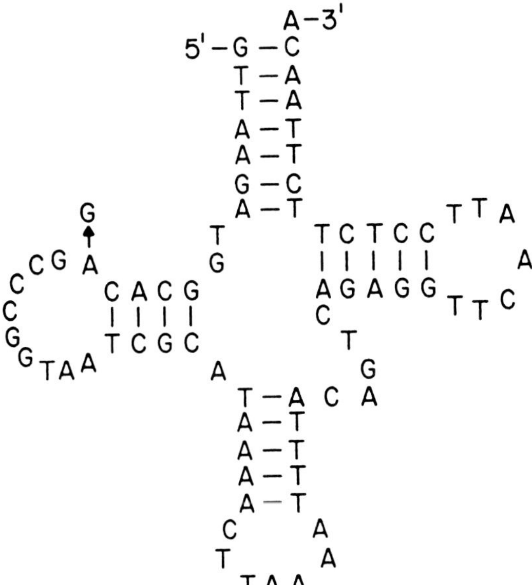

Figure 8–7. The MELAS point mutation of transfer RNA (tRNA) for leucine of mitochondrial DNA occurs at nucleotide 3243 and consists of an adenine (A) to guanine (G) substitution (*arrow*).

Recently, the mutation that causes MERRF was found in the extraocular muscles of elderly, healthy individuals.[33a] Taken together with other evidence of a common deletion of mtDNA that accumulates with aging, it appears that deletions and point mutations of mtDNA are part of the age-related impairment of mitochondrial function in the elderly.

In one family with PEO and ragged red fibers and with features overlapping with MELAS, an identical mutation of tRNA[Leu] was identified.[17]

Pathogenesis

As with the MERRF syndrome, a point mutation in the tRNA gene for leucine impairs protein synthesis by disrupting translation.[24a] Disruption in translation appears to be a common molecular mechanism by which mitochondrial disorders produce clinical disease. This is exemplified in KSS, MERRF, and MELAS.

Treatment

MELAS has no specific treatment. Supportive care is essential for the strokelike episodes, and appropriate anticonvulsants are necessary for seizures.

SUCCINATE DEHYDROGENASE (COMPLEX II) DEFICIENCY

Although defects in complex II of the respiratory chain have been reported in patients with clinical and laboratory features of a mitochondrial encephalomyopathy,[4,40,41] recent studies cast doubt on the specificity of these biochemical findings.[3] On the other hand, a disorder of muscle metabolism with lifelong exercise intolerance appears to be specific for succinate dehydrogenase deficiency.[18] Although the biochemical defect was only recently recognized, similar patients had been described in previous decades.[26,28]

Clinical Features

Succinate dehydrogenase deficiency presents in childhood as a disorder of exercise tolerance. Physical exertion, even of a modest degree, causes exhaustion associated with shortness of breath and palpitations. If activity persists, rhabdomyolysis may occur, with painful, stiff, and swollen muscles and myoglobinuria. Following severe rhabdomyolysis, weakness and fatigue may persist for many months. Permanent weakness is uncommon.

Physical examination usually appears normal, except following episodes of rhabdomyolysis, when weakness and tenderness occur. Calf enlargement has been reported in several patients.[26] Exercise-induced dyspnea and tachycardia can be demonstrated by having patients climb a flight of stairs.

Laboratory Features

The diagnosis of succinate dehydrogenase deficiency must be established by muscle biopsy, where ragged red fibers are seen. Reduced succinate dehydrogenase activity can be demonstrated. Biochemical analysis reveals marked impairment of succinate oxidation. Additional, nonspecific abnormalities may include elevation of the CK level and a myopathic EMG, especially during episodes of muscle breakdown.

Genetics

Succinate dehydrogenase is the only enzyme of the respiratory chain in which all subunits are encoded entirely by nuclear DNA. A cluster of families has been found with autosomal recessive inheritance.[26,28]

Pathogenesis

Succinate dehydrogenase deficiency interrupts the citric acid cycle because of impaired oxidation of succinate. This defect results in decreased oxygen extraction during exercise and to excess production of lactate and especially of pyruvate.

Treatment

No specific treatment has been found to overcome this metabolic defect. Patients should be advised not to exceed their exercise limitations.

CYTOCHROME *c* OXIDASE (COMPLEX IV) DEFICIENCY

The established clinical syndromes of cytochrome *c* oxidase (COX) deficiency include two infantile myopathies[9,10,31,55,62] and a disorder predominantly affecting the brain (subacute necrotizing encephalopathy, also referred to as Leigh's disease (Table 8–7).[6,27] The brain disorder is reviewed here because it can be diagnosed by muscle biopsy.

Fatal Infantile Myopathy

CLINICAL FEATURES

A fatal form of COX deficiency presenting primarily as a myopathy occurs in the neonatal period.[9,31,55] Usually these patients appear normal at birth, but hypotonia and generalized weakness develop during the first few weeks of life. The weakness then rapidly progresses to respiratory failure requiring ventilatory assistance. Primary brain involvement does not occur, but pneumonia may lead to hypoxia and seizures. Nearly all patients have shown a renal tubular defect leading to aminoaciduria, referred to as the De Toni-Fanconi-Debré syndrome. In rare

Table 8–7 SYNDROMES WITH CYTOCHROME *c* OXIDASE (COX) DEFICIENCY

FATAL INFANTILE MYOPATHY
 Hypotonia
 Weakness
 Respiratory distress
 Renal tubular defect: glycosuria, amino aciduria, etc.
 Mitochondrial myopathy with selective absence of subunits VII a, b of COX

BENIGN INFANTILE MYOPATHY
 Hypotonia
 Weakness
 Respiratory insufficiency
 Spontaneous recovery by age 2–3 years
 Mitochondrial myopathy with selective absence of subunits VII a, b and II of COX

LEIGH'S SYNDROME
 Hypotonia
 Episodic vomiting and feeding problems
 Loss of motor and verbal skills
 Hearing and visual loss
 Spasticity
 Muscle biopsy normal except for COX deficiency with absence of all COX subunits

instances, cardiomyopathy occurs. Progressive weakness usually leads to death by 1 year of age, although this may vary with medical management.

LABORATORY FEATURES

The CK level may be mildly elevated, and serum lactic acid levels are raised. As mentioned, a generalized renal tubular defect results in proteinuria, glycosuria, and generalized aminoaciduria. The muscle biopsy demonstrates COX deficiency histochemically (Fig. 8–8). Muscle fibers also show focal deposits of oxidative enzyme staining (NADH and SADH), as well as excessive lipid droplets. Electron microscopy reveals enlarged mitochondria with concentric whorls, crystalline inclusions, and disarray of cristae (see Fig. 8–8D to F).

Immune staining, using a battery of antibodies to the subunits of COX, can be used to distinguish this fatal infantile myopathy from other forms of COX deficiency.[52] The selective loss of subunits VII a,b represents a defect in a nuclear-encoded polypeptide of the respiratory chain.

GENETICS

Fatal infantile COX deficiency occurs in sporadic cases and in siblings,[31] suggesting autosomal recessive inheritance. Parents of affected patients do not have symptoms, and their muscle biopsies are normal.[9]

PATHOGENESIS

Antibody studies show a selective loss of the nuclear-DNA-encoded subunits VII a,b of COX in all muscle fibers; antibodies against other subunits of COX are normal. Therefore, a defect in the nuclear gene encoding subunits VII a and b is the probable cause of COX deficiency. These findings are consistent with an autosomal recessive disease presenting very early in life and affecting all muscle fibers, in contrast to disorders involving mtDNA, where heteroplasmy is common.

Benign Infantile Myopathy

CLINICAL FEATURES

The initial clinical neuromuscular manifestations of benign infantile my-

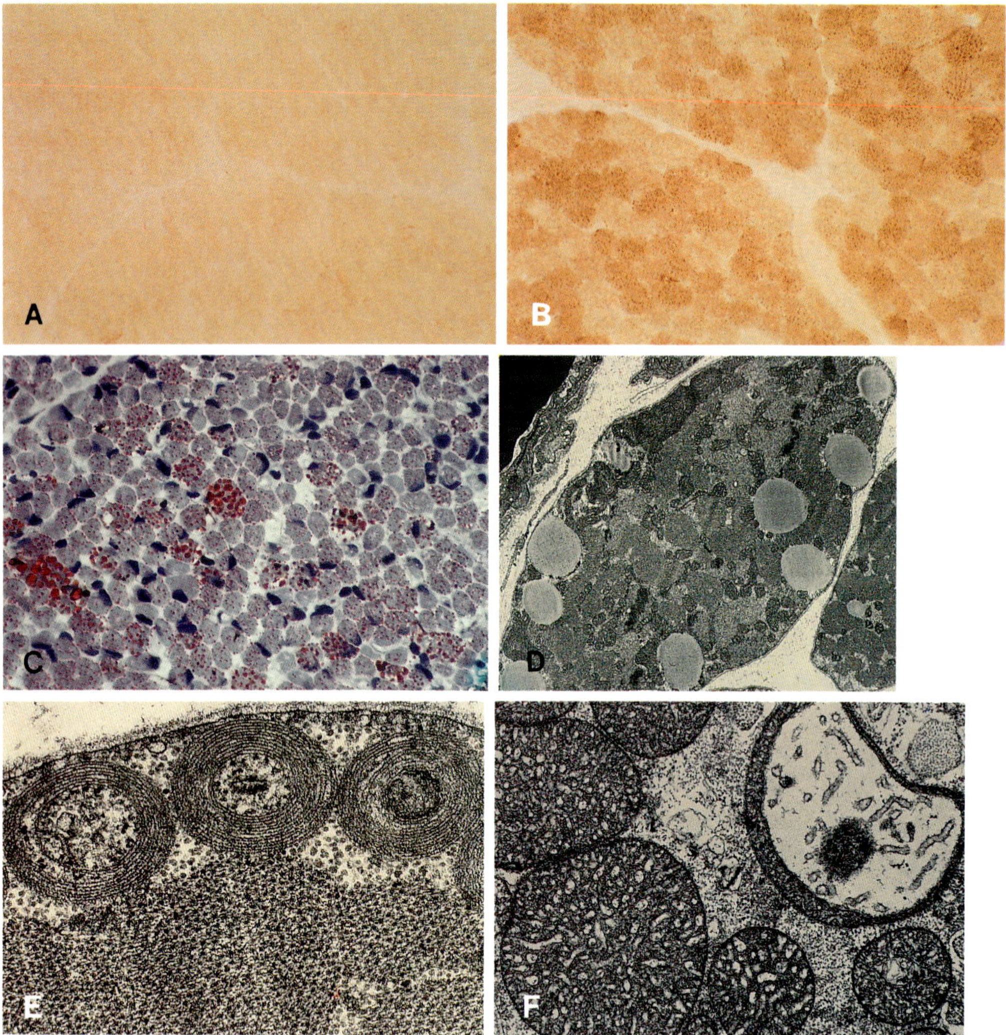

Figure 8–8. Cytochrome *c* oxidase (COX) deficiency of skeletal muscle. (*A*) COX deficiency with absent staining of muscle (cytochrome oxidase reaction). (*B*) normal COX staining of muscle (cytochrome oxidase reaction). (*C*) excess lipid droplets in COX deficiency (oil red O). (*D*) electron micrograph showing excess lipid droplets in COX deficiency. (*E*) mitochondria with concentric whorls. (*F*) mitochondria with disarray of cristae.

opathy due to COX deficiency are indistinguishable from the fatal form.[10,62] At birth or in the neonatal period, patients develop hypotonia, severe weakness, and respiratory insufficiency requiring assisted ventilation. In contradistinction to the fatal form, however, patients with the benign infantile COX myopathy have no renal tubular defect. A more important distinction is the spontane-

ous recovery. Improvement begins during the first year of life, and the children are normal by age 2 to 3 years.

LABORATORY FEATURES

The CK level is elevated and patients have lactic acidosis. No aminoaciduria occurs. The initial muscle biopsy changes resemble those of fatal infantile myopathy due to COX deficiency. Gradually, however, muscle COX activity returns, concomitant with an improvement in clinical symptoms.

The benign form of infantile myopathy due to COX deficiency can be distinguished from the fatal form by immune staining. As in the fatal form, the nuclear-encoded subunits VII a,b are absent but, in addition, subunit II of mtDNA is also absent.[52] Immune staining of these subunits returns to normal as the clinical condition improves.

GENETICS

No familial cases of benign infantile COX myopathy have been reported. All cases have been sporadic, and the inheritance pattern has not been established.

PATHOGENESIS

The spontaneous return of COX activity is difficult to explain, especially in view of defects in both nuclear- and mitochondrial-encoded subunits of COX. A defect in a regulatory developmental protein encoded by either nuclear or mitochondrial DNA cannot explain the observed phenomena.[52]

Leigh's Syndrome (Subacute Necrotizing Encephalomyelopathy)

In 1951, Leigh described a patient, normal until 6 months of age, who then became somnolent, with poor suck, hearing loss, optic atrophy, and spasticity.[27] The patient rapidly worsened and died, and the autopsy showed necrotic and spongiform lesions typical of Wernicke's encephalopathy. The disease remains poorly understood, but subsequent work has demonstrated metabolic abnormalities related to the pyruvate dehydrogenase complex in some cases,[7] to COX deficiency in others,[11] and to a point mutation within the ATPase gene in mtDNA in still others.[51a] Muscle biopsy plays an important role in the diagnosis of the COX-deficient form of Leigh's syndrome.

CLINICAL FEATURES

Leigh's syndrome typically has its onset in the first year of life. It may begin in the first few weeks, but more often children will develop normally for the first few months before regressing. Hypotonia then develops, accompanied by a poor suck and recurrent vomiting. Later, visual and hearing loss occur, and seizures may develop. In some cases onset of symptoms of Leigh's syndrome may be delayed until after walking begins. In these patients, ataxia and loss of intellectual development may accompany muscle weakness. Nystagmus and feeding problems are also present in this group. The rate of progression varies. Leigh's original patient died shortly after onset, but insidious or intermittent progression for several years can occur.[7]

LABORATORY FEATURES

Elevated lactate and pyruvate levels occur in the cerebrospinal fluid and less often in the blood.[6,7,52] Nonspecific EEG changes occur, along with abnormalities in auditory, visual, and somatosensory evoked potentials, reflecting the distribution of central nervous system lesions. CT and MRI scans show lesions in the basal ganglia, thalamus, and brainstem.

Defects in pyruvate metabolism are associated with some cases of Leigh's syndrome.[7] The urine of some patients contains an inhibitor that interferes with the catalytic conversion of thiamine pyrophosphate to thiamine triphosphate.[38] A defect in the regulation of the thiamine-dependent pyruvate dehydrogenase complex has been observed in cultured fibroblasts.[7]

Other patients with Leigh's syndrome have COX deficiency.[11] In this group, the muscle biopsy is important in diagnosis. Although the muscle histology by light and electron microscopy appears normal, histochemical staining for COX is markedly reduced and can be substantiated biochemically.[11] Immune staining differentiates the fatal and benign infantile COX-deficient myopathies from Leigh's syndrome, in which all subunits of COX, both mitochondrial- and nuclear-encoded polypeptides, are absent (see Table 8–7).

GENETICS

Most cases of Leigh's syndrome, are sporadic, but the disorder also occurs in siblings, suggesting an autosomal recessive inheritance.[11] A mutation at the nucleotide 8993 of mtDNA appears to be a relatively common cause of the syndrome.[7a,44a] An X-linked pattern of inheritance has also been suggested.[30b]

PATHOGENESIS

The cause of COX deficiency in Leigh's syndrome remains unknown. The absence of all subunits of COX, both mitochondrial- and nuclear-encoded, and the presence of autosomal recessive inheritance suggests a disorder not directly related to mtDNA. Tissue culture studies demonstrate that COX-deficient fibroblasts from patients with Leigh's syndrome can be corrected by a nuclear-DNA-encoded factor.[32] Collectively these studies provide evidence in favor of an abnormality in the assembly of the COX complex that is due to an abnormality in a nuclear-encoded protein.

OTHER SYNDROMES

MNGIE Syndrome

Findings in patients with this syndrome include *m*yopathy, *n*europathy, *g*astrointestinal disease with *i*ntestinal pseudoobstruction, and *e*ncephalopathy manifested as a leukodystrophy.[11a] The term "MNGIE" has been criticized because PEO, lactic acidosis, and other features can also occur.[50a]

Mitochondrial DNA Depletion Syndrome

A marked decrease in mtDNA in one or more tissues has been attributed to an abnormality in mtDNA replication that shows autosomal recessive inheritance.[11] Severe myopathy accompanied by a variable degree of renal and hepatic dysfunction usually results in respiratory failure in infancy. The diagnosis depends on the identification of ragged red fibers on muscle biopsy and then the demonstration of a decrease in mtDNA.[11a]

Leber's Optic Atrophy

Patients with this syndrome have progressive, acute or subacute, bilateral loss of vision. Other manifestations include ataxia, neuropathy, and cardiac conduction abnormalities. Myopathy is not a feature, but ragged red fibers are present on muscle biopsy.

SUMMARY

The mitochondrial myopathies were initially characterized by their distinctive morphologic abnormalities on muscle biopsy: ragged red fibers evident on modified Gomori trichrome; and enlarged, overly abundant, or abnormal-appearing mitochondria on electron microscopy. Subsequently, characterization of various clinical disorders indicated that specific oxidative enzymes were deficient in a number of cases. Many early reports of "specific biochemical defects" were, however, simply the result of a general abnormality in protein translation. It remained for genetic studies to define both the true nature of the defect and to account for the inheritance of the disorders.

Mitochondrial DNA is maternally transmitted via ovarian cytoplasm. Mitochondrial proteins are encoded by both mitochondrial DNA and by nuclear DNA. Although many questions remain to be answered and new diseases will be discovered, thus far there are four distinct genetic mechanisms for clinical disease production in mitochondrial myopathies. First, the sporadic disorder, Kearns-Sayre syndrome, results from a variety of deletions of somatic mitochondrial DNA. Second, autosomal dominant cases of PEO demonstrate multiple, large-scale mtDNA deletions, a finding which favors a mutation of a nuclear gene involved in mtDNA replication. Third, single base substitutions in mitochondrial DNA result in defective protein translation by RNA. The maternally transmitted disorders MERRF and MELAS result from this disorder of the mitochondrial genome. Finally, specific gene lesions of either the mitochondrial or nuclear genome result in abnormal or absent proteins, as occurs in cases of cytochrome oxidase deficiency.

Identification of the gene lesion permits specific diagnosis of many mitochondrial myopathies. More will doubtless be defined in the near future. Many of the clinical problems of patients with mitochondrial myopathies can be treated or prevented with supportive measures. Biochemical and genetic strategies for disease arrest or improvement are already on the horizon.

REFERENCES

1. Anderson S, Bankier AT, Barrell BG, et al: Sequence and organization of the human mitochondrial genome. Nature 290:457, 1981.
2. Askansas V, Engel WK, Britton DE, et al: Reincarnation in cultured muscle of mitochondrial abnormalities: Two patients with epilepsy and lactic acidosis. Arch Neurol 35:801, 1978.
3. Barohn RJ, Clanton T, Sahenk Z, and Mendell JR: Recurrent respiratory insufficiency and depressed ventilatory drive complicating mitochondrial myopathies. Neurology 40:103, 1990.
4. Behbehani AW, Goebel H, Osse G, et al: Mitochondrial myopathy with lactic acidosis and deficient activity of muscle succinate cytochrome-c-oxidoreductase. Eur J Pediatr 143:67, 1984.
4a. Bendahan D, Desnuelle C, Vanuxem D, et al: 31P NMR spectroscopy and ergometer exercise test as evidence for muscle oxidative performance improvement with coenzyme Q in mitochondrial myopathies. Neurology 42:1203, 1992.
5. Berenberg RA, Pellock JM, DiMauro S, et al: Lumping or splitting? "Ophthalmoplegia-plus" or Kearns-Sayre syndrome? Ann Neurol 1:37, 1977.
5a. Brockington M, Sweeney MG, Hammans SR, et al: A tandem duplication in the D-loop of human mitochondrial DNA is associated with deletions in mitochondrial myopathies. Nat Genet 4:67, 1993.
6. DeVivo DC, DiMauro S, and Rapin I: Mitochondrial disorders. In: Rudolph AM (ed): Pediatrics, ed 18. Appleton & Lange, Norwalk, CT, 1987, p 1736.
7. DeVivo DC, Haymond MW, Obert KA, et al: Defective activation of the pyruvate dehydrogenase complex in subacute necrotizing encephalomyelopathy (Leigh disease). Ann Neurol 6:483, 1979.
7a. de Vries BD, van Engelen BG, Gabreels FJ, et al: A second missense mutation in the mitochondrial ATPase 6 gene in Leigh's syndrome. Ann Neurol 34:410, 1993.
8. DiMauro S, Bonilla E, Zeviani M, et al: Mitochondrial myopathies. Ann Neurol 17:521, 1985.
9. DiMauro S, Mendell JR, Sahenk Z, et al: Fatal infantile mitochondrial myopathy and renal dysfunction due to cytochrome-c-oxidase deficiency. Neurology 30:795, 1980.
10. DiMauro S, Nicholson JF, Hays AP, et al: Benign infantile mitochondrial myopathy due to reversible cytochrome c oxidase deficiency. Ann Neurol 14:226, 1983.
11. DiMauro S, Servidei S, Zeviani M, et al: Cytochrome c oxidase deficiency in Leigh syndrome. Ann Neurol 22:498, 1987.

11a. DiMauro S, Tonin P, and Servidei S: Metabolic myopathies. In Vinken PJ, Bruyn GW, and Klawans HL (eds): Myopathies. Elsevier Science, London, 1992, p 479.

12. Drachman DA: Ophthalmoplegia plus: the neurodegenerative disorders associated with progressive external ophthalmoplegia. Arch Neurol 18:654, 1968.

13. Driscoll PF, Larsen PD, and Gruber AB: MELAS syndrome involving a mother and two children. Arch Neurol 44:971, 1987.

13a. Egger J and Wilson J: Mitochondrial inheritance in a mitochondrially mediated disease. N Engl J Med 309:142, 1983.

13b. Fang W, Huang CC, Lee CC, et al: Ophthalmologic manifestations in MELAS syndrome. Arch Neurol 50:977, 1993.

13c. Fang W, Huang CC, Chu NS, et al: Myoclonic epilepsy with ragged red fibers (MERRF) syndrome: Report of a Chinese family with mitochondrial DNA point mutation in tRNA (Lys) gene. Muscle Nerve 17:52, 1994.

14. Folkers K, Wolaniuk J, Simonen R, et al: Biochemical rationale and the cardiac response of patients with muscle disease to therapy with coenzyme Q_{10}. Proc Natl Acad Sci USA 82:4513, 1985.

15. Fukuhara N: Myoclonus epilepsy and mitochondrial myopathy. In Cerri C and Scarlato G (eds): Mitochondrial pathology in muscle disease. Piccin Editore, Padua, 1983, p 87.

16. Fukuhara N, Tokiguchi S, Shirakawa K, et al: Myoclonus epilepsy associated with ragged-red fibers (mitochondrial abnormalities): Disease entity or a syndrome? Light-and-electron-microscopic studies of two cases and review of literature. J Neurol Sci 47:117, 1980.

17. Goto Y, Nonaka I, and Horai S: A mutation in the tRNA[Leu(UUR)] gene associated with the MELAS subgroup of mitochondrial encephalomyopathies. Nature 348:651, 1990.

18. Haller RG, Henriksson KG, Jorfeldt L, et al: Muscle succinate dehydrogenase deficiency: Exercise pathophysiology

of a novel mitochondrial myopathy. Neurology 40 (Suppl 1):413, 1990.

18a. Hammans SR, Sweeney MG, Brockington M, et al: The mitochondrial DNA transfer RNA (Lys)A—>G(8344) mutation and the syndrome of myoclonic epilepsy and ragged red fibres (MERRF). Relationship of clinical phenotype to proportion of mutant mitochondrial DNA. Brain 116:617, 1993.

19. Hart ZH, Chang CH, Perrin EVD, et al: Familial poliodystrophy, mitochondrial myopathy, and lactic acidemia. Arch Neurol 34:180, 1977.

20. Holliday PL, Climie ARW, Giloy J, and Mahmud MZ: Mitochondrial myopathy and encephalopathy: Three cases. A deficiency of NADH-CoQ dehydrogenase? Neurology 33:1619, 1983.

21. Holt IJ, Harding AE, and Morgan-Hughes JA: Deletions of muscle mitochondrial DNA in patients with mitochondrial myopathies. Nature 331:717, 1988.

22. Iannaccone ST, Griggs RC, Markesbery WR, and Joynt RJ: Familial progressive external ophthalmoplegia and ragged-red fibers. Neurology 24:1033, 1974.

23. Kearns TP and Sayre GP: Retinitis pigmentosa, external ophthalmoplegia, and complete heart block. Arch Ophthal 60:280, 1958.

24. Kobayashi Y, Momoi MY, Tominaga K, et al: A point mutation in the mitochondrial tRNALeu(UUR) gene in MELAS (mitochondrial myopathy, encephalopathy, lactic acidosis and stroke-like episodes). Biochem Biophys Res Commun 173:816, 1990.

24a. Koga Y, Davidson M, Schon EA, et al: Fine mapping of mitochrondrial RNAs derived from the mtDNA region containing a point mutation associated with MELAS. Nucleic Acids Res 21:657, 1993.

24b. Koo B, Becker LE, Chuang S, et al: Mitochondrial encephalomyopathy, lactic acidosis, stroke-like episodes (MELAS): Clinical, radiological, pathological, and genetic observations. Ann Neurol 34:25, 1993.

25. Kuriyama M, Umezaki H, Fukuda Y, et al: Mitochondrial encephalomyopathy

with lactate-pyruvate elevation and brain infarctions. Neurology 34:72, 1984.

26. Larsson LE, Linderholm H, Müller R, et al: Hereditary metabolic myopathy with paroxysmal myoglobinuria due to abnormal glycolysis. J Neurol Neurosurg Psychiatry 27:361, 1964.

27. Leigh D: Subacute necrotizing encephalomyelopathy in an infant. J Neurol Neurosurg Psychiatry 14:216, 1951.

28. Linderholm H, Müller R, Ringqvist T, and Sörnäs R: Hereditary abnormal muscle metabolism with hyperkinetic circulation during exercise. Acta Med Scand 185:153, 1969.

29. Lombes A, Mendell JR, Nakase H, et al: Myoclonic epilepsy and ragged-red fibers with cytochrome oxidase deficiency: Neuropathology, biochemistry, and molecular genetics. Ann Neurol 26:20, 1989.

30. Luft R, Ikkos D, Palmieri G, et al: A case of severe hypermetabolism of nonthyroid origin with a defect in the maintenance of mitochondrial respiratory control: A correlated clinical, biochemical and morphological study. J Clin Invest 41:1776, 1962.

30a. Macmillan C, Lach B, Shoubridge ER: Variable distribution of mutant mitochondrial DNA (tRNA(Leu[3243])) in tissues of symptomatic relatives with MELAS: The role of mitotic segregation. Neurology 43:1586, 1993.

30b. Matthews PM, Marchington DR, Squier M, et al: Molecular genetic characterization of an X-linked form of Leigh's syndrome. Ann Neurol 33:652, 1993.

31. Minchom PE, Dormer RL, Hughes IA, et al: Fatal infantile mitochondrial myopathy due to cytochrome *c* oxidase deficiency. J Neurol Sci 60:453, 1983.

32. Miranda AF, Ishii S, DiMauro S, and Shay JW: Cytochrome *c* oxidase deficiency in Leigh's syndrome: genetic evidence for a nuclear DNA-encoded mutation. Neurology 39:697, 1989.

32a. Moraes CT, Ciacci F, Silvestri G, et al: Atypical clinical presentation associated with the MELAS mutation at position 3243 of human mitochondrial DNA. Neuromuscul Disord 3:43, 1993.

33. Moraes CT, DiMauro S, Zeviani M, et al: Mitochondrial DNA deletions in progressive external ophthalmoplegia and Kearns-Sayre syndrome. N Engl J Med 320:1293, 1989.

33a. Munscher C, Rieger T, Muller-Hocker J, et al: The point mutation of mitochondrial DNA characteristic for MERRF disease is found also in healthy people of different ages. FEBS Lett 317:27, 1993.

34. Ogasahara S, Yorifuji S, Nishikawa Y, et al: Improvement of abnormal pyruvate metabolism and cardiac conduction with coenzyme Q_{10} in Kearns-Sayre syndrome. Neurology 35:372, 1985.

35. Olson W, Engel WK, Walsh GO, et al: Oculocraniosomatic neuromuscular disease with "ragged-red" fibers. Arch Neurol 26:193, 1972.

36. Pavlakis SG, Phillips PC, DiMauro S, et al: Mitochondrial myopathy, encephalopathy, lactic acidosis, and strokelike episodes: a distinctive clinical syndrome. Ann Neurol 16:481, 1984.

37. Pearce GW: Electron microscopy in the study of muscular dystrophy. Ann N Y Acad Sci 138:138, 1966.

38. Pincus JH, Cooper JR, Piros K, and Turner V: Specificity of the urine inhibitor test for Leigh's disease. Neurology 24:885, 1974.

39. Rich A and RajBhandary UL: Transfer RNA: molecular structure, sequence, and properties. Annu Rev Biochem 45:805, 1976.

40. Riggs JE, Schochet SS, Fakadej AV, et al: Mitochondrial encephalomyopathy with decreased succinate-cytochrome *c* reductase activity. Neurology 34:48, 1984.

41. Rivner MH, Shamsnia M, Swift TR, et al: Kearns-Sayre syndrome and complex II deficiency. Neurology 39:693, 1989.

42. Rosing HS, Hopkins LC, Wallace DC, et al: Maternally inherited mitochondrial myopathy and myoclonic epilepsy. Ann Neurol 17:228, 1985.

43. Rowland LP: Molecular genetics, pseu-

dogenetics and clinical neurology. Neurology 33:1179, 1983.

44. Rowland LP, Hays AP, DiMauro S, et al: Diverse clinical disorders associated with morphological abnormalities of mitochondria. In Cerri C and Scarlato G (eds): Mitochondrial pathology in muscle diseases. Piccin Editore, Padua, 1983, p 141.

44a. Santorelli FM, Shanske S, Macaya A, et al: The mutation at nt 8993 of mitochondrial DNA is a common cause of Leigh's syndrome. Ann Neurol 34:827, 1993.

45. Seibel P, Degoul F, Romero N, et al: Identification of point mutations by mispairing PCR as exemplified in MERRF disease. Biochem Biophys Res Commun 173:561, 1990.

46. Shapira Y, Cederbaum SD, Cancilla PA, et al: Familial poliodystrophy, mitochondrial myopathy and lactate acidemia. Neurology 25:614, 1975.

47. Shoffner JM, Lott MT, Lezza AMS, et al: Myoclonic epilepsy and ragged-red fiber disease (MERRF) is associated with a mitochondrial DNA tRNA^{Lys} mutation. Cell 61:931, 1990.

48. Shy GM and Gonatas NK: Human myopathy with giant abnormal mitochondria. Science 145:493, 1964.

49. Shy GM, Gonatas NK, and Perez M: Two childhood myopathies with abnormal mitochondria: I. Megaconial myopathy. II. Pleoconial myopathy. Brain 89:133, 1966.

50. Shy GM, Silberberg DH, Appel SH, et al: A generalized disorder of nervous system, skeletal muscle and heart resembling Refsum's disease and Hurler's syndrome, I. Clinical, pathologic and biochemical characteristics. Am J Med 42:163, 1967.

50a. Simon LT, Horoupian DS, Dorfman LJ, et al: Polyneuropathy, ophthalmoplegia, leukoencephalopathy, and intestinal pseudo-obstruction: POLIP syndrome. Ann Neurol 28:349, 1990.

51. Skoglund RR: Reversible alexia, mitochondrial myopathy, and lactic acidemia. Neurology 29:717, 1979.

51a. Tatuch Y, Christdoulou J, Feigenbaum A, et al: Heteroplasmic mtDNA mutation (T → G) at 8993 can cause Leigh disease when the percentage of abnormal mtDNA is high. Am J Hum Genet 50:852, 1992.

51b. Tokunaga M, Mita S, Sakuta R, et al: Increased mitochondrial DNA in blood vessels and ragged-red fibers in mitochondrial myopathy, encephalopathy, lactic acidosis, and stroke-like episodes (MELAS). Ann Neurol 33:275, 1993.

52. Tritschler HJ, Bonilla E, Lombes A, et al: Differential diagnosis of fatal and benign cytochrome *c* oxidase-deficient myopathies of infancy: An immunohistochemical approach. Neurology 41:300, 1991.

53. Trounce I, Byre E, and Marzuki S: Decline in skeletal muscle mitochondrial respiratory chain function: Possible factor in aging. Lancet 1:637, 1989.

54. Tsairis P, Engel WK, and Kark P: Familial myoclonic epilepsy syndrome associated with skeletal muscle mitochondrial abnormalities [abstract]. Neurology 23:408, 1973.

55. van Biervliet JP, Bruinvis L, Ketting D, et al: Hereditary mitochondrial myopathy with lactic acidemia, a DeToni-Fanconi-Debré syndrome, and a defective respiratory chain in voluntary striated muscles. Pediatr Res 11:1088, 1977.

56. Wallace DC: Report of the Committee on human mitochondrial DNA. Cytogenet Cell Genet 51:612, 1989.

57. Wallace DC, Zheng X, Lott MT, et al: Familial mitochondrial encephalomyopathy (MERRF): Genetic, pathophysiological, and biochemical characterization of a mitochondrial DNA disease. Cell 55:601, 1988.

58. Yiannikas C, McLeod JG, Pollard JD, and Bauerstock J: Peripheral neuropathy associated with mitochondrial myopathy. Ann Neurol 20:249, 1986.

59. Zeviani M, Amati P, Bresolin N, et al: Rapid detection of the A → G$^{(8344)}$ mutation of mtDNA in Italian families with myoclonus epilepsy and ragged-red fibers (MERRF). Am J Hum Genet 48:203, 1991.

60. Zeviani M, Bresolin N, Gellera C, et al: Nucleus-driven multiple large-scale

deletions of the human mitochondrial genome: A new autosomal dominant disease. Am J Hum Genet 47:904, 1990.

61. Zeviani M, Moraes CT, DiMauro S, et al: Deletions of mitochondrial DNA in Kearns-Sayre syndrome. Neurology 38:1339, 1988.

62. Zeviani M, Peterson P, Servidei S, et al:

Benign reversible muscle cytochrome *c* oxidase deficiency: A second case. Neurology 37:64, 1987.

63. Zeviani M, Servidei S, Gellera C, et al: An autosomal dominant disorder with multiple deletions of mitochondrial DNA starting at the D-loop region. Nature 339:309, 1989.

Chapter 9

PERIODIC PARALYSIS AND MYOTONIA

PERIODIC PARALYSIS

Patients often complain of episodic weakness, but most patients complaining of weakness in fact mean fatigue (see pp. 20–21). Documented episodic paralysis is uncommon. This chapter focuses on the primary periodic paralysis, because these disorders are probably caused by specific disease of the muscle cell. It should be emphasized that patients with episodic weakness often have secondary forms of periodic paralysis in which the paralysis results from a systemic electrolyte disturbance. These conditions are summarized in this chapter; some of the major conditions are also noted in Chapter 10. We have grouped periodic paralyses with myotonic disorders in this chapter because patients with these disorders often have both episodic weakness and myotonia. Moreover, there is evidence that both groups of diseases result from hereditary defects of ion channels in the sarcolemma. It is now apparent that certain myotonic disorders without paralysis are caused by genetic defects at the same chromosomal locus as one or more of the forms of periodic paralysis.

The defects responsible for the periodic paralyses result in striking alterations in potassium levels or in the response to agents altering potassium metabolism. These alterations of potassium metabolism are the result of the periodic paralyses, rather than the primary defect. Nevertheless, factors altering potassium levels are important in diagnosis and treatment.

CLASSIFICATION OF PERIODIC PARALYSIS

Table 9–1 lists many of the conditions that can be associated with an episode of weakness. Most of these disorders can be recurrent. Several are considered in greater detail in Chapter 10. Only those conditions with either hypokalemia or hyperkalemia are likely to be confused with a primary periodic paralysis. The most frequent secondary disorders that simulate hypokalemic periodic paralysis are renal tubular acidosis, aldosterone-producing adenomas of the adrenal gland, and villous adenomas of the colon.[112] The only sec-

Table 9–1 SECONDARY CAUSES OF EPISODIC PARALYSIS

HYPOKALEMIC
Primary hyperaldosteronism (Conn's syndrome)
Renal tubular acidosis
Juxtaglomerular apparatus hyperplasia (Bartter's syndrome)
Villous adenoma
Alcoholism
Diuretics, licorice, *p*-aminosalicylic acid, amphotericin B, corticosteroids

HYPERKALEMIC
Potassium load (e.g., oral supplements, salt substitutes)
Potassium-sparing diuretics — spironolactone, triamterene
Hyporeninemic hypoaldosteronism — diabetic, other renal disease; secondary to indomethacin, ibuprofen
Addison's disease
Chronic renal failure
Isolated aldosterone deficiency
Chronic heparin therapy
Rhabdomyolysis (e.g., McArdle's syndrome)
Ileostomy complicated by tight stoma syndrome

NORMOKALEMIC
Guanidine
Sleep paralysis
Myasthenia gravis, multiple sclerosis, Eaton-Lambert syndrome
Transient ischemic attacks

Table 9–2 CLASSIFICATION OF THE PRIMARY PERIODIC PARALYSES

HYPOKALEMIC
Familial and sporadic (localized to dihydropyridine receptor, chromosome 1q)
Thyrotoxic

POTASSIUM-SENSITIVE (Most disorders localize to the alpha-subunit of sodium channel on chromosome 17q)
Hyperkalemic (familial and sporadic)
Normokalemic
Myotonic (includes some atypical myotonia congenita)
Paramyotonia
   Paramyotonia congenita
   Potassium-sensitive (paralysis periodica paramyotonica)
Associated with cardiac arrhythmias (Andersen's syndrome not localized to chromosome 17q)

ondary disorders that frequently cause hyperkalemic periodic paralysis are conditions that cause hyporeninemic hypoaldosteronism.[131] This disorder usually occurs in diabetic patients with renal disease and impaired renin production.

Table 9–2 lists the primary periodic paralyses, which are divided into two major groups. There is general agreement on these major categories, but a substantial proportion of patients have features that are not typical of any of them. Whether the subdivisions in Table 9–2 are justified remains to be determined by further characterization of the genetic defects. The distinctions between these subgroups listed are useful, however, because there is usually homogeneity within kindreds, as well as reproducible, differing responses to provocative and therapeutic modalities.[112]

In the past, overlaps in clinical features between so-called hyperkalemic periodic paralysis and normokalemic periodic paralysis,[97,112] and between hyperkalemic periodic paralysis and the paramyotonias,[72] have led to controversy. The fact that certain of these disorders (if not all) are allelic (i.e., involve the same gene) has greatly simplified their nosology.[100,101] Normal function can be restored by treatment for virtually all patients, but each case must be fully evaluated to provide the basis for effective treatment.

All types of periodic paralyses have certain similarities (Table 9–3); hypo-

Table 9–3 SIMILAR CLINICAL FEATURES OF THE PERIODIC PARALYSES

HISTORY
Onset by third decade
Attacks of limb weakness; sparing of bulbar, ocular, respiratory muscles
Attacks provoked by rest following exercise
Greater severity in males
Oliguria preceding and during attacks
Family history (most cases) — autosomal dominant

EXAMINATION
Eyelid myotonia
Normal sensation
Normal strength between attacks (for initial 5- to 10-year period)
Untreated cases eventually develop "fixed" proximal weakness
Hyporeflexia during attacks

kalemic and potassium-sensitive periodic paralysis are *not* mirror images of each other.[41] Thus, all periodic paralyses are characterized by episodic attacks of limb weakness; all forms begin by the third decade and are more severe in males in a given family; in all disorders, attacks typically occur after the rest that follows exercise; and in all disorders, strength is usually normal between attacks for the first 5 to 10 years of the disorder, but progressive, proximal "fixed" weakness during attack-free intervals occurs if the disease is not treated.[112]

Hypokalemic Periodic Paralysis

This disorder results from mutations in the dihydropyridine receptor on chromosome 1q and is the most homogeneous of the periodic paralyses (Table 9–4). Attacks usually begin within the second decade, almost invariably before age 30. In contrast, potassium-sensitive periodic paralysis usually begins within the first decade. The attack frequency in hypokalemic periodic paralysis is often lower than in other forms of periodic paralysis; attacks may be as infrequent as once or twice a year. On the other hand, attacks can occur daily. Although some attacks may last only 1 to 4 hours, most last longer — up to 24 hours or more in patients with severe disease. Death from respiratory muscle paralysis and cardiac arrhythmias has been reported.[123] Cranial muscles are involved occasionally, but ocular muscles are usually spared.

Myotonia in hypokalemic periodic paralysis has been confined to the eyelids[107] (see pp. 26–29). Myotonia of the limbs has not been demonstrated by electromyography (EMG), and its presence on EMG makes another form of periodic paralysis likely.

Thyrotoxic Periodic Paralysis

Attacks of thyrotoxic periodic paralysis (TPP) resemble those of primary hypokalemic periodic paralysis in their clinical features, but TPP differs markedly from the primary disorder in that TPP occurs sporadically, most frequently in Asian adults, although it can occur in all races.[67] Despite the higher incidence of thyrotoxicosis in women, less than 5% of the cases of TPP occur in women.[91] As many as 10% of thyrotoxic Asian males may develop TPP; the proclivity for an individual to develop periodic paralysis when thyrotoxic may be transmitted as an autosomal dominant disorder.[78] Attacks abate when thyrotoxicosis resolves but will recur if thyroid hormone levels become elevated again.[90] Not surprisingly, the diagnosis of thyrotoxicosis is sometimes clinically inapparent in these patients; those with more obvious signs of hyperthyroidism would have come to medical attention earlier. Attacks of hypokalemic periodic paralysis presenting in adulthood thus demand thorough evaluation of the patient for occult hyperthyroidism. TPP may be associated with progressive muscle weakness and with cardiac arrhythmias, probably as a result of the thyrotoxicosis.[83,106]

Table 9–4 DISTINGUISHING CLINICAL FEATURES OF THE PERIODIC PARALYSES

	Hypokalemic	Potassium-sensitive (hyperkalemic)	Paramyotonia
Age of onset	5–35	Before age 10	Before age 10
Attack duration (typical)	>2 h	<2 h	2–24 h
Attack severity	Often severe	Seldom severe	Seldom severe
Attacks precipitated by	Carbohydrate ingestion	Fasting	Cold
Muscle hypertrophy	Absent	Present	Often present
Sensory symptoms	Absent	Present	Absent

Potassium-Sensitive Periodic Paralysis (Hyperkalemic Periodic Paralysis)

The gene locus for potassium-sensitive periodic paralysis has been defined,[34] and consequently the classification of these disorders has been clarified. Many disorders characterized by potassium sensitivity localize to chromosome 17q and are related to abnormalities of the alpha-subunit of the sodium channel.[34,100,101] Plasma potassium levels and the effect of potassium administration on the strength of patients with periodic paralysis remain important in evaluating patients and planning their treatment.

Patients who had hyperkalemia rather than hypokalemia during attacks of periodic paralysis were first recognized in 1955.[121] In 1956, Gamstorp[37] described a large kindred of patients and introduced the term *adynamia episodica hereditaria*. This disorder is more heterogeneous than hypokalemic periodic paralysis. The potassium level may be normal, elevated, or occasionally even low in spontaneous attacks of weakness,[37] so that the disease is defined by the patient's response to potassium rather than by the absolute potassium level during attacks. Inheritance is commonly autosomal dominant, but sporadic cases resulting from new mutations have been identified.[32,116] Potassium-sensitive periodic paralysis is earlier in onset than hypokalemic periodic paralysis, and the majority of patients begin to have symptoms within the first decade. Attacks are brief and mild in most instances, usually lasting anywhere from 30 minutes to 4 hours.

Attacks of weakness are precipitated by rest following exercise or by fasting. Weakness is usually in proximal leg or shoulder-girdle muscles, but distal muscles may be more affected following strenuous activity, and unilateral weakness may occur following selective strenuous activity. During attacks of weakness, involved muscles are flaccid and hyporeflexic. Although Chvostek's sign can often be elicited, and paresthesias may be present in the hands or feet, sensory examination is usually normal.

Myotonia is prominent on both clinical and electromyographic evaluation in many patients with potassium-sensitive periodic paralysis.[138,139] The extent of the myotonia is variable within families, but it can usually be elicited in all patients in a kindred if it is severe in one member. Some families show no evidence of myotonia, so the disorder in kindreds with myotonia has been termed *myotonic periodic paralysis*,[138] to distinguish it from the disorder shown by other patients with potassium-sensitive periodic paralysis. Because a myotonic disorder that lacks paralytic attacks is allelic to potassium-sensitive periodic paralysis, the differences between these disorders reflect the nature of the sodium channel defect.[100]

Progressive, persistent (interattack) weakness is not as severe or frequent in potassium-sensitive periodic paralysis as in hypokalemic periodic paralysis, but it has been noted in numerous reports.[93] Creatine kinase levels are often elevated during attacks of weakness and may be persistently elevated even during attack-free intervals. The potassium level is often relatively elevated (while still within the normal range) during sequential studies of patients without weakness. These findings suggest that mild, recurrent, clinically inapparent attacks may be occurring more than once during the day in patients with potassium-sensitive periodic paralysis.[66]

Potassium-Sensitive Periodic Paralysis with Cardiac Arrhythmias

Cardiac arrhythmias are not common in periodic paralysis but have been noted in hypokalemic periodic paralysis,[65] thyrotoxic periodic paralysis,[83,106] potassium-sensitive periodic paralysis,[131b] and in a family with a disorder termed "normokalemic periodic paralysis."[4] The most striking cardiac dysrhythmia associated with periodic paralysis occurs in a distinctive syndrome that was first characterized in 1971.[4] Patients with this distinctive disorder have potassium-sensitive periodic paralysis and frequent ectopic ventricular premature beats (most commonly bigeminy or a bidirectional tachycardia),[4,92] as well as characteristic dysmorphic features consisting of short stature, hypertelorism, low-set ears, mandibular hypoplasia, and clinodactyly (Fig. 9–1). In reported cases the family history reveals autosomal dominant inheritance, although in certain kindreds the disorder may not be recognized in mildly affected patients. One of the patients had only two episodes of slight leg weakness.[92] Because the characteristic phenotype was not recognized until Andersen's report,[4] some of the earlier cases of periodic paralysis with bidirectional tachycardia or bigeminy may have had the same disorder.[57]

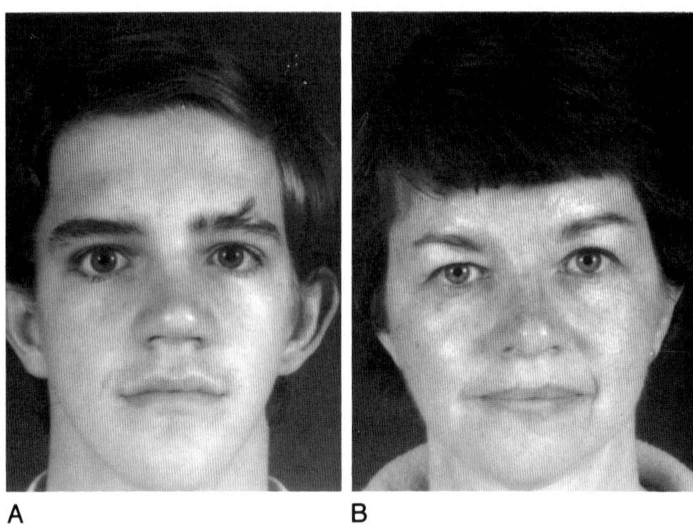

A   B

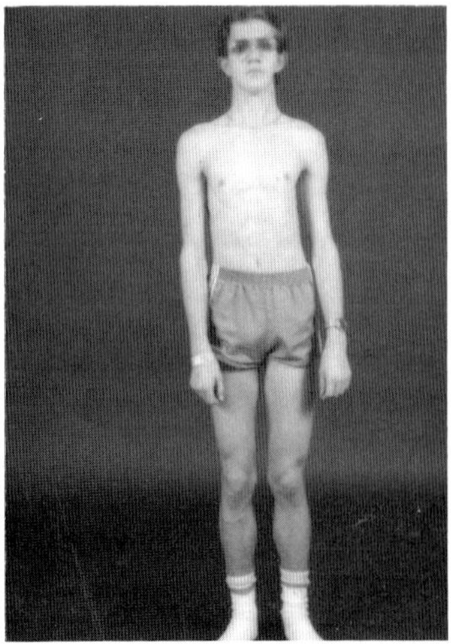

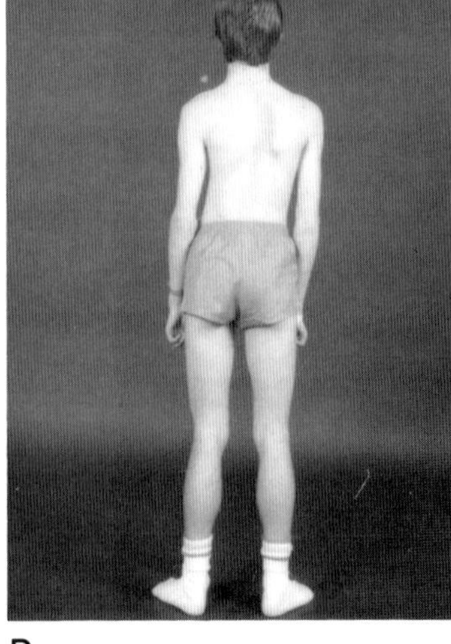

C   D

Figure 9–1. Patients with potassium-sensitive periodic paralysis and cardiac arrhythmia. (*A*) A 16-year-old with characteristic facial features: low-set ears, hypoplastic mandible. This patient had frequent attacks of weakness, persistent interattack weakness, and ventricular ectopy. (From Tawil et al.[131b] Reprinted with permission from Annals of Neurology 35: 326–330, 1994.) (*B*) Mother of patient in A. She had only two episodes of weakness, slight proximal weakness, and ventricular ectopy. (*C*) The patient has proximal weakness and atrophy. (*D*) Scoliosis was prominent.

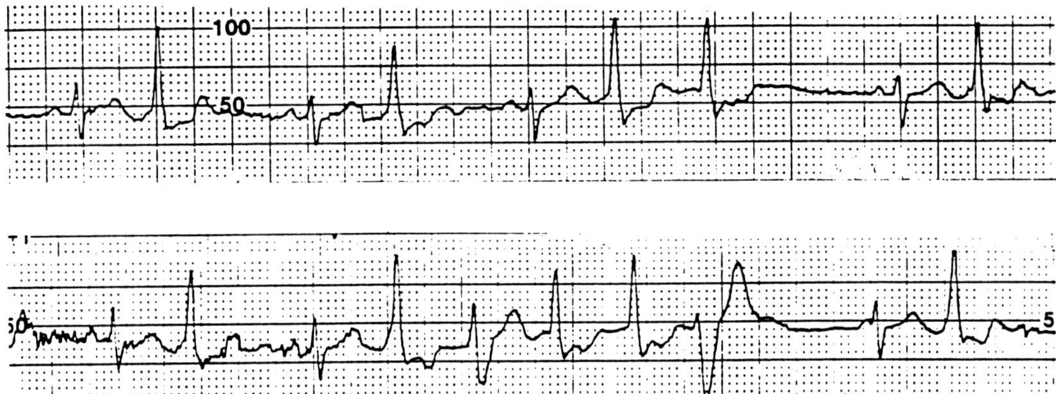

Figure 9–2. Holter monitoring of patient with potassium-sensitive periodic paralysis and cardiac arrhythmias, showing ventricular ectopy: bigeminy (*top tracing*) and ventricular tachycardia (*bottom tracing*). The patient was asymptomatic during numerous episodes of ventricular tachycardia.

Cardiac arrhythmia detected by physical examination is often the presenting manifestation of the disorder (Fig. 9–2). Severe scoliosis is occasionally present.[92] The cardiac dysrhythmia and periodic paralysis mirror each other's behavior in terms of the response to provocative and therapeutic tests. That is, raising plasma potassium precipitates weakness but normalizes the electrocardiogram. Lowering potassium improves strength but exacerbates the electrocardiographic abnormalities.[92]

It may be an oversimplification to classify the disorder of periodic paralysis with cardiac arrhythmias along with the potassium-sensitive periodic paralyses, because arrhythmias have also been described in cases of hypokalemic periodic paralysis. Moreover, this disorder is not linked to the sodium channel locus on chromosome 17q[131b]. On the other hand, it is unclear from the literature whether the arrhythmias associated with euthyroid hypokalemic periodic paralysis were seen in untreated patients or only occurred after treatment was initiated.[112] Because parenteral administration of potassium diluted in glucose or saline can actually cause levels of plasma potassium to *fall*, the arrhythmias reported in several instances could be the result of treatment rather than the primary disease.[112]

The Paramyotonic Paralyses

Eulenburg[31] originally described paramyotonia in 1886, and noted the autosomal dominant inheritance, paradoxical myotonia (myotonia that worsens with activity — see p. 29), exacerbation of myotonia by cold and attacks of weakness that are provoked by cold, or occur without cold exposure. Since that time it has become clear that there are two clinically distinct disorders with these features.[7,111] Both disorders appear, however, to be allelic on chromosome 17q and to involve distinct mutations of the alpha-subunit of the sodium channel.[27] Except for the characteristic cold provocation of weakness and paradoxical myotonia, the clinical features of both disorders resemble those of other periodic paralyses.

PARAMYOTONIA CONGENITA

In this disorder, attacks of weakness are associated with and precipitated by lowering plasma potassium.[111] The occurrence of this form of paramyotonia in descendants of Eulenberg's original "paramyotonia congenita" family justifies the Eulenberg designation.[111]

POTASSIUM-SENSITIVE PARAMYOTONIA (PARALYSIS PERIODICA PARAMYOTONICA)

In this disorder, attacks are precipitated by potassium administration. This potassium-sensitivity accounts for the reported overlap between "paramyotonia congenita" and potassium-sensitive (hyperkalemic) periodic paralysis.[42,86,133] All patients with paramyotonia congenita should be challenged with glucose and insulin, as well as with oral potassium, to adequately characterize their condition as either paramyotonia congenita or paralysis periodica paramyotonica. Although the two disorders are probably allelic, their treatments are usually different (see below).

Other Forms of Periodic Paralysis

NORMOKALEMIC PERIODIC PARALYSIS

A few patients have been reported to have episodic weakness in which there is a normal plasma potassium level during the attacks and a failure of a potassium or glucose-insulin challenge to provoke weakness.[82] Most cases described as "normokalemic periodic paralysis," however, have been potassium-sensitive.[97,137] Only a single kindred has proved resistant to the effects, both of lowering the serum potassium with glucose and insulin, and of oral potassium loading.[82] Although genetic studies have not yet been reported, in general, this term does not identify a distinct form of periodic paralysis. In all probability, it is allelic to other potassium-sensitive disorders.

ATYPICAL MYOTONIA CONGENITA

A form of myotonia congenita with pain (see p. 343) shows a periodic worsening of myotonia that correlates with changes in plasma potassium level; potassium administration worsens symptoms, and carbohydrate loads improve symptoms. While this disorder is allelic to other potassium-sensitive disorders that are associated with periodic paralysis,[100] in these patients potassium levels remain in the normal range, and actual weakness does not occur. Autosomal recessive myotonia congenita, on the other hand, is characterized by true and fluctuating weakness (see p. 343). A similar, if not identical, disorder termed *myotonia fluctuans* is also allelic to hyperkalemic periodic paralysis.[64a]

OTHER DISORDERS

In rare instances, periodic weakness has been associated with muscle destruction and with prolonged, severe weakness with only gradual resolution.[112] These cases differ so markedly from periodic paralysis as to pose little difficulty in differential diagnosis.[112]

COINCIDENTAL DISEASES

The occurrence of permanent weakness in cases of periodic paralysis has been attributed to coincidental disease such as spinal muscular atrophy, or to a "progressive" myopathy or muscular dystrophy. Whether such weakness is distinct from the characteristic weakness of untreated or inadequately treated periodic paralysis is unclear. One patient with potassium-sensitive periodic paralysis presented a clinical picture of facioscapulohumeral muscular dystrophy. The family history included other patients with weakness in a facioscapulohumeral distribution but without episodic paralysis.[55] Treatment prevented attacks and improved, but did not totally alleviate, the weakness.

MISTAKEN DIAGNOSIS

One large kindred whose disorders were termed "periodic paralysis" by evaluating physicians responded to acetazolamide, the usual treatment for hypokalemic periodic paralysis. In subsequent studies, however, this disorder proved to be an intermittent ataxia that was acetazolamide-responsive.[46] The intermittent inability to walk resulted from ataxia, not weakness. This serendipitous finding was the result of the misdiagnosis of periodic paralysis. More than 30 similar families have subsequently been identified, and most cases have responded to acetazolamide.[70]

EVALUATION OF THE PATIENT WITH EPISODIC WEAKNESS

During an Episode of Weakness

CLINICAL FINDINGS

The clinical findings during an attack of weakness are similar in all types of periodic paralysis. Weakness is usually proximal and generally symmetric. Weakness precipitated by rest following exercise may be more marked in the exercised muscles. Sensation is normal. Reflexes are depressed or absent. In certain forms of periodic paralysis, especially potassium-sensitive periodic paralysis and the paramyotonias, myotonia may be prominent and Chvostek's sign strongly positive (Table 9–5).

STUDIES TO OBTAIN

It is important to obtain as much information as possible if the patient is seen during an attack of weakness. Serial electrolyte determinations (every 15–30 minutes) will indicate both the absolute level of potassium and sequential changes. Because potassium levels are often normal in potassium-sensitive periodic paralysis and occasionally normal in the hypokalemic form, the direction of serum potassium change during worsening or improving strength is important. Careful quantitation of function testing, such as the ability to rise from the floor or from a chair, often provides better documentation of weakness than does formal, manual muscle

Table 9–5 EVALUATION OF THE PATIENT WITH EPISODIC WEAKNESS

Patient seen *during* episode
  Physical examination (special attention to reflexes, myotonia, Chvostek's sign)
  Sequential potassium levels (every 15–30 min)
  Creatine kinase
  Electrocardiogram
  Sequential tests of respiratory and muscle function
  Exclude other disorders — hypercalcemia, hypocalcemia, hypophosphatemia, hypermagnesemia; rhabdomyolysis

Patient seen in *attack-free* interval
  Exclude other disorders — thyroid, adrenal
  Electromyography – myotonia
  Muscle biopsy — occasionally may be pathognomonic in hypokalemic paralysis; supportive of diagnosis in other forms
  Serial serum potassium levels — often elevated in potassium-sensitive periodic paralysis
  Genetic studies
    Specific molecular defect
    Linkage analysis (if defect not defined)

testing. The electrocardiogram should be monitored for cardiac arrhythmia and for T-wave changes characteristic of hypokalemia (flattening, with the appearance of U waves) or hyperkalemia (peaked T waves). Respiratory failure is unusual during attacks of hypokalemic periodic paralysis and very rare in other forms, but respiratory function may be reduced, and sequential testing of strength is an excellent means of quantitating duration and severity of the attack.

Body Potassium Distribution and the Regulation of Blood Potassium. The response of patients with periodic paralysis to provocative and therapeutic agents must be considered in the context of normal potassium distribution and regulation.[10,23] Muscle is the major reservoir of potassium (Fig. 9–3). Muscle and other cellular membranes respond to a variety of hormones, substrates, and electrolytes with either potassium uptake or potassium release (Table 9–6), to regulate the plasma potassium (less than 1% of

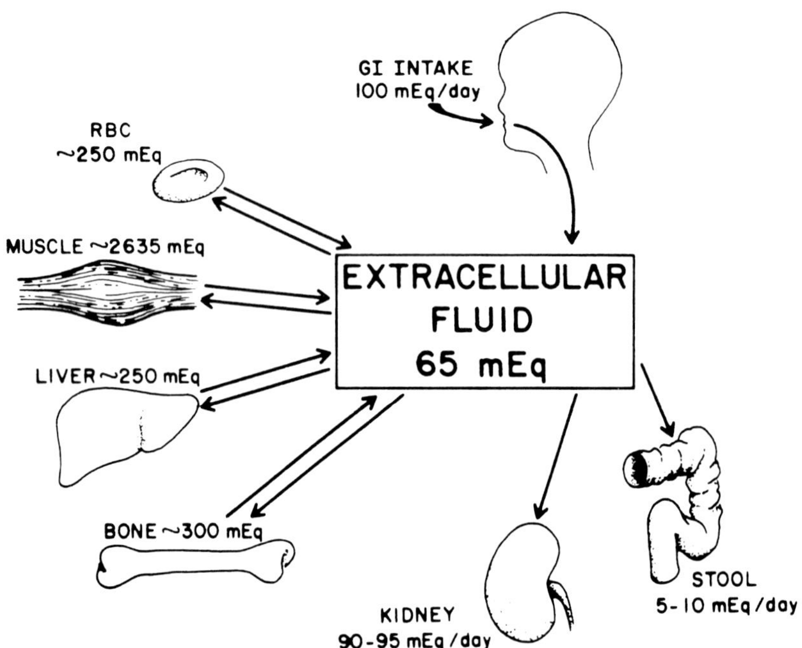

Figure 9–3. Body potassium distribution. Plasma or serum potassium is only a small fraction of total body potassium. Red blood cells, muscle, and other tissues are the major repositories of potassium. (From DeFronzo RA, et al.[23] Modified with permission from the Annual Review of Medicine, Vol. 33, © 1982 by Annual Reviews Inc.)

the potassium in the body). Because the major repository of potassium is muscle, patients with periodic paralysis who develop atrophy have a decrease in total body potassium that reflects the degree of muscle wasting.[45]

The prostacyclin-renin-aldosterone system is a major regulator of renal potassium handling. The kidney produces prostacyclin (prostaglandin I_2),[87] which stimulates renin production by the juxtaglomerular apparatus. Renin, in turn, promotes the formation in the liver of angiotensin I, which is then converted to angiotensin II by angiotensin converting enzyme. Angiotensin II is a potent pressor and also stimulates production of aldosterone by the adrenals. Aldosterone regulates extracellular fluid volume and has both renal and extrarenal effects on potassium metabolism. An increase in aldosterone secretion can result in hypokalemia (and resulting weakness), and the administration of potassium stimulates aldosterone secretion.[88]

The diagnostic characterization of periodic paralysis usually depends on evaluation of plasma potassium levels during spontaneous or provoked attacks of weakness. The usual "normal" range of potassium has been defined by many laboratories as approximately 3.5 to 5.3 mEq/L, but many factors can

Table 9–6 EFFECTS OF HORMONES, SUBSTRATES, AND ELECTROLYTES ON PLASMA POTASSIUM

Lower Potassium	Elevate Potassium
Insulin	Glucagon
Catecholamines	Mannitol
Aldosterone (prostacyclin, renin, angiotensin)	Glucose (insulinopenic subjects)
Glucose	Acidosis
Sodium	
Alkalosis	

affect routine potassium determinations.[10,88] For example:

- Tourniquet-induced stasis elevates potassium levels.[88]
- Whole-body or forearm exercise elevates potassium levels.[25,56]
- Morning levels of potassium may be lower than evening levels.[84]
- Food intake affects potassium levels both directly and by stimulating insulin release.[23]
- Hemolysis of erythrocytes can elevate plasma potassium, but the elevation is not important unless the degree of hemolysis is sufficient to discolor the plasma.

It is likely that a much "tighter" range of normal values is obtained if subjects are studied under controlled conditions. In one study of normal subjects, the range of venous plasma potassium was 3.85 to 4.17 mEq/L (4.01 $\pm$ 0.05 mEq/L, mean $\pm$ SEM).[114]

EXCLUDING THYROTOXIC PERIODIC PARALYSIS

Thyrotoxicosis must be excluded in all patients with hypokalemic periodic paralysis who have no family history. As already mentioned, the diagnosis is often occult. The thyroxine (T_4) and thyrotropin (TSH) levels should be obtained (and triiodothyronine E (T_3) if T_4 is normal). T_3 toxicosis occurs predominantly in older patients and is usually associated with goiter.

DIFFERENTIAL DIAGNOSIS

Patients presenting with an initial attack of weakness may not have a definite history of repeated, spontaneous attacks. For that reason, other causes of acute weakness need to be considered, including hypercalcemia, hypocalcemia, hypophosphatemia, hypermagnesemia, and rhabdomyolysis.[20] In addition, nonneuromuscular neurologic diseases such as multiple sclerosis, spinal cord ischemia, transverse myelitis, and brainstem lesions can produce quadriparesis; however, the sensory symptoms and signs in such patients usually point to a central nervous system origin of paralysis rather than a muscular one.

Conversion disorders and malingering can simulate periodic paralysis. Psychogenic weakness is usually accompanied by other, nonanatomic findings, however, and is notable for preserved reflexes. The patient with quadriplegia from periodic paralysis is invariably hyporeflexic or areflexic.

OTHER LABORATORY STUDIES

Muscle biopsy and serum enzyme tests are not very helpful for diagnosis during attacks of paralysis but may be useful to exclude other disorders (see below). In severe attacks of all forms of periodic paralysis, the creatine kinase level is often elevated, and biopsy may disclose vacuoles within muscle fibers, as well as necrotic fibers.

Electrodiagnostic studies are markedly abnormal *during attacks* of periodic paralysis and help to confirm the diagnosis but often do not help to distinguish between the different types of paralysis. Sensory-nerve conduction studies are normal, but motor-nerve conduction studies become distinctly abnormal, with reduced compound muscle action potential (CMAP) amplitudes that correlate with the degree of weakness.[40] Serial studies may objectively document the fall in evoked CMAP as paralysis increases and the subsequent increase in CMAP amplitude as clinical recovery ensues. Repetitive stimulation of the motor nerve during attacks of paralysis may increase CMAP amplitude by as much as 400%.[16] The most significant increases in CMAP size occur with prolonged (and uncomfortable) stimulation for 1 to 2 minutes at 10 Hz, but a substantial rise (up to 50%) is also seen with a brief train of four supramaximal stimuli at 25 Hz.[49] Contractile force increases in proportion to CMAP amplitude as a consequence of improved impulse propagation. Unfortunately, the improvement after repetitive stimulation is only transient.[16]

Electromyographic (EMG) studies during an attack reveal a reduction in the duration and amplitude of motor unit potentials, a change that becomes more pronounced as weakness increases. As weakness becomes severe, fewer motor units are recruited, and ultimately the muscle becomes completely silent.[16,40,49] With recovery, a small number of units appear; recruitment gradually increases until the duration and size of motor unit potentials are finally normal.[16,40] EMG changes are similar in all types of periodic paralysis, with one exception: In patients with potassium-sensitive periodic paralysis who have myotonia, the myotonic discharges are evident early in the attack and are of diagnostic importance. The myotonic discharges disappear as weakness increases, and return with clinical recovery.

During Attack-Free Intervals

Most patients with the complaint of intermittent weakness present for evaluation when they are without symptoms (see Table 9–5). The patient's history will usually suggest a diagnosis of periodic paralysis, and the clinical features may indicate the most likely form. Examination discloses weakness, atrophy, and hyporeflexia only in patients with repeated, untreated or inadequately treated attacks. Myotonia (see Chapter 2, pp. 26–29) may be elicited in many patients with all forms of periodic paralysis except hypokalemic periodic paralysis, where myotonia is confined to the eyelids.[107] Confirmatory studies are always indicated, since these studies help both to refine the diagnosis and to predict the best treatment.

Specific molecular diagnosis is now possible for the majority of patients with periodic paralysis[34,99a,99b,99c] and should eventually replace many other diagnostic tests (see p. 332). Serum enzymes, electrodiagnostic studies, and muscle biopsy may provide helpful information, particularly if there is doubt as to whether actual paralysis is occurr-

ing. The creatine kinase level is often elevated, even during attack-free intervals.

Between attacks, EMG may be helpful diagnostically in two respects. First, in patients who develop fixed weakness, a myopathic pattern is observed. Second, the finding of myotonic discharges in a patient with episodic weakness suggests the diagnosis of potassium-sensitive periodic paralysis. The other condition associated with episodic weakness and myotonic discharges is paramyotonia congenita. The latter condition is relatively easy to characterize because: (1) cold provokes attacks; (2) cooling the muscle to 20°C eliminates both myotonic discharges and voluntary activity and results in a fall in evoked CMAP amplitude; and (3) delayed muscle relaxation outlasts myotonic discharges.[15,35,127,133]

THE EXERCISE TEST

Another approach for evaluating patients between attacks takes advantage of the changes in CMAP produced by exercise. Thus, while motor- and sensory-nerve conduction studies are usually normal between attacks, exercise may provoke diagnostically helpful abnormalities in the evoked CMAP and twitch. Testing is based on the observation that, as described above, repetitive nerve stimulation or a strong voluntary muscle contraction is followed by a substantial increase in CMAP amplitude during attacks, with a subsequent decline of CMAP size.[79]

The test involves supramaximal motor nerve stimulation of the ulnar nerve, taking care to immobilize the hand. The CMAP is recorded with surface electrodes over the belly and tendon of the hypothenar muscle.[79] At least three control CMAPs are recorded at 1-minute intervals. Then the patient executes a maximum voluntary contraction for 2 to 5 minutes, with brief rests (3–4 seconds) every 15 seconds. CMAP is recorded at 1-minute intervals during exercise and recovery. In control subjects, only small CMAP changes

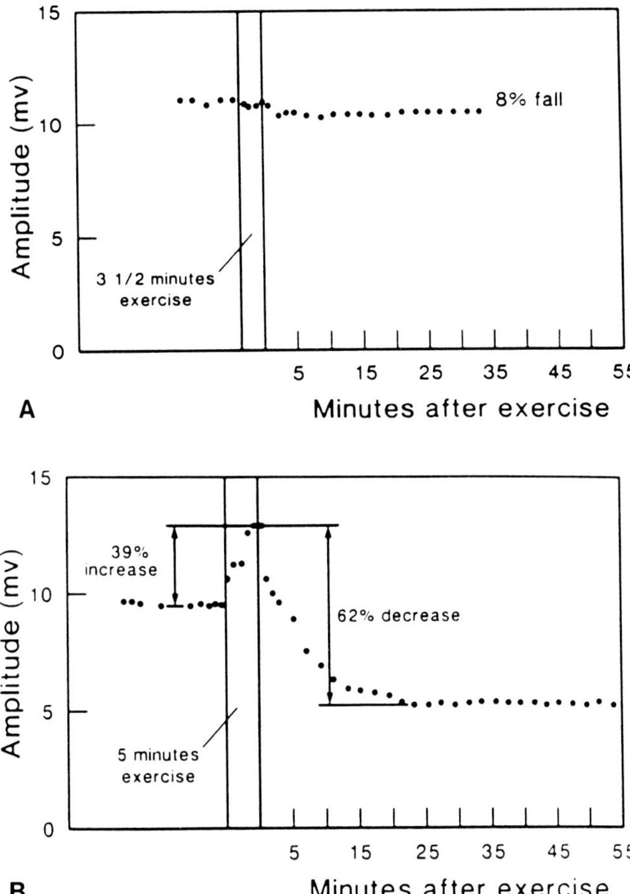

Figure 9–4. The amplitude of hypothenar compound muscle action potential recorded before, during, and after maximal voluntary contraction of hypothenar muscles. (*A*) Normal subject. (*B*) Patient with periodic paralysis. Dots indicate amplitude in response to a single stimulus.

occur: Amplitude increases immediately after exercise (mean 11%, range 0%–27%) and decreases after 5 minutes of recovery (mean 15%, range 0%–30%). Most patients with periodic paralysis, on the other hand, show a greater-than-normal increase in CMAP size after exercise (Fig. 9–4). Of 21 patients in whom clinical diagnosis was definitive, the mean increase was 35%, with a range of 0% to 300%. Findings were abnormal on this part of the test for all patients with potassium-sensitive periodic paralysis, 7 of 13 with the hypokalemic disorder, and 6 of 9 with secondary paralysis.[79] The subsequent decline in CMAP amplitude (mean decrease 48%) is maximal during the first 20 minutes after the cessation of exercise. An abnormal exercise response

occurs in approximately 70% of patients. The test does not help to distinguish between different types of periodic paralysis.

Test results for patients with paramyotonia congenita (as well as myotonia congenita and myotonic dystrophy) show a different pattern of abnormalities, in which CMAP amplitude is reduced both during and immediately after exercise. For periodic paralysis patients, on the other hand, increased CMAP amplitude is found after exercise, with a later decline.

BIOPSY FINDINGS

Muscle biopsy is often remarkably abnormal during attack-free intervals and may provide findings characteristic

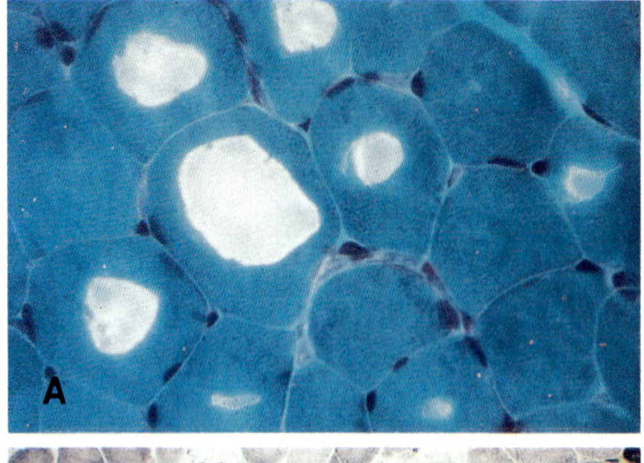

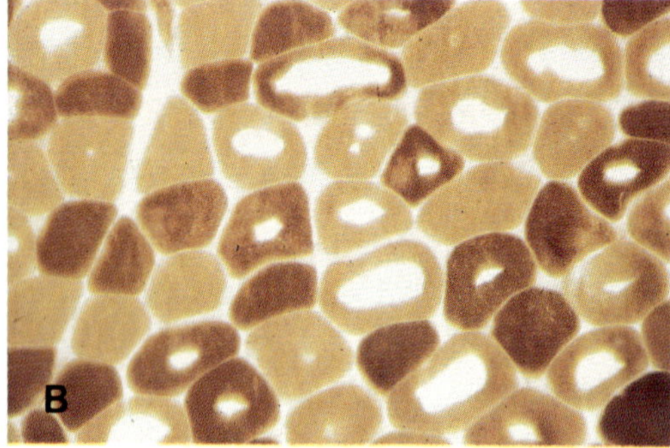

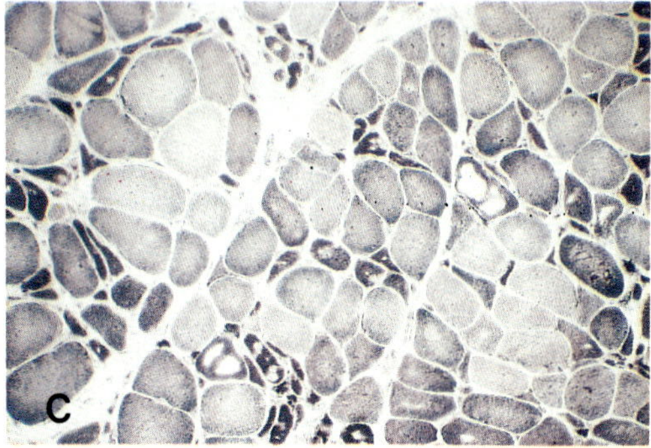

Figure 9–5. Biopsy findings in hypokalemic paralysis. (*A*) Vacuoles are typical of periodic paralysis; in hypokalemic periodic paralysis, vacuoles are characteristically large and central (trichrome). (*B*) ATPase 9.4 shows vacuoles in both type-1 and type-2 fibers (ATPase 9.4). (*C*) Oxidative-enzyme–positive atrophic fibers are prominent in patients with persistent weakness. Vacuoles can be seen in many fibers (NADH-tetrazolium reductase).

of a specific diagnosis. It seldom affords a definitive diagnosis, however, and is often unnecessary if molecular or provocative tests are diagnostic.

Hypokalemic Periodic Paralysis. Hypokalemic periodic paralysis is characterized on light microscopy by the presence of distinctive, large, central vacuoles (Fig. 9–5A,B). A single vacuole may fill the bulk of the fiber, or multiple vacuoles may be present. The vacuoles are seen more frequently in patients with long-standing weakness,[29] but they can also occur in a large number of fibers in a muscle of normal strength.[44] Muscle fiber necrosis and focal degeneration of myofibers is also noted in some biopsies. The biopsy of muscles that are weak often shows marked atrophy, with angular fibers suggesting chronic denervation (Fig. 9–5C).[13]

Potassium-Sensitive Periodic Paralysis. In potassium-sensitive periodic paralysis, light microscopy shows vacuolar changes, but the vacuoles are smaller, less numerous, and often peripheral.[29] The extent of fiber necrosis

and focal degeneration is similar to that in hypokalemic periodic paralysis. A spectrum of myopathic changes occurs with long-standing weakness.[11] For the variant of potassium-sensitive periodic paralysis associated with ventricular arrhythmias, a characteristic biopsy shows numerous tubular aggregates[131b] (Fig. 9–6), but vacuoles have not been observed.

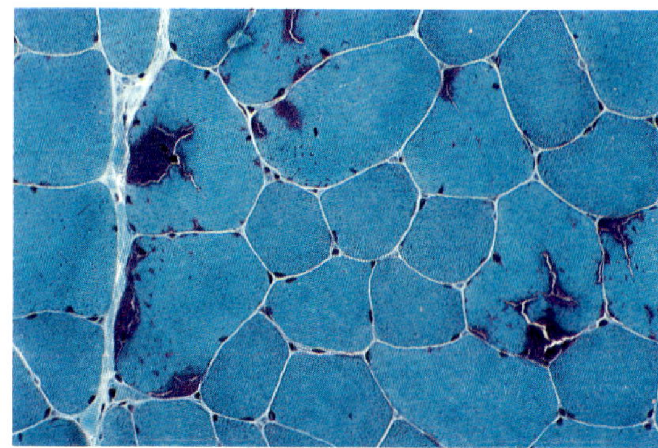

Figure 9–6. Biopsy findings in potassium-sensitive periodic paralysis with cardiac arrhythmias, showing prominent tubular aggregates in many muscle fibers (trichrome).

The muscle biopsy findings of patients with the two forms of paramyotonia congenita have not been as extensively described as other forms of periodic paralysis. Vacuolar changes tend to be less frequent than in other forms of periodic paralysis.[111] A spectrum of myopathic features occurs, and such features are more marked in patients with permanent weakness.[111]

PROVOCATIVE TESTING

Inaccurate or inadequate characterization of the diagnosis precludes successful treatment of periodic paralysis. Even if the diagnosis is clear by molecular and clinical testing, the patient's response to hypokalemic and hyperkalemic challenges may provide information useful for determining treatment (Table 9–7). For example, some patients with hypokalemic periodic paralysis become weak at "normal" levels of potassium,[134] certain patients with potassium-sensitive periodic paralysis become weak with hypokalemia,[61] and most, if not all, patients with periodic myotonia experience clinical changes that correlate with changes in plasma potassium.[136]

Hypokalemic Challenge. Caution is necessary with all provocative testing. A physician must be present during testing; strength, electrocardiogram, and electrolytes must be serially monitored (see Table 9–7). Patients with a history of severe weakness should usually be given intravenous glucose or insulin in reduced dosage.

Hyperkalemic Challenge. Potassium must not be administered to patients with renal insufficiency or with insulinopenic diabetes, and potassium administration may be hazardous in patients with other concomitant diseases (see Table 9–7). Initial doses of potassium chloride should be small, and careful monitoring is essential.

Cold Provocation Testing. Patients having a history of cold-induced weakness or myotonia must be challenged with caution. The maximum

Table 9–7 HYPOKALEMIC AND HYPERKALEMIC CHALLENGE OF PATIENTS SUSPECTED OF HAVING PERIODIC PARALYSIS

FOR HYPOKALEMIC PERIODIC PARALYSIS

Initial
Oral glucose load 1.5 g/kg (maximum 100 g)—over 3 min

Monitor
Strength in 2–4 muscles every 30 min
Electrolytes (Na$^+$, K$^+$, Cl$^-$) and CO$_2$ every 30 min for 3 h; then hourly to 5 h
Electrocardiogram every 30 min

If no weakness or adverse effects from oral load and if no medical contraindication (e.g., cardiac failure)
IV glucose load 3 g/kg (maximum 200 g) in water (2 g/5 mL) infused over 1 h. If not weak at 30 min, 0.1 U/kg insulin IV. If not weak at 60 min, repeat insulin.

Monitor
Strength (see above) every 15 min for 2 h
Electrolytes and CO$_2$ every 30 min and when the patient becomes weak
Electrocardiogram every 15 min throughout study
Anticipate hypoglycemia at 75–150 min

FOR POTASSIUM-SENSITIVE PERIODIC PARALYSIS

Potassium loading (*only if renal and cardiac function are normal*)
Initial testing—0.05 g/kg KCl in sugar-free liquid over 3 min
If negative, subsequent testing with 0.10–0.15 g/kg KCl may be performed
Monitor electrolytes (Na$^+$, K$^+$, Cl$^-$ and HCO$_3^-$), electrocardiogram, strength in 2–4 muscles every 15 min for 2 h; then every 30 min for 2 h
Weakness is characteristically seen at 90–180 min

IV = intravenously.

challenge we have employed is immersion of the arm for 30 minutes in water maintained at 10°C.[111] Strength and myotonia are evaluated at 5, 10, 15, and 30 minutes, and if abnormalities occur, then at 30- to 60-minute intervals until strength returns to normal. The cold immersion is terminated when weakness is first documented. Abnormalities usually appear within 5 to 15 minutes. Use of a hand dynamometer (e.g., Jamar [Asinow Engineering Company, Santa

Monica, CA]) is helpful for documentation of weakness. It is also helpful for the examiner to perform a similar immersion and testing of his or her own arm for comparison. Some subjective or objective clinical signs of muscle stiffness may occur even in normal subjects, but normal subjects do not lose strength.

PATHOGENESIS OF THE PERIODIC PARALYSES

The genetic defect responsible for the majority of patients with potassium-sensitive periodic paralysis has been localized to chromosome 17q,[34,101] and consists of single base substitution in the gene for the alpha-subunit of the sodium channel in the sarcolemma.[99,117] Similarly, the gene lesion responsible for hypokalemic periodic paralysis is a mutation in the dihydrophyridine receptor on chromosome 1q.[34a,99c]

Figure 9–7 depicts the alpha-subunit of the sodium channel, showing four homologous domains, each with six membrane-spanning segments, and the point mutations identified in patients having potassium-sensitive periodic paralysis. DNA analysis from leucocytes or muscle now permits specific diagnosis of this disorder.

Additional mutations of the sodium channel gene will likely be found in patients with various forms of potassium-sensitive periodic paralyses and paramyotonic disorders. Specific point mutations have been defined in the sodium channel gene in paramyotonia congenita.[98] Variations in the phenotype are likely to correspond to different alterations of the sodium channel as a result of mutations at specific sites.

Once linkage to chromosome 1q was established,[34a] a candidate gene, the dihydropyridine receptor gene, was studied for mutations. Thus far, several mutations have been identified in this gene; the presence of de novo mutations in a sporadic case also has been documented.[99c]

Hypokalemic Periodic Paralysis

RELATIONSHIP TO
POTASSIUM LEVEL

The plasma potassium level invariably falls during paralytic attacks in hypokalemic periodic paralysis. Levels are usually below 3.0 mEq/L, and levels

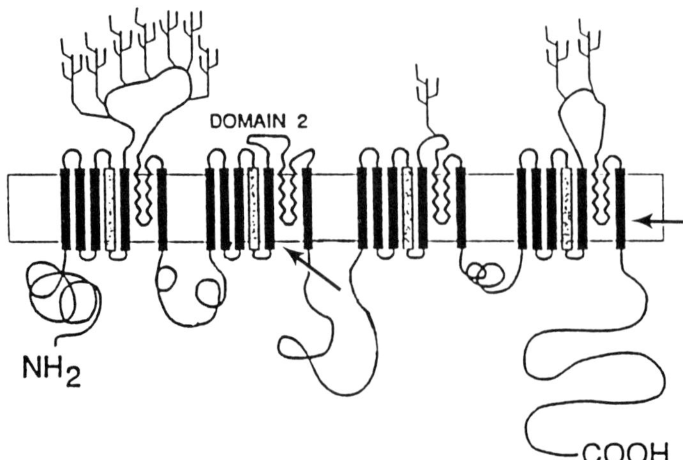

Figure 9–7. Sodium channel model showing four homologous domains, each with six membrane-spanning segments. Arrows show the approximate sites of point mutations in segment 5 of domain 2 (C to T transition resulting in a methionine to threonine substitution) and segment 6 of domain 4 (A to G substitution causing a methionine to valine change) identified in patients with potassium-sensitive periodic paralysis. (From Ptacek et al.[99b] Reprinted by permission of The New England Journal of Medicine 328:482, 1993.)

below 2.0 mEq/L are not uncommon.[112] Severe hypokalemia is associated with profound weakness in patients who are hypokalemic for other reasons,[41] but in hypokalemic periodic paralysis, weakness often persists even after the potassium level has returned to normal.[112] Moreover, in certain patients, plasma potassium need not fall to abnormal levels even during severe attacks.[134] It thus seems likely that the fall in potassium is the *result*, not the *cause*, of the attacks.[36]

There is excellent evidence for abnormal uptake of potassium by muscle in patients with hypokalemic periodic paralysis.[142] Prior to and during an attack of weakness, urinary potassium excretion falls,[102,142] and excessive muscle uptake can be demonstrated by studying arteriovenous differences across forearm skeletal muscle during both attacks and attack-free intervals.[142,49] Using intra-arterial infusions of insulin, Zierler[142] showed that muscle is abnormally sensitive to the effect of insulin on potassium uptake. The basis for this increase in muscle sensitivity to insulin is not known.

MUSCLE MEMBRANE DEFECT

Hypokalemic periodic paralysis is caused by mutations in the voltage-sensitive dihydropyridine receptor.[99c] The mutations thus far identified occur in the fourth putative membrane-spanning segment of the receptor's fourth domain. Dihydropyridine receptors are involved with excitation-contraction coupling and voltage-gated calcium conductance. The portion of the receptor containing mutations functions as a voltage sensor for the calcium channel. Work currently in progress should clarify the basis for the episodic electrical inexcitability and associated changes in potassium levels that occur with attacks of paralysis.[99c]

The muscle cell membrane is therefore the site of abnormality in hypokalemic periodic paralysis. Muscle fibers become electrically inexcitable during attacks of weakness[120]; the resting membrane potential is decreased during and between attacks.[36] Studies of "skinned" muscle fibers established that the muscle contractile apparatus responds normally to directly applied calcium, indicating an abnormal sarcolemma.[30] Muscle fibers are slightly depolarized in normal extracellular potassium but markedly depolarized with lowered external potassium concentrations.[36,119] Potassium and chloride conductances are normal; an increase in sodium conductance with an increased sodium permeability is likely.[135] A similar conclusion was supported by studies showing an increased intracellular sodium concentration.[51]

Thyrotoxic Periodic Paralysis

Although thyroid hormone administration does not exacerbate familial hypokalemic periodic paralysis, a defect in muscle probably permits the development of periodic paralysis in thyrotoxic patients.[29] The evidence that beta-adrenergic blocking agents improve thyrotoxic myopathy and periodic paralysis suggests that an abnormal sensitivity to catecholamines may underlie the defect in this disorder.[106]

Studies of muscle membrane in thyrotoxic periodic paralysis have been limited, but they show evidence of increased muscle uptake of potassium during attacks.[122] In vitro studies of muscle suggest a decrease in calcium pump activity,[130] which is possibly related to a thyroid-induced defect in oxidative phosphorylation. Studies of erythrocytes from two patients with thyrotoxic periodic paralysis have shown abnormalities of sodium or potassium influx, suggesting a disturbance of the sodium-potassium pump.[75]

Potassium-Sensitive Periodic Paralysis

SODIUM CHANNEL ABNORMALITY

Electrophysiologic studies on intercostal muscles from patients with potassium-sensitive periodic paralysis suggest a functional abnormality in the sodium channel.[36,120] These observations prompted the search for the gene locus of the alpha-subunit of the sodium channel.[34] As mentioned, the gene defect has been characterized,[99,117] but the structure-function relationships remain to be determined.

RELATIONSHIP TO POTASSIUM LEVEL

The plasma potassium level rises during many attacks of potassium-sensitive periodic paralysis but often remains within the normal range.[4,37,114] Furthermore, the plasma potassium level may later become subnormal even while weakness persists,[37,112] and it seldom reaches the level of potassium (>6.5 mEq/L) that is associated with weakness in patients without periodic paralysis.[23] It is the *response* to potassium and the persistent abnormalities in potassium regulation that best characterize the disorder. In fact, the sustained elevation of potassium observed in many patients is often diagnostically helpful during attack-free intervals (Fig. 9–8).[66]

MUSCLE MEMBRANE DEFECT

As in hypokalemic periodic paralysis, the membrane potential has been noted to be low both during and between attacks.[36,120] In vitro studies point to an abnormally increased muscle membrane sodium permeability, which then leads to the passive efflux of potassium from muscle.[4] Because potassium efflux from muscle is continuously abnormal, as evidenced by both in vivo[66] and in vitro[62] data, an additional, intermittent factor has been considered. Abnormalities in the secretion of corticotropin (ACTH),[124] insulin,[94] and catecholamines have been noted, but none has been observed consistently.[4]

TREATMENT OF PERIODIC PARALYSIS

All forms of periodic paralysis are amenable to treatment, and patients' symptoms can usually be alleviated. Emergency treatment is often necessary for acute attacks of hypokalemic periodic paralysis but is seldom required for potassium-sensitive or paramyotonic paralysis. Prophylactic treat-

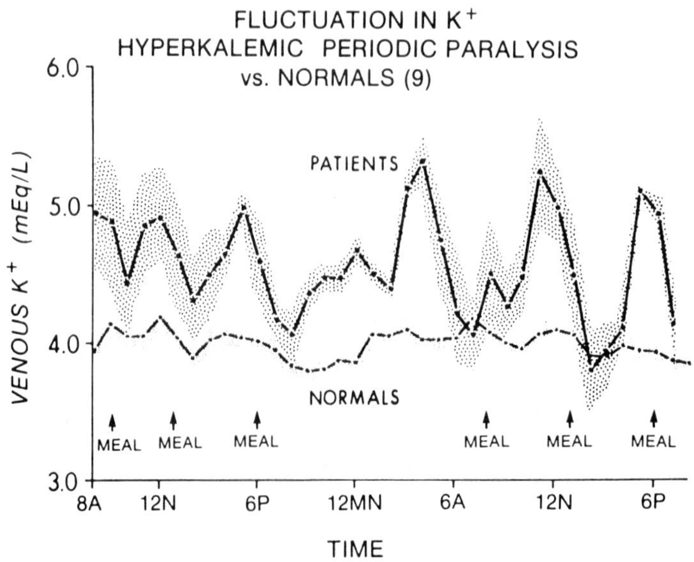

Figure 9–8. Plasma venous K+ (mEq per liter) determined hourly throughout a 36-hour period. Patient data are the mean ± SEM of duplicate studies in two patients with hyperkalemic periodic paralysis. Normal data are the mean ± SEM for nine normal subjects. Meals (*arrows*) were at identical times for all studies. (From Lewis et al,[66] with permission.)

ment to prevent attacks is indicated for patients with all forms of periodic paralysis in whom attacks are frequent, as such treatment may prevent progressive weakness. When persistent weakness has already developed, it can be improved, but severe weakness is seldom completely reversible.

Hypokalemic Periodic Paralysis

ACUTE ATTACKS

The treatment is similar to that of hypokalemia from any cause, except that patients with hypokalemic periodic paralysis have a pathologically greater uptake of potassium in muscle in response to insulin, catecholamines, and possibly other hormones. This sensitivity of periodic paralysis muscle to insulin makes the means of potassium administration particularly important.[142] Administration should be oral if at all possible. Only when patients have nausea or vomiting, or are unable to swallow, should intravenous treatment be considered (Table 9–8).

Table 9–8 TREATMENT OF ACUTE ATTACKS OF WEAKNESS: HYPOKALEMIC PERIODIC PARALYSIS

Preferred
  Oral potassium salts (0.25 mEq/kg body
    weight until weakness improves, every 30
    min)
  Avoid carbohydrate-containing foods
  Avoid IV fluids
*If patient's condition precludes oral potassium
  administration* (e.g., vomiting)
  Intravenous potassium—requires serial
    electrocardiogram monitoring and
    sequential serum potassium measurements.
    Potassium dosage must be decreased for
    patients with renal disease.
  KCl bolus (0.05–0.1 mEq KCL/kg body weight)
  KCl in 5% mannitol (20–40 mEq/L)—avoid
    glucose or NaCl-containing diluents (see text)

All patients
  Gentle exercise of involved muscles often
    hastens recovery

Hazards of Parenteral Potassium. Intravenous potassium administration poses special hazards in periodic paralysis. In normal subjects, the administration of potassium using glucose or physiologic saline as a diluent is often associated with a *fall* in plasma potassium.[33,58] Such a fall, accompanied by greater weakness, has also been observed in patients with periodic paralysis who were given large doses of intravenous potassium with 5% glucose as a diluent.[48] Use of 5% mannitol as a diluent, however, produces a prompt rise in potassium and an improvement in strength (Fig. 9–9).[48] Mannitol also has been shown to increase plasma potassium in normal subjects when given intravenously (see Table 9–6).[85] The potential hazards of intravenous potassium administration have led us to administer bolus potassium chloride rather than continuous infusions of potassium.

Side Effects. Besides those attributable to diluents used in intravenous treatment, other side effects of potassium administration include gastrointestinal irritation and ulceration with oral potassium preparations, and peripheral vein inflammation and pain with intravenous administration.[60]

PROPHYLACTIC TREATMENT

Dietary modification with a low-carbohydrate, low-sodium diet may decrease the severity of attacks but is seldom sufficient to eliminate them. Acetazolamide is the treatment of choice to prevent paralytic attacks in hypokalemic periodic paralysis and is effective in 90% of patients (Table 9–9).[108] Acetazolamide prevents and improves interattack weakness.[44] A few patients, however, not only fail to respond to acetazolamide, but their condition may even be worsened by it.[134] Triamterene has proved effective in such patients.[134] Spironolactone has also been useful in some patients. Another carbonic anhydrase inhibitor, dichlorphenamide, is effective in pre-

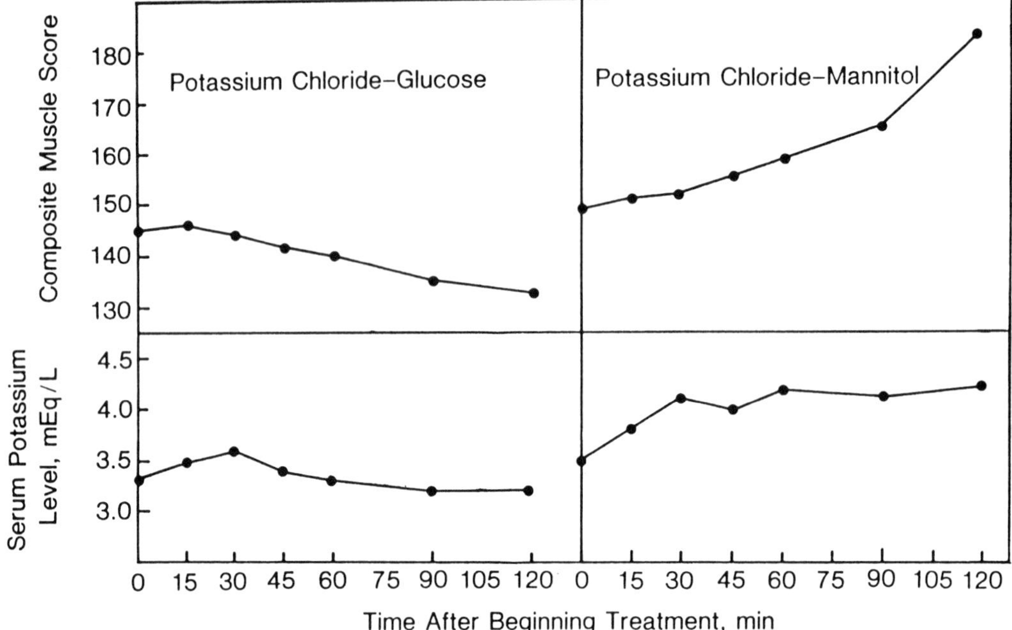

Figure 9–9. Muscle strength and serum potassium levels during intravenous treatment of similar attacks of weakness with either a potassium chloride-glucose solution (50 mEq of potassium chloride per liter of 5% glucose) or a potassium chloride-mannitol solution (35 mEq of potassium chloride per liter of 5% mannitol). Solutions were administered at a rate of 250 mL/h. (From Griggs et al: Intravenous treatment of hypokalemic periodic paralysis. Arch Neurol 40:539, 1983. Copyright © 1983, American Medical Association.)

venting attacks and may be more effective than acetazolamide in treating persistent interattack weakness.[22]

Acetazolamide is well tolerated. The usual toxic effects of acetazolamide are those of any sulfonamide, and include rash, hepatotoxicity, and hematologic toxicity.[71] These side effects have not been reported in patients with periodic

Table 9–9 PREVENTION OF ATTACKS: HYPOKALEMIC PERIODIC PARALYSIS

Diet — avoidance of carbohydrate, sodium loads
Oral potassium supplements — 0.25–0.5
  mEq/kg body weight, taken at bedtime

Carbonic anhydrase inhibitors
  Acetazolamide — 125–1500 mg/d
  Dichlorphenamide — 50–150 mg/d

*Patients unresponsive to carbonic anhydrase
  inhibitors*
  Triamterene — 25–100 mg/d (*caution with
    potassium supplements*)
  Spironolactone — 25–100 mg/d (*caution with
    potassium supplements*)

paralysis but should be considered, particularly as therapy is being introduced. The only common complication of acetazolamide therapy is the formation of renal calculi, which occurs in approximately 10% of patients treated for prolonged periods. Renal failure has never occurred, however, and symptoms related to the calculi are uncommon. Patients taking acetazolamide should be monitored with an annual ultrasound or roentgenographic study for renal calculi, which can be removed by lithotripsy.[131a] Slight side effects that are frequent in patients at the beginning of treatment include nausea, anorexia, mild weight loss, and dysgeusia for carbonated beverages.[112,113] Sulfonamides should not be given to patients taking acetazolamide, because sulfonamide calculi may form. Patients do not become refractory to acetazolamide for this indication, as they characteristically do when acetazolamide is used for treatment of seizures.[113]

Dichlorphenamide toxicity is, in general, similar to that of acetazolamide, although the number of patients who have been followed on long-term dichlorphenamide therapy is not large enough to indicate the risk of forming renal calculi with chronic use.

Thyrotoxic Periodic Paralysis

Thyrotoxic periodic paralysis should be treated by conventional management for thyrotoxicosis. Acetazolamide is not beneficial for attack prevention and is associated with severe side effects.[89] Beta-adrenergic blocking agents are rapidly effective in preventing paralytic attacks and improving persistent interattack weakness in these patients.[18] Thyroid ablation by medical or surgical means results in permanent remission of thyrotoxic periodic paralysis,[112] but readministration of thyroid hormone or recurrence of hyperthyroidism is associated with the return of paralytic attacks.[90]

Potassium-Sensitive Periodic Paralysis

ACUTE ATTACKS

Most individual attacks are mild and do not require treatment (Table 9–10). Patients frequently discover that carbohydrate-containing food and fluid promptly improve weakness. Such food (e.g., orange juice) frequently contains high concentrations of potassium, however, which one would theoretically wish to avoid. We recommend foods (e.g., glucose-containing candy) containing simple carbohydrates that are low in potassium. The beta-adrenergic agonist salbutamol is effective, and when used as an inhalant, it is convenient and relatively safe.[9] It is important to identify these patients whose condition is associated with cardiac arrhythmias,[131b] because administration of adrenergic agents is potentially hazardous. The usual measures to lower plasma potassium are effective (see Table 9–10). Hyperkalemic weakness sufficient to justify intravenous as opposed to oral therapy is much more frequent in secondary causes of hyperkalemic paralysis than in primary, potassium-sensitive periodic paralysis. The electrocardiogram must be monitored if patients are receiving intravenous treatment to lower potassium levels.

PROPHYLACTIC TREATMENT

Although individual attacks are characteristically mild, they should be prevented in an effort to forestall permanent weakness (Table 9–11). The beneficial effect of acetazolamide in preventing attacks of periodic paralysis was first noted in potassium-sensitive periodic paralysis,[76] and this drug is occasionally the most effective preventative. Thiazide therapy is equally effective, however, has fewer short-term side effects, and is usually our choice for management.[61] Recent evidence that

Table 9–10 TREATMENT OF ATTACKS OF POTASSIUM-SENSITIVE PERIODIC PARALYSIS

SLIGHT TO MODERATE ATTACKS
  Dietary
    Simple carbohydrate ingestion
    Avoid potassium-containing foods
  β-adrenergic agents
    Salbutamol inhalation (contraindicated if
      cardiac arrhythmia present)

SEVERE ATTACKS*
  IV treatment of hyperkalemia
    Sodium bicarbonate
    Glucose-insulin
    Calcium gluconate

*Uncommon.

Table 9–11 PREVENTION OF ATTACKS: POTASSIUM-SENSITIVE PERIODIC PARALYSIS

Chlorothiazide—250–1000 mg/d (may require supplemental potassium)
Acetazolamide—125–1000 mg/d
Dichlorphenamide—50–150 mg/d

chlorothiazide may accelerate atherosclerotic cardiovascular disease by its effect on plasma lipoproteins argues against its long-term use,[96] but newer agents that do not increase cholesterol, such as indapamide,[81] have not been studied in periodic paralysis. Thiazides are also associated with a number of rare, idiosyncratic side effects, including rash, vasculitis, and hematologic and hepatic toxicity.[2] The major side effect encountered with thiazide treatment of potassium-sensitive periodic paralysis is the lowering of plasma potassium levels, which result in hypokalemic weakness. Potassium administration improves this weakness. This paradoxical effect further emphasizes the inappropriateness of the term "hyperkalemic periodic paralysis."[61,112] Despite the various concerns about thiazide treatment, it remains the preferred agent.

Careful, sequential follow-up of patients with hyperkalemic periodic paralysis is important, because the mildness of attacks often leads patients to ignore them. Such patients may be at risk for progressive weakness that will become irreversible if not recognized and treated relatively early in its course.[112]

Potassium-Sensitive Periodic Paralysis with Cardiac Arrhythmias

This disorder is difficult to treat. The lowering of potassium with thiazide diuretics prevents attacks but worsens cardiac arrhythmias. Because life-threatening ventricular arrhythmias are present in many such patients and sudden death is frequent,[131b] it is difficult to justify agents that increase cardiac irritability. The tricyclic antidepressant imipramine has been reported to be effective in decreasing ventricular irritability.[131b]

Acetazolamide or dichlorphenamide administration has decreased attack frequency and severity. These agents lower potassium slightly, but the administration of low-dose potassium appears to prevent the worsening of cardiac arrhythmias. Persistent weakness has been noted to improve when attacks are prevented.[131b]

The Paramyotonias

ACUTE ATTACKS

Patients with paramyotonia seldom seek treatment during attacks. Attacks are so clearly related to precipitating exposure to cold or exercise that patients characteristically adjust their activities and exposure to cold to cope with their symptoms. If treatment is necessary, the diametrically opposite responses of the two forms of periodic paralysis to potassium bears emphasis, as agents raising or lowering potassium may produce profound effects in these patients. Patients with paramyotonia congenita will often become weak with hypokalemia,[111] whereas myotonia is alleviated. On the other hand, patients with paralysis periodica paramyotonica become weak with potassium administration or elevation and improve with lowering of potassium.

PROPHYLACTIC TREATMENT

The orally absorbed methylated lidocaine derivatives mexiletine and tocainide are effective for treatment of both paramyotonia congenita and paralysis periodica paramyotonica.[118,125] Both the cold-induced and exercise-induced exacerbation of myotonia and precipitation of generalized weakness respond to treatment.[118] The major side effects of mexiletine are diarrhea and abdominal cramps; it is also associated with rash. Agranulocytosis is a major untoward side effect of tocainide.[39] The frequency of this side effect is uncertain, but its occurrence has led to recommendations that it not be used for cardiac arrhythmias and myotonia.[39] We have chosen to use mexiletine as the initial treatment in many patients with paramyotonia and myotonia. The paramyotonias do not usually respond well to other treatments for myotonia such as quinine, procainamide, and phenytoin.

Both acetazolamide and chlorothiazide have prevented attacks of weakness and alleviated myotonic symptoms in paralysis periodica paramyotonica[111]; acetazolamide has occasionally been of dramatic benefit. Patients with paramyotonia congenita, on the other hand, have developed severe weakness with acetazolamide administration, perhaps because of the hypokalemia it induced.[111] In general it is expected that the potassium-sparing drugs would be beneficial for prophylaxis of paralysis in paramyotonia congenita, and kaliuretic agents, in paralysis periodica myotonica.[111] Further study of these disorders is indicated.

Mechanism of Action of Acetazolamide in Periodic Paralysis

The basis for acetazolamide action in periodic paralysis has been the subject of a number of studies.[52,114,115,141] With all forms of periodic paralysis, some patients exhibit a paradoxical response to this agent, an observation that suggests some commonality in underlying defect. Acetazolamide is kaliuretic and produces a metabolic acidosis.[74] It lowers plasma potassium in normal subjects (Fig. 9-10) and in patients with hypokalemic periodic paralysis.[114,134] This lowering of potassium may account for the precipitation of hypokalemic paralytic attacks by acetazolamide in approximately 10% of patients with hypokalemic periodic paralysis.[134] Its therapeutic effect in some patients

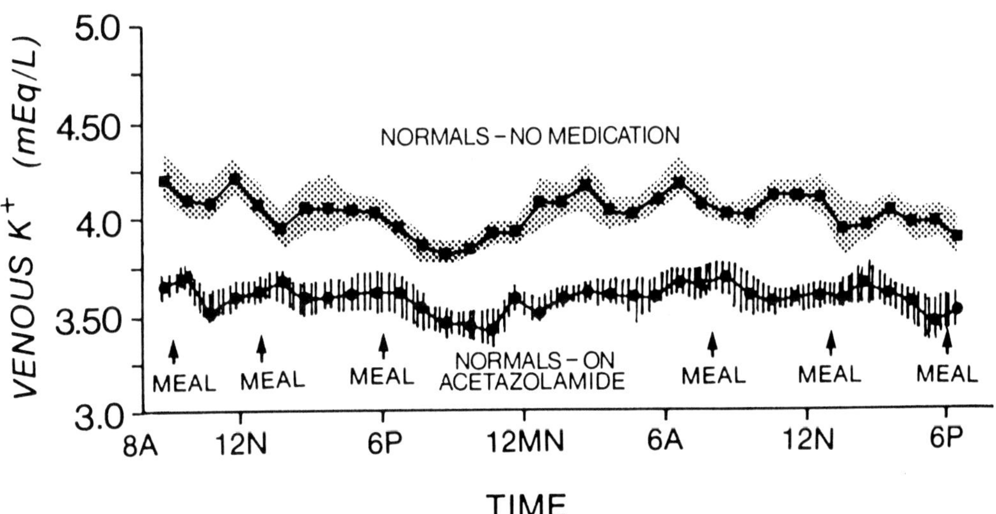

Figure 9–10. Fluctuation of plasma potassium in normals with and without acetazolamide. Plasma venous K+ (mEq per liter) determined hourly throughout a 36-hour period. Data are the mean ± SEM for eight normal subjects on no medication and seven normal subjects on acetazolamide. Meals (*arrows*) were at identical times for all studies. (From Riggs et al,[114] with permission.)

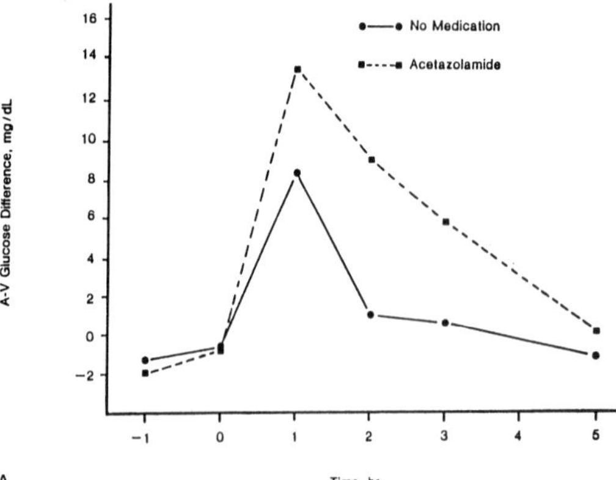

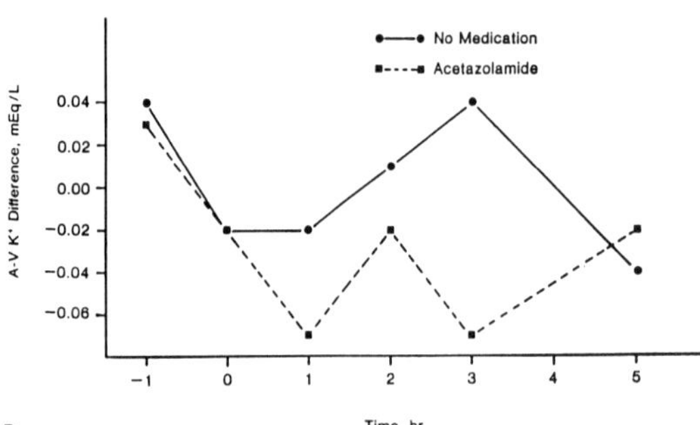

Figure 9–11. (*A*) Mean arterialized-minus-venous (A-V) glucose differences in eight untreated and acetazolamide-treated normal subjects, determined 1 hour before and during a 5-hour oral glucose tolerance test (glucose load, 1.5 g/kg). (*B*) Mean arterialized-minus-venous potassium (A-V K^+) differences during the same study. (From Riggs et al: Dissociation of glucose and potassium arterial-venous differences across the forearm by acetazolamide: A possible relationship to acetazolamide's beneficial effect in hypokalemic periodic paralysis. Arch Neurol 41:35–38, 1984. Copyright © 1984, American Medical Association.)

may be produced by metabolic acidosis,[108,141] as it prevents the intracellular movement of potassium, augments glucose uptake in normal subjects (Fig. 9–11),[52,140] and may prevent the pathologic ingress of potassium into muscle in patients with hypokalemic paralysis. Induction of metabolic acidosis with ammonium chloride prevents attacks of hypokalemic periodic paralysis.[140]

When carbonic anhydrase inhibitors were first recognized to be effective treatment for periodic paralysis, evidence indicated an absence of carbonic anhydrase in skeletal muscle.[73] More recently, it has been shown that a sulfonamide-resistant carbonic anhydrase is present in substantial concentrations in skeletal muscle in animals[54] and in humans.[95] Three isozymes (CA I, CA II, and CA III) have been found in skeletal muscle, with CA III constituting up to 20% of noncontractile muscle protein. Diseased muscle may have an alter-

ation in carbonic anhydrase enzyme activity.[95] Acetazolamide inhibits only CA I. At this point, therefore, it is unlikely that direct carbonic anhydrase inhibition in muscle contributes to the therapeutic effectiveness of carbonic anhydrase inhibitors in periodic paralysis and myotonia.

It is now feasible to directly study the effects of acidosis, potassium concentration, and other factors in mutant and normal sodium and calcium channels.[16a,99a,99b] Such studies should help characterize the basis for acetazolamide's benefit.

MYOTONIA

CLINICAL FEATURES AND SYMPTOMS OF MYOTONIA

Myotonias have in common the distinctive clinical phenomenon of delayed relaxation of the skeletal muscle following either voluntary contraction or the contraction resulting from muscle percussion (see Fig. 2–6 to 2–10; pp. 26–29). Clinical myotonia is accompanied by repetitive electrical muscle activity reflected as action potentials on electromyography. The clinical elicitation of myotonia is discussed in Chapter 2. Because action myotonia and percussion myotonia are not equally expressed in the different myotonic disorders, a specific search for each type of myotonia is necessary. Certain disorders have a characteristic distribution of myotonia. Most notable is myotonic dystrophy, where myotonia is not elicitable in muscles that are clinically less affected.[126]

Slight myotonia is often asymptomatic. Facial myotonia usually causes embarrassment when lid closure produces sustained orbicularis oculi myotonia and a persistent inability to open the eyelids (see Fig. 2–9). The resulting "squint" may persist for minutes. Eyelid myotonia produces a "frightened," staring expression that is similarly embarrassing. Generalized limb myotonia is often more disabling (see Fig. 2–6), as sudden muscle contraction may cause virtually complete immobility. Good exercise performance is often possible in such patients, however, because their myotonia improves with repeated activity (warm-up), although performance may be severely limited in cold weather. Patients may lose balance and fall if they suddenly or unexpectedly initiate activity. Extraocular muscle myotonia is less common; it may induce double vision or limit eye-hand coordination in sporting events. Patients with myotonia usually complain of "stiffness" but may occasionally describe their symptom as "cramps" or "charley horses." Pain is not usually a feature of myotonia, except in variant forms of myotonia congenita.[136]

Some rare patients with clinical features of myotonia do not have EMG myotonia. These conditions are considered in Chapter 2 (p. 27). Likewise, EMG myotonia is occasionally seen without clinical accompaniment, although in most such instances the abnormal EMG activity is not typical of the classic "dive bomber" pattern (see Chapter 2).

CLASSIFICATION OF MYOTONIA

Table 9–12 lists the major disorders associated with myotonia. Myotonic dystrophy is the commonest, outnumbering all other conditions by approximately 10 to 1; it is followed in frequency by the various forms of myotonia congenita.

Myotonic Dystrophy

This disorder is the most frequent cause of myotonia but has been considered in detail in Chapter 4. Myotonia is helpful in diagnosis but is frequently asymptomatic. Weakness rather than myotonia is usually responsible for the symptoms of hand stiffness, and alleviation of myotonia is seldom helpful in improving function. Myotonia in myotonic dystrophy occurs most prominently in muscles that are symptomatically the weakest.[126] On the other hand,

Table 9–12 CLASSIFICATION OF DISORDERS ASSOCIATED WITH CLINICAL MYOTONIA

Myotonic dystrophy
Myotonia congenita
  Autosomal dominant (Thomsen's disease)
  Autosomal recessive (Becker's disease)
Sodium-channel (alpha-subunit) defects
  Autosomal dominant (painful, periodic variant)
  Paramyotonia congenita
  Potassium-sensitive (paralysis periodica paramyotonica)
  Potassium-sensitive (hyperkalemic) periodic paralysis
Isaac's syndrome: myokymia, hyperhidrosis, distal wasting
Chondrodystrophic myotonia
Drugs
  Clofibrate
  Diazocholesterol
  2,4-Dichlorphenoxyacetate (2,4-D)

as weakness progresses and muscle atrophy occurs, myotonia sometimes can no longer be elicited.

Myotonia Congenita

AUTOSOMAL DOMINANT MYOTONIA CONGENITA

Clinical Features. Autosomal dominant myotonia congenita is also known as Thomsen's disease.[17,126] Symptoms of myotonia are usually noted in infancy and are more troublesome in males than females. The severity of disease symptoms often lessens when patients reach the third and fourth decade. Symptoms are worsened with cold and improved by warm-up. The severity of symptoms fluctuates, but shows no obvious correlations with weather, dietary intake, stress, or exercise. On physical examination, strength is always normal. Muscle bulk is either normal or moderately increased; hypertrophy may develop particularly in the masseter muscles (producing a characteristic facial appearance, as in Fig. 2–15), proximal arm muscles, thighs, and calves. The extensor digitorum brevis muscle also is often enlarged. Muscle stretch reflexes and the sensory examination are normal.

Laboratory Studies. The creatine kinase (CK) level is occasionally slightly elevated, possibly because of the enlarged muscle mass. Other than myotonic discharges, the EMG is usually normal. Even with minimal needle movement or muscle contraction, profuse myotonic discharges may make it difficult to evaluate motor unit potentials in some patients.

Repetitive nerve stimulation or exer-

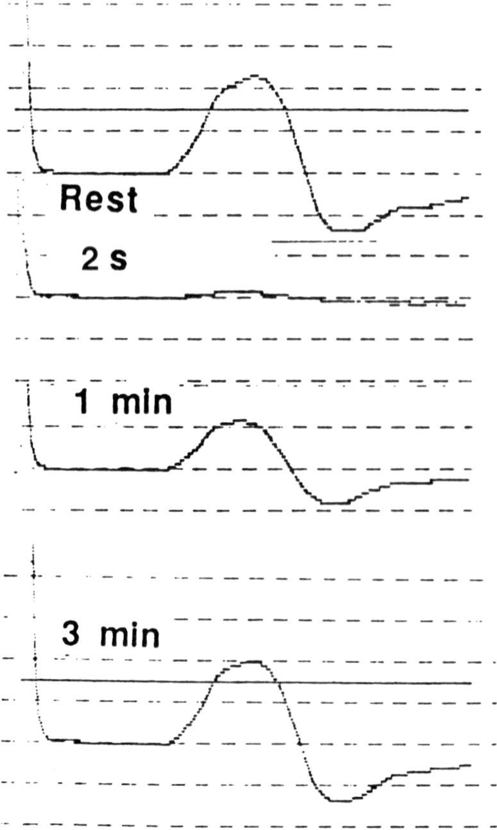

Figure 9–12. Evoked muscle action potentials from tibialis anterior at rest (*top*). The compound muscle action potential was reduced immediately (2 seconds) after a 10-second maximum voluntary contraction (not shown), with partial recovery demonstrated at 1 minute and 3 minutes.

cise may produce substantial changes in muscle membrane function; these may be useful in diagnosis. Decremental responses to repetitive nerve stimulation are common, particularly at high frequencies (>30 Hz).[126] Similar changes can be produced with exercise testing using a 10-second maximum voluntary contraction of immobilized muscles. The CMAP amplitude is reduced immediately after exercise and recovers within 2 to 4 minutes (Fig. 9–12).[3,126] Cooling has no significant effect on the results of this test in patients with myotonia congenita.

Finally, other family members should be studied to help determine the pattern of inheritance, because asymptomatic family members may have myotonic discharges. Muscle biopsy shows no evidence for muscle destruction, but a distinctive lack of type 2B fibers has been recognized in both autosomal dominant and autosomal recessive forms of disease.[21] A generalized enlargement of muscle fibers has also been noted.[21]

AUTOSOMAL RECESSIVE MYOTONIA CONGENITA

Clinical Features. The autosomal recessive form of myotonia was first described by Becker and now bears his name.[8] In certain cases, the clinical features are indistinguishable from those of Thomsen's disease.[50] In some, slight distal weakness and atrophy with contractures of distal joints have been observed.[8,50,128] In others, there is transient weakness that resolves with exercise; this weakness can be severe and disabling.[128] Symptoms may appear later (age 4–12 years) and be more severe in the legs with this condition than in Thomsen's disease.[126] The CK level is often elevated to 2 to 4 times normal. Nerve conduction studies give normal results, but repetitive nerve stimulation or short exercise testing may demonstrate substantial reduction in CMAP amplitude (see Fig. 9–12), which recovers rapidly. The CMAP amplitude may be reduced by up to 80% of resting amplitude, a reduction that corresponds to the frequent transient paresis

in such patients.[126,128] EMG evidence of myopathy correlates with the moderate weakness that affects many patients with this condition. Myotonic discharges are usually present in both proximal and distal muscles. Occasionally, heterozygous individuals may have myotonic discharges.[128]

Genetics. Sporadic cases of myotonia congenita presumably have this recessive form of myotonia. Cases with two or more siblings within one kindred but without affected parents have been identified.[128] It remains unclear whether all sporadic cases represent autosomal recessive myotonia congenita or whether some may be mutations of autosomal dominant myotonia. Spontaneous mutations of autosomal dominant myotonia occurring *de novo* and exhibiting subsequent transmission consistent with an autosomal dominant pattern have not yet been documented.

PAINFUL VARIANT OF MYOTONIA CONGENITA

Both autosomal dominant and autosomal recessive forms of myotonia congenita are usually painless,[17,128] but one autosomal dominant variant of myotonia congenita is characterized by muscle pain and periodic worsening of myotonia.[136] The treatment for this variant is different than for other forms (see below). This form of myotonia congenita can be identified both by the clinical features and by muscle biopsy: Type 2B muscle fibers were present in multiple patients in two separate families,[136] whereas they are absent in the other forms of myotonia congenita.[21] The gene lesion for this atypical form of myotonia congenita has been localized to the alpha-subunit of the sodium channel, and it is thus allelic to hyperkalemic periodic paralysis.[99a] Other cases of "sodium-channel myotonia" have also been studied.[64a]

Paramyotonia Congenita

The paramyotonias are considered earlier in this chapter, under the periodic paralyses. Myotonia in these disorders is markedly exacerbated by cold. In many instances this myotonia is paradoxical (see Fig. 2–9; p. 29) and *worsens* with repeated activity rather than "warming up."

DIFFERENTIAL DIAGNOSIS

Numerous other causes of sustained muscle contraction or of impaired muscle relaxation can resemble myotonia (see Table 9–12). All are infrequent and are distinguishable from myotonia on both clinical and electrophysiologic evaluation.

A number of common conditions that do not cause myotonia can occasionally be interpreted as suggesting myotonia, based on either history or examination. For example, muscle cramps are painful muscle contractions that result from paroxysmal discharges of nerve (see Chapter 2; pp. 26–27). Cramps are readily distinguished from myotonia by EMG. Increases in muscle tone from central nervous system disease result in spasticity or rigidity on a central basis. Accompanying neurologic signs usually indicate the basis for the abnormal muscle tone. Dystonia, particularly when focal and paroxysmal, is often painless and can suggest a primary muscular rigidity. The sustained postures that are adopted distinguish dystonia clinically from myotonia, and the EMG activity is that of entire motor units, as opposed to muscle fiber hyperactivity.

PATHOGENESIS OF MYOTONIA

The gene lesions responsible for most diseases that cause myotonia are being defined as this book goes to press. Defects of both the chloride channel[38a,57a] and sodium channel[64a,99a,99b] cause the various forms of myotonia congenita. Paramyotonia congenita results from a defect in the sodium channel. The gene product is still poorly characterized for myotonic dystrophy.[33a] Studies currently in progress in many laboratories are using in vitro systems to define the molecular pathomechanisms responsible for myotonia in each disorder.[17a,64a]

Myotonia Congenita

Myotonia congenita in humans is virtually identical to an animal model of goat myotonia congenita[69]; autosomal dominant genetic transmission occurs in both disorders. Extensive study of myotonic goat intercostal muscle, together with more limited studies in humans, suggests that an abnormal decrease in chloride permeability is a major defect in myotonic muscle.[14] Myotonic discharges would be expected with a decrease in chloride conductance,[1a,6,12] and computer models of muscle membrane function predict that such a decrease in chloride conductance and permeability will result in repetitive, propagated action potentials.[6,12] Studies of experimental, drug-induced myotonia have confirmed this prediction.[59] This model is also consistent with the observed increase in myotonia predicted by increases in extracellular potassium.[26]

Chloride conductance is indeed abnormal in patients with myotonia congenita.[53] Two different techniques have been used to study the pathogenesis of myotonia: (1) electrophysiologic investigation of whole intercostal muscle fibers removed on biopsy, and (2) resealed fiber segments from biopsy of limb muscles. The latter method permits patch-clamp analysis of sodium currents.[53] Studies of autosomal dominant myotonia congenita (Thomsen's disease) show normal chloride conductance but abnormal inactivation of sodium channels, resulting in reopening. Similar abnormal gating of the sodium channel is also present in most other forms of myotonia.[53] Although in vitro work suggests an abnormality in sodium channel function, autosomal dominant myotonia congenita is not allelic to other sodium channel disorders.

Instead, it results from a mutation of a chloride channel locus on chromosome 7.[1,38a] Similarly, autosomal recessive myotonia congenita is likely to be the result of a chloride channel defect.[57a,99b]

Myotonic Dystrophy

In myotonic dystrophy, the myotonic phenomenon is similar, but direct evidence shows that it does not result from an alteration in chloride permeability.[68] Instead, there are numerous abnormalities of muscle membrane function that include alterations in the sodium pump[77] and membrane sodium-potassium adenosine triphosphatase (ATPase) activity.[5] Cultured myotonic muscle has been found to be hyperexcitable and to have decreased muscle membrane potentials,[80] but this observation has not been confirmed by all workers.[129] Preliminary evidence suggests an abnormality in the calcium-activated potassium channel in mammalian muscle: In a single study, binding of the bee-venom toxin (apamin) by myotonic but not by normal muscle has been observed.[105] Recent work has shown that the gene defect in myotonic dystrophy results in an abnormality of a protein kinase that may in turn affect cell membrane responses to normal signals (see Chapter 4).[33a,99b]

Paramyotonia Congenita

In paramyotonia congenita, EMG study shows that the frequency of myotonic discharge is less than in myotonia congenita and myotonic dystrophy, and the waxing and waning character responsible for the "dive-bomber" sound is infrequently seen.[110] Muscle cooling in the absence of action will produce repetitive motor unit discharges that reflect cold-induced muscle depolarization.[64] With increased cooling of muscle, myotonia disappears and complete muscle depolarization and paralysis occur.[110] Studies of intercostal muscle have suggested that abnormal

function of the sodium channel causes this depolarization.[63,109] Genetic studies have confirmed this defect and defined the locus to the alpha-subunit of the sodium channel.[101] Both cold and exercise provoke attacks of muscle weakness. In both forms of paramyotonia, potassium uptake by muscle occurs during attacks. In contrast, normal subjects release potassium.[86] This influx of potassium into muscle also contrasts with the situation in potassium-sensitive periodic paralysis, in which potassium is released from muscle during spontaneous paralytic attacks.[86] It is not clear whether *spontaneous* attacks in the paramyotonias are associated with potassium uptake or with potassium release, but in most patients, the majority of attacks, if not all, are associated either with cold or exercise provocation. It has been hypothesized that in paramyotonia congenita, muscle sodium channels remain abnormally open at rest, and that this abnormal open state is markedly increased with cooling.[86,120] The sodium-potassium pump is probably normal and accounts for the increased potassium uptake.

TREATMENT OF MYOTONIC DISORDERS

Table 9–13 lists agents that have been used successfully in the treatment of myotonia. For myotonia congenita, quinine and procainamide are usually the most satisfactory treatment. They can be taken intermittently when symptoms are troublesome. Thus, a patient can take quinine shortly before engaging in physical activity or when the weather is cold. In patients requiring chronic antimyotonic treatment, phenytoin is often the agent of choice in view of its relatively low incidence of side effects.[41]

In patients with cardiac conduction abnormalities, such as occur in myotonic dystrophy, phenytoin is theoretically preferable, because both quinine and procainamide slow conduction

Table 9–13 TREATMENT OF MYOTONIA

MYOTONIA CONGENITA
　Quinine (200–1200 mg/d)
　Procainamide (125–1000 mg/d)
　Phenytoin (300–400 mg/d usually necessary
　　to achieve a therapeutic level of 10–20 μg/mL)
　Acetazolamide (125–750 mg/d)
　Mexiletine (150–1000 mg/d)
　Others—corticosteroids, verapamil, diazepam

MYOTONIC DYSTROPHY (treatment seldom
　indicated)
　Phenytoin—usually necessary to achieve
　　therapeutic level

PARAMYOTONIA
　Paramyotonia congenita
　　Mexiletine (150–1000 mg/d)
　　Spironolactone, acetazolamide (see text)
　Potassium-sensitive paramyotonia (paralysis
　　periodica paramyotonica)
　　Mexiletine (150–1000 mg/d)
　　Chlorothiazide (250–1000 mg/d)
　　Spironolactone, acetazolamide

through the atrioventricular (AV) node.[43] Phenytoin, on the other hand, speeds conduction through the AV node.[43] Even in the patient who already has a cardiac pacemaker, procainamide use may be hazardous, because it can decrease response to the pacemaker-generated impulse.[38] Fortunately, myotonia congenita is not associated with an increased incidence of cardiac conduction abnormalities.

In some patients, particularly those with Becker's myotonia congenita, therapy with quinine, procainamide, or phenytoin is ineffective.[126] Side effects may also dictate alternative therapy. In these situations, one of the other agents listed on Table 9–13 may be necessary. Acetazolamide has been found to be effective in patients with atypical myotonia,[47,136] as well as in patients with paramyotonia.[112] Tocainide and mexiletine are also effective in some patients with myotonia congenita and have the added benefit of preventing weakness in paramyotonia.[126] The toxicity of these agents was discussed on p. 338.

Occasionally patients do not respond to the foregoing agents. Other agents that can be tried for treatment of myotonia include corticosteroids, adrenocorticotropic hormone, and calcium channel blockers.[36,41,50] The long-term hazards of corticosteroids limit their usefulness. Occasional patients have also responded to diazepam or thiazides.

Mechanism of Action

The basis for the therapeutic effect of phenytoin and other therapeutic agents in myotonia is not fully understood. Phenytoin may produce its effect by stabilizing muscle membranes[41]; it has been shown to decrease net sodium influx during membrane excitation. Similarly, procainamide and quinine also are believed to stabilize muscle membranes.[41] The effect of acetazolamide is probably related, in part, to the modest kaliuresis and slight decline in serum potassium level it produces.[47] Myotonia is increased by potassium administration,[136] and diminishes in correlation with a fall in serum potassium level (Fig. 9–13).

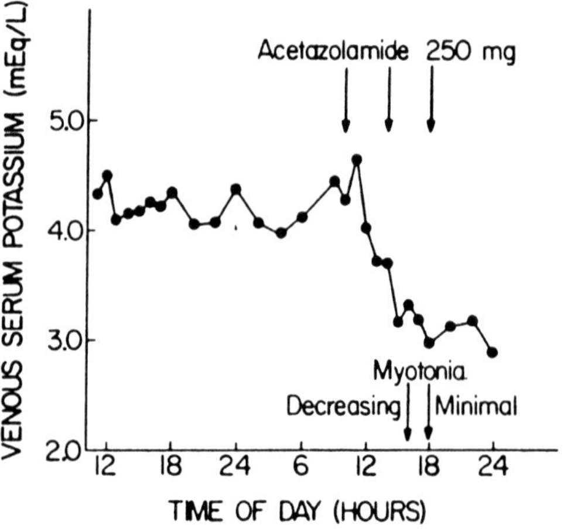

Figure 9–13. Effect of acetazolamide (doses shown by *upper arrows*) on venous potassium in a patient with periodic painful myotonia. As potassium declined, myotonia improved (*lower arrows*). (From Griggs et al.[47] Reprinted with permission from Annals of Neurology 3:531–537, 1978.)

Agents Exacerbating Myotonia

In myotonia congenita, succinylcholine and anticholinesterase agents should be avoided, since they aggravate myotonia.[132] If muscle relaxation is necessary during anesthesia, *d*-tubocurarine is preferable. Myotonia is not prevented by curare, but is not exacerbated by it either.[50] Because potassium administration exacerbates myotonia,[47] intravenous and oral potassium supplementation should be given only with caution and with careful clinical observation.

Hyperthermic responses to general anesthesia have been noted in patients with myotonic disorders.[104] It is unclear whether patients with myotonia congenita or myotonic dystrophy are likely to develop true malignant hyperpyrexia.[41] Nonetheless, it seems prudent not to use succinylcholine and to avoid general anesthesia when possible.

SUMMARY

The *periodic paralyses* and paramyotonia congenita are rare disorders characterized by the onset of episodic weakness, usually in childhood or adolescence. Patients are initially of normal strength between attacks, but if attacks are not treated, progressive interattack weakness develops, usually a decade or more after the onset of attacks. There are many different types of periodic paralysis, and the specific diagnosis is established by the clinical history and by the careful, serial documentation of electrolyte levels during attacks. Provocative testing is usually necessary if the attacks are infrequent and is also helpful in planning therapy. For all forms of periodic paralysis, attacks of weakness can be prevented by appropriate treatment in nearly all patients.

Most forms of periodic paralysis have been shown to be inherited as autosomal dominant disorders. It has been determined that the genetic defect in potassium-sensitive periodic paralysis is located on chromosome 17 and is due to single base substitutions in different domains of the gene coding for the alpha-subunit of the sodium channel.

The *myotonic disorders* are characterized by complaints of muscle stiffness and occasionally pain. Weakness is not usually present, although it can be severe in myotonic dystrophy. Moderate weakness is also present in the autosomal recessive form of myotonia congenita. The genetic defect that causes myotonia has been defined for potassium-sensitive periodic paralysis and for myotonic dystrophy, although the gene product abnormality remains unclear for the latter. Preliminary evidence suggests that defects in the gene coding for the chloride channel will account for both autosomal dominant and autosomal recessive myotonia congenita. Atypical, painful, or fluctuating myotonias result from mutations in the alpha-subunit of the sodium channel. Most of the disorders show autosomal dominant inheritance. Symptoms of myotonia can usually be alleviated by treatment, and the weakness of autosomal recessive myotonia often responds to adequate treatment of the myotonia.

REFERENCES

1. Abdalla JA, Casley WL, Hudson AJ, et al: Linkage analysis of candidate loci in autosomal dominant myotonia congenita. Neurology 42:1561, 1992.
1a. Adrian RH and Marshall MW: Action potentials reconstructed in normal and myotonic muscle fibres. J Physiol 258:125, 1976.
2. Ames RP: Negative effects of diuretic drugs on metabolic risk factors for coronary heart disease: Possible alternative drug therapies. Am J Cardiol 51:632, 1983.
3. Aminoff MJ, Layzer RB, Satya-Murti S, and Faden AI: The declining electrical response of muscle to repetitive nerve stimulation in myotonia. Neurology 27:812, 1977.
4. Andersen ED, Krasilnikoff PA, and Overvad H: Intermittent muscular

weakness, extrasystoles, and multiple developmental anomalies. Acta Paediat Scand 60:559, 1971.

5. Appel SH and Roses AD: Membranes and myotonia. In Rowland LP (ed): Pathogenesis of Human Muscular Dystrophies. Excerpta Medica, Amsterdam, 1977.

6. Barchi RL: Myotonia. An evaluation of the chloride hypothesis. Arch Neurol 32:175, 1975.

7. Becker PE: Genetic approaches to the nosology of muscle diseases: Myotonias and similar diseases. Birth Defects 7:52, 1971.

8. Becker PE: Syndromes associated with myotonia: Clinical-genetic classification. In Rowland LP (ed): Pathogenesis of Human Muscular Dystrophies. Excerpta Medica, Amsterdam, 1977, p. 699.

9. Bendheim PE, Reale EO, and Berg BO: β-Adrenergic treatment of hyperkalemic periodic paralysis. Neurology 35:746, 1985.

10. Bia MJ and DeFronzo RA: Extrarenal potassium homeostasis. Am J Physiol 240:F257, 1981.

11. Bradley WG: Adynamia episodica hereditaria: Clinical, pathological and electrophysiological studies in an affected family. Brain 92:345, 1969.

12. Bretag AH: Myotonia and chloride. Arch Neurol 33:304, 1976.

13. Brooke MH and Engel WK: The histographic analysis of human muscle biopsies with regard to fiber types. 3: Myotonias, myasthenia gravis, and hypokalemic periodic paralysis. Neurology 19:469, 1969.

14. Bryant SH: Cable properties of external intercostal muscle fibres from myotonic and nonmyotonic goats. J Physiol 204:539, 1969.

15. Burke D, Skuse NF, and Lethlean K: Contractile properties of the abductor digiti minimi muscle in paramyotonia congenita. J Neurol Neurosurg Psychiatry 37:894, 1974.

16. Campa JF and Sanders DB: Familial hypokalemic periodic paralysis. Local recovery after nerve stimulation. Arch Neurol 31:110, 1974.

16a. Cannon SC, Brown RH, Corey DP: Theoretical reconstruction of myotonia and paralysis caused by incomplete inactivation of sodium channels. Biophys J 65:270, 1993.

17. Caughey JE and Myrianthopoulos NC: Dystrophia Myotonica and Related Disorders. Charles C Thomas, Springfield, IL, 1963.

17a. Chahine M, George AL, Zhou M, et al: Sodium channel mutations in paramyotonia congenita uncoupled inactivation from activation. Neuron 12:1, 1994.

18. Conway MJ, Seibel JA, and Eaton RP: Thyrotoxicosis and periodic paralysis: improvement with beta blockade. Ann Intern Med 81:332, 1974.

19. Deleted in proof.

20. Corbett AJ: Electrolyte disorders affecting muscle. Semin Neurol 3:248, 1983.

21. Crews J, Kaiser KK, and Brooke MH: Muscle pathology of myotonia congenita. J Neurol Sci 28:449, 1976.

22. Dalakas MC and Engel WK: Treatment of "permanent" muscle weakness in familial hypokalemic periodic paralysis. Muscle Nerve 6:182, 1983.

23. DeFronzo RA, Bia M, and Smith D: Clinical disorders of hyperkalemia. Annu Rev Med 33:521, 1982.

24. Delwaide PJ and Penders CA: Paramyotonie familiale et crises parétiques avec hypokaliémie. Rev Neurol (Paris) 125:287, 1971.

25. Don BR, Sebastian A, Cheitlin M, Christiansen M, and Schambelan M: Pseudohyperkalemia caused by fist clenching during phlebotomy. N Engl J Med 322:1290, 1990.

26. Durelli L, Mutani R, Fassio F, and Delsedime M: The effects of the increase of arterial potassium upon the excitability of normal and dystrophic myotonic muscles in man. J Neurol Sci 55:249, 1982.

27. Ebers GC, George AL, Barchi RL, et al: Paramyotonia congenita and hyperkalemic periodic paralysis are linked to the adult muscle sodium channel gene. Ann Neurol 30:810, 1991.

28. Engel AG: Evolution and content of vacuoles in primary hypokalemic periodic paralysis. Mayo Clin Proc 45:774, 1970.

29. Engel AG: Periodic paralysis. In Engel AG, Banker BQ (eds): Myology. McGraw-Hill, New York, 1986, p 1843.

30. Engel AG and Lambert EH: Calcium activation of electrically inexcitable muscle fibers in primary hypokalemic periodic paralysis. Neurology 19:851, 1969.

31. Eulenburg A: Ueber eine familiare, durch 6 generationen verfolgbare form congenitaler paramyotonie. Neurologische Centralblatt 5:265, 1886.

32. Fenech FF and Soler NG: Hyperkalaemic periodic paralysis starting at age 48. BMJ 2:472, 1968.

33. Fisch C, Shields JP, Ridolfo SA, and Feigenbaum H: Effect of potassium on conduction and ectopic rhythms in atrial fibrillation treated with digitalis. Circulation 18:98, 1958.

33a. Fischbeck KH: The mechanism of myotonic dystrophy. Ann Neurol 35:255, 1994.

34. Fontaine B, Khurana TS, Hoffman EP, et al: Hyperkalemic periodic paralysis and the adult muscle sodium channel α-subunit gene. Science 250:1000,1990.

34a. Fontaine B, Vale-Santos J, Jurkat-Rott K, et al: Mapping of the hypokalaemic periodic paralysis (HypoPP) locus to chromosome 1q31-32 in three European families. Nature Genetics 6:267, 1994.

35. French EB and Kilpatrick R: A variety of paramyotonia congenita. J Neurol Neurosurg Psychiatry 20:40, 1957.

36. Furman RE and Barchi RL: Pathophysiology of myotonia and periodic paralysis. In Asbury AK, McKhann GM, and McDonald WI (eds): Diseases of the Nervous System. WB Saunders, Philadelphia, 1986, p 208.

37. Gamstorp I and Wohlfart G: A syndrome characterized by myokymia, myotonia, muscular wasting and increased perspiration. Acta Psychiatr Neurologica Scand 34:181, 1959.

38. Gay RJ and Brown DF: Pacemaker failure due to procainamide toxicity. Am J Cardiol 34:728, 1974.

38a. George AL, Crackower MA, Abdalla JA, Hudson AJ, Ebers GC: Molecular basis of Thomsen's disease (autosomal dominant myotonia congenita). Nature Genetics 3:305, 1993.

39. Gertz MA, Garton JP, and Jennings WH: Aplastic anemia due to tocainide. N Engl J Med 314:583, 1986.

40. Gordon AM, Green JR, and Lagunoff D: Studies on a patient with hypokalemic familial periodic paralysis. Am J Med 48:185, 1970.

41. Griggs RC: The myotonic disorders and the periodic paralyses. In Griggs RC and Moxley RT (eds): Advances in Neurology, vol 17, Raven Press, New York, 1977, p 143.

42. Griggs RC: Periodic paralysis. In Wilson JD, Braunwald E, Isselbacher KJ, et al (eds): Harrison's Principles of Internal Medicine, ed 12. McGraw-Hill, New York, 1991, p 2121.

43. Griggs RC, Davis RJ, Anderson DC, Dove JT: Cardiac conduction in myotonic dystrophy. Am J Med 59:37, 1975.

44. Griggs RC, Engel WK, and Resnick JS: Acetazolamide treatment of hypokalemic periodic paralysis. Ann Intern Med 73:39, 1970.

45. Griggs RC, Forbes G, Moxley RT, and Herr BE: The assessment of muscle mass in progressive neuromuscular disease. Neurology 33:158, 1983.

46. Griggs RC, Moxley RT, Lafrance RA, and McQuillen J: Hereditary paroxysmal ataxia: Response to acetazolamide. Neurology 28:1259, 1978.

47. Griggs RC, Moxley RT, Riggs JE, and Engel WK: Effects of acetazolamide on myotonia. Ann Neurol 3:531, 1978.

48. Griggs RC, Resnick J, and Engel WK: Intravenous treatment of hypokalemic periodic paralysis. Arch Neurol 40:539, 1983.

49. Grob D, Johns RJ, and Liljestrand Ä: Potassium movement in patients with familial periodic paralysis. Rela-

tionship to the defect in muscle function. Am J Med 23:356, 1957.

50. Harper PS: Myotonic Dystrophy. WB Saunders, Philadelphia, 1979, pp 54–69.

51. Hofmann WW and Smith RA: Hypokalemic periodic paralysis studied in vitro. Brain 93:445, 1970.

52. Hoskins B, Maren TH, Vroom FQ, and Jarrell MA: Acetazolamide and potassium flux in red blood cells: Studies in patients with hyperkalemic periodic paralysis. Arch Neurol 31:187, 1974.

53. Iaizzo PA, Franke C, Hatt H, et al: Altered sodium channel behaviour causes myotonia in dominantly inherited myotonia congenita. Neuromuscular Disorders 1:47, 1991.

54. Jeffrey S, Carter ND, and Smith A: Immunocytochemical localization of carbonic anhydrase isozymes I, II, and III in rat skeletal muscle. J Histochem Cytochem 34:513, 1986.

55. Jozefowicz R, Megahed M, Hyser C, and Griggs RC: Facioscapulohumeral muscular dystrophy with potassium-sensitive periodic paralysis. unpublished material, 1994.

56. Kjeldsen K, Norgaard, and Hau C: Exercise-induced hyperkalaemia can be reduced in human subjects by moderate training without change in skeletal muscle Na, K-ATPase concentration. Eur J Clin Invest 20:642, 1990.

57. Klein R, Ganelin R, Marks JF, Usher P, and Richards C: Periodic paralysis with cardiac arrhythmia. J Pediatr 62:371, 1963.

57a. Koch MC, Ricker K, Otto M, et al: Linkage data suggesting allelic heterogeneity for paramyotonia congenita and hyperkalemic periodic paralysis on chromosome 17. Human Genetics 88:71, 1991.

57b. Koch MC, Steinmeyer K, Lorenz C: The skeletal muscle chloride channel in dominant and recessive human myotonia. Science 257:797, 1992.

58. Kunin AS, Surawicz B, and Sims EAH: Decrease in serum potassium concentrations and appearance of cardiac arrhythmias during infusion of potassium with glucose in potassium-depleted patients. N Engl J Med 266:228, 1962.

59. Kwieciński H, Lehmann-Horn F, and Rüdel R: Drug-induced myotonia in human intercostal muscle. Muscle Nerve 11:576, 1988.

60. Lawson DH: Adverse reactions to potassium chloride. Q J Med 43:433, 1974.

61. Layzer RB, Lovelace RE, and Rowland LP: Hyperkalemic periodic paralysis. Arch Neurol 16:455, 1967.

62. Lehmann-Horn F, Rüdel R, Ricker K, Lorković H, Dengler R, and Hopf HC: Two cases of adynamia episodica hereditaria: In vitro investigation of muscle cell membrane and contraction parameters. Muscle Nerve 6:113, 1983.

63. Lehmann-Horn F, Rüdel R, Dengler R, Lorkovic H, Haass A, and Ricker K: Membrane defects in paramyotonia congenita with and without myotonia in a warm environment. Muscle Nerve 4:396, 1981.

64. Lehmann-Horn F, Rüdel R, and Ricker K: Membrane defects in paramyotonia congenita (Eulenburg). Muscle Nerve 10:633, 1987.

64a. Lerche H, Heine R, Pika U, et al: Human sodium channel myotonia: Slowed channel inactivation due to substitutions for a glycine within the III-IV linker. J Physiol 470:13, 1993.

65. Levitt LP, Rose LI, and Dawson DM: Hypokalemic periodic paralysis with arrhythmia. N Engl J Med 286:253, 1972.

66. Lewis ED, Griggs RC, and Moxley RT: Regulation of plasma potassium in hyperkalemic periodic paralysis. Neurology 29:1131, 1979.

67. Linder MA: Periodic paralysis associated with hyperthyroidism: Report of three cases. Ann Intern Med 43:241, 1955.

68. Lipicky RJ: Studies in human myotonic dystrophy. In Rowland LP (ed): Pathogenesis of Human Muscular Dystrophies. Excerpta Medica, Amsterdam, 1977, pp 729–738.

69. Lipicky RJ and Bryant SH: Sodium, potassium, and chloride fluxes in intercostal muscle from normal goats

and goats with hereditary myotonia. J Gen Physiol 50:89, 1966.

70. Livingstone IR, Gardner-Medwin D, and Pennington RJT: Familial intermittent ataxia with possible X-linked recessive inheritance. J Neurol Sci 64:89, 1984.

71. Lombroso CT and Forxythe I: A long-term follow-up of acetazolamide (Diamox) in the treatment of epilepsy. Epilepsia 1:493, 1959.

72. Magee KR: Paramyotonia congenita. Association with cutaneous cold sensitivity and description of peculiar sustained postures after muscle contraction. Arch Neurol 14:590, 1966.

73. Maren TH: Carbonic anhydrase: Chemistry, physiology, and inhibition. Physiol Rev 47:595, 1967.

74. Maren TH: Use of inhibitors in physiological studies of carbonic anhydrase. Am J Physiol 232:F291, 1977.

75. Marx A, Ruppersberg JP, Pietrzyk C, and Rüdel R: Thyrotoxic periodic paralysis and the sodium/potassium pump. Muscle Nerve 12:810, 1989.

76. McArdle B: Adynamia episodica hereditaria and its treatment. Brain 85:121, 1962.

77. McComas AJ and Mrozek K: The electrical properties of muscle fibre membranes in dystrophia myotonica and myotonia congenita. J Neurol Neurosurg Psychiatry 31:441, 1968.

78. McFadzean AJS and Yeung R: Familial occurrence of thyrotoxic periodic paralysis. BMJ 1:760, 1969.

79. McManis PG, Lambert EH, and Daube JR: The exercise test in periodic paralysis. Muscle Nerve 9:704, 1986.

80. Merickel M, Gray R, Chauvin P, and Appel S: Cultured muscle from myotonic muscular dystrophy patients: Altered membrane electrical properties. Proc Natl Acad Sci USA 78:648, 1981.

81. Meyer-Sabellek W, Gotzen R, Heitz J, et al: Serum lipoprotein levels during long-term treatment of hypertension with indapamide. Hypertension 7 (6 pt 2):II 170, 1985.

82. Meyers KR, Gilden DH, Rinaldi CF, and Hansen JL: Periodic muscle weakness, normokalemia, and tubular aggregates. Neurology 22:269, 1972.

83. Miller D, delCastillo J, and Tsang TK: Severe hypokalemia in thyrotoxic periodic paralysis. Am J Emerg Med 7:584, 1989.

84. Moore-Ede MC, Meguid MM, Fitzpatrick GF, Boyden CM, and Ball MR: Circadian variation in response to potassium infusion. Clin Pharmacol Ther 23:218, 1978.

85. Moreno M, Murphy C, and Goldsmith C: Increase in serum potassium resulting from the administration of hypertonic mannitol and other solutions. J Lab Clin Med 73:291, 1969.

86. Moxley RT, Ricker K, Kingston WJ, and Böhlen R: Potassium uptake in muscle during paramyotonic weakness. Neurology 39:952, 1989.

87. Nadler JL, Lee FO, Hsueh W, and Horton R: Evidence of prostacyclin deficiency in the syndrome of hyporeninemic hypoaldosteronism. N Engl J Med 314:1015, 1986.

88. Nardone DA, McDonald WJ, and Girard DE: Mechanisms in hypokalemia: clinical correlation. Medicine 57:435, 1978.

89. Norris FH: Use of acetazolamide in thyrotoxic periodic paralysis. N Engl J Med 286:893, 1972.

90. Okihiro MM and Nordyke RA: Hypokalemic periodic paralysis: Experimental precipitation with sodium liothyronine. JAMA 198:949, 1966.

91. Okinaka S, Shizume K, Iino S, et al: The association of periodic paralysis and hyperthyroidism in Japan. J Clin Endocrinol Metab 17:1454, 1957.

92. Deleted in proof.

93. Pearson CM: The periodic paralyses: differential features and pathological observations in permanent myopathic weakness. Brain 87:341, 1964.

94. Peters BH and Samaan NA: Periodic hypoinsulinemia and hyperglycemia in myotonic periodic paralysis [abstract]. Neurology 22:426, 1972.

95. Peyronnard JM, Charron LF, Messier JP, Lavoie J, Faraco-Cantin F, and Dubreuil M: Histochemical localiza-

tion of carbonic anhydrase in normal and diseased human muscle. Muscle Nerve 11:108, 1988.

96. Pollare T, Lithell H, and Berne C: A comparison of the effects of hydrochlorothiazide and captopril on glucose and lipid metabolism in patients with hypertension. N Engl J Med 321:868, 1989.

97. Poskanzer DC and Kerr DNS: A third type of periodic paralysis, with normokalemia and favourable response to sodium chloride. Am J Med 31:328, 1961.

98. Ptáček LJ, George AL Jr, Barchi RL, et al: Mutations in an S4 segment of the adult skeletal muscle sodium channel cause paramyotonia congenita. Neuron 8:891, 1992.

99. Ptáček LJ, George AL, Griggs RC, et al: Identification of a mutation in the gene causing hyperkalemic periodic paralysis. Cell 67:1021, 1991.

99a. Ptáček LJ, Griggs RC, Tawil R, et al: Sodium channel mutations in acetazolamide-responsive myotonia congenita, paramyotonia congenita and hyperkalemic periodic paralysis. Neurology, in press.

99b. Ptáček LJ, Johnson KJ, Griggs RC: Genetics and physiology of the myotonic muscle disorders. N Engl J Med 328:482, 1993.

99c. Ptáček LJ, Tawil R, Griggs RC, et al: Dihydropyridine receptor mutations cause hypokalemic periodic paralysis. Cell 77:1, 1994.

100. Ptáček LJ, Tawil R, Griggs RC, Storvik D, and Leppert M: Linkage of atypical myotonia congenita to a sodium channel locus. Neurology 42:431, 1992.

101. Ptáček LJ, Trimmer JS, Agnew WS, et al: Paramyotonia congenita and hyperkalemic periodic paralysis map to the same sodium channel locus [abstract]. Neurology 41:1163, 1991.

102. Pudenz RH, McIntosh JF, and McEachern D: The role of potassium in familial periodic paralysis. JAMA 3:2253, 1938.

103. Pun KK, Wong CK, Tsui EYL, Tam SCF, Kung AWC, and Wang CCL: Hypokalemic periodic paralysis due to the Sjögren syndrome in Chinese patients. Ann Intern Med 110:405, 1989.

104. Ravin M, Newmark Z, and Saviello G: Myotonia dystrophica—an anesthetic hazard: Two case reports. Anesth Analg 54:216, 1975.

105. Renaud JF, Desnuelle C, Schmid-Antomarchi H, Hugues M, Serratrice G, and Lazdunski M: Expression of apamin receptor in muscles of patients with myotonic muscular dystrophy. Nature 319:678, 1986.

106. Resnick JS, Dorman JD, and Engel WK: Thyrotoxic periodic paralysis. Am J Med 47:831, 1969.

107. Resnick JS and Engel WK: Myotonic lid lag in hypokalaemic periodic paralysis. J Neurol Neurosurg Psychiatry 30:47, 1967.

108. Resnick JS, Engel WK, Griggs RC, and Stam AC: Acetazolamide prophylaxis in hypokalemic periodic paralysis. N Engl J Med 278:582, 1968.

109. Ricker K, Camacho LM, Grafe P, Lehmann-Horn F, and Rüdel R: Adynamia episodica hereditaria: What causes the weakness? Muscle Nerve 12:883, 1989.

110. Ricker K, Hertel G, Langscheid K, and Stodieck G: Myotonia not aggravated by cooling: Force and relaxation of the adductor pollicis in normal subjects and in myotonia as compared to paramyotonia. J Neurol 216:9, 1977.

111. Riggs JE: The periodic paralyses. Neurol Clin North Am 6:485, 1988.

112. Riggs JE and Griggs RC: Diagnosis and treatment of the periodic paralyses. Clin Neuropharmacol 4:123, 1979.

113. Riggs JE and Griggs RC: Carbonic anhydrase inhibitors. In Frey HH and Janz D (eds): Handbook of Experimental Pharmacology: Antiepileptic Drugs. Springer-Verlag, New York, 1985, pp 595–600.

114. Riggs JE, Griggs RC, Moxley RT, and Lewis ED: Acute effects of acetazolamide in hyperkalemic periodic paralysis. Neurology 31:725, 1981.

115. Riggs JE, Griggs RC, and Moxley RT: Dissociation of glucose and potas-

sium arterial-venous differences across the forearm by acetazolamide: A possible relationship to acetazolamide's beneficial effect in hypokalemic periodic paralysis. Arch Neurol 41:35, 1984.

116. Riggs JE, Moxley RT, Griggs RC, and Horner FA: Hyperkalemic periodic paralysis: An apparent sporadic case. Neurology 31:1157, 1981.

117. Rojas CV, Wang J, Schwartz LS, Hoffman EP, Powell BR, and Brown RH Jr: A met-to-val mutation in the skeletal muscle Na$^+$ channel alpha-subunit in hyperkalemic periodic paralysis. Nature 354:387, 1991.

118. Rüdel R, Dengler R, Ricker K, Haass A, and Emser W: Improved therapy of myotonia with the lidocaine derivative tocainide. J Neurol 222:275, 1980.

119. Rüdel R, Lehmann-Horn F, Ricker K, and Küther G: Hypokalemic periodic paralysis: In vitro investigation of muscle fiber membrane parameters. Muscle Nerve 7:110, 1984.

120. Rüdel R and Ricker K: The primary periodic paralyses. Trends Neurosci 8:467, 1985.

121. Sagild AU and Helweg-Larsen HF: Det kliniske billede ved arvelige transitoriske muskellammelser. Periodisk adynami og periodisk paralyse. Nord Med 53:981, 1955.

122. Shizume K, Shishiba Y, Sakuma M, Yamauchi H, Nakao K, and Okinaka S: Studies on electrolyte metabolism in idiopathic and thyrotoxic periodic paralysis. Metabolism 15:138, 1966.

123. Smith WA: Periodic paralysis: report of two fatal cases. J Nerv Ment Dis 90:210, 1939.

124. Streeten DHP, Dalakos TG, and Fellerman H: Studies on hyperkalemic periodic paralysis: Evidence of changes in plasma Na and Cl and induction of paralysis by adrenal glucocorticoids. J Clin Invest 50:142, 1971.

125. Streib EW: Successful treatment with tocainide of recessive generalized congenital myotonia. Ann Neurol 19:501, 1986.

126. Streib EW: AAEE minimonograph #27: Differential diagnosis of myotonic syndromes. Muscle Nerve 10:603, 1987.

127. Subramony SH, Malhotra CP, and Mishra SK: Distinguishing paramyotonia congenita and myotonia congenita by electromyography. Muscle Nerve 6:374, 1983.

128. Sun SF and Streib EW: Autosomal recessive generalized myotonia. Muscle Nerve 6:143, 1983.

129. Tahmoush AJ, Askanas V, Nelson PG, and Engel WK: Electrophysiologic properties of aneurally cultured muscle from patients with myotonic muscular atrophy. Neurology 33:311, 1983.

130. Takagi A, Schotland DL, DiMauro S, and Rowland LP: Thyrotoxic periodic paralysis. Function of sarcoplasmic reticulum and muscle glycogen. Neurology 23:1008, 1973.

131. Tan SY and Burton M: Hyporeninemic hypoaldosteronism: An overlooked cause of hyperkalemia. Arch Intern Med 141:30, 1981.

131a. Tawil R, Moxley RT, and Griggs RC: Acetazolamide-induced nephrolithiasis: Implications for treatment of neuromuscular disorders. Neurology 43:1105, 1993.

131b. Tawil R, Ptáček LJ, Pavlakis SG, et al: Andersen's syndrome: Potassium-sensitive periodic paralysis, ventricular ectopy, and dysmorphic features. Ann Neurol 35:326, 1994.

132. Thiel RE: The myotonic response to suxamethonium. Br J Anaesth 39:815, 1967.

133. Thrush DC, Morris CJ, and Salmon MV: Paramyotonia congenita: A clinical, histochemical and pathological study. Brain 95:537, 1972.

134. Torres CF, Griggs RC, Moxley RT, and Bender AN: Hypokalemic periodic paralysis exacerbated by acetazolamide. Neurology 31:1423, 1981.

135. Troni W, Doriguzzi C, and Mongini T: Interictal conduction slowing in muscle fibers in hypokalemic periodic paralysis. Neurology 33:1522, 1983.

136. Trudell RG, Kaiser KK, and Griggs RC: Acetazolamide-responsive myo-

tonia congenita. Neurology 37:488, 1987.

137. Tyler FH, Stephens FE, Gunn FD, and Perkoff GT: Studies in disorders of muscle. VII. Clinical manifestations and inheritance of a type of periodic paralysis without hypopotassemia. J Clin Invest 30:492, 1951.

138. Van Der Meulen JP, Gilbert GJ, and Kane CA: Familial hyperkalemic paralysis with myotonia. N Engl J Med 264:1, 1961.

139. Van't Hoff W: Familial myotonic periodic paralysis. Q J Med 31:385, 1962.

140. Viskoper RJ, Licht A, Fidel J, and Chaco J: Acetazolamide treatment in hypokalemic periodic paralysis: A metabolic and electromyographic study. Am J Med Sci 266:119, 1973.

141. Vroom FQ, Jarrell MA, and Maren TH: Acetazolamide treatment of hypokalemic periodic paralysis. Arch Neurol 32:385, 1975.

142. Zierler KL and Andres R: Movement of potassium into skeletal muscle during spontaneous attack in family periodic paralysis. J Clin Invest 36:730, 1957.

ENDOCRINE MYOPATHIES
ELECTROLYTE DISTURBANCES
CHRONIC RENAL FAILURE
MALIGNANCY
NUTRITIONAL AND
  GASTROINTESTINAL DISEASE
DRUGS AND OTHER TOXINS

Many systemic diseases cause muscle weakness. The management of these disorders varies according to the organ system affected. Although the effects of the systemic disorder may be the overproduction or underproduction of an essential hormone that directly affects muscle, the myopathies of systemic disease should be distinguished from "primary" disorders of muscle. In order not to simply reiterate information that can be found in standard textbooks of medicine, our approach is as follows: (1) to emphasize important points in recognizing clinical manifestations of myopathies in systemic diseases; (2) to provide insights into known treatments; and (3) to provide useful references for further reading, such as Layzer's *Neuromuscular Manifestations of Systemic Disease* in this series.

There is a major distinction between the constitutional symptoms of fatigue and weakness characterizing common conditions such as chronic heart failure, lung disease, liver disease, and renal disease and the readily demonstrable muscle weakness justifying the term "myopathy." Any serious systemic illness causing inactivity and poor nutrition may result in moderate weakness, but patients with such disorders usually demonstrate remarkably good manual muscle strength, muscle function, and motor testing, albeit briefly.

ENDOCRINE MYOPATHIES

Patients with endocrine dysfunction frequently complain of fatigue and weakness. These symptoms are often referred to as a "myopathy" despite lack of defined histologic or electrophysiologic criteria fulfilling such a diagnosis. In fact, many of these patients show only muscle atrophy without muscle degeneration. Despite recognition of this problem in nomenclature, terms like "thyrotoxic myopathy" and "steroid myopathy" have become so ingrained in the medical literature that it has become customary to refer to these disorders as myopathies.

Thyroid Disorders

Abnormalities of the thyroid gland cause a wide array of muscle disorders (Table 10–1). These conditions are related to the important role of thyroid hormones in the metabolism of carbohydrates and lipids, as well as in accelerating protein synthesis and enzyme production. Thyroid hormones also stimulate calorigenesis in muscle, increase muscle demand for vitamins, and enhance muscle sensitivity to circulating catecholamines.[71]

Table 10–1 NEUROMUSCULAR DISORDERS ASSOCIATED WITH THYROID DISEASE

HYPOTHYROIDISM
 Neuropathy
  Diffuse, sensorimotor peripheral neuropathy
  Entrapment neuropathy—especially carpal
   tunnel syndrome
 Neuromuscular junction disorders
  Possibly increased incidence of myasthenia
   gravis
  Myasthenic syndrome
 Myopathy
  Children—Debré Kocher-Sémélaigne
   syndrome associated with cretinism
  Adult—muscle cramping, asymptomatic
   hyper-CK-emia, hypertropic myopathy
   (Hoffman's syndrome) with progressive
   proximal weakness

HYPERTHYROIDISM
 Neuropathy (?)
  Cramps and fasciculations
  Motor neuron disease (possible association)
 Neuromuscular junction disorder
  Increased incidence of myasthenia gravis
 Myopathy
  Proximal weakness
  Periodic paralysis
  Bulbar syndrome
  Ophthalmoplegia

HYPOTHYROIDISM

Incidence of Symptoms. Hypothyroid patients have frequent muscle complaints (Table 10–2), but definite muscle weakness occurs in only about 30% to 40% of patients.[147] The prevalence may be higher with more severe or chronic hypothyroidism.[77] Muscle cramps, pain, and stiffness occur in at least one third of cases.[55,178] The so-called myotonoid features, characterized by slow muscle contraction and relaxation, occur in 25% of patients.[146] Proximal weakness in hypothyroid myopathy develops insidiously over months.

Clinical and Laboratory Features (Table 10–2). Myxedema occasionally presents with a painful myopathy that can simulate polymyalgia or polymyositis. In such patients the muscle complaints so dominate the clinical picture that other signs of hypothyroidism may be overlooked.[67] The elevated crea-

tine kinase (CK) level (10-fold to 100-fold times normal) may lead to a misdiagnosis of other muscle diseases, especially "polymyositis."[38,78] The diagnosis of hypothyroidism is made by thyroxine level. Low circulating thyroxine levels establish that hypothyroidism is present; *free* thyroxine is the most reliable measure. The distinction between primary and secondary hypothyroidism is made by thyrotropin (TSH) level. TSH levels are elevated in primary hypothyroidism and low in hypothalamic-pituitary failure.

Specific Syndromes. Within the large group of patients with hypothyroid myopathy, several distinct syndromes have been described. About 20% of severely hypothyroid children, especially boys, have the Debré-Kocher-Sémélaigne syndrome, which is characterized by weakness, slowness of movement, and striking muscle hypertrophy causing an "infant Hercules" appearance.[116] Hypothyroidism and growth retardation are more severe in these patients than in other hypothyroid children.[116] A similar picture in adult hypothyroidism, Hoffman's syndrome, results in prominent muscle enlargement and weakness accompanied by muscle stiffness and "myotonoid" features.[79] The cause of the muscle en-

Table 10–2 ADULT HYPOTHYROID MYOPATHY—CLINICAL AND LABORATORY FEATURES

HISTORY
 Muscle pain, cramps, spasms, stiffness
 Slight functional loss; major fatigue
 Paresthesias

EXAMINATION
 Slight proximal weakness
 Muscle enlargement (occasionally)
 Hyporeflexia with delayed relaxation of reflexes

LABORATORY
 CK level—markedly elevated
  (10-fold–100-fold)
 Biopsy—often normal; fiber atrophy; rarely
  shows sarcoplasmic replacement by
  PAS*-positive material
 EMG—often normal; occasionally myopathic

*PAS = periodic acid-Schiff.

largement in these two syndromes has not been determined, and no distinctive light or ultrastructural pathologic findings have been noted.[3]

Pathogenesis of Myopathy. Many pathogenic mechanisms at multiple sites in the motor unit can contribute to weakness in hypothyroidism. Evidence of peripheral nerve dysfunction exists in most patients, and neuromuscular transmission defects also occur.[119] In a few cases a striking accumulation of myxoid material occurs within muscle fibers,[104] and a disturbance of glycogen metabolism has been demonstrated.[104] Muscle histology is usually normal, however, or shows only slight neurogenic atrophy. Most importantly, weakness recovers with appropriate treatment.

HYPERTHYROIDISM

Incidence of Symptoms. Thyrotoxicosis from any cause may result in muscle atrophy and weakness. Thyrotoxic patients present because of muscle weakness in only 4% to 5% of cases, but the majority will describe weakness when asked and have weakness on clinical examination.[141,146] Although thyrotoxicosis occurs more commonly in women, the myopathy affects both sexes equally, indicating a greater susceptibility in men.[146] A progressive disorder of extraocular muscles associated with proptosis frequently accompanies thyrotoxicosis from Graves' disease. Other neuromuscular disorders occurring less often in association with hyperthyroidism include periodic paralysis (see Chapter 9), myasthenia gravis,[141] spastic paraparesis,[49] and bulbar palsy.[164]

Clinical Features. Proximal weakness and atrophy with preserved and often brisk reflexes characterize thyrotoxic myopathy (Table 10–3). Fasciculations occur and may be so prominent as to suggest amyotrophic lateral sclerosis. The arms may be more affected than the legs, and prominent shoulder-girdle atrophy associated with scapular wing-

Table 10–3 HYPERTHYROID MYOPATHY — CLINICAL AND LABORATORY FEATURES

HISTORY
Insidious onset
Proximal, painless weakness
Occasional patients have pain, cramps, and
  bulbar and ocular muscle weakness

EXAMINATION
Proximal weakness with prominent atrophy;
  scapular winging
Fasciculations (uncommon)
Reflexes brisk to hyperactive

LABORATORY
CK level — normal or low
Biopsy — normal (majority) *or* atrophy of type
  2 > type 1 fibers
EMG — myopathy; occasionally fasciculations,
  fibrillations

ing is distinctive (Fig. 10–1).[145] Distal muscle involvement occurs in about 20% of patients and occasionally may be an isolated manifestation.[141] Bulbar, respiratory, and even esophageal muscles may occasionally be affected, causing dysphagia, dysphonia, aspiration, and at times respiratory compromise.[164] When bulbar involvement occurs, it is usually accompanied by chronic proximal limb weakness, but it may occasionally present acutely in the absence of a generalized thyrotoxic myopathy.[100] Differentiating the acute bulbar form of thyrotoxic myopathy from coincidental myasthenia gravis requires special care.[142,162]

Laboratory Studies. The diagnosis is usually made by the finding of an elevated thyroxine (T_4) level; occasionally only the triiodothyronine (T_3) level is raised. The usual diagnostic studies for neuromuscular disease are not specific. Serum CK levels are often low in thyrotoxic myopathy,[38] probably related to increased clearance of the enzyme from blood.[75] About 90% of patients show electromyographic abnormalities. In proximal muscles, the pattern is most often myopathic, with decreased duration and increased polyphasia of motor

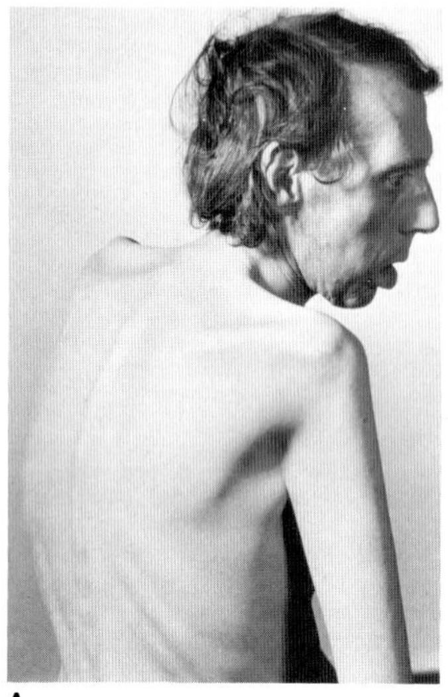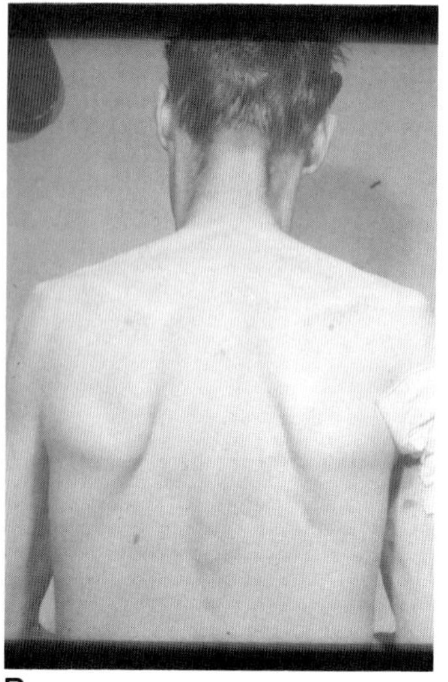

A B

Figure 10–1. Prominent shoulder-girdle atrophy and scapular winging in thyrotoxic myopathy. (*A*) Posterolateral view. (*B*) Posterior view. (Courtesy of I.D. Ramsay.)

unit action potentials.[141,146] Fasciculations, fibrillations, and positive sharp waves may be seen, especially in distal muscles.[141] The electrodiagnostic features correlate with the degree of weakness and atrophy but not with the severity of thyrotoxicosis.[23]

The majority of patients have normal muscle biopsies. About one fourth of patients show nonspecific changes consisting of atrophy of both fiber types, slight fatty infiltration, and connective tissue proliferation.[84,177]

Recognition: Pitfalls in Diagnosis. Severe weakness as a manifestation of hyperthyroidism occurs infrequently because of the widespread screening of patients for thyroid hormone levels. Therefore, hyperthyroid-induced weakness more likely occurs in settings masking the diagnosis, such as in patients on beta-blocker drug therapy, and in trained athletes in whom a pulse rate in the hyperthyroid state may only be in the range of 70 to 90 per minute because the normal resting pulse is 36 to 48 per minutes. Changes induced by propanolol cause particular problems in interpretation with regard to thyroid abnormalities. Propranolol drug therapy causes an elevated T_4 level without a change in thyroid function.[110] The situation may be further complicated be-

cause propranolol can cause weakness and myotonia in its own right.[18] Furthermore, the antithyroid agent propylthiouracil, used in the treatment of thyrotoxicosis, occasionally causes a collagen-disease–like illness, producing a myositis.[158] T_3 toxicosis may cause both myopathy and periodic paralysis. This condition usually presents after age 40 and has an associated goiter. T_3 toxicosis can be difficult to recognize because T_4 levels may be normal in such patients.

Case History

A 30-year-old physician noted the gradual onset of fatigue and weight loss over a 6-week period. He developed weakness of the legs, making stair-climbing difficult. Muscle fasciculations and cramps occurred in all four extremities.

On examination he was tachycardiac, diaphoretic, and anxious. No abnormality of the thyroid gland was found. Motor examination demonstrated slight proximal weakness, atrophy, and occasional fasciculations. Reflexes were hyperactive.

Laboratory studies disclosed an elevated T_4, depressed TSH, and normal thyroglobulin. Radioactive iodine uptake by the thyroid gland was markedly depressed. A diagnosis of subacute thyroiditis (de Quervain's thyroiditis) was made. With propranolol treatment, symptoms resolved, and T_4 returned to normal over the ensuing 3 months.

Comment: This patient's symptoms of thyrotoxicosis were unusually insidious. Although absence of thyroid pain was atypical, laboratory findings of elevated T_4 and depressed radioactive iodine uptake by the thyroid gland supported the diagnosis of thyroiditis. The normal thyroglobulin level made factitious hyperthyroidism unlikely. Muscular symptoms and signs resulted from transient elevation of T_4 levels; these symptoms improved following the institution of treatment with beta-blockers. Over the ensuing months, the thyroiditis and thyrotoxicosis resolved spontaneously, and the patient remained normal after the withdrawal of beta-blockade medication. Short-term or permanent hypothyroidism can often develop after the transient hyperthyroidism but did not in this case.

Pathogenesis. Thyrotoxicosis-induced weakness and muscle wasting probably result from increased muscle catabolism.[25] Points favoring this pathogenic mechanism include increased urinary creatine levels[26] and 3-methyl-histidine[179] excretion, and increased synthesis of muscle protein.[40,54] The observation that beta-blockade improves strength in patients with thyrotoxic muscle wasting[134] suggests that thyroid hormone may alter the catecholamine responsiveness of skeletal muscle.[71]

Therapy. Successful treatment of thyrotoxicosis improves the myopathy, usually over a period of months.[23,146] Improvement in strength precedes the reversal of muscle atrophy, and a full recovery of the muscle weakness can be anticipated. Propanolol reverses many of the systemic signs and symptoms of hyperthyroidism and improves proximal strength,[134] as well as relieving the bulbar weakness of acute thyrotoxic myopathy.[73,176]

Thyrotoxicosis is associated with other autoimmune disorders that characteristically produce weakness. Coincidental myasthenia gravis and pernicious anemia should be considered in thyrotoxic patients. Recognizing myasthenia is particularly important be-cause treatment of thyrotoxicosis with beta-blockers may produce dramatic exacerbation of myasthenic weakness.

Parathyroid Disorders

The wide use of serum calcium in routine screening laboratory studies has resulted in earlier detection of patients with hypoparathyroidism or hyperparathyroidism. The myopathy may be overlooked, however, in a setting of another disorder like renal disease, which may dominate the clinical picture.

HYPOPARATHYROIDISM

Clinical Features. Patients with hypocalcemia from any cause may have symptoms of tetany secondary to peripheral nerve hyperexcitability with resulting muscle spasms and paresthesias; patients may also develop seizures (Table 10–4). Hypocalcemic tetany may occasionally have associated muscle weakness (see illustrative case) with elevated serum CK and minor histologic changes on muscle biopsy.[86,157]

Case History

A 21-year-old student nurse presented with a 2-month history of episodes of leg weakness during which her "legs would tighten up and her knees buckle beneath her." If the episodes occurred while she was observed, she would attempt to hide them by pretending to stop and tie her shoelaces. On one occasion the feeling in her legs made it difficult to cross a busy street. The periods of

---

Table 10–4 NEUROMUSCULAR MANIFESTATIONS OF CHRONIC HYPOCALCEMIA

TETANY
  Paresthesias, muscle pain
  Carpal and pedal spasms
  Carpal tunnel syndrome

WEAKNESS
  Proximal distribution (mild)

Hyporeflexia or areflexia

weakness varied from a few seconds to half an hour; 10 to 20 episodes occurred on some days, with none on others. When the CK level was found to be 2900 IU/mL, she was referred for evaluation of episodic weakness.

Physical examination found slight proximal weakness on formal muscle testing (4+ range) in arms and legs. Functional testing was normal. Muscle stretch reflexes were absent. Sensory examination was normal.

The electrocardiogram showed a marked prolongation of the Q-T interval, and serum calcium was then found to be 4.8 mg/100 mL (normal 8.6–10.4 mg/100 mL); serum phosphorus was 6.8 mg/100 mL (normal 2.5–4.5 mg/100 mL). Reexamination of the patient disclosed pathologically brisk Chvostek signs and markedly positive Trousseau signs.

Subsequent laboratory evaluation showed basal ganglia calcification, as indicated by computed tomography (CT) scan and normal parathyroid hormone levels but a brisk increase in urinary cyclic adenosine monophosphate (AMP) levels with exogenous parathyroid hormone. Electromyography (EMG) detected fasciculations in muscles of both upper and lower extremities and fibrillations in the tibialis anterior muscle but normal motor unit potentials and a normal interference pattern in all muscles. Muscle biopsy showed moderate fiber type grouping (see Chapter 2, pp. 56–57).

A diagnosis of pseudohypoparathyroidism was made. Oral calcium and vitamin D treatment resulted in complete resolution of her clinical findings and all laboratory abnormalities. (Neuromuscular studies and CT scans were not repeated.)

Comment: This patient had clinical signs and symptoms of tetany, which produced intermittent weakness. The fivefold elevation of the CK level led to an initial suspicion of "polymyositis," but the abnormal value presumably reflected sustained muscle contraction and secondary injury from tetany. Chronic hypocalcemia causes *areflexia*, although the mechanism has not been elucidated; reflexes returned to normal with treatment.

Pathogenesis. Neuromuscular symptoms in hypocalcemic states probably result from dysfunction of nerve rather than muscle.[87] Electrophysiologic studies have demonstrated that the hyperexcitability of tetany reflects peripheral nerve depolarization, as documented by the double-cuff studies of Kugelburg.[87] There is little evidence from electrophysiologic or histologic studies favoring primary muscle damage or myopathy.

HYPERPARATHYROIDISM

Clinical and Laboratory Features. Primary hyperparathyroidism commonly presents with proximal weakness.[89] Muscle atrophy and *hyperreflexia* are usual, and fasciculations may occur. Secondary hyperparathyroidism, particularly that associated with osteomalacia, usually has associated muscle weakness and may be easily overlooked as a cause of myopathy because the calcium level may be normal or depressed. An elevated alkaline phosphatase level points to the diagnosis of secondary hyperparathyroidism. Hypophosphatemia, low blood levels of vitamin D, and other factors contribute to the clinical picture.[89]

In hyperparathyroidism, the laboratory features include a muscle biopsy that typically shows type 2 muscle fiber atrophy (Fig. 10–2), and a mixed picture of myopathy and neuropathy by needle EMG examination. The results of nerve conduction studies are usually normal unless coincidental renal dis-

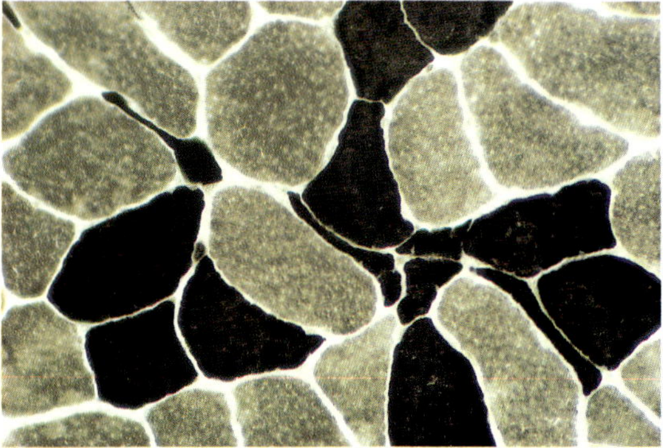

Figure 10–2. Muscle biopsy demonstrating preferential atrophy of type 2 fibers (dark), which appear small and angular. ATPase stain pH 9.4.

ease is present. CK levels may be normal or slightly elevated.[89,98,128] In primary hyperparathyroidism, weakness resolves with appropriate treatment, but when chronic renal disease is also present, achieving normal calcium homeostasis may be very difficult.

Pathogenesis. The mechanism responsible for muscle weakness in hyperparathyroidism and osteomalacia has not been elucidated. Multiple factors have been considered, because the causes for osteomalacia and hyperparathyroidism are heterogeneous.[98] Parathyroid hormone excess has been considered, but levels vary greatly in the known conditions, some of which (for example, antacid abuse) have normal parathyroid levels. Serum calcium and phosphorous levels also show very little correlation with clinical manifestations of myopathy in these syndromes.[48,98,160] Vitamin D directly affects muscle, independent of calcium and phosphorous; relative vitamin D deficiency may be important in producing weakness.[136] Vitamin D increases muscle adenosine triphosphate (ATP) concentration and accelerates amino acid incorporation into muscle protein.[17] In addition, skeletal muscle appears to have a receptor for binding 25-hydroxy vitamin D_3.[17] Vitamin D influences both the uptake of calcium by sarcoplasmic reticulum[138] and the concentration of troponin C, important in calcium binding by the *troponin complex*; these functions are decreased in vitamin D–deficient animals. Muscle contractility is also diminished in vitamin D–deficient animals.

Adrenal Disorders

CUSHING SYNDROME AND CORTICOSTEROID ATROPHY

Clinical and Laboratory Features. Corticosteroid myopathy is the most common endocrine-related muscle disease. A long-standing elevated level of adrenocorticosteroids from any cause results in muscle atrophy and weakness.[114] On the other hand, weakness as a presenting complaint occurs infrequently from *endogenous* hypercortisolism. Weakness can result from hypokalemia,[174] as well as from the corticosteroid-induced muscle atrophy.[76,114] Virtually every synthetic glucocorticoid can produce muscle atrophy, but evidence suggests that accelerated muscle damage occurs with the 9-alpha-fluorinated glucocorticoids.[2,5,137] Daily prednisone doses exceeding 30 mg/d increase vulnerability to corticosteroid-induced weakness to a greater extent than do lower doses or alternate-day regimens.[20] Corticosteroid-induced weakness, however, does not necessarily correlate with duration of treatment and drug dosage, because of individual sensitivity. Moreover, corticosteroids have a more profound weakness-inducing effect in women.[24] Recently, an acute myopathy leading to prolonged paralysis attributable to a combination of steroids and vecuronium treatment has been described.[3a,34a]

Corticosteroid-related weakness usually affects proximal muscles. Muscle stretch reflexes initially remain intact. The CK level is normal or reduced, and muscle biopsy shows fiber atrophy; this is typically greater for type 2 than type 1 fibers (see Fig. 10–2). The EMG shows no abnormalities except in severely affected patients, in whom a myopathic change may be observed. The recently described steroid-vecuronium syndrome is notable for a high CK level and extensive loss of myosin, producing core-like lesions on muscle biopsy.[34a]

Some degree of muscle atrophy will occur in all patients receiving exogenous corticosteroid medication for treatment of underlying disease, especially in doses exceeding 30 mg prednisone daily or its equivalent. Corticosteroid-induced muscle atrophy does not in itself contravene the use of corticosteroids for treatment of an active inflammatory or immune-mediated disorder. Rather, conditions exaggerating this atrophy should be minimized whenever possible. Such conditions include malnutrition, disuse, pain, other endocrinopathy, neuropathy, and systemic disorders involving the liver, kidney, lung, and heart. In patients with any of these additional factors, atrophy can occur in as little as 1 week.[74]

Prevention and Treatment. Corticosteroid atrophy from exogenous steroids can often be avoided if patients are kept active. Exercise increases strength and reverses corticosteroid atrophy,[69,70] and pain relief through the use of analgesic and nonsteroidal anti-inflammatory agents can be beneficial in maintaining activity.

Pathogenesis. The effect of corticosteroids on muscle may be related to altered lipid metabolism,[114] or to changes in mitochondrial function and oxidative phosphorylation.[174] Diminished capillary numbers have been noted but are not clearly related to muscle weakness.[5] An important mechanism of corticosteroid-induced muscle atrophy may be decreased synthesis of muscle protein.[53,126] Recent evidence indicates a *decrease* rather than an increase in muscle protein catabolism,[53] so that muscle atrophy may reflect a depression of muscle protein synthesis that outweighs the corresponding decrease in catabolism.[53,113,126] Recent experimental studies demonstrate that corticosteroids cause a preferential depletion of myosin, particularly in denervated muscle. This depletion is most prominent in type 2B fibers.[151] Selective fiber-type atrophy also raises the possibility that an altered neural influence, such as a change in the rate of firing, could contribute to the effect of corticosteroids on muscle.

NELSON'S SYNDROME

Nelson's syndrome develops after total bilateral adrenalectomy (for many years the standard treatment for Cushing's disease). Following adrenalectomy, the pituitary (usually an adenoma) continues to produce high levels of adrenocorticotrophin (ACTH). A myopathy occurs in patients with Nelson's syndrome, suggesting that high serum ACTH levels directly affect muscle independent of excess glucocorticoids. ACTH may not be the cause of weakness, however, because patients with this condition receive replacement glucocorticoid therapy. Other features of Nelson's syndrome, in addition to the muscle weakness, include easy fatigability and generalized hyperpigmentation.[139] EMG studies show a myopathic pattern with increased insertional activity, positive waves, and pseudomyotonic discharges.[139] The muscle biopsy demonstrates increased lipid in both type 1 and type 2 fibers, especially in a subsarcolemmal location. Serum CK levels remain normal.

It is of interest that Nelson's syndrome has not been reported since 1968. In all likelihood this reflects recent observations that pituitary adenomas producing hypersecretion of ACTH cause most cases of adrenal hyperplasia; such lesions are now detected early by MRI imaging and successfully removed through transphenoidal resection.[169]

ADRENAL INSUFFICIENCY

Adrenal insufficiency commonly causes muscle fatigue.[29] Objective weakness occurs less commonly and is typically mild. If the patient has severe weakness, disorders associated with adrenal insufficiency such as panhypopituitarism, hyperthyroidism, or myasthenia gravis should be considered. Patients with myopathy in adrenal insufficiency usually have severe electrolyte disturbances.[111] When adrenal gland destruction results in a deficiency of both glucocorticoids and mineralocorticoids, hyperkalemia can result and produce severe quadriparesis.[172] A picture simulating periodic paralysis may occur if intermittent hyperkalemia develops.[12] Severe weakness from mineralocorticoid deficiency can occur even in patients taking high doses of glucocorticoids.[72]

CORTICOSTEROID WITHDRAWAL

Corticosteroid withdrawal in patients who have been on long-term treatment occasionally produces a distinctive syndrome of myalgias, arthralgias, joint effusions, rash, and subjective weakness. Splenomegaly may even occur. This constellation of findings, termed Slocumb's pseudorheumatism, can be particularly difficult to recognize in the patient who has been receiving corticosteroid treatment for an underlying joint or muscle inflammatory disease.[159]

Acromegaly

CLINICAL AND LABORATORY FEATURES

Muscle weakness in acromegaly develops insidiously and represents a relatively late manifestation of the endocrinopathy. Patients usually show mild, proximal upper- and lower-extremity muscle weakness without muscle atrophy, although occasional patients manifest more severe weakness.[132] The muscles often appear enlarged but have decreased force generation. The serum CK level may be normal or mildly elevated.[97,102,163] EMG changes are moderate and typical of myopathy, consisting of small motor unit potentials of diminished amplitude and duration.[97,132,163] The muscle biopsy may be normal or may show a small number of necrotic muscle fibers.[97,102,132]

PATHOGENESIS

The duration of acromegaly rather than serum growth hormone levels correlates with the presence of myopathy.[115,132] Experimental growth hormone administration in rats leads to muscle hypertrophy[16] and increased protein synthesis.[140] Despite increased muscle size, there is muscle weakness, which can be reversed by lowering the levels of growth hormone.[132] There is recent evidence that administration of recombinant growth hormone to hu-

man subjects increases muscle mass and muscle protein synthesis (C. Thornton, unpublished). At this point, it is unclear why weakness occurs in acromegaly.

Diabetes

DIFFERENTIAL DIAGNOSIS OF PROXIMAL WEAKNESS IN DIABETICS

A generalized myopathy does not occur in diabetes. Diabetics with proximal weakness frequently have a coincidental disorder. However, proximal weakness in diabetics most commonly results from proximal diabetic neuropathy,[4] also commonly referred to as diabetic amyotrophy.[51] Both of these terms are misleading because the disorder affects both the proximal and distal muscles of the leg and occurs secondary to multifocal ischemic lesions in the proximal nerve trunks, lumbosacral plexus, and nerve roots.[10,144] The clinical syndrome occurs with abrupt onset of unilateral pain in the hip and low back, followed by asymmetric proximal and distal leg weakness reaching a nadir in days to weeks. In some cases, however, the course has been documented to be stepwise or insidiously progressive, with bilateral leg involvement. An alternate form of proximal diabetic neuropathy has been reported with relatively painless, bilateral lower-extremity weakness. This disorder has been attributed to a neuropathy selectively affecting the distal intramuscular nerves of the proximal lower-extremity muscles because of metabolic abnormalities.[28]

Another type of neuropathy, distinct from the common distal symmetric diabetic neuropathy, also causes proximal and distal weakness in diabetics. This disorder, chronic inflammatory demyelinating polyneuropathy, represents a chronic form of Guillain-Barré syndrome and occurs with increased frequency in diabetics.[31] The disorder has an immune-mediated basis and responds to corticosteroid treatment, plasmapheresis,[9] and intravenous immunoglobulin infusion.[171]

THIGH INFARCTION IN DIABETES MELLITUS

Ischemic infarction of the thigh muscles represents the only myopathic syndrome occurring in diabetes mellitus. The condition occurs most often in younger, poorly controlled diabetic patients with long-standing disease and is usually associated with other end-organ complications (retinopathy, nephropathy, neuropathy). Symptoms develop acutely with pain and swelling in one thigh; the syndrome may progress to affect both thighs.[7] The muscles most frequently involved are the vastus lateralis, thigh adductors, and biceps femoris (hamstrings). Pain, tenderness, and edema of the thigh occur, often with an associated, palpable mass. MRI scan shows an image with high signal intensity in the affected muscle (Fig. 10–3). Biopsy of muscle shows infarction, with large areas of muscle necrosis, hemorrhage, and inflammatory infiltration in surrounding viable tissue (Fig. 10–4); connective tissue and fatty infiltration occur subsequently. Small and medium-sized arteries have thickened media, and arterioles may be occluded by calcium, fibrin, or lipid.[92] Although the infarction tends to resolve spontaneously over several weeks, recurrence in the same or contralateral thigh may be seen. Treatment consists of immobilization of the involved limb; surgical intervention and even muscle biopsy should be avoided.[7] Diagnosis by MRI or CT is favored.[92]

In summary, because myopathy does not occur in diabetes, and because most patients with proximal neuropathy resulting from diabetes have associated pain, *painless proximal weakness in a diabetic should prompt consideration of a coincidental disorder.*

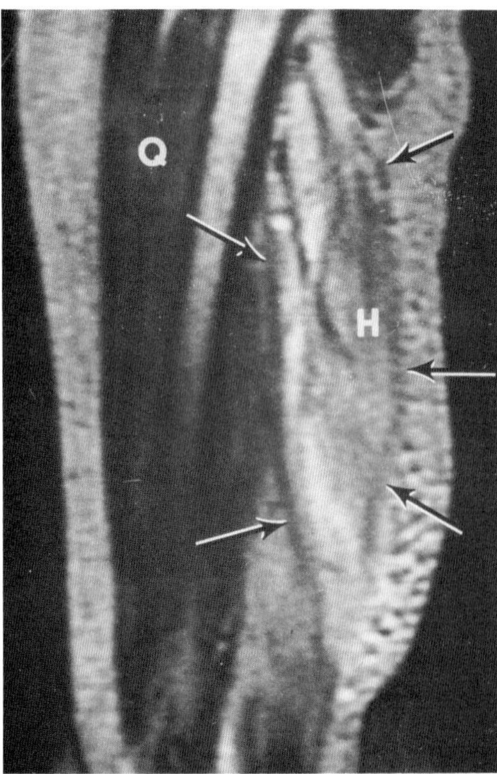

Figure 10–3. Diabetic thigh infarction. T_2-weighted MRI showing high signal intensity in the hamstring muscle (H) and surrounding tissue planes. The quadriceps muscle (Q) is not affected in this case.

HYPOGLYCEMIA

Hypoglycemia can complicate the course of insulin-treated diabetes and, when recurrent or severe, may produce profound muscle atrophy as a result of injury to anterior horn cells.[65] There is little evidence, however, that hypoglycemia produces primary muscle damage.

FLIER'S SYNDROME

Flier's syndrome, a distinctive condition associated with diabetes, presents with complaints of muscle pain, cramps, and fatigue.[45] The initial report, which involved a brother and sister, suggested a hereditary basis,[45] but most subsequent reports have been sporadic. Patients have acanthosis nigricans (Fig. 10–5) and progressive enlargement of the hands and feet. They may complain of weakness, but examination usually reveals normal strength.

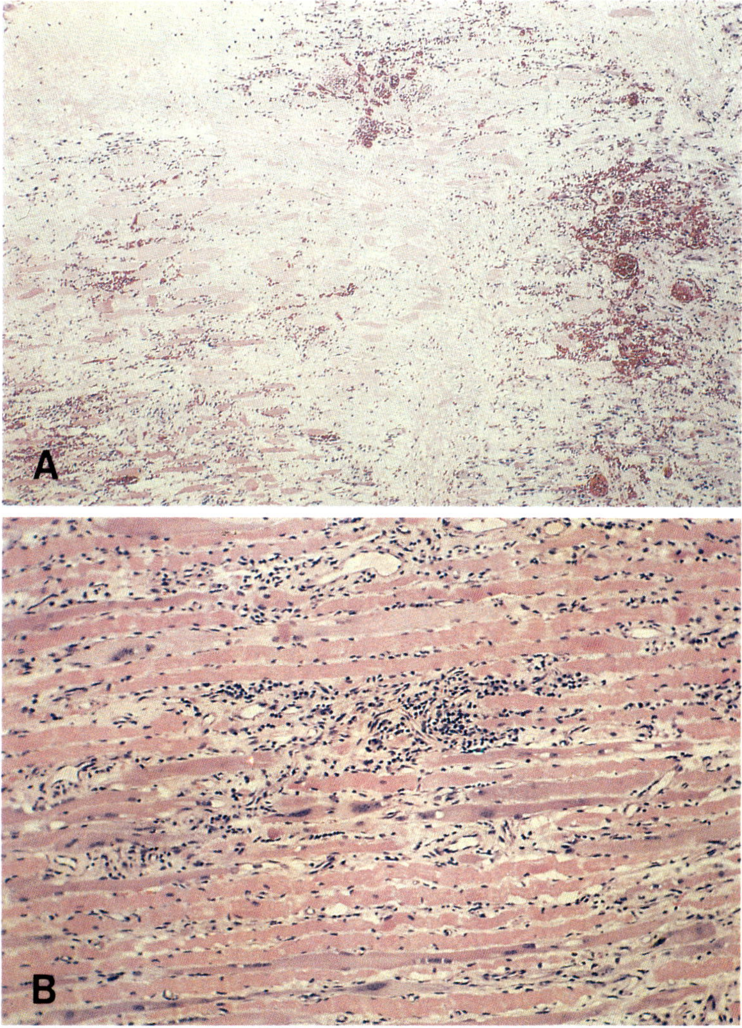

Figure 10–4. Muscle biopsy in diabetic thigh infarction from the hamstring muscle shown in Figure 10–3. (*A*) Area of muscle from the center of the infarct demonstrating focal areas of hemorrhage and sparse, pale-staining necrotic fibers (H&E stain). (*B*) Section of muscle immediately adjacent to necrotic area, showing inflammatory infiltration and regenerating muscle fibers (blue staining with large nuclei) (H&E stain).

CK levels are moderately elevated (two to fivefold). A distinctive form of glucose intolerance with marked insulin resistance occurs. Phenytoin often alleviates the symptoms of muscle pain.[108] Muscle histology is relatively unremarkable, and the basis for the muscle pain is not known.

Pheochromocytoma

Patients with pheochromocytomas usually experience weight loss and may appear to have muscle atrophy. This weight loss is presumably the consequence of hypermetabolism from catecholamine excess. Strength is typically

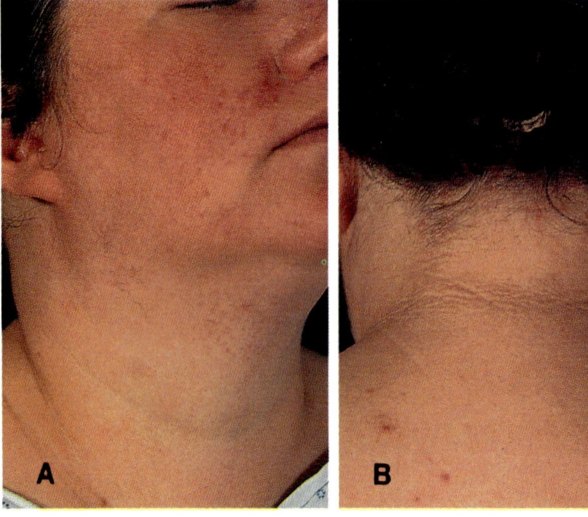

Figure 10–5. (*A* and *B*) Acanthosis nigricans. Velvety, hyperpigmented, slightly raised, maculopapular lesions located about the neck posterior and anterior. Similar lesions were present in the axillae and antecubital fossae.

normal despite muscle atrophy. In rare instances, marked elevations occur in CK levels; these may be accompanied by muscle weakness and inflammation.[15] Myoglobinuria has been reported.[125]

ELECTROLYTE DISTURBANCES

Major elevation or depression of blood levels of potassium, sodium, calcium, magnesium, and phosphorus can each cause muscle weakness varying in degree from mild to severe. Muscle cramps occur commonly with electrolyte disturbances. Only in the case of potassium and of phosphorus, however, is it likely that weakness occurs as a direct result of an abnormality within the muscle fiber (see Chapter 9). Most cases of weakness occurring with altered sodium levels are related to central nervous system abnormalities.[82] Those associated with calcium can usually be attributed to peripheral nerve mechanisms,[87] and magnesium-induced weakness occurs because of alterations in neuromuscular junction physiology.[44] In rare instances, chronic magnesium deficiency is associated with a mitochondrial myopathy. A diagnosis of muscle weakness secondary to most electrolyte disturbances is seldom overlooked because of the widespread availability and routine analysis of serum electrolyte levels. Because magnesium levels are not obtained on a routine basis, however, hypomagnesemia or hypermagnesemia is often unrecognized.

Hypokalemia

Hypokalemia is the most common disturbance of electrolytes that produces muscle weakness. Because most conditions associated with hypokalemia can occur episodically, the differential diagnosis of hypokalemic weakness is considered with the periodic paralyses in Chapter 9 (p. 327). The most common causes of recurrent or persistent hypokalemic weakness are the use of diuretics, chronic diarrhea (often associated with laxative abuse), and chronic renal tubular acidosis.[117] Acute hypokalemic weakness is common in patients with alcoholism, hepatic disease, and in the context of fluid replacement of diabetes mellitus. Iatrogenic hypokalemia is frequent during the course of treating alcoholic patients admitted to the hospital. Nearly 50% of such alcoholic patients are hypokalemic on admission, and the subsequent administration of intravenous fluids with inadequate potassium replacement often exacerbates the mild baseline hypokalemia and weakness. (See Chapter 9, p. 335 for discussion of appropriate intravenous potassium replacement.)

The clinical picture of hypokalemic myopathy is usually that of painless proximal weakness. Muscle pain and cramps are present in some patients and may occasionally be severe. Diminished muscle tone and lost muscle stretch reflexes occur when severe weakness is present; sensory symptoms and signs occur only if there are other electrolyte abnormalities such as hypocalcemia. Laboratory evaluation shows an elevated CK level that parallels the severity of weakness. Muscle biopsy demonstrates vacuolar changes in patients with severe weakness; muscle fiber necrosis is often evident.[101] Clinical and laboratory abnormalities resolve rapidly with replacement of potassium and correction of hypokalemia. If rhabdomyolysis has been severe, EMG may show evidence of active myopathy, including fibrillations. Patients with marked weakness from hypokalemia may have a normal EMG. Where EMG abnormalities such as fibrillations are the result of acute muscle destruction, they resolve rapidly following correction of the electrolyte abnormalities. In many patients with hypokalemic weakness, a myopathic pattern reflects associated conditions such as malnutrition.

Hyperkalemia

Severe hyperkalemia causes limb weakness that can reach total quadriparesis and respiratory paralysis.[35] Life-threatening cardiac dysfunction and cardiac arrest often develop. The causes of hyperkalemia commonly associated with weakness are listed in Table 9–1. Renal insufficiency and acidosis are present in most patients developing severe hyperkalemia. Acidosis aggravates hyperkalemia by causing a shift of potassium from intracellular to extracellular fluid compartments. The

use of salt substitutes, or prescription of nonsteroidal anti-inflammatory agents, potassium-sparing diuretics, beta-blockers, and other medications is often the superimposed factor leading to severe hyperkalemia. Hyperkalemic weakness does not produce muscle destruction comparable to that seen in hypokalemia; therefore, CK levels are usually normal, and muscle biopsy does not usually show vacuolar change or rhabdomyolysis.

The need for urgent and aggressive treatment of hyperkalemia in order to prevent cardiac dysfunction has precluded the study of patients with hyperkalemic paralysis (other than periodic paralysis) during severe weakness.[35] There is frequently evidence for neuromuscular irritability, as evidenced by a Chvostek sign; myotonic lid lag also has been observed.[143] In experimental models of hyperkalemia, there is evidence that muscle remains excitable; this leads to the suggestion that hyperkalemia induces weakness by affecting nerve rather than muscle.[168] Treatment of hyperkalemia is considered in detail in Chapter 9 (p. 337).

Hyponatremia

Patients with severe hyponatremia often report fatigue and weakness.[82] Examination usually demonstrates normal strength. In acute hyponatremia, patients often have muscle fasciculations and cramps, but muscle damage occurs only in the context of generalized seizures.

Hypernatremia

Hypernatremia is seldom associated with muscle symptoms. Rapid correction of hypernatremia with intravenous fluids can be associated with seizures. Patients with active and repeated seizures frequently have evidence of muscle destruction, including marked elevations in CK level. A single report of severe hypernatremia in children described profound weakness and myoglobinuria.[124]

Hypocalcemia and Hypercalcemia

Disordered calcium metabolism is associated with muscle weakness. The most frequently encountered causes are parathyroid disorders. Hypocalcemia is associated with both chronic and intermittent weakness. The diagnosis of chronic hypocalcemia may occasionally be overlooked because of an unexpected *decrease* in muscle stretch reflexes, despite evidence for increased neuromuscular irritability, as evidenced by Chvostek and Trousseau signs. With correction of hypocalcemia, reflexes gradually return to normal.

Equally surprising is the finding that severe, chronic hypercalcemia is associated with muscle weakness and *hyper*reflexia. This hyperreflexia can even occur with spasticity and pathologic reflexes (see pp. 360–361). This hyperreflexia with chronic hypercalcemia contrasts with the depression of reflexes observed when acute hypercalcemia is produced by the intravenous infusion of calcium.

Hypophosphatemia

Severe, sustained hypophosphatemia (serum phosphate < 0.4 mM/L) is often associated with evidence of rhabdomyolysis and myoglobinuria.[83] Hypophosphatemia of this severity occurs only in the setting of acute illnesses such as diabetic ketoacidosis, acute alcoholism, or intravenous hyperalimentation with phosphate-poor preparations.[83] In these situations, acute paralysis with areflexia may be observed. Recovery occurs with phosphate repletion. Less severe, chronic hypophosphatemia is associated with muscle weakness in patients who are taking phosphate-binding antacids, in chronic alcoholics, and in patients with chronic diarrhea. Neuromuscular symptoms in these more chronic causes of hypophosphatemia are not well understood.[80]

The diagnosis of hypophosphatemia as a cause of neuromuscular symptoms is confounded by the effects of hyperventilation on phosphate levels.[82] Thus, patients who have been intubated because of chronic lung disease or other acute processes and are overventilated often have transient hypophosphatemia. Moderate to severe hypophosphatemia can even be produced by hyperventilation in the office setting.[58] Unless phosphate levels are below 1.0 mM/L on repeat determinations, therefore, hypophosphatemia should not be implicated as the sole cause of neuromuscular symptoms. On the other hand, phosphate repletion should be undertaken in patients with persistent weakness and low phosphate levels.[60]

The cause of muscle destruction in patients with severe hypophosphatemia may be difficult to interpret because of the other accompanying abnormalities.[83] Furthermore, other signs and symptoms of hypophosphatemia, such as paresthesias and depressed muscle stretch reflexes, suggest that nerve dysfunction occurs in addition to muscle changes.

Magnesium-Related Disorders

Hypomagnesemia is associated with neuromuscular signs of tetany.[46] Most patients with hypomagnesemia are also hypocalcemic, however, and may have other electrolyte abnormalities. Therefore, it may be difficult to attribute the tetany associated with hypomagnesemia to a single causative factor.

The clinical picture of hypermagnesemia contrasts with that of low magnesium. Severe, generalized weakness and respiratory insufficiency occur frequently with elevated magnesium. Hypermagnesemia is usually the result of orally administered magnesium-containing cathartics in a setting of renal insufficiency. The use of parenteral magnesium for treatment of eclampsia can also produce hypermagnesemia. If the disorder is recognized and respiratory support provided promptly, patients usually recover fully.[112]

CHRONIC RENAL FAILURE

A myopathy distinct from uremic polyneuropathy has been attributed to chronic renal failure.[47,66,99] Many factors related to chronic renal failure can contribute to development of myopathy, especially abnormalities in calcium and phosphorus homeostasis related to abnormal bone metabolism and secondary hyperparathyroidism. In addition, the reduction in liver synthesis of 1,25-dihydroxyvitamin D_3 in chronic renal failure leads to decreased intestinal absorption of calcium. Further accentuations of hyperphosphatemia secondary to decreased renal phosphate clearance result in hypocalcemia, which then leads to secondary hyperparathyroidism. Renal osteodystrophy results from the compensatory hyperparathyroidism, which in turn leads to osteomalacia due to reduced calcium availability, and to osteitis fibrosa due to excess parathyroid hormone.[98]

Many disorders that cause uremia may produce myopathy or other neuromuscular diseases (Table 10-5). Most neuromuscular complications of renal failure, except for gangrenous calcification, will not be associated with marked elevation of CK or evidence from biopsy of muscle breakdown; thus, the presence of these laboratory features should promote a search for a coincidental disorder or raise the possibility of drug toxicity.

Clinical and Laboratory Findings

Patients with the myopathy of chronic renal failure have a clinical picture identical to that associated with hyperparathyroidism and osteomalacia. Proximal muscle weakness and bone pain are accompanied by normal CK levels and by atrophy of type 2 muscle fibers.[47,98] Some patients have been responsive to vitamin D in high doses[47,66]; others, especially those undergoing chronic hemodialysis, are resistant to vitamin D treatment.[47,68] In the latter group, the lack of response to vitamin D may be due to a contaminant in the dialysate, common to certain geographic areas, which can be removed by water purification. The contaminant may be aluminum, which can cause a vitamin D–resistant osteomalacia when given to rats.[41]

ISCHEMIC MYOPATHY IN UREMIA

Gangrenous calcification represents a separate, rare, and sometimes fatal complication of chronic renal failure.[56,149] In this condition, widespread arterial calcification (Fig. 10-6) involves the media and external elastic lamina, with subsequent intimal proliferation in small subcutaneous and intramuscular arteries, a condition which results in ischemia. Extensive skin necrosis may occur, along with a painful myopathy and myoglobinuria.[149] Newer peritoneal and hemodialysis techniques for control of uremia have significantly reduced the incidence of this complication.

Table 10-5 CAUSES OF WEAKNESS IN THE UREMIC PATIENT

NEUROPATHY
Sensorimotor from uremia

NEUROMUSCULAR JUNCTION DEFECTS
Aminoglycoside toxicity

MYOPATHY
Cachexia—from nephrotic syndrome; generalized inanition
Electrolyte disturbances (hypercalcemia, hyperkalemia, hypermagnesemia)
Associated with metabolic bone disease (abnormal vitamin D metabolism)
Metastatic calcification producing muscle infarcts

OTHER
Aluminum-related; drug toxicity

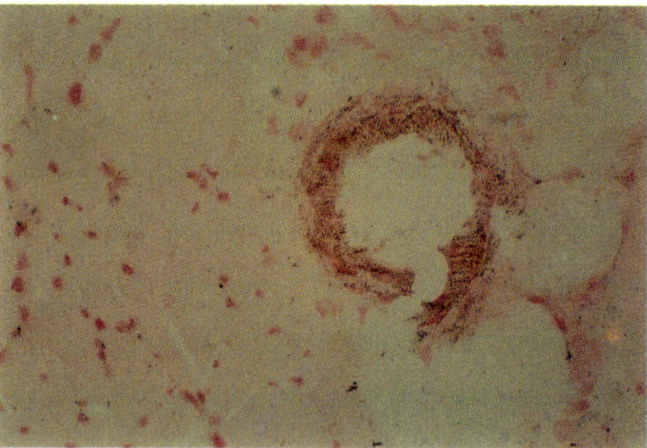

Figure 10–6. Chronic renal failure demonstrating calcification of intramuscular artery. A fine granular pattern (brown staining) can be seen throughout the arterial wall in a Von Kossa stain for calcium. The break in the blood vessel wall is artifactual.

MALIGNANCY

Generalized Myopathy

Only rarely do patients with malignancy have widespread, direct tumor invasion of muscle with pain, swelling, and muscular weakness.[39] Usually only leukemias and lymphomas invade muscle. More commonly, patients with malignancy have variable degrees of generalized muscle atrophy, which may be profound in some patients. This muscle atrophy is usually multifactorial, the result of impaired nutrition, decreased activity, or a hypermetabolic state induced by malignancy. The peptide cachectin, a compound virtually identical to tumor necrosis factor, is produced by many tumors. Cachectin can accelerate muscle degradation and is a potential cause of muscle wasting.[14]

Carcinomatous Myopathy

The term "carcinomatous myopathy" (or neuromyopathy) has been used to explain the frequent occurrence of muscle atrophy in patients with malignancy.[167] In patients with severe weakness, a more specific cause can often be found. The following disorders should be considered:

- Dermatomyositis, which may be associated with occult malignancy.[8]
- Hormone-producing tumors resulting in hypercalcemia.
- Corticosteroid atrophy from ectopic ACTH production.
- The carcinoid syndrome, which occasionally produces a mild myopathy.[173]
- The Lambert-Eaton syndrome (LES), often associated with malignancy (particularly small-cell carcinoma of the lung) may cause severe proximal weakness. LES may be mistaken for a myopathy, but it represents a disorder of the distal nerve terminal. Other features pointing to LES include dry mouth and areflexia. A diagnosis depends on repetitive nerve stimulation studies showing a decrementing response at low rates of stimulation and a facilitating response at high frequency (see Chapter 2; Fig. 2–31). Studies demonstrate the site of pathology to be clearly presynaptic, with immunoglobulin deposition resulting in impaired release of acetylcholine at the nerve terminal.[94] This disorder can be treated with immunosuppression with prednisone and azathioprine,[118] by tumor removal,[27] by plasma exchange,[118] and (in preliminary work) by 3,4-diaminopyridine.[105]

NUTRITIONAL AND GASTROINTESTINAL DISEASE

Malnutrition typically results in muscle wasting. Even when wasting is severe, however, muscle function tends to be preserved unless a specific deficiency occurs or unless peripheral neuropathy develops.[50] Inadequate intake of vitamins, carbohydrate and protein substrate, and minerals such as calcium or magnesium leads to neuromuscular abnormalities. In catabolic states, muscle protein provides fuel for other tissues[57]; this catabolism falls to low levels if malnutrition or starvation persists.[131] Patients with inadequate fat stores are more vulnerable to protein catabolism.[96]

Despite the long-standing clinical impression[36] that strength is preserved in chronic malnutrition, recent evidence indicates that critically ill, hospitalized patients improve substantially with careful protein-calorie treatment by means of intravenous alimentation.[131]

Treatment of obesity with any gastric restriction approach such as gastric resection, gastric stapling, or intragastric balloon may lead to neuromuscular symptoms including fatigue, cramps, myalgias, and weakness. A specific cause of the symptoms (e.g., vitamin B_{12} deficiency, hypokalemia, or vitamin D deficiency) can be defined in the majority of patients. In a few, however, no cause can be found, and the severity of symptoms may require reversal of the gastric volume-restricting procedure.

DRUGS AND OTHER TOXINS

Numerous medications and toxic substances are associated with muscle dysfunction. The mechanisms by which drugs and toxins produce myopathy include:
- Direct toxic effect (e.g., colchicine)
- Local toxic effect when injected into muscle (e.g., meperidine)

Table 10-6 DRUGS AND TOXINS THAT PRODUCE ACUTE RHABDOMYOLYSIS

Direct toxic effect (postulated)
  Alcohol
  Cocaine
  Cyclosporine
  Isoniazid
  Lovastatin
  Zidovudine
Depression of consciousness
  Alcohol
  Opiates
  Other sedatives
Effects on systemic metabolism
  Hypokalemic myopathy
    Alcohol
    Drugs producing renal tubular acidosis
Malignant hyperthermia (see Chapter 7)
    Anesthetics
    Depolarizing muscle relaxants

Table 10-7 DRUGS AND TOXINS THAT CAUSE MYOPATHY

COMMONLY ENCOUNTERED
  Self-administered—alcohol, cocaine, heroin (other opiates), pentazocine
  Iatrogenic—corticosteroids,* thyroid hormone,* colchicine, clofibrate, zidovudine,* cyclosporine, lovastatin, niacin,* gemfibrozil, agents producing hypokalemia (e.g., diuretics)

UNCOMMONLY ENCOUNTERED IATROGENIC AGENTS
  Rifampin
  Penicillamine
  Amiodarone
  Ipecac

*Occasionally obtained without prescription.

- Production of a systemic endocrine, metabolic, or immunologic disorder that causes weakness (e.g., hypokalemia)
- Depression of consciousness with resulting pressure on limbs and ischemic necrosis of muscles (e.g., heroin).

Severe muscle destruction produces rhabdomyolysis (Table 10-6). Recognition of a drug-related toxic myopathy requires awareness of both the distinctive syndromes produced by drugs and toxins, and a high index of suspicion for use of surreptitious drugs.

Agents Directly Toxic to Muscle

Certain toxic drugs so commonly affect muscle that they should be considered as the cause of muscle symptoms in any patient presenting with muscle pain or weakness (Table 10-7). Self-administered agents such as alcohol, cocaine, and opiates are frequently associated with weakness. The prescribed medications most commonly associated with toxic myopathy include colchicine, clofibrate, zidovudine, cyclosporine, and lovastatin.

ALCOHOL

Alcohol produces muscle weakness by several different mechanisms (Table 10-8) and presents with three different clinical pictures:

Table 10–8 TYPES OF ALCOHOL-RELATED NEUROMUSCULAR DISEASE

MYOPATHY
  Direct toxic effect
    Acute necrotizing myopathy
    Myopathy with tubular aggregates
    Acute rhabdomyolysis (may also result from
      electrolyte imbalance or coma)
    Abnormal glycogenolysis
  Electrolyte disturbance
    Hypokalemia
    Hypophosphatemia
    Hypocalcemia
    Hypomagnesemia
  Seizure-induced rhabdomyolysis
  Coma-induced rhabdomyolysis
  Cachexia or malnutrition

NEUROPATHY
  Related to coincidental vitamin deficiency
  Rhabdomyolysis and coma-induced
    plexopathies

1. Acute rhabdomyolysis in the patient with seizures or obtundation
2. Acute, painful muscle weakness
3. Chronic, progressive weakness

Rhabdomyolysis. Acute rhabdomyolysis causes severe weakness and myoglobinuria in alcoholics. Causes include alcohol-withdrawal seizures and obtundation that leads to sustained pressure on dependent parts of the body, thereby occluding blood flow. Other mechanisms implicated as a cause of rhabdomyolysis in the alcoholic include hypokalemia[101,152] and hypophosphatemia,[81] but the contribution of these factors remains unclear. Studies attempting to implicate potassium and phosphate by serum measurements will be inaccurate because both ions can be "auto-corrected" by their liberation following acute muscle destruction.

Acute, Painful Myopathy. Patients with alcoholism can develop sudden, severe muscle pain.[129,130] Weakness may be present, but the muscle pain and "cramps" dominate the picture.[129] Impaired glycogen metabolism has been demonstrated by magnetic resonance spectroscopy,[19] by exercise testing showing impaired exercise-induced lactate production,[129] and by muscle

biopsy.[63] Some alcoholics with acute myopathy demonstrate extensive tubular aggregates on biopsy (see Chapter 2, Fig. 2–49); these aggregates may also be present in alcoholics without symptoms.[30]

Chronic Alcoholic Myopathy. The existence of an alcohol-induced chronic myopathy causing slowly progressive weakness remains controversial. Although chronic alcoholics clearly have impaired muscle function,[170] weakness in many patients is accounted for by myelopathy[154] or peripheral neuropathy.[11] Furthermore, cachexia from malnutrition and disuse may cause type 2 fiber atrophy.[64] These findings suggest a multifactorial process and justify a strong recommendation to the patient that alcohol consumption be stopped. *Severe* progressive muscle weakness should rarely be attributed to the direct effects of alcohol alone.

Pathogenesis of Alcoholic Myopathy. Considerable controversy remains as to whether alcohol itself directly damages muscle.* Convincing evidence indicates that chronic alcoholics have both weakness and muscle damage,[63,170] but a direct relationship to alcohol toxicity (as opposed to periodic or chronic malnutrition, episodic disturbances of electrolyte levels, or recurrent stupor) has not been established. Short-term alcohol ingestion in humans has produced muscle damage.[161] Similarly, chronic administration of alcohol in animal studies has also produced evidence for alcohol toxicity.[153] On the other hand, other animal studies (in the rat) showed that alcohol alone was not associated with muscle damage; caloric restriction in addition to alcohol administration was required to produce muscle damage.[62]

HORMONES

Pharmacologic doses of corticosteroids or ACTH produce drug-induced myopathy (see pp. 361–362). Surrepti-

---

*References 11,63,64,153,154,161,170.

tious ingestion of thyroid hormone in large amounts will produce thyrotoxic myopathy (see pp. 357–358).

ZIDOVUDINE

Patients with human immunodeficiency virus (HIV-1) infection may develop one or more types of myopathy.[90] Myopathy may appear before or after the development of acquired immunodeficiency syndrome (AIDS) (see Chapter 5). Following the introduction of zidovudine therapy for treatment of AIDS, the number of patients with myopathy increased rapidly, and it has become apparent that this drug produces a dose-related myopathy.[13,33,106] Patients develop proximal weakness and pain. Muscle biopsy shows a distinctive pathologic alteration of skeletal muscle resembling ragged red fibers (Fig. 10–7),[33] with evidence favoring mitochondrial dysfunction.[106] The weakness of some AIDS patients treated with zidovudine has improved with stopping the drug or dosage reduction. In a few patients, zidovudine may be reintroduced at a lower dosage without return of weakness.[107] The presence of an inflammatory myopathy in some patients with HIV has made it difficult to assign observed abnormalities of CK levels or EMG to either the HIV infection or zidovudine. Muscle biopsy evidence of inflammation suggests that muscle symptoms are caused by HIV-I infection; ragged red fibers suggest zidovudine toxicity.[34] However, either decreasing zidovudine or treating the patient with prednisone may be necessary.[158a]

COCAINE

Evidence strongly indicates that a direct toxic effect of cocaine accounts for rhabdomyolysis in many drug abusers.[85] Support for a direct myotoxic effect of cocaine or a contaminant, as opposed to a pressure-induced cause from coma (see pp. 277–278), comes from a large series of cases reported from a single institution.[150a] An ischemic pathogenesis related to vasoconstriction seems likely because of the marked vasoconstriction produced in coronary vessels causing myocardial infarction,[91] in cerebral vessels causing brain infarction,[52] and demonstrated in cases of muscle infarction.[181] Whether cocaine-induced vascular changes represent a direct effect of cocaine or result from impurities in street drugs has not been clarified.

COLCHICINE

The anti-inflammatory drug colchicine can cause proximal weakness that

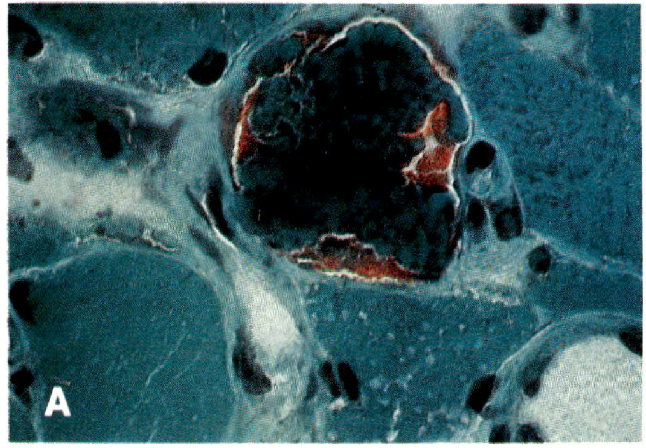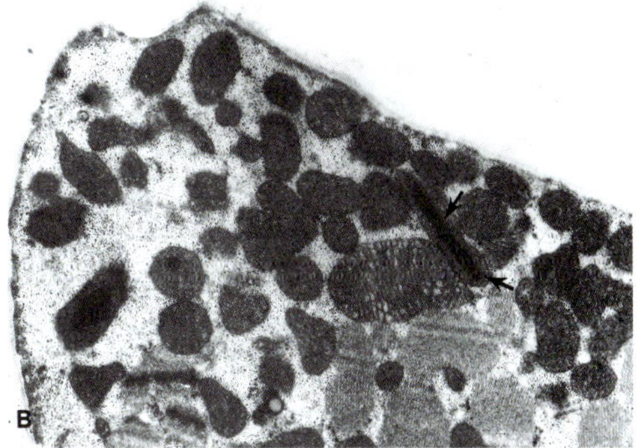

Figure 10–7. Zidovudine myopathy. (A) Muscle fiber with subsarcolemmal accumulation of red-staining material resembles a ragged red fiber (modified trichrome). (B) Electron micrograph of muscle fiber with subsarcolemmal accumulation of mitochondria, some having paracrystalline inclusions (*arrow*). (Courtesy of Marinos Dalakas, MD, National Institutes of Health, Bethesda, Maryland.)

is associated with evidence of myopathy from EMG, CK levels, and muscle biopsy.[88,150] Sensory abnormalities suggest a peripheral neuropathy, accounting for the term "neuromyopathy" (or "myoneuropathy") in reference to colchicine toxicity.[58,150,180] Patients taking unusually large doses of colchicine or patients with renal insufficiency[150] have a greater likelihood of developing neuromuscular toxicity. Weakness remits with discontinuation of colchicine.[150,180]

CHLOROQUINE

The antimalarial agent chloroquine has been used frequently to treat conditions associated with myopathies, especially systemic lupus erythematosus and sarcoidosis. Chloroquine administration causes a vacuolar myopathy,[156] which may complicate the underlying condition (Fig. 10–8). Chloroquine also causes other neuromuscular complications, including neuropathy and myasthenia gravis.[156] These abnormalities are reversible upon discontinuation of the drug.

VINCRISTINE

The widespread use of this vinca alkaloid in treatment of lymphoproliferative disorders exposes many patients to the well-described, highly predictable neuropathy.[59] Occasional patients develop a myopathy; this possibility should be considered in patients with muscle pain and tenderness.[22] The neuropathy rarely causes pain. Administration of vincristine to animals causes a vacuolar myopathy similar in appearance to that caused by chloroquine.[21]

CHOLESTEROL-LOWERING AGENTS

Clofibrate, lovastatin, gemfibrozil, and niacin have all been implicated as causes of myopathy. Lovastatin alone or in combination with gemfibrozil has caused acute rhabdomyolysis and myoglobinuria.[165] Currently, use of clofibrate has diminished, whereas use of the other three agents is increasing.

Lovastatin. This agent has been approved for use since 1987 and is now being administered to millions of patients. Lovastatin potently inhibits 3-hydroxy-3-methylglutaryl coenzyme A (HMG-CoA) reductase and reduces the blood concentration of low-density lipoproteins while raising that of high-density lipoproteins. Elevation of CK level occurs in more than 1% of patients, and roughly half of these develop clinical myopathy with muscle pain and weakness.[164a,165] CK values often reach levels of 1000 times normal. The concomitant use of cyclosporine,[121] nicotinic acid,[148]

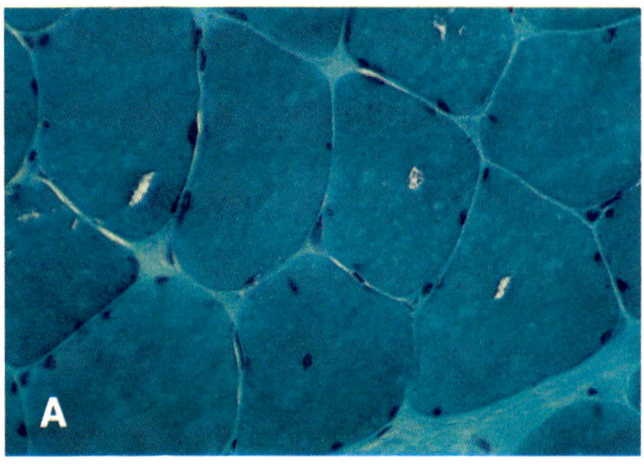

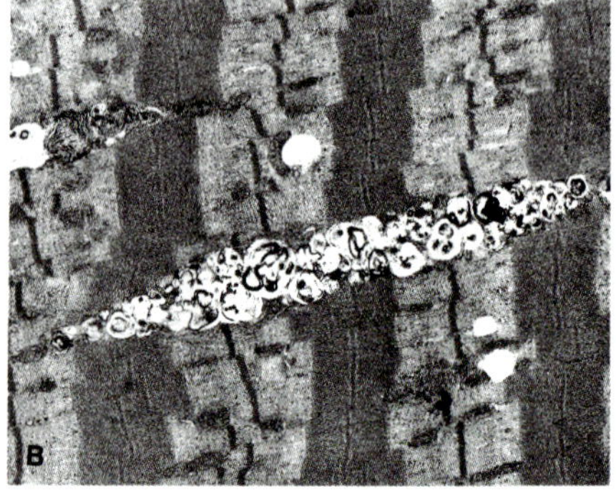

Figure 10–8. Chloroquine myopathy. (A) Muscle fibers show atypical vacuoles (modified trichrome). (B) Electron micrograph shows whorls of membranous material within vacuoles (A and B).

and gemfibrozil[99,133] may potentiate the toxicity of lovastatin. Lovastatin rhabdomyolysis may also occur without the use of other cholesterol-lowering agents. Other HMG-CoA reductase inhibitors are under development. One new agent, simvastatin, also causes rhabdomyolysis,[37] suggesting that myolysis may be a side effect of therapy directed against HMG-CoA reductase.

Niacin. Niacin (a generic term that includes nicotinic acid) lowers cholesterol and is now prescribed for that purpose. Over-the-counter forms provide easy availability of a potentially toxic agent. Doses of over 1 g/d have been reported to cause a myopathy characterized by weakness and muscle pain.[95] Niacin also causes asymptomatic enzyme elevations (aspartate aminotransferase, alanine aminotransferase) and can cause rash, urticaria, and hyperpigmentation.[43] The syndrome resolves promptly on cessation of the agent. The diagnosis may be overlooked when a patient denies taking "medication," believing harmless vitamins are not drugs.[127] Niacin is also an HMG-CoA reductase inhibitor, and the mechanism of myopathy induction is probably similar to that of the other drugs interfering with cholesterol synthesis.

Cyclosporine. This agent is used to treat both transplant patients and those with autoimmune disorders, including neuromuscular diseases such as myasthenia gravis, multiple sclerosis, and chronic inflammatory demyelinating polyneuropathy. Rarely, cyclosporine causes myalgia, myotonia, weakness, and elevated CK levels.[32,120] In most instances where severe rhabdomyolysis occurred, other agents were used, such as an HMG-CoA reductase inhibitor. Cyclosporine myotoxicity may relate to its cholesterol-lowering effect.

Agents Producing Myotonia

Propranolol, cyclosporine, iodides, clofibrate, and penicillamine have all caused myotonia in small numbers of patients.[166] In most instances, the myotonia is not clinically apparent but can be demonstrated on EMG. Each of the foregoing agents, except iodides, also has been associated with clinical muscle weakness without myotonia.

Agents Producing Myopathy Indirectly

A large number of drugs can induce weakness by causing hypokalemia or hyperkalemia (see Chapter 9, p. 319). Much less commonly, hypophosphatemia, hypocalcemia, and hypercalcemia can produce weakness as a result of the administration of various agents (see p. 319).

Agents Producing an Inflammatory Myopathy

PENICILLAMINE

Convincing evidence suggests that penicillamine produces an inflammatory myopathy.[61] Although most patients reported have had an underlying collagen disease, discontinuation and rechallenge has demonstrated that the inflammatory myopathy results from penicillamine.[155] Interestingly, one patient with rheumatoid arthritis developed a penicillamine-related neuromuscular disease in association with widespread fasciculations. The fasciculations remitted when penicillamine was discontinued and recurred upon reintroduction.[135] Penicillamine also causes a reversible myasthenia gravis associated with elevated acetylcholine receptor antibodies.[166]

CIMETIDINE

The histamine H_2-receptor antagonist cimetidine has been reported to cause "polymyositis" and a vasculitis.[109,175] In one carefully described patient, weakness progressed for 6 months, with markedly elevated serum

CK levels and biopsy demonstration of muscle inflammation, in the setting of a severe nephropathy.[175]

Agents Producing Localized Toxicity

Intramuscular injections may produce focal muscle damage as a result of the needle trauma.[42] In addition, a number of agents produce local pain and swelling and may lead to permanent muscle fibrosis and damage. Three agents in particular produce severe damage with fibrosis and joint contractures: pentazocine, meperidine, and heroin.[1,6,103,123,181] It is usually the self-administered abuse of these agents that leads to muscle damage. The self-administration of pentazocine into hip and shoulder-girdle muscles produces a distinctive syndrome of proximal atrophy and contractures in association with severe induration of muscle and overlying connective tissue. Patients with this condition have a characteristic appearance, with abduction of the arms as shown in Fig. 10–9. Intramus-

cular antibiotic administration in infants can also cause muscle fibrosis.[122]

SUMMARY

Many systemic diseases result in muscle pain, weakness, or fatigue. Patients with severe debilitating chronic illness also develop muscle atrophy. Diagnosis and treatment of most myopathies resulting from endocrine, metabolic, and toxic disorders can be accomplished only by recognition of the underlying disease.

A few patients elude diagnosis because atypical features of their systemic disorder obscures the diagnosis. Hyperthyroidism, hypothyroidism, and hypocalcemia, as well as toxic myopathies caused by agents that seldom cause myopathy (e.g., chloroquine, colchicine, and vincristine), are notable for their insidious onset in occasional patients.

Often, the most challenging aspect of patient evaluation is discerning whether weakness is caused by the systemic disease or by a different process, either related or coincidental. Diabetes,

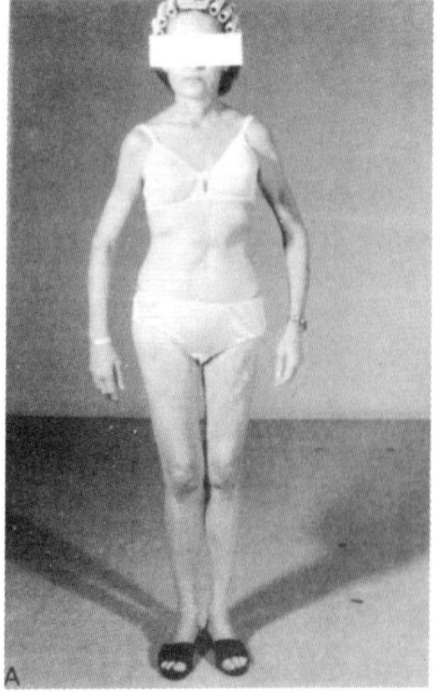 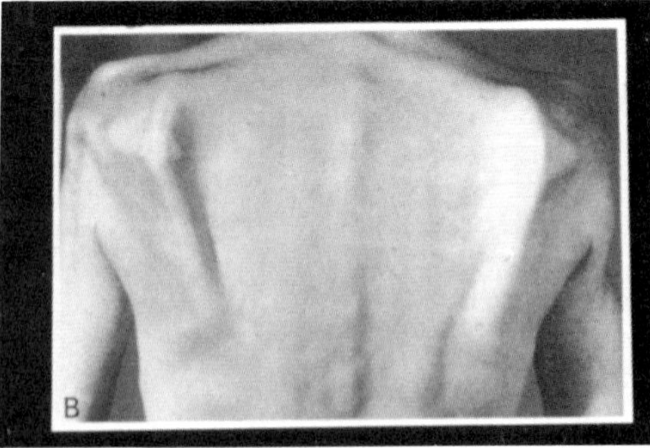

Figure 10–9. Pentazocine myopathy: A 43-year-old woman with a 5-year history of progressive proximal muscle weakness, associated with repeated self-administration of IM pentazocine. Note the abduction contractures in deltoid muscles, severe wasting of supraspinatus, infraspinatus, biceps, and triceps, and patchy areas of fibrosis in quadriceps. Biopsy of left quadriceps showed dense fibrous tissue with very occasional muscle fibers. Surgical release of fibrous bands in deltoids and tensor fasciae latae on both sides corrected the joint contractures. (From Baker.[6] Reprinted with permission from Seminars in Neurology 3:265–273, 1983, Thieme Medical Publishers, Inc.)

for example, is notable for the absence of myopathy, so that the diabetic with severe weakness often has a treatable, coincidental neuromuscular disease such as chronic inflammatory demyelinating polyneuropathy or an inflammatory myopathy. Similarly, severe weakness in the alcoholic or uremic patient often stems from a coexisting process.

Awareness of the expected neuromuscular findings in patients with systemic diseases is absolutely essential in order to identify the patient with coincidental disease. EMG and muscle biopsy findings are seldom specific in endocrine, metabolic, or toxic myopathies. Diagnosis usually depends on the clinical evaluation and on specific laboratory tests assessing the nature and severity of the underlying disease.

REFERENCES

1. Aberfeld DC, Bienenstock H, Shapiro MS, Namba T, and Grob D: Diffuse myopathy related to meperidine addiction in a mother and daughter. Arch Neurol 19:384, 1968.
2. Afifi AK, Bergman RA, and Harvey JC: Steroid myopathy: Clinical, histologic and cytologic observations. The Johns Hopkins Medical Journal 123:158, 1968.
3. Afifi AK, Najjar SS, Mire-Salman J, and Bergman RA: The myopathology of the Kocher-Debré-Sémélaigne syndrome. J Neurol Sci 22:445, 1974.
3a. Al-Lozi MT, Pestronk A, Yee WC, Flaris N, and Cooper J: Rapidly evolving myopathy with myosin-deficient muscle fibers. Ann Neurol 35:273, 1994.
4. Asbury AK: Proximal diabetic neuropathy. Ann Neurol 2:179, 1977.
5. Askari A, Vignos PJ, and Moskowitz RW: Steroid myopathy in connective tissue disease. Am J Med 61:485, 1976.
6. Baker PCH: Drug-induced and toxic myopathies. Semin Neurol 3:265, 1983.
7. Banker BQ and Chester CS: Infarction of thigh muscle in the diabetic patient. Neurology 23:667, 1973.
8. Barnes BE: Dermatomyositis and malignancy. Ann Intern Med 84:68, 1976.
9. Barohn RJ, Kissel JT, Warmolts JR, and Mendell JR: Chronic inflammatory demyelinating polyradiculoneuropathy: Clinical characteristics, course, and recommendations for diagnostic criteria. Arch Neurol 46:878, 1989.
10. Barohn RJ, Sahenk Z, Warmolts JR, and Mendell JR: The Bruns-Garland syndrome (Diabetic Amyotrophy): Revisited 100 years later. Arch Neurol 48:1130, 1991.
11. Behse F and Buchthal F. Alcoholic neuropathy: Clinical, electrophysiological, and biopsy findings. Ann Neurol 2:95, 1977.
12. Bell H, Hayes WL, and Vosburgh J: Hyperkalemic paralysis due to adrenal insufficiency. Arch Intern Med 115:418, 1965.
13. Bessen LJ, Greene JB, Louie E, Seitzman P, and Weinberg H: Severe polymyositis-like syndrome associated with zidovudine therapy of AIDS and ARC. N Engl J Med 318:708, 1988.
14. Beutler B and Cerami A: Cachectin and tumour necrosis factor as two sides of the same biological coin. Nature 320:584, 1986.
15. Bhatnagar D, Carey P, and Pollard A: Focal myositis and elevated creatine kinase levels in a patient with phaeochromocytoma. Postgrad Med J 62:197, 1986.
16. Bigland B and Jehring B: Muscle performance in rats, normal and treated with growth hormone. J Physiol 116:129, 1952.
17. Birge SJ and Haddad JG: 25-hydroxycholecalciferol stimulation of muscle metabolism. J Clin Invest 56:1100, 1975.
18. Blessing W and Walsh JC: Myotonia precipitated by propranolol therapy. Lancet 1:73, 1977.
19. Bollaert PE, Robin-Lherbier B, Escanye JM, et al: Phosphorus nu-

clear magnetic resonance evidence of abnormal skeletal muscle metabolism in chronic alcoholics. Neurology 39:821, 1989.

20. Bowyer SL, LaMothe MP, and Hollister JR: Steroid myopathy: Incidence and detection in a population with asthma. J Allergy Clin Immunol 76:234, 1985.

21. Bradley WG: The neuromyopathy of vincristine in the guinea pig: An electrophysiological and pathological study. J Neurol Sci 10:133, 1970.

22. Bradley WG, Lassman LP, Pearce GW, and Walton JN: The neuromyopathy of vincristine in man: Clinical, electrophysiological and pathological studies. J Neurol Sci 10:107, 1970.

23. Buchthal F: Electrophysiological abnormalities in metabolic myopathies and neuropathies. Acta Neurol Scan 46 (Suppl 43):129, 1970.

24. Bunch TW, Worthington JW, Combs JJ, Ilstrup DM, and Engel AG: Azathioprine with prednisone for polymyositis. A controlled, clinical trial. Ann Intern Med 92:365, 1980.

25. Carter WJ, Van Der Weijden BWS, and Faas FH: Effect of experimental hyperthyroidism on protein turnover in skeletal and cardiac muscle. Metabolism 29:910, 1980.

26. Carter WJ, Van Der Weijden BWS, and Faas FH: Effect of experimental hyperthyroidism on skeletal-muscle proteolysis. Biochem J 194:685, 1981.

27. Chalk CH, Murray NMF, Newsom-Davis J, O'Neill JH, and Spiro SG: Response of the Lambert-Eaton myasthenic syndrome to treatment of associated small-cell lung carcinoma. Neurology 40:1552, 1990.

28. Chokroverty S: Proximal nerve dysfunction in diabetic proximal amyotrophy. Electrophysiology and electron microscopy. Arch Neurol 39:403, 1982.

29. Christy NP: Iatrogenic Cushing's syndrome. In Christy NP (ed): The Human Adrenal Cortex. Harper & Row, New York, 1971, p 395.

30. Chui LA, Neustein H, and Munsat TL: Tubular aggregates in subclinical alcoholic myopathy. Neurology 25:405, 1975.

31. Cornblath DR, Drachman DB, and Griffin JW: Demyelinating motor neuropathy in patients with diabetic polyneuropathy. Ann Neurol 22:126, 1987.

32. Costigan DA: Acquired myotonia, weakness and vacuolar myopathy secondary to cyclosporine. Muscle Nerve 12:761, 1989.

33. Dalakas MC, Illa I, Pezeshkpour GH, Laukaitis J, Cohen B, and Griffin JL: Mitochondrial myopathy caused by long-term zidovudine therapy. N Engl J Med 322:1098, 1990.

34. Dalakas MC, Pezeshkpour GH, and Flaherty M: Progressive nemaline (rod) myopathy associated with HIV infection. N Engl J Med 317:1602, 1987.

34a. Danon MJ and Carpenter S: Myopathy with thick filament (myosin) loss following prolonged paralysis with vecuronium during steroid treatment. Muscle Nerve 14:1131, 1991.

35. DeFronzo RA, Bia M, and Smith D: Clinical disorders of hyperkalemia. Annu Rev Med 33:521, 1982.

36. Denny-Brown D: Neurological conditions resulting from prolonged and severe dietary restriction. (Case reports in prisoners-of-war, and general review). Medicine 26:41, 1947.

37. Deslypere JP and Vermeulen A: Rhabdomyolysis and simvastatin. Ann Intern Med 114:342, 1991.

38. Docherty I, Harrop JS, Hine KR, Hopton MR, Matthews HL, and Taylor CJ: Myoglobin concentration, creatine kinase activity, and creatine kinase B subunit concentrations in serum during thyroid disease. Clin Chem 30:42, 1984.

39. Doshi R and Fowler T: Proximal myopathy due to discrete carcinomatous metastases in muscle. J Neurol Neurosurg Psychiatry 46:358, 1983.

40. Edwards RHT, Khaleeli AA, and Mills KR: Muscle function in endocrine and metabolic myopathy. Semin Neurol 3:294, 1983.

41. Ellis HA, McCarthy JH, and Herring-

ton J: Bone aluminum in haemodialysed patients and in rats injected with aluminum chloride: Relationship to impaired bone mineralisation. J Clin Pathol 32:832, 1979.

42. Engel WK: Focal myopathic changes produced by electromyographic and hypodermic needles: Needle myopathy. Arch Neurol 16:509, 1967.

43. Etchason JA, Miller TD, Squires RW, et al: Niacin-induced hepatitis: A potential side effect with low-dose time-release niacin. Mayo Clin Proc 66:23, 1991.

44. Ferdinandus J, Pederson JA, and Whang R: Hypermagnesemia as a cause of refractory hypotension, respiratory depression, and coma. Arch Intern Med 141:669, 1981.

45. Flier JS, Young JB, and Landsberg L: Familial insulin resistance with acanthosis nigricans, acral hypertrophy, and muscle cramps. N Engl J Med 303:970, 1980.

46. Flink EB: Magnesium deficiency: Etiology and clinical spectrum. Acta Medica Scandinavica (Suppl) 647:125, 1981.

47. Floyd M, Ayyar DR, Barwick DD, Hudgson P, and Weightman D: Myopathy in chronic renal failure. Q J Med 43:509, 1974.

48. Frame B, Heinze EG, Block MA, and Manson GA: Myopathy in primary hyperparathyroidism: Observations in three patients. Ann Intern Med 68:1022, 1968.

49. Garcia CA and Fleming RH: Reversible corticospinal tract disease due to hyperthyroidism. Arch Neurol 34:647, 1977.

50. Gardiner PF, Montanaro G, Simpson DR, and Edgerton VR: Effects of glucocorticoid treatment and food restriction on rat hindlimb muscles. Am J Physiol 238:E124, 1980.

51. Garland H: Diabetic amyotrophy. Br Med J 2:1287, 1955.

52. Golbe LI and Merkin MD: Cerebral infarction in a user of free-base cocaine ("crack"). Neurology 36:1602, 1986.

53. Goldberg AL, and Goldspink DF: Influence of food deprivation and adrenal steroids on DNA synthesis in various mammalian tissues. Am J Physiol 228:310, 1975.

54. Goldberg AL, Tischler M, DeMartino G, and Griffin G: Hormonal regulation of protein degradation and synthesis in skeletal muscle. Fed Proc 39:31, 1980.

55. Golding DN: Hypothyroidism presenting with musculoskeletal symptoms. Ann Rheum Dis 29:10, 1970.

56. Goodhue WW, Davis JN, and Porro RS: Ischemic myopathy in uremic hyperparathyroidism. JAMA 221:911, 1972.

57. Goodman MN, Lowell B, Belur E, and Ruderman NB: Sites of protein conservation and loss during starvation: Influence of adiposity. Am J Physiol 246:E383, 1984.

58. Gorman JM, Cohen BS, Liebowitz MR, et al: Blood gas changes and hypophosphatemia in lactate-induced panic. Arch Gen Psychiatry 43:1067, 1986.

59. Gottschalk PG, Dyck PJ, and Kiely JM: Vinca alkaloid neuropathy: Nerve biopsy studies in rats and in man. Neurology 18:875, 1968.

60. Gravelyn TR, Brophy N, Siegert C, and Peters-Golden M: Hypophosphatemia-associated respiratory muscle weakness in a general inpatient population. Am J Med 84:870, 1988.

61. Halla JT, Fallahi S, and Koopman WJ: Penicillamine-induced myositis: Observations and unique features in two patients and review of the literature. Am J Med 77:719, 1984.

62. Haller RG and Drachman DB: Alcoholic rhabdomyolysis: An experimental model in the rat. Science 208:412, 1980.

63. Haller RG and Knochel JP: Skeletal muscle disease in alcoholism. Med Clin North Am 68:91, 1984.

64. Hanid A, Slavin G, Mair W, et al: Fibre type changes in striated muscle of alcoholics. J Clin Pathol 34:991, 1981.

65. Harrison MJG: Muscle wasting after prolonged hypoglycaemic coma: Case report with electrophysiological data. J Neurol Neurosurg Psychiatry 39:465, 1976.

66. Henderson RG, Russell RGG, Ledingham JGG, et al: Effects of 1,25-dihydroxycholecalciferol on calcium absorption, muscle weakness, and bone disease in chronic renal failure. Lancet 1:379, 1974.

67. Hochberg MC, Koppes GM, Edwards CQ, Barnes HV, and Arnett FC: Hypothyroidism presenting as a polymyositis-like syndrome. Arth Rheum 19:1363, 1976.

68. Hodsman AB, Sherrard DJ, Wong EGC, et al: Vitamin-D-resistant osteomalacia in hemodialysis patients lacking secondary hyperparathyroidism. Ann Intern Med 94:629, 1981.

69. Horber FF, Hoopeler H, Scheidegger JR, Grünig BE, Howard H, and Frey FJ: Impact of physical training on the ultrastructure of midthigh muscle in normal subjects and in patients treated with glucocorticoids. J Clin Invest 79:1181, 1987.

70. Horber FF, Scheidegger JR, Grünig BE, and Frey FJ: Evidence that prednisone-induced myopathy is reversed by physical training. J Clin Endocrinol Metab 61:83, 1985.

71. Ingbar SH: The thyroid gland. In Wilson JD and Foster DW (eds): Textbook of Endocrinology, ed 7. WB Saunders, Philadelphia, 1985, p 682.

72. Jacobs TP, Whitlock RT, Edsall J, and Holub DA: Addisonian crisis while taking high-dose glucocorticoids: An unusual presentation of primary adrenal failure in two patients with underlying inflammatory diseases. JAMA 260:2082, 1988.

73. Kammer GM and Hamilton CR: Acute bulbar muscle dysfunction and hyperthyroidism: A study of four cases and review of the literature. Am J Med 56:464, 1974.

74. Kaplan PW, Rocha W, Sanders DB, D'Souza B, and Spock A: Acute steroid-induced tetraplegia following status asthmaticus. Pediatrics 78:121, 1986.

75. Karlsberg RP and Roberts R: Effect of altered thyroid function on plasma creatine kinase clearance in the dog. Am J Physiol 235:E614, 1978.

76. Khaleeli AA, Edwards RHT, Gohil K, et al: Corticosteroid myopathy: A clinical and pathological study. Clin Endocrinol (Oxf) 18:155, 1983.

77. Khaleeli AA, Griffith DG, and Edwards RHT: The clinical presentation of hypothyroid myopathy and its relationship to abnormalities in structure and function of skeletal muscle. Clin Endocrinol (Oxf) 19:365, 1983.

78. Kingston WJ: Endocrine myopathies. Semin Neurol 3:258, 1983.

79. Klein I, Parker M, Shebert R, Ayyar DR, and Levey GS: Hypothyroidism presenting as muscle stiffness and pseudohypertrophy: Hoffman's syndrome. Am J Med 70:891, 1981.

80. Knochel JP: The pathophysiology and clinical characteristics of severe hypophosphatemia. Arch Intern Med 137:203, 1977.

81. Knochel JP: Hypophosphatemia in the alcoholic. Arch Intern Med 140:613, 1980.

82. Knochel JP: Neuromuscular manifestations of electrolyte disorders. Am J Med 72:521, 1982.

83. Knochel JP: The clinical status of hypophosphatemia: An update. N Engl J Med 313:447, 1985.

84. Korényi-Both A, Korényi-Both I, and Kayes BC: Thyrotoxic myopathy: Pathomorphological observations of human material and experimentally induced thyrotoxicosis in rats. Acta Neuropathol (Berl) 53:237, 1981.

85. Krohn KD, Slowman-Kovacs S, and Leapman SB: Cocaine and rhabdomyolysis. Ann Intern Med 108:639, 1988.

86. Kruse K, Scheunemann W, Baier W, and Schaub J: Hypocalcemic myopathy in idiopathic hypoparathyroidism. Eur J Pediatr 138:280, 1982.

87. Kugelberg E: Activation of human nerves by hyperventilation and hypocalcemia: Neurologic mechanisms of symptoms of irritation in tetany. Arch Neurol Psychiatry 60:153, 1948.

88. Kuncl RW, Cornblath DR, Avila O, and Duncan G: Electrodiagnosis of human colchicine myoneuropathy. Muscle Nerve 12:360, 1989.

89. Lafferty FW: Primary hyperparathyroidism. Changing clinical spectrum, prevalence of hypertension, and discriminant analysis of laboratory tests. Arch Intern Med 141:1761, 1981.

90. Lange DJ, Britton CB, Younger DS, and Hays AP: The neuromuscular manifestations of human immunodeficiency virus infections. Arch Neurol 45:1084, 1988.

91. Lange RA, Cigarroa RG, Yancy CW, et al: Cocaine-induced coronary-artery vasoconstriction. N Engl J Med 321:1557, 1989.

92. Lauro GR, Kissel JT, and Simon SR: Idiopathic muscular infarction in a diabetic patient. J Bone Joint Surg 73A:301, 1991.

93. Lazaro RP and Kirshner HS: Proximal muscle weakness in uremia: Case reports and review of the literature. Arch Neurol 37:555, 1980.

94. Leys K, Lang B, Johnston I, and Newsom-Davis J: Calcium channel autoantibodies in the Lambert-Eaton myasthenic syndrome. Ann Neurol 29:307, 1991.

95. Litin SC and Anderson CF: Nicotinic acid-associated myopathy: A report of three cases. Am J Med 86:481, 1989.

96. Lowell BB and Goodman MN: Protein sparing in skeletal muscle during prolonged starvation: Dependence on lipid fuel availability. Diabetes 36:14, 1987.

97. Lundberg PO, Osterman PO, and Stålberg E: Neuromuscular signs and symptoms in acromegaly. In Walton JN, Canal N, and Scarlato G (eds): International Congress on Muscle Disease, Milan 1969. Excerpta Medica, Amsterdam, 1970, p 531.

98. Mallette LE, Patten BM, and Engel WK: Neuromuscular disease in secondary hyperparathyroidism. Ann Intern Med 82:474, 1975.

99. Marais GE and Larson KK: Rhabdomyolysis and acute renal failure induced by combination lovastatin and gemfibrozil therapy. Ann Intern Med 112:228, 1990.

100. Marks P, Anderson J, and Vincent R: Thyrotoxic myopathy presenting with dysphagia. Postgrad Med J 56:669, 1980.

101. Martin JB, Craig JW, Eckel RE, and Munger J: Hypokalemic myopathy in chronic alcoholism. Neurology 21:1160, 1971.

102. Mastaglia FL, Barwick DD, and Hall R: Myopathy in acromegaly. Lancet 2:907, 1970.

103. Mastaglia FL, Gardner-Medwin D, and Hudgson P: Muscle fibrosis and contractures in a pethidine addict. BMJ 4:532, 1971.

104. McDaniel HG, Pittman CS, Oh SJ, and DiMauro S: Carbohydrate metabolism in hypothyroid myopathy. Metabolism 26:867, 1977.

105. McEvoy KM, Windebank AJ, Daube JR, and Low PA: 3,4-Diaminopyridine in the treatment of Lambert-Eaton myasthenic syndrome. N Engl J Med 321:1567, 1989.

106. Mhiri C, Baudrimont M, Bonne G, et al: Zidovudine myopathy: A distinctive disorder associated with mitochondrial dysfunction. Ann Neurol 29:606, 1991.

107. Miller RG, Carson PJ, Moussavi RS, Green AT, Baker AJ, and Weiner MW: Fatigue and myalgia in AIDS patients. Neurology 41:1603, 1991.

108. Minaker KL, Flier JS, Landsberg L, et al: Phenytoin-induced improvement in muscle cramping and insulin action in three patients with the syndrome of insulin resistance, acanthosis nigricans, and acral hypertrophy. Arch Neurol 46:981, 1989.

109. Mitchell GG, Magnusson AR, and Weiler JM: Cimetidine-induced cutaneous vasculitis. Am J Med 75:875, 1983.

110. Mooradian A, Morley JE, Simon G, and Shafer RB: Propranolol-induced

hyperthyroxinemia. Arch Intern Med 143:2193, 1983.

111. Mor F, Green P, and Wysenbeek AJ: Myopathy in Addison's disease. Ann Rheum Dis 46:81, 1987.

112. Mordes JP and Wacker WEC: Excess magnesium. Pharmacol Rev 29:273, 1978.

113. Moxley RT, Lorenson M, Griggs RC, et al: Decreased breakdown of muscle protein after prednisone therapy in Duchenne dystrophy (DD) [abstract]. J Neurol Sci (Suppl) 98:419, 1990.

114. Müller R and Kugelberg E: Myopathy in Cushing's syndrome. J Neurol Neurosurg Psychiatry 22:314, 1959.

115. Nagulesparen M, Trickey R, Davies MJ, and Jenkins JS: Muscle changes in acromegaly. BMJ 2:914, 1976.

116. Najjar SS: Muscular hypertrophy in hypothyroid children. The Kocher-Debré-Semelaigne syndrome: A review of 23 cases. J Pediatr 85:236, 1974.

117. Nardone DA, McDonald WJ, and Girard DE: Mechanisms in hypokalemia: Clinical correlation. Medicine 57:435, 1978.

118. Newsom-Davis J and Murray NMF: Plasma exchange and immunosuppressive drug treatment in the Lambert-Eaton myasthenic syndrome. Neurology 34:480, 1984.

119. Nickel SN, Frame B, Bebin J, Tourtellotte WW, Parker JA, and Hughes BR: Myxedema neuropathy and myopathy: A clinical and pathological study. Neurology 11:125, 1961.

120. Noppen M, Velkeniers B, Dierckx R, Bruyland M, and Vanhaelst L: Cyclosporine and myopathy [letter]. Ann Intern Med 107:945, 1987.

121. Norman DJ, Illingworth DR, Munson J, and Hosenpud J: Myolysis and acute renal failure in a heart-transplant recipient receiving lovastatin. N Engl J Med 318:46, 1988.

122. Norman MG, Temple AR, and Murphy JV: Infantile quadriceps-femoris contracture resulting from intramuscular injections. N Engl J Med 282:964, 1970.

123. Oh SJ, Rollins JL, and Lewis I: Pentazocine-induced fibrous myopathy. JAMA 231:271, 1975.

124. Opas LM, Adler R, Robinson R, and Lieberman E: Rhabdomyolysis with severe hypernatremia. J Pediatr 90:713, 1977.

125. Oristrell-Salvá J and Miradacanals A: Phaeochromocytoma and rhabdomyolysis. BMJ 288:1198, 1984.

126. Pacy PJ and Halliday D: Muscle protein synthesis in steroid-induced proximal myopathy: A case report. Muscle Nerve 12:378, 1989.

127. Palumbo PJ: Rediscovery of crystalline niacin. Mayo Clin Proc 66:112, 1991.

128. Patten BM, Bilezikian JP, Mallette LE, Prince A, Engel WK, and Aurbach GD: Neuromuscular disease in primary hyperparathyroidism. Ann Intern Med 80:182, 1974.

129. Perkoff GT, Dioso MM, Bleisch V, and Klinkerfuss G: A spectrum of myopathy associated with alcoholism. I. Clinical and laboratory features. Ann Intern Med 67:481, 1967.

130. Perkoff GT, Hardy P, and Velez-Garcia E: Reversible acute muscular syndrome in chronic alcoholism. N Engl J Med 274:1277, 1966.

131. Pichard C and Jeejeebhoy KN: Muscle dysfunction in malnourished patients. Q J Med 69:1021, 1988.

132. Pickett JBE, Layzer RB, Levin SR, Schneider V, Campbell MJ, and Sumner AJ: Neuromuscular complications of acromegaly. Neurology 25:638, 1975.

133. Pierce LR, Wysowski DK, and Gross TP: Myopathy and rhabdomyolysis associated with lovastatin-gemfibrozil combination therapy. JAMA 264:71, 1990.

134. Pimstone N, Marine N, and Pimstone B: Beta-adrenergic blockade in thyrotoxic myopathy. Lancet 2:1219, 1968.

135. Pinals RS: Diffuse fasciculations induced by D-penicillamine. J Rheumatol 10:809, 1983.

136. Pleasure D, Wyszynski B, Sumner D, et al: Skeletal muscle calcium metab-

olism and contractile force in vitamin D-deficient chicks. J Clin Invest 64:1157, 1979.

137. Pleasure DE, Walsh GO, and Engel WK: Atrophy of skeletal muscle in patients with Cushing's syndrome. Arch Neurol 22:118, 1970.

138. Pointon JJ, Francis MJO, and Smith R: Effect of vitamin D deficiency on sarcoplasmic reticulum function and troponin C concentration of rabbit skeletal muscle. Clin Sci 57:257, 1979.

139. Prineas J, Hall R, Barwick DD, and Watson AJ: Myopathy associated with pigmentation following adrenalectomy for Cushing's syndrome. Q J Med 37:63, 1968.

140. Prysor-Jones RA and Jenkins JS: Effect of excessive secretion of growth hormone on tissues of the rat, with particular reference to the heart and skeletal muscle. J Endocrinol 85:75, 1980.

141. Puvanendran K, Cheah JS, Naganathan N, and Wong PK: Thyrotoxic myopathy: A clinical and quantitative analytic electromyographic study. J Neurol Sci 42:441, 1979.

142. Puvanendran K, Cheah JS, Naganathan N, Yeo PPB, and Wong PK: Neuromuscular transmission in thyrotoxicosis. J Neurol Sci 43:47, 1979.

143. Radó JP, Marosi J, Takó J, and Dévényi I: Hyperkalemic intermittent paralysis associated with spironolactone in a patient with cardiac cirrhosis. Am Heart J 76:393, 1968.

144. Raff MC, Sangalang V, and Asbury AK: Ischemic mononeuropathy multiplex associated with diabetes mellitus. Arch Neurol 18:487, 1968.

145. Ramsay ID: Muscle dysfunction in hyperthyroidism. Lancet 2:931, 1966.

146. Ramsay I: Thyroid disease and muscle dysfunction. Year Book Medical, Chicago, 1974.

147. Rao SN, Katiyar BC, Nair KRP, and Misra S: Neuromuscular status in hypothyroidism. Acta Neurol Scand 61:167, 1980.

148. Reaven P and Witztum JL: Lovastatin, nicotinic acid, and rhabdomyolysis. Ann Intern Med 109:597, 1988.

149. Richardson JA, Herron G, Reitz R, and Layzer R: Ischemic ulcerations of skin and necrosis of muscle in azotemic hyperparathyroidism. Ann Intern Med 71:129, 1969.

149a. Riggs JE, Klingberg WG, Flink EB, Schochet SS Jr, Balian AA, and Jenkins JJ: Cardioskeletal mitochondrial myopathy associated with chronic magnesium deficiency. Neurology 42:128, 1992.

150. Riggs JE, Schochet SS, Gutmann L, Crosby TW, and DiBartolomeo AG: Chronic human colchicine neuropathy and myopathy. Arch Neurol 43: 521, 1986.

150a. Roth D, Alarcon FJ, Fernandez JA, Preston RA, and Bourgoignie JJ: Acute rhabdomyolysis associated with cocaine intoxication. N Engl J Med 319:673, 1988.

151. Rouleau G, Karpati G, Carpenter S, Soza M, Prescott S, and Holland P: Glucocorticoid excess induces preferential depletion of myosin in denervated skeletal muscle fibers. Muscle Nerve 10:428, 1987.

152. Rubenstein AE and Wainapel SF: Acute hypokalemic myopathy in alcoholism. Arch Neurol 34:553, 1977.

153. Rubin E, Katz AM, Lieber CS, Stein EP, and Puszkin S: Muscle damage produced by chronic alcohol consumption. Am J Pathol 83:499, 1976.

154. Sage JI, Van Uitert RL, and Lepore FE: Alcoholic myelopathy without substantial liver disease: A syndrome of progressive dorsal and lateral column dysfunction. Arch Neurol 41: 999, 1984.

155. Schraeder PL, Peters HA, and Dahl DS: Polymyositis and penicillamine. Arch Neurol 27:456, 1972.

156. Sghirlanzoni A, Mantegazza R, Mora M, Pareyson D, and Cornelio F: Chloroquine myopathy and myasthenia-like syndrome. Muscle Nerve 11:114, 1988.

157. Shane E, McClane KA, Olarte MR, and Bilezikian JP: Hypoparathyroid-

ism and elevated muscle enzymes. Neurology 30:192, 1980.

158. Shergy WJ and Caldwell DS: Polymyositis after propylthiouracil treatment for hyperthyroidism. Ann Rheum Dis 47:340, 1988.

158a. Simpson DM, Citak K, Godfrey E, Godbold J, and Wolfe DE: HIV or zidovudine myopathy? [reply] Neurology 44:362, 1994.

159. Slocumb CH: Rheumatoid arthritis. In Brown J and Pearson CM (eds): Clinical Uses of Adrenal Steroids. McGraw-Hill, New York, 1962, p 30.

160. Smith R and Stern G: Muscular weakness in osteomalacia and hyperparathyroidism. J Neurol Sci 8:511, 1969.

161. Song SK and Rubin E: Ethanol produces muscle damage in human volunteers. Science 175:327, 1972.

162. Stern LZ and Fagan JM: The endocrine myopathies. In Vinken PJ and Bruyn GW (eds): Handbook of Clinical Neurology. North Holland, Amsterdam, Vol 40, 1979, p 235.

163. Stern LZ, Payne CM, and Hannapel LK: Acromegaly: Histochemical and electron microscopic changes in deltoid and intercostal muscle. Neurology 24:589, 1974.

164. Sweatman MCM and Chambers L: Disordered oesophageal motility in thyrotoxic myopathy. Postgrad Med J 61:619, 1985.

164a. Thompson PD, Gadaleta PA, Yurgalevitch S, Cullinane E, and Herbert PN: Effects of exercise and lovastatin on serum creatine kinase activity. Metabolism 40:1333, 1991.

165. Tobert JA: Efficacy and long-term adverse effect pattern of lovastatin. Am J Cardiol 62:28J, 1988.

166. Torres CF, Griggs RC, Baum J, and Penn AS: Penicillamine-induced myasthenia gravis in progressive systemic sclerosis. Arthritis Rheum 23:505, 1980.

167. Trojaborg W, Frantzen E, and Andersen J: Peripheral neuropathy and myopathy associated with carcinoma of the lung. Brain 92:71, 1969.

168. Troni W, Bruatto S, and Genero O: Electromyographic study on experimental hyperkalemia. I: Electrophysiological alterations. Acta Neurol (Napoli) 33:381, 1978.

169. Tyrrell JB, Brooks RM, Fitzgerald PA, Cofoid PB, Forsham PH, and Wilson CB: Cushing's disease: Selective trans-sphenoidal resection of pituitary microadenomas. N Engl J Med 298:753, 1978.

170. Urbano-Marquez A, Estruch R, Navarro-Lopez F, et al: The effects of alcoholism on skeletal and cardiac muscle. N Engl J Med 320:409, 1989.

171. Vermeulen M, van der Meché FGA, Speelman JD, Weber A, and Busch HFM: Plasma and gamma-globulin infusion in chronic inflammatory polyneuropathy. J Neurol Sci 70:317, 1985.

172. Vilchez JJ, Cabello A, Benedito J, and Villarroya T: Hyperkalemic paralysis, neuropathy and persistent motor neuron discharges at rest in Addison's disease. J Neurol Neurosurg Psychiatry 43:818, 1980.

173. Vinik AI, Thompson N, Eckhauser F, and Moattari AR: Clinical features of carcinoid syndrome and the use of somatostatin analogue in its management. Acta Oncologica 28:389, 1989.

174. Walsh G, DeVivo D, and Olson W: Histochemical and ultrastructural changes in rat muscle: Occurrence following adrenal corticotrophic hormone, glucocorticoids, and starvation. Arch Neurol 24:83, 1971.

175. Watson AJS, Dalbow MH, Stachura I, et al: Immunologic studies in cimetidine-induced nephropathy and polymyositis. N Engl J Med 308:142, 1983.

176. Weinstein R, Schwartzman R, and Levey GS: Propranolol reversal of bulbar dysfunction and proximal myopathy in hyperthyroidism. Ann Intern Med 82:540, 1975.

177. Wiles CM, Young A, Jones DA, and Edwards RHT: Muscle relaxation rate, fibre-type composition and energy turnover in hyper- and hypothyroid patients. Clin Sci 57:375, 1979.

178. Wilson J and Walton JN: Some muscular manifestations of hypothyroidism. J Neurol Neurosurg Psychiatry 22:320, 1959.

179. Yates RO, Connor H, and Woods HF: Muscle protein breakdown in thyrotoxicosis assessed by urinary 3-methylhistidine excretion. Ann Nutr Metab 25:262, 1981.

180. Younger DS, Mayer SA, Weimer LH, Alderson LM, Seplowitz AH, and Lovelace RE: Colchicine-induced myopathy and neuropathy. Neurology 41:943, 1991.

181. Zamora-Quezada JC, Dinerman H, Stadecker MJ, and Kelly JJ: Muscle and skin infarction after free-basing cocaine (crack). Ann Intern Med 108:564, 1988.

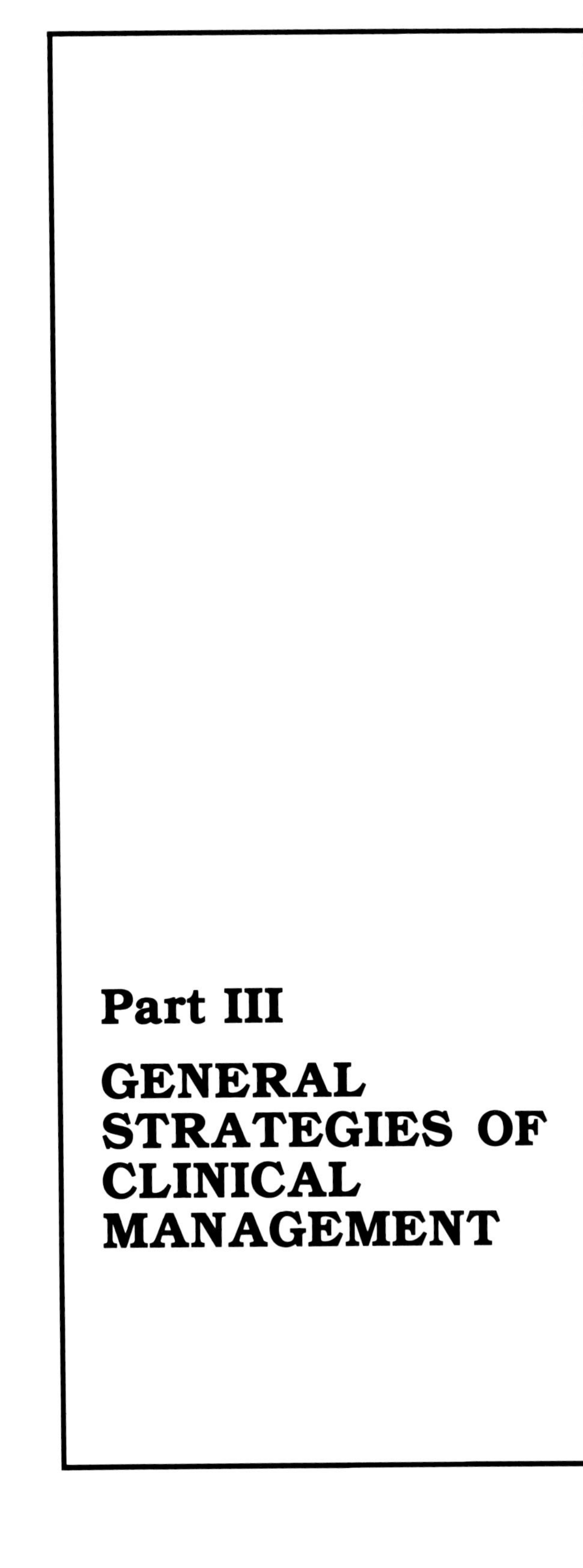

Part III

GENERAL
STRATEGIES OF
CLINICAL
MANAGEMENT

Chapter 11

MUSCLE PAIN AND FATIGUE

PATHOGENESIS OF MUSCLE PAIN
PAIN ARISING FROM BONE AND JOINT DISORDERS
MYOPATHIES ASSOCIATED WITH MUSCLE PAIN
OTHER NEUROLOGIC CONDITIONS WITH MUSCLE PAIN
FIBROMYALGIA (FIBROSITIS)
DISORDERS ASSOCIATED WITH MUSCLE FATIGUE

Muscle pain and fatigue are universal human experiences. When patients present with myalgia or fatigue as a chief complaint, it is sometimes difficult to determine whether these symptoms represent an underlying muscle disease. In general, the most common cause of muscle pain is trauma or unaccustomed exercise. Similarly, fatigue is an extremely common problem, the major complaint of approximately 25% of patients presenting to adult primary care clinics.[39] In a population-based survey in the United States, 14% of men and 20% of women rated themselves as significantly fatigued.[16] Clearly the vast majority of patients who present with myalgia and excessive fatigue do not have one of the muscular disorders described thus far in this text. Nonetheless, many patients complain persistently of myalgia, excessive fatigue, or both, and these complaints may prompt an evaluation for neuromuscular disease. In this chapter we outline the physiologic basis for muscle pain and fatigue, provide a framework for evaluating patients with these symptoms, and suggest strategies for management. Although considerable controversy surrounds the precise classification of patients with debilitating myalgia or fatigue, the approach described in this chapter is useful in clinical practice.

PATHOGENESIS OF MUSCLE PAIN

Painful stimuli from skeletal muscle are transmitted by small afferent nerve fibers, which are either thinly myelinated (group III or A delta) or unmyelinated (group IV or C).[47] Freely branching and unencapsulated, these nerve endings are distributed throughout skeletal muscle, particularly in tendons and fascia. There are generally two types of pain receptors within muscle, and these are receptive either to chemical change or to mechanical alteration. Some of these nociceptors respond to a variety of chemical stimuli, whereas others respond to chemical, thermal, and mechanical stimuli. The activity of these receptors is influenced by histamine, potassium ion, hydrogen ion, bradykinin, 5-hydroxytryptamine, tumor necrosis factor, and various lymphokines. Aspirin reduces their responsiveness. These same receptors are also important in modulating cardiovascular responses during exercise and in regulating motor unit discharge frequencies.[80]

Pain during Exercise

Intense muscle exertion can produce pain due to:
• Ischemia during sustained, high-intensity muscle contraction

- Tearing muscle fibers ("a pulled muscle")
- Rupturing a muscle tendon (see Fig. 2-4)
- Inducing a true muscle cramp
- Claudication of muscle in individuals with impaired circulation from vascular disease
- Exhausting fuel supply and producing contracture in patients with metabolic defects (myophosphorylase deficiency, carnitine palmitoyl transferase deficiency, and so on).

During most types of exercise, there is little muscle pain, which is surprising when one considers that blood flow declines to a nadir when the force of a sustained muscle contraction exceeds 40% of the maximum voluntary contraction[9,29,69] (Fig. 11-1). In normal muscle, ischemia probably accounts for much of the pain that occurs during high-intensity exercise. The precise mechanisms underlying this type of pain are not entirely clear. Ischemia alone produces relatively little muscle pain unless it is very long-standing. Similarly, pre-exercise ischemia does not influence muscular endurance during ischemia. Accumulating metabolites appear to play a major role in the production of ischemic pain, but the belief that lactic acid is the major cause of ischemic pain is no longer tenable. Patients with myophos-

phorylase deficiency experience substantial pain during ischemic exercise and have no lactic acid buildup. Similarly, the clearance of lactic acid is much slower than the resolution of pain during the recovery period after ischemic exercise. Recent evidence suggests that lymphokines may contribute to this pain, and changes in potassium ion, hydrogen ion, and possibly other substances also may be important.[24]

Pain after Exercise

After unaccustomed exercise, normal individuals often have pain and soreness of muscles, especially during active movement. This pain begins after a delay of several hours and persists from 12 hours up to 5 days.[52] The muscles are tender to palpation and may be uncomfortable at rest. Demonstrable weakness[19,52] and evidence of muscle destruction[50,51] accompany the pain and soreness, particularly after vigorous training.

ECCENTRIC VERSUS CONCENTRIC MUSCLE CONTRACTION

The nature of the muscle contraction is an important determinant of the extent of muscle pain and damage. Muscle

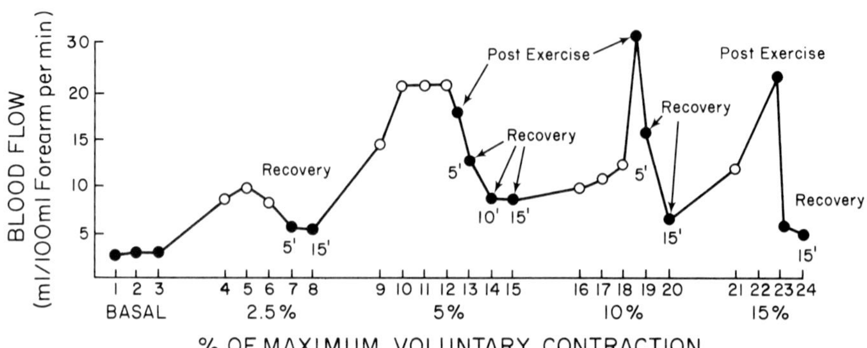

Figure 11-1. Effect of muscle contraction on forearm blood flow in a normal subject. Blood flow was measured by strain gauge plethysmography. The subject gripped a dynamometer with increasing levels of force. Blood flow increased with low levels of contraction but decreased at levels greater than 15% of maximum voluntary contraction. Open circles (during contraction); closed circles (at rest or recovery). Blood flow is decreased by sustained contraction.

contraction can occur as the muscle shortens (*concentric* contraction), or as it lengthens (*eccentric* contraction). Chair-stepping provides a useful paradigm illustrating concentric versus eccentric contraction. In stepping up onto a chair with one leg, the leg muscles that participate in the force of lifting contract *concentrically.* In stepping down from the chair, the leg muscles supporting the leg must lengthen as they contract *eccentrically.* The difference in stress placed on muscle fibers in concentric compared with eccentric contraction is clinically important.

Eccentric contraction is more likely than concentric contraction to produce muscle soreness,[52] histologic evidence of muscle damage,[51] and abnormalities of creatine kinase (CK) level (see Fig. 7–15).[50] Indeed, even brief periods (20 minutes) of eccentric leg exercise can produce 10-fold to 100-fold elevations of CK levels.[19] Eccentric contraction may be especially damaging to diseased muscle.[76] The basis for postexertional muscle soreness may be an increase in intramuscular fluid pressure caused by muscle fiber breakdown and edema.[20]

Muscle Cramps

Intense pain accompanies true muscle cramps (defined in Chapter 2, p. 22), which are experienced quite commonly in the gastrocnemius muscles. The pain of muscle cramps is characterized by acute onset; short duration; a strong, hard, palpable muscular contraction; and immediate relief by stretching the muscle. Cramps that recur frequently in other muscles, such as the hamstrings or any of the muscles of the upper extremity or chest wall, usually signify an underlying denervating disease, especially motor neuron disease, peripheral neuropathy, or nerve root disease. Some patients with a predominance of type 2 fibers, however, may present with either unexplained cramps or exertional myalgia,[70] and some patients have a hereditary predisposition to muscle cramps.[59] Other definable causes of

muscle spasm and abnormal contraction are considered in Chapter 2.

PAIN ARISING FROM BONE AND JOINT DISORDERS

Muscle pain is common even when the actual cause is a joint, bone, or tendinous disorder. Nonmuscular disorders may present with muscle pain because of a misperception of the location of pain. A misleading complaint of "muscle pain" may make localization of the site of pathology very difficult. In fact, muscular atrophy may develop because nonmuscular pain hinders exercise or daily activities. For example, with polymyalgia rheumatica, despite typical complaints of "muscle pain and stiffness" in the shoulder or hip-girdle musculature, radionuclide scanning shows inflammation of the joints and increased joint fluid[54]; it is likely, therefore, that this pain arises from *joints* rather than *muscles* (see also Chapter 5). Examples of contiguous joint or bone diseases that produce muscle atrophy and muscle pain are listed in Table 11–1. Failure to recognize the underlying condition may result in a mistaken diagnosis of myopathy.

Coincidental abnormalities of muscle may also point to the wrong location. Pain associated with certain conditions, especially metabolic bone disease and

Table 11–1 IMPORTANT CAUSES OF MUSCLE PAIN OF NONMUSCULAR ORIGIN

JOINT DISEASE
  Rheumatoid arthritis
  Systemic lupus erythematosus
  Scleroderma
  Polymyalgia rheumatica
  Joint hypermobility syndromes (common)
    Ehlers-Danlos syndrome (relatively
     uncommon)
  Gout

BONE DISEASE
  Osteomalacia
  Primary and secondary hyperparathyroidism
  Myeloproliferative disorders

rheumatoid arthritis, can cause disuse, which may lead to visible muscle atrophy as well as abnormal muscle histologic and electrophysiologic findings. These biopsy and electromyographic (EMG) changes result from two factors: (1) coincidental but not necessarily important abnormalities of nerve and (2) changes in the muscle resulting from disuse. Such findings as atrophy of type 1 or type 2 muscle fibers, moth-eaten fibers (multifocal loss of oxidative enzyme staining in individual muscle fibers), inflammatory cell infiltrates, and small, angular fibers that appear dark on staining with NADH-tetrazolium reductase, are frequent and nonspecific.[11] These abnormalities do not cause the muscle pain but rather result from underlying joint or bone disease.

MYOPATHIES ASSOCIATED WITH MUSCLE PAIN

Some of the myopathies considered earlier in this volume may produce pain (Table 11–2). The suggested diagnostic approach to the patient with muscle pain is outlined below (see Table 11–6). In one series, roughly one third of patients with muscle pain had a definable cause.[45]

Table 11–2 OCCURRENCE OF MUSCLE PAIN IN MYOPATHIES

MUSCULAR DYSTROPHIES
  Facioscapulohumeral — stretch injuries
  Limb-girdle, Becker's — exertional pain
  Others (less common) — muscle damage
  secondary to overuse

INFLAMMATORY MYOPATHIES (seldom a presenting complaint except in childhood dermatomyositis)

METABOLIC MYOPATHIES (e.g., deficiency of myophosphorylase [McArdle's disease]; phosphofructokinase deficiency)

MITOCHONDRIAL MYOPATHIES

MYOTONIA CONGENITA (ATYPICAL)

Tubular Aggregates and Cylindrical Spirals

In one group of patients, exertional muscle pain has been associated with the finding of numerous tubular aggregates in the muscle biopsy (Fig. 11–2).[7a,10,41,53] Small numbers of tubular aggregates are a nonspecific finding in many normal subjects and in many different diseases. Large numbers are not common, however, and the larger numbers found in these cases suggest that they may be related to the muscle pain, although the mechanism remains unknown. In several cases, tubular aggregates occurred in association with cylindrical spirals (Fig. 11–3), further

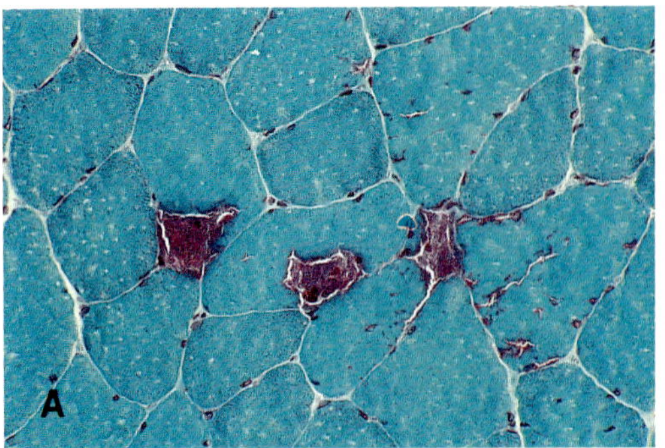
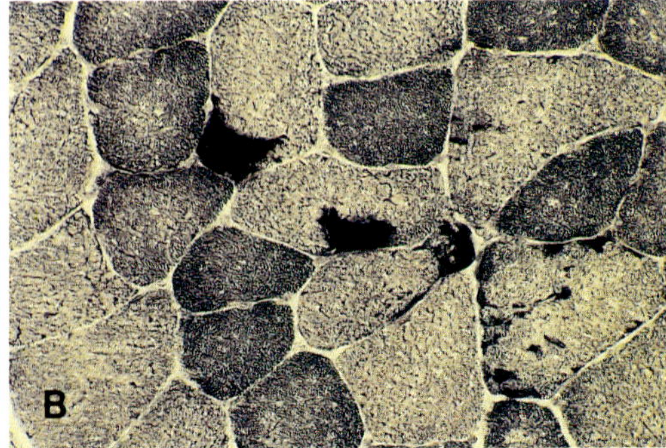

Figure 11–2. Tubular aggregates in biceps muscle of patient complaining of exercise-induced myalgias. (A) Modified trichrome shows four contiguous muscle fibers with red-staining material characteristic of tubular aggregates. (B) NADH tetrazolium reductase stain demonstrates dark-staining material corresponding to tubular aggregates. Note that tubular aggregates are found exclusively in type-2 (light-staining) fibers.

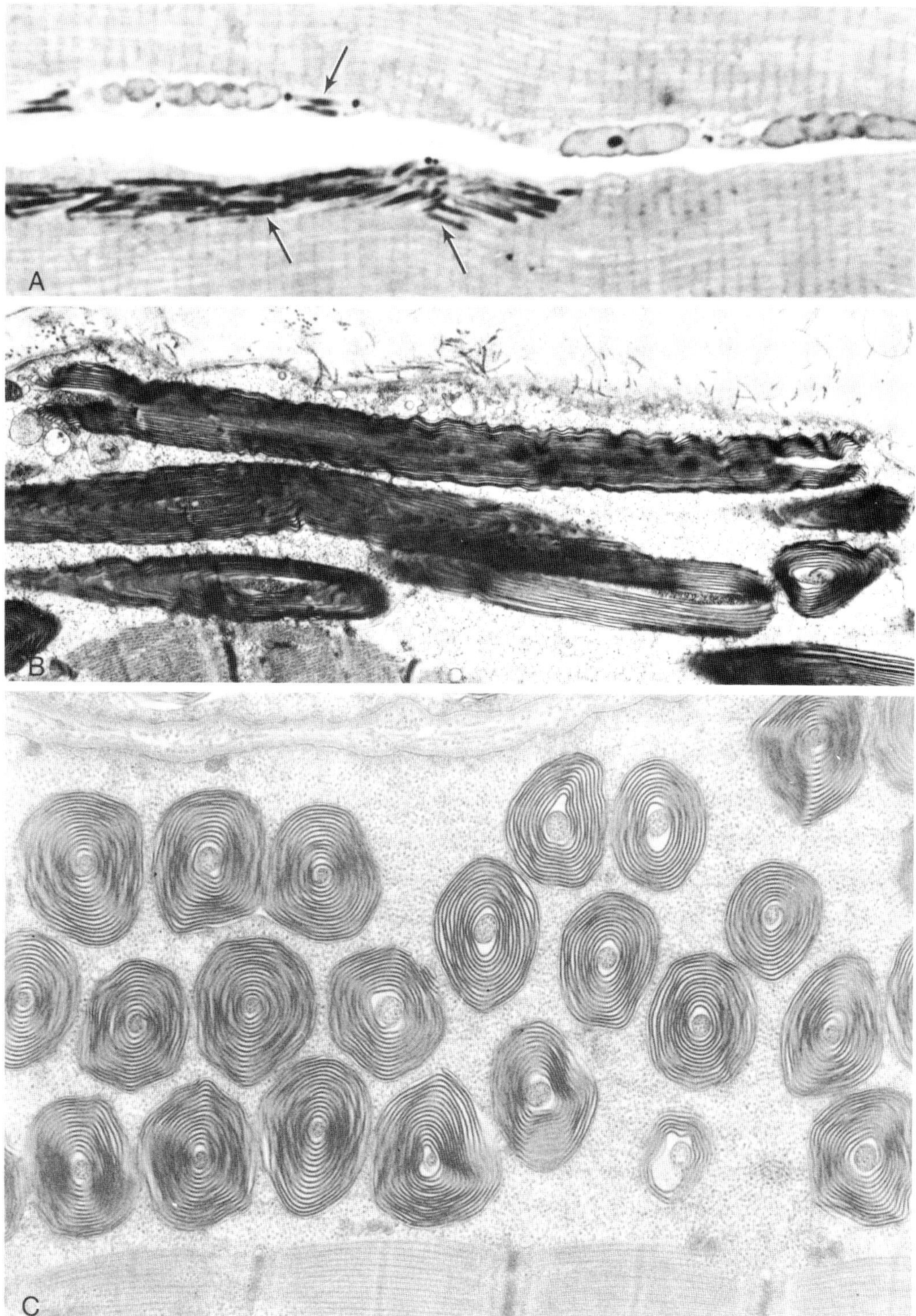

Figure 11–3. Cylindrical spirals as seen in light and electron micrographs. (*Top*) Plastic-embedded 1-mm thick section of muscle showing cylindrical spirals in two adjacent muscle fibers (*arrows*). (*Middle*) Electron micrograph of cylindrical spirals seen in the longitudinal axis. (*Bottom*) Cross-sections of cylindrical spirals.

distinguishing this subset of patients with muscle pain.[18,53]

Familial X-linked Myalgia and Cramps

Recognition of this condition resulted from discovery of the gene defect causing Duchenne dystrophy. In contrast to Duchenne dystrophy, where dystrophin is absent (see Chapter 4, pp. 103–104), patients with X-linked myalgia and cramps have dystrophin of lower molecular weight without reduction in amount. A DNA deletion accounts for this abnormal protein.[27] Patients present with exercise-induced myalgia and muscle cramps but not weakness, and the serum CK level is elevated. Although the condition is rare, its existence has raised the possibility that some patients with unexplained muscle pain may represent undefined allelic variants of a muscular dystrophy or other hereditary myopathy.

Eosinophilic Myopathies

A small number of patients with constant and diffuse muscle pains but normal strength have eosinophilic infiltrates of muscle (Fig. 11–4).[60,64] Peripheral eosinophilia is not necessarily present. Eosinophilic polymyositis, diffuse fasciitis with eosinophilia, and the eosinophilia myalgic syndrome with ingestion of tryptophan are more extensively discussed in Chapter 5.

OTHER NEUROLOGIC CONDITIONS WITH MUSCLE PAIN

Restless Legs Syndrome

Patients with this condition usually present after age 30 and may have a positive family history.[73] Patients experience an intensely uncomfortable feeling in their legs, especially the calf muscles and hamstrings. Symptoms develop almost exclusively during sitting or lying down, and may be described as "painful," although patients seldom seek or respond to analgesic medication.[74] Activity relieves the abnormal sensation. Detailed studies of peripheral nerve histology and function usually show no consistent pathology, although similar symptoms have been described in association with neuropathies of known cause, such as uremia. Symptoms can be alleviated by opiates, phenothiazines or clonazepam, but chronic use of neuroleptics should be avoided if possible because of the frequent occurrence of side effects.[75] In se-

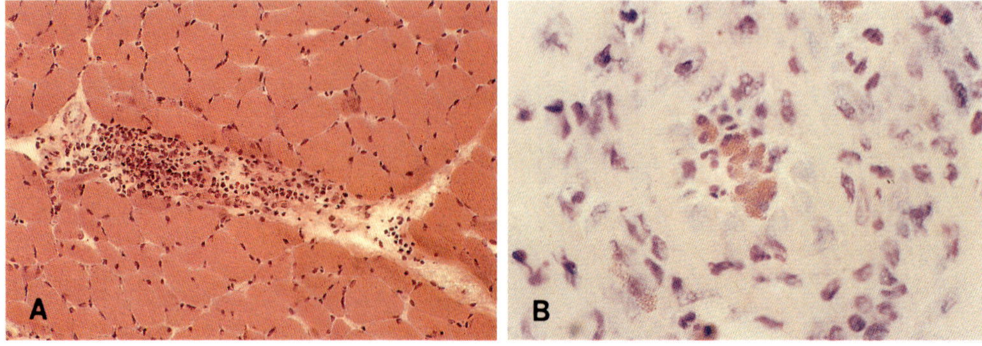

Figure 11–4. Eosinophilic perimyositis in biceps muscle. (A) The inflammation can be seen to be restricted to the perimysial connective tissue (H&E stain). (B) At high power (oil immersion) with special stains, many of the inflammatory cells can be identified as eosinophils in the center of the field (Giemsa stain).

vere cases, dopaminergic agents such as bromocriptine or L-dopa may be effective and appropriate.[74]

Upper Motor Neuron Disease

Patients with well-characterized upper motor neuron disorders such as multiple sclerosis occasionally complain of severe muscle pain. In addition, severe exertional fatigue is common (see p. 26). The neurologic findings of spasticity, hyperreflexia, Babinski signs, or other pathologic reflexes indicate the presence of central nervous system disease.

Focal Dystonias

Focal dystonias such as "writer's cramp" may present with aching or even severe "pain" with sustained activity. The causes of the pain, and even of the dystonia, are poorly understood, but evidence for an abnormality of reciprocal inhibition exists in many patients.[55]

FIBROMYALGIA (FIBROSITIS)

A disorder that has become known as fibromyalgia or fibrositis is much more common as a cause of muscle pain than are any of the specific myopathies. Not all authorities accept this diagnostic label, preferring to deal with symptoms as a pain syndrome, without a specific diagnosis.[5a,17a,21,30] We regard the syndrome as clinically homogeneous,[5] and the diagnosis to be as useful as that of any other syndrome wherein pathophysiology is still uncertain. Important reasons for making the diagnosis include avoiding repeated and expensive evaluations; avoiding the trap of attributing symptoms to a coincidental laboratory abnormality; providing credibility to the patient's symptoms by avoiding a pejorative or psychiatric label; prescribing appropriate treatment; and avoiding medication shown to be ineffective, particularly prednisone.[25,63] The American College of Rheumatology, in a multicenter trial using modern epidemiologic techniques,[8,79] has defined a syndrome with characteristic symptoms and signs presented by large numbers of patients.

The term "fibrositis" has been used for decades to describe patients with multifocal muscle pain and tenderness. Although Gowers first used the term more than a century ago, the subject still engenders confusion and controversy.[28] The entity of fibrositis (now more commonly called fibromyalgia), however, cannot be ignored or avoided, as indicated by the proliferation of articles, editorials, and reviews of the topic.[5a,25,57a,63,71,78,81] The following case history highlights some of the issues in this syndrome.

Case History

A 27-year-old woman, in the second year of her medical residency, reported a 12-month history of diffuse myalgia, particularly affecting the neck and shoulder muscles. Two months after a whiplash injury in a motor vehicle accident, the severity of symptoms was substantially increased. She continued to carry out all of her work-related responsibilities but noted increasing difficulty. She slept poorly and frequently awoke with a worsening of neck pain. The pain did not radiate into the arms, and no paresthesias occurred. The pain was worsened after exercise so that she had stopped all athletic activity for 2 months. She had generalized headache that worsened as the day wore on and had intermittent episodes of diarrhea and abdominal cramping, which were diagnosed as irritable bowel syndrome. Although she was under the stress of a residency training program, she was not anxious or depressed.

The general physical examination revealed tightness and multifocal tenderness throughout the cervical paraspinal muscles and the muscles of the shoulder girdle, particularly the trapezius bilaterally. Several trigger points were located both medial and superior to the scapula on both sides. Definite, less severe tenderness was also elicited over thigh, calf, and humeral muscles. The range of motion of the cervical spine was limited because of pain and tenderness. The results for the rest of the general physical and neurologic examinations were normal. Tests of muscular strength and endurance were normal, as were roentgenograms of the cervical spine and numerous blood studies.

The patient was treated with amitriptyline, beginning with 25 mg and gradually increasing to 75 mg each night. Within 1 week she was sleeping better, and within 4 weeks the neck pain improved substantially. Gradually she was able to return to a program of endurance exercise training and over the next 6 months showed substantial but incomplete improvement of her symptoms.

Comment: This patient satisfied the major diagnostic criteria for fibromyalgia (Table 11–3): generalized muscle pain involving three or more anatomic sites for at least 3 months and at least six typical and reproducible tender points on examination. She also had at least four of the minor criteria. The worsening after trauma and during stress is common. No systemic condition was identified that could cause her symptoms. Finally, she responded to a moderate dose of amitriptyline, which is subtherapeutic as treatment for depression. Moreover, she never appeared depressed and did not have vegetative symptoms of depression.

Clinical Features

It has been estimated that 5% of patients seen in a general medical clinic, and 12% of new patients referred to rheumatologists, have fibromyalgia.[5] In the United States the prevalence has been estimated at 3 to 6 million people.[25] Women account for 73% to 88% of patients, and the median age of onset of symptoms is in the early 30s. The average age of medical presentation, however, is considerably later, ranging from 34 to 53 years, which suggests that many patients live with the symptoms for a long interval prior to seeking medical attention.[25]

Fibromyalgia is a syndrome that consists of chronic, diffuse, musculoskeletal aching and soreness in association with a disturbed sleep pattern, fatigue, morning stiffness, and often some affective disturbance.[25,36] Both muscle pain and joint pain are common, and many patients report subjective swelling of hands or knees, although this is rarely objectively demonstrable. By definition, the history must indicate a duration of at least 3 months, and pain is most commonly located around the neck and shoulders. Some patients, however, also complain of pain at the ribs, elbows, buttocks, hips, and knees. Many patients also have headache, irritable bowel syndrome, and Raynaud's phenomenon. The symptoms usually begin gradually, occasionally in childhood or adolescence. Most patients report no identifiable precipitating event, but some attribute symptoms to recent trauma or intense stress.

As noted, the diagnosis depends on two major criteria: (1) the history of widespread pain for at least 3 months, and (2) the demonstration of pain and trigger points in at least 11 of 18 sites on digital palpation with a pressure of 4 kg (Fig. 11–5).[8] These criteria were sufficient to identify patients with fibro-

---

Table 11–3 PROPOSED CRITERIA FOR PRIMARY FIBROMYALGIA

MAJOR CRITERIA
1. Three or more areas of pain, aching, or stiffness lasting 3 mo or longer
2. Exclusion of other causes of muscle pain
3. Tender points (5 of 40 specific proposed areas; see Fig. 11–5)

MINOR CRITERIA
1. Exercise-related symptoms
2. Subjective subcutaneous swelling
3. Areas of cutaneous numbness
4. Change in symptoms with weather
5. Aggravation in symptoms by anxiety or stress
6. Disturbed sleep
7. Fatigue or tiredness
8. Anxiety
9. Chronic headache
10. Irritable bowel syndrome

Presence of three major and at least three of the minor criteria supports the diagnosis (modified from Yunus et al,[81]).

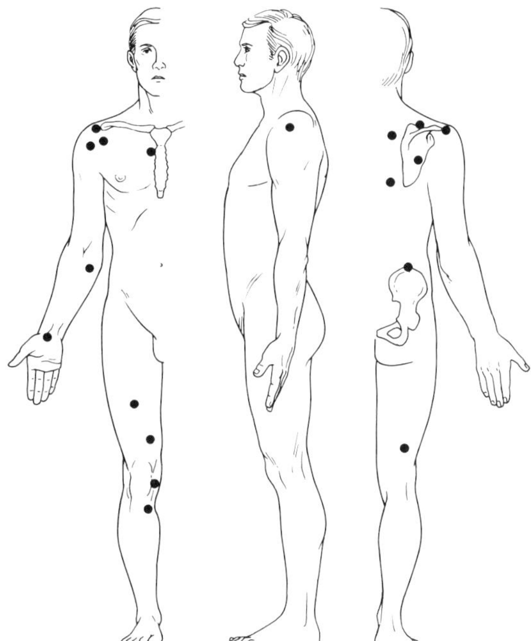

Figure 11–5. Nineteen sites of anatomic tenderness observed in fibromyalgia patients as compared to controls ($P < 0.001$). (Modified from Simms et al,[63] page 185, with permission.)

myalgia syndrome with a sensitivity of 88.4% and a specificity of 81.1% in a multicenter North American controlled trial.[79] The diagnostic criteria are summarized in Table 11–3. The rest of the physical and neurologic findings are normal in these patients.

Laboratory Findings

In general, the results of all radiographic and other laboratory screening tests are normal.[25] Occasionally the serum CK level is elevated because of minor trauma or unaccustomed exercise. Usually a repeat determination is normal after 5 days without exercise.

Similarly, fibromyalgia patients show minor abnormalities on EMG and magnetic resonance imaging and muscle biopsy results are indistinguishable from those of controls.[19a,38a,68] The finding of myoadenylate deaminase deficiency (MADD) poses special problems. The symptoms of the fibromyalgia syndrome have been attributed to such a deficiency (Fig. 7–14), but this relationship is still controversial (see Chapter 7,

p. 274).[62] In addition, the relative nonspecificity of many serologic studies, including antinuclear antibody determinations and rheumatoid factor tests, means that as many as 10% to 15% of patients will have "positive" results on these studies.

Pathophysiology

Various hypotheses have been offered to explain the development of the fibromyalgia syndrome. A great deal of attention was initially focused on nonspecific abnormalities in muscle biopsies, including type 2 atrophy and motheaten type 1 fibers, but these abnormalities probably are secondary to the disuse and deconditioning present in most of these patients. Thus, although some fibromyalgia patients were moderately weaker than controls, this weakness is likely to be a detraining effect.[33]

A disturbed sleep pattern is conspicuous, and most patients have nonrestorative sleep. Many studies have documented abnormal electroencephalographic (EEG) patterns during sleep.

The disturbed sleep pattern and the response to tricyclic medications has led some to hypothesize that disturbed serotonin pathways in the central nervous system may cause the syndrome.[47a,48] The analgesic effect of amitriptyline is probably separate from its antidepressant effect, however, and it has relatively little activity on serotonergic neurons. More recent attention has focused on substance P and endorphins, but no convincing data, or even a theory, have emerged.

Finally, there has been speculation that fibromyalgia may be an autoimmune disorder. It shares many diagnostic commonalities with chronic fatigue syndrome,[24a,37,47a] a disorder in which the theory of an autoimmune disturbance has received wide attention. Some have proposed that hypoxia and impaired microcirculation occur within the areas of painful muscle, but this too has not been established. Moreover, in patients with fibromyalgia, there is a normal oxygen uptake during muscular exercise.[62a]

Treatment

Unfortunately the natural history of this condition is not fully elaborated. There are no longitudinal, prospective studies of a large population of fibromyalgia patients. In general, however, long-term follow-up in single cases for over 40 years,[13] and a retrospective evaluation of a series of patients[5,13] indicate that the disease persists unabated but with fluctuations of severity.[13] Thus, many patients do have extremely long-standing and refractory symptoms. In spite of this, most patients are able to continue in gainful employment, with no higher rate of unemployment than the national average.[15] Patients should be spared a rigorous and extensive diagnostic evaluation, and they should be reassured that there is no serious underlying cause for their symptoms.

Despite the definition of fibromyalgia as chronic or persistent (3 months or longer), most treatment strategies have only been studied in short-term therapeutic trials. Few studies include a follow-up period of even 12 months, so there is little or no information on long-term efficacy.[17] Symptomatic treatment strategies producing benefit in controlled studies include tricyclic antidepressants such as amitriptyline in a daily dose of 10 to 75 mg[14]; combinations of amitriptyline with nonsteroidal anti-inflammatory agents such as naproxen, in doses of 500 mg twice a day[7]; and the muscle relaxant cyclobenzaprine (Flexeril), 10 to 40 mg daily.[6]

Hypnotics provide short-term benefits for the sleep disturbances, but their long-term value has not been established.[25] Fluoxetine hydrochloride (Prozac), which blocks serotonin uptake, improved sleep in an uncontrolled study.[22] Reassurance and an end to the relentless search for an alternative diagnosis remain important goals of management. Most fibromyalgia patients do not have an affective disorder, but psychiatric management may be indicated for those who do.[36] For all patients, an attempt should be made to achieve reconditioning through physical activity[43] and to modify disturbed sleep patterns whenever possible.

DISORDERS ASSOCIATED WITH MUSCLE FATIGUE

As emphasized in Chapter 2, patients most often refer to fatigue when they use the term "weakness." Such fatigue without weakness, termed asthenia, is only rarely a sign of myopathy. In contrast, patients with true muscle weakness usually do not complain of fatigue. Nonetheless, some rare neuromuscular diseases can cause notable fatigue associated with varying degrees of weakness, as can central nervous system diseases (Table 11–4). Fatigue also commonly accompanies many systemic diseases including cardiac, pulmonary, and renal disorders, blood dyscrasias of all types, and cancer. The following case illustrates some of the issues in the

Table 11–4 NEUROLOGIC CONDITIONS ASSOCIATED WITH SUBSTANTIAL MUSCLE FATIGUE

NEUROMUSCULAR DISEASE
Neuromuscular junction disorders
  Myasthenia gravis and Eaton-Lambert syndrome
Myopathies
  Mitochondrial disorders
  Glycolytic defects

CENTRAL NERVOUS SYSTEM DISORDERS—
invariably accompanied by neurologic findings

diagnosis and management of a representative patient with disabling fatigue.

Case History

A 36-year-old woman had a 2-year history of chronic weakness and fatigue. Besides easy muscular fatigability, her symptoms of fatigue included mental exhaustion and poor concentration. She had a low energy level and frequently needed to nap in the afternoon. On wakening in the morning she felt as though she had no energy whatsoever. In the past she had pursued active exercise, but she had been unable to perform any athletic activity for more than 18 months. She had occasional headache, intermittent low-grade fever and chills, swollen glands, and a marked disturbance of sleep pattern, as well as migratory arthralgia and myalgia involving all four limbs. She had no disturbance of appetite or bowel pattern and no affective symptoms.

In the past she was extraordinarily athletic, and outstandingly productive in her work as a court reporter. More than a year prior to evaluation, she became unable to work because of the profound weakness and fatigue. She had seen numerous physicians for evaluation and had undergone extensive testing without receiving a diagnosis.

The general physical examination was completely normal and a full neurologic examination disclosed no abnormality. She easily performed 20 deep knee bends and could hold her right arm outstretched for 3 minutes.

The serum CK and lactate levels, erythrocyte sedimentation rate, VDRL test for syphilis, levels of thyroxine and thyroid stimulating hormone, routine chemistry panel, and complete blood count (CBC) were all normal. Repetitive nerve stimulation and quantitative electromyography all gave normal results.

Comment: This patient satisfies the major criteria for chronic fatigue syndrome—debilitating fatigue persisting for more than 6 months with no other explanation for the symptoms. In addition, she has nine of the minor criteria establishing the diagnosis. Like many patients, she had gone through a series of evaluations without receiving any explanation of her symptoms. She subsequently improved on moderate doses of amitriptyline and a graduated program of endurance exercise.

Chronic Fatigue Syndrome

CLINICAL FEATURES

Currently used terms for this disorder of excessive fatigue include chronic fatigue syndrome, myalgic encephalomyelitis, and the postviral fatigue syndrome. The syndrome has also been referred to as epidemic neuromyasthenia, Iceland disease, and the Royal Free Hospital syndrome.[1] "Chronic fatigue syndrome" remains the preferable term, as it implies no specific cause.[61] The condition involves a constellation of perceived symptoms, but excessive muscle fatigue represents the major feature. Additional symptoms include myalgias, paresthesias, headache, dizziness, diaphoresis, and fainting spells. Other symptoms attributed to the disorder, such as impaired concentration, memory disturbances, and emotional lability, imply origin in the central nervous system.[77] Some viral infections incriminated include infectious mononucleosis (Epstein-Barr virus), influenza, Coxsackie virus, and varicella.[34,44,67]

Diagnostic criteria for chronic fatigue syndrome have been developed (Table 11–5).[32,49] Both major criteria—new onset of debilitating fatigue for more than 6 months and exclusion of other known medical causes of fatigue—and

Table 11–5 CHRONIC FATIGUE SYNDROME: DIAGNOSTIC CRITERIA

MAJOR CRITERIA
New debilitating fatigue that reduces activity below 50% and does not resolve with bed rest—
persisting for at least 6 mo
No other cause—requires thorough search (history, examination, laboratory)

MINOR CRITERIA
Mild fever (oral temperature between 37.6°C and 38.6°C, if measured by the patient) or chills
Sore throat
Painful lymph nodes in the anterior or posterior cervical and axillary distribution
Myalgia
Prolonged (≥24 h) fatigue after exercise previously well tolerated
Generalized headaches (of a type, severity, or pattern different from headaches the patient may
have had in the premorbid state)
Migratory arthralgia
Neuropsychologic complaints (photophobia, transient visual scotomata, forgetfulness, excessive
irritability, confusion, difficulty thinking, inability to concentrate, depression)
Sleep disturbance (hypersomnia or insomnia)
Symptom complex initially developing over a few hours to a few days

PHYSICAL CRITERIA (documented by physician on two occasions 1 mo apart)
Low-grade fever (oral temperature between 37.6°C and 38.6°C, or rectal temperature between
37.8°C and 38.8°C)
Nonexudative pharyngitis
Palpable or tender anterior or posterior cervical or axillary lymph nodes

Modified from reference 32 and 49. See text.

at least six of the minor criteria must be satisfied to fulfill the diagnostic definition.

Convincing evidence exists for the hysterical origin of many clustered or epidemic cases,[44] but not for all cases exhibiting this syndrome. A consensus conference concluded that many cases were not hysterical.[32] A publication from the National Institutes of Health has presented suggested research criteria for the diagnosis.[49] The "Myalgic Encephalomyelitis Association," a self-help group, has perpetuated the term for which it is named.[1]

Patients with this disorder all have excessive fatigability. In most patients, fatigue follows physical exercise and may be associated with myalgia. It has been assumed that the fatigue is muscular in origin,[2,3,58] but more recent studies suggest that muscle function is normal (see below).[2a,12,22a,35,42,65] Although many patients do complain of excessive fatigability on exercise, compared with their previous performance, a large proportion feel a subjective sense of fatigue that is independent of physical exertion. Moreover, many patients complain of *mental* fatigue, including difficulty in concentration and impaired memory, which is aggravated by intense cognitive activity.[28a,77] Thus, in many patients, the fatigue is a matter of subjective perception, involving skeletal muscle only in part. Many patients also have some anxiety or depression, as well as a tendency to somatization. Most describe feeling both reduced energy and excessive mental fatigue, as well as increased fatigability with exercise. Many also have a disturbed sleep pattern.[43a,47b] The results of physical and neurologic examinations of such patients are virtually always normal.[40]

LABORATORY FINDINGS

Laboratory features, including serum CK and lactate levels, thyroid function, blood counts, and metabolic screens, are entirely normal. EMG studies often demonstrate low-frequency discharges of motor units with intermittent recruitment, a profile indicating incomplete effort. Routine EMG and nerve conduction studies disclose no other definite abnormality. Using superimposed maximal nerve stimulation on a maximal voluntary contraction, it is possible to demonstrate added force of isometric contraction in some patients, a finding which further supports the conclusion that there is incomplete voluntary effort.[22a,35,65]

Muscle biopsies in patients with chronic fatigue show no morphologic abnormality or disturbance of carnitine, glycolytic, or mitochondrial enzymes.[11,12,19b] Early and excessive lactic acid formation during exercise has been noted and could reflect physical deconditioning,[2] but more recent studies did not confirm these findings.[2a,35] Coincidental but unimportant nerve root disease, or other antecedent conditions, may lead to inappropriate diagnosis and treatment of patients if they are subjected to repeated or extensive EMG studies.

PATHOPHYSIOLOGY

This group of patients was previously thought to have chronic infection with Epstein-Barr virus,[31,34,38,39,67] but more recent studies have found little evidence to support a pathogenic role for this virus in chronic fatigue syndrome.[23,66] Although a number of other reports have raised a question about human herpes virus, enteroviruses, or human retroviruses, no convincing evidence supports a causative role for any of these agents.[10a,19c]

Similarly, studies of immune function have shown no consistent abnormality.[61] Some patients have had evidence of subtle and diffuse dysfunction: partial hypogammaglobulinemia, partial hypergammaglobulinemia, elevated levels of autoantibodies (particularly antithyroid antibodies and antinuclear antibodies), elevated levels of circulating immune complexes, elevated ratios of helper-suppressor T cells, reduced in vitro synthesis of interleukin 2 and interferon by cultured lymphocytes, in-creased levels of antibodies to at least six viruses, and deficient functional activity of natural killer cells.[61] These and other findings have led may investigators to pursue the possibility that immune system abnormalities may be important in the development of this syndrome. Most of these abnormalities affect only a minority of patients, however, and the magnitude of the abnormal findings is indeed small compared with those found in classic immunologic disorders. Thus, the role of immune system dysfunction is still uncertain.

Many patients with chronic fatigue syndrome have cognitive complaints and difficulty with both concentration and memory function on formal testing.[28a] Standard visual, auditory, and somatosensory evoked potential studies have been entirely normal,[57] but latencies of the cognitive evoked potentials were prolonged, particularly for the P300 response.[57] Also, reaction times from the onset of a tone to the pressing of a button were significantly prolonged in these patients compared with control subjects. These results were interpreted as indicating deficits in attention and slower information processing; similar findings have not been observed in patients with depression.[56]

Most studies that have attempted to quantify muscular fatigability in patients with chronic fatigue syndrome have demonstrated normal muscular endurance and function. For example, measurements of isometric strength and endurance were normal in 20 patients with a postviral fatigue syndrome.[42] In a study of 30 patients with chronic fatigue syndrome, intermittent tetanic stimulation of the adductor pollicis muscle disclosed normal endurance and recovery patterns during fatiguing exercise.[65] During exhaustive bicycle exercise, some patients with chronic fatigue syndrome discontinued the exercise well before reaching maximal predicted heart rate, suggesting "central" fatigue. In other words, it appears that these patients' perception of fatigue somehow differs in a way that limits their effort in muscular activation.[22a]

Magnetic stimulation applied to the scalp and electrical stimulation of the cervical spinal cord have been used to evoke responses from hand muscles to evaluate central motor conduction in patients with chronic fatigue syndrome. Both before and after fatiguing exercise, central motor conduction times were normal, and amplitudes of the evoked responses were preserved even after fatiguing exercise.[72]

In a recent study, the response of these patients to systemic exercise was normal, but voluntary activation of the tibialis anterior was significantly lower during maximal sustained exercise.[35] Muscle metabolism, neuromuscular transmission, and muscle membrane function were all normal. This failure of activation was well in excess of that found in control subjects and suggests an important central component of muscle fatigue in patients with chronic fatigue syndrome. The finding of central fatigue, particularly during prolonged fatiguing exercise, is consistent with the reports of abnormal cognitive potentials, which point to problems with concentration and attention in these patients. The functional integrity of central motor pathways appears to be preserved, but other factors in central fatigue have not been subjected to systematic study. In summary, most evidence suggests that the major source of fatigue in patients with chronic fatigue syndrome resides outside of the motor control system.

TREATMENT

Fortunately, spontaneous improvement characterizes the natural history of this disorder in at least half the patients. No specific treatment has yet been found, in spite of several prospective, randomized, double-blind, placebo-controlled trials with a number of therapeutic agents, including acyclovir, intravenous immunoglobulin, and magnesium sulfate.[61] Management basically has three aspects. First, the reassurance that there is no serious neuromuscular disorder, and that most patients do improve with time, is often critical. The second part of the program should include a gradual increase in physical activity to reverse the deconditioning that takes place in all patients. Finally, antidepressant medication such as amitriptyline is often beneficial, in low to moderate doses, usually lower than those needed to treat depression.

SUMMARY

In patients with a normal examination and CK level, muscle pain and fatigue usually are not the result of a myopathy. When objective signs of weakness are present, however, a myopathy can often be identified (Table 11–6).

By far the most common condition associated with muscle pain is fibromyalgia. The most common disorder asso-

---

Table 11–6 EVALUATION OF MUSCLE PAIN AND FATIGUE

Assess strength and endurance
Evaluate trigger points
Laboratory determinations: CBC, ESR, CK, K^+, Ca^{2+}, phosphate, T_4, TSH
Electrodiagnostic studies

Normal results	High CK or myopathic EMG

Consider evaluation for:
   Immunologic disorders
   Cardiac, pulmonary, other systemic disease
   Depression
	Forearm exercise testing
	   (lactate, ammonia)
	Muscle biopsy

CBC = complete blood count; ESR = erythrocyte sedimentation rate; T_4 = thyroxine; TSH = thyroid-stimulating hormone.

ciated with fatigue is the chronic fatigue syndrome. Emotional disturbances are present in many patients with fibromyalgia or the chronic fatigue syndrome; frankly psychotic behavior and severe personality disorders are uncommon. The severity of the symptoms, particularly when they appear *de novo* in previously healthy individuals, more than explains the depression, anxiety, and other psychiatric symptoms. Symptomatic and supportive management is helpful in some but not all patients.

It is often difficult to determine whether a patient with muscle pain or fatigue really has a pathologic disorder. Our current understanding of fibromyalgia and the chronic fatigue syndrome is disappointing, and many argue that these disorders do not really fit the medical model. Nonetheless, clinicians interested in neuromuscular disorders will see many patients with these symptoms and must formulate a plan for evaluation and management. The two syndromes are closely related and indeed overlap significantly.[24a,37] While we await a more satisfactory understanding of their pathophysiology, a compassionate and supportive approach to these patients is often helpful.

REFERENCES

1. Archer MI: The post-viral syndrome: A review. J R Coll Gen Pract 37:212, 1987.
2. Arnold DL, Bore PJ, Radda GK, Styles P, and Taylor DJ: Excessive intracellular acidosis of skeletal muscle on exercise in a patient with a post-viral exhaustion/fatigue syndrome. A ^{31}P nuclear magnetic resonance study. Lancet 1:1367, 1984.
2a. Barnes PR, Taylor DJ, Kemp GJ, Radda GK: Skeletal muscle bioenergetics in the chronic fatigue syndrome. J Neurol Neurosurg Psychiatry 56:679, 1993.
3. Behan PO and Behan WMH: Postviral fatigue syndrome. Crit Rev Neurobiol 4:157, 1988.
4. Bengtsson A, Henriksson KG, and Larsson J: Reduced high-energy phosphate levels in the painful muscles of patients with primary fibromyalgia. Arthritis Rheum 29:817, 1986.
5. Bennett RM: Fibromyalgia. JAMA 257:2802, 1987.
5a. Bennett RM: Fibromyalgia and the facts: Sense or nonsense. Rheum Dis Clin North Am 19:45, 1993.
6. Bennett RM, Gatter RA, Campbell SM, Andrews RP, Clark SR, and Scarola JA: A comparison of cyclobenzaprine and placebo in the management of fibrositis. A double-blind controlled study. Arthritis Rheum 31:1535, 1988.
7. Bennett RM, Clark SR, Goldberg L, et al: Aerobic fitness in patients with fibrositis. Arthritis Rheum 32:454, 1989.
7a. Beyenburg S and Zierz S: Chronic progressive external ophthalmoplegia and myalgia associated with tubular aggregates. Acta Neurol Scand 87:397, 1993.
8. Boissevain MD and McCain GA: Toward an integrated understanding of fibromyalgia syndrome, I. Medical and pathophysiological aspects. Pain 45:227, 1991.
9. Boska MD, Moussavi RS, Carson PJ, Weiner MW, and Miller RG: The metabolic basis of recovery after fatiguing exercise of human muscle. Neurology 40:240, 1990.
10. Bove KE, Iannaccone ST, Hilton PK, and Samaha, F: Cylindrical spirals in a familial neuromuscular disorder. Ann Neurol 7:550, 1980.
10a. Bowles NE, Bayston TA, Zhang HY, et al: Persistence of enterovirus RNA in muscle biopsy samples suggests that some cases of chronic fatigue syndrome result from a previous, inflammatory viral myopathy. Jornal de Medico 24:145, 1993.
11. Brooke MH and Kaplan H: Muscle pathology in rheumatoid arthritis, polymyalgia rheumatica, and polymyositis. Arch Pathol 94:101, 1972.
12. Byrne E and Trounce I: Chronic fatigue and myalgia syndrome: Mitochondrial and glycolytic studies in skeletal mus-

cle. J Neurol Neurosurg Psychiatry 50:743, 1987.

13. Calabro JJ: Fibromyalgia (fibrositis) in children. Am J Med 81:(Suppl 3A):57, 1986.

14. Carette S, McCain GA, Bell DA, and Fam AG: Evaluation of amitriptyline in primary fibrositis. A double-blind, placebo-controlled study. Arthritis Rheum 29:655, 1986.

15. Cathey MA, Wolfe F, Kleinheksel SM, and Hawley DJ: Socioeconomic impact of fibrositis: A study of 81 patients with primary fibrositis. Am J Med 81(Suppl 3A):78, 1986.

16. Chen MK: The epidemiology of self-perceived fatigue among adults. Prev Med 15:74, 1986.

17. Clark S, Tindall E, and Bennett R: A double blind crossover trial of prednisone vs placebo in the treatment of fibrositis. J Rheumatol 12:980, 1985.

17a. Cohen ML and Quintner JL: Fibromyalgia syndrome, a problem of tautology. Lancet 342:906, 1993.

18. Danon MJ, Carpenter S, and Harati Y: Muscle pain associated with tubular aggregates and structures resembling cylindrical spirals. Muscle Nerve 12:265, 1989.

19. Davies CTM and White MJ: Muscle weakness following eccentric work in man. Pflüegers Arch 392:168, 1981.

19a. Drewes AM, Andreasen A, Schroder HD, Hogsaa B, and Jennum P: Pathology of skeletal muscle in fibromyalgia: A histo-immunochemical and ultrastructural study. Br J Rheumatol 6:479, 1993.

19b. Edwards RH, Gibson H, Clague JE, and Helliwell T: Muscle histopathology and physiology in chronic fatigue syndrome. Ciba Found Symp 173:102, 1993.

19c. Folks TM, Heneine W, Khan A, et al: Investigation of retroviral involvement in chronic fatigue syndrome. Ciba Found Symp 173:160, 1993.

20. Friden J, Sfakianos PN, and Hargens AR: Muscle soreness and intramuscular fluid pressure: Comparison between eccentric and concentric load. J Appl Physiol 61:2175, 1986.

21. Gatter RA: Pharmacotherapeutics in fibrositis. Am J Med 81(Suppl 3A):63, 1986.

22. Geller SA: Treatment of fibrositis with fluoxetine hydrochloride (Prozac). Am J Med 87:594, 1989.

22a. Gibson H, Carroll N, Clague JE, and Edwards RH: Exercise performance and fatigability in patients with chronic fatigue syndrome. J Neurol Neurosurg Psychiatry 56:993, 1993.

23. Gold D, Bowden R, Sixby J, et al: Chronic fatigue: A prospective clinical and virologic study. JAMA 264:48, 1990.

24. Goldberg AL, Kettelhut IC, Furuno K, Fagan JM, and Baracos V: Activation of protein breakdown and prostaglandin E_2 production in rat skeletal muscle in fever is signaled by a macrophage product distinct from interleukin 1 or other known monokines. J Clin Invest 81:1378, 1988.

24a. Goldenberg DL: Fibromyalgia, chronic fatigue syndrome, and myofascial pain syndrome. Curr Opin Rheumatol 5:199, 1993.

25. Goldenberg DL: Fibromyalgia syndrome: An emerging but controversial condition. JAMA 257:2782, 1987.

26. Goldenberg DL, Felson DT, and Dinerman H: A randomized, controlled trial of amitriptyline and naproxen in the treatment of patients with fibromyalgia. Arthritis Rheum 29:1371, 1986.

27. Gospe SM, Lazaro RP, Lava NS, Grootscholten PM, Scott MO, and Fischbeck KH: Familial X-linked myalgia and cramps: A nonprogressive myopathy associated with a deletion in the dystrophin gene. Neurology 39:1277, 1989.

28. Gowers WR: Lumbago: Its lesson and analogues. BMJ 117, 1904.

28a. Grafman J, Schwartz V, Dale JK, et al: Analysis of neuropsychological functioning in patients with chronic fatigue syndrome. J Neurol Neurosurg Psychiatry 56:684, 1993.

29. Griggs RC, Matthews SM, and Rennie MJ: The metabolic response to graded isometric forearm exercise in overnight-fasted man. J Physiol 332:39P, 1982.

30. Hadler NM: A critical reappraisal of the fibrositis concept. Am J Med 81(Suppl 3A):26, 1986.

31. Hellinger WC, Smith TF, Van Scog RE, et al: Chronic fatigue syndrome and the diagnostic utility of antibody to Epstein-Barr virus early antigen. JAMA 260:971, 1988.

32. Holmes GP, Kaplan JE, Gantz NM, et al: Chronic fatigue syndrome: A working case definition. Ann Intern Med 108:387, 1988.

33. Jacobsen S and Danneskiold-Samsoe B: Isometric and isokinetic muscle strength in patients with fibrositis syndrome. Scand J Rheumatol 16:61, 1987.

34. Jones JF, Ray CG, Minnich LL, Hicks MJ, Kibler R, and Lucas DO: Evidence for active Epstein-Barr virus infection in patients with persistent, unexplained illnesses: Elevated anti-early antigen antibodies. Ann Intern Med 102:1, 1985.

35. Kent-Braun JA, Sharma KR, Weiner MW, Massie B, and Miller RG: Central basis of muscle fatigue in chronic fatigue syndrome. Neurology 43:125, 1993.

36. Kirmayer LJ, Robbins JM, and Kapusta MA: Somatization and depression in fibromyalgia syndrome. Am J Psychiatry 145:950, 1988.

37. Komaroff AL and Goldenberg D: The chronic fatigue syndrome: Definition, current studies and lessons for fibromyalgia research. J Rheumatol 16 (Suppl 19):23, 1989.

38. Koo D: Chronic fatigue syndrome: A critical appraisal of the role of Epstein-Barr virus. West J Med 150:590, 1989.

38a. Kravis MM, Munk PL, McCain GA, Vellet AD, and Levin MF: MR imaging of muscle and tender points in fibromyalgia. J Magn Reson Imaging 3:669, 1993.

39. Kroenke K, Wood DR, Mangelsdorff D, Meier NJ, and Powell JB: Chronic fatigue in primary care: Prevalence, patient characteristics, and outcome. JAMA 260:929, 1988.

40. Lane TJ, Matthews DA, and Manu P: The low yield of physical examinations and laboratory investigations of patients with chronic fatigue. Am J Med Sci 299:313, 1990.

41. Lazaro RP, Fenichel GM, Kilroy AW, Saito A, and Fleischer S: Cramps, muscle pain, and tubular aggregates. Arch Neurol 37:715, 1980.

42. Lloyd AR, Hales JP, and Gandevia SC: Muscle strength, endurance and recovery in the post-infection fatigue syndrome. J Neurol Neurosurg Psychiatry 51:1316, 1988.

43. McCain GA: Role of physical fitness training in the fibrositis/fibromyalgia syndrome. Am J Med 81(Suppl 3A):73, 1986.

43a. McCluskey DR: Pharmacological approaches to the therapy of chronic fatigue syndrome. Ciba Found Symp 173:280, 1993.

44. McEvedy CP and Beard AW: Concept of benign myalgic encephalomyelitis. BMJ 1:11, 1970.

45. Mills KR and Edwards RHT: Investigative strategies for muscle pain. J Neurol Sci 58:73, 1983.

46. Mills KR, Newham DJ, and Edwards RHT: Force, contraction frequency and energy metabolism as interactive determinants of ischaemic muscle pain. Pain 14:149, 1982.

47. Mills KR, Newham DF, and Edwards RHT: Muscle pain. In Wall PD and Melzack R (eds): Textbook of Pain. Churchill Livingstone, New York, 1984, p 319.

47a. Moldofsky H: Fibromyalgia, sleep disorder and chronic fatigue syndrome. Ciba Found Symp 173:262, 1993.

47b. Morriss R, Sharpe M, Sharpley AL, et al: Abnormalities of sleep in patients with the chronic fatigue syndrome. Br Med J 306:1161, 1993.

48. Moldofsky H: Sleep and musculoskeletal pain. Am J Med 81(Suppl 3A):85, 1986.

49. National Institute of Allergy and Infectious Diseases: Chronic fatigue syndrome: A pamphlet for physicians. NIH Publication No 90-484, October, 1990.

50. Newham DJ, Jones DA, and Edwards RHT: Large delayed plasma creatine kinase changes after stepping exercise. Muscle Nerve 6:380, 1983.

51. Newham DJ, McPhail G, Mills KR,

and Edwards RHT: Ultrastructural changes after concentric and eccentric contractions of human muscle. J Neurol Sci 61:109, 1983.

52. Newham DJ, Mills KR, Quigley BM, and Edwards RHT: Pain and fatigue after concentric and eccentric muscle contractions. Clin Sci 64:55, 1983.

53. Niakan E, Harati Y, and Danon MJ: Tubular aggregates: Their association with myalgia. J Neurol Neurosurg Psychiatry 48:882, 1985.

54. O'Duffy JD, Wahner HW, and Hunder GG: Joint imaging in polymyalgia rheumatica. Mayo Clin Proc 51:519, 1976.

55. Panizza ME, Hallett M, and Nilsson J: Reciprocal inhibition in patients with hand cramps. Neurology 39:85, 1989.

56. Patterson JV, Michalewski HJ, and Starr A: Latency variability of the components of auditory event-related potentials to infrequent stimuli in aging, Alzheimer-type dementia and depression. Electroencephalogr Clin Neurophysiol 71:450, 1988.

57. Prasher D, Smith A, and Findley L: Sensory and cognitive event-related potentials in myalgic encephalomyelitis. J Neurol Neurosurg Psychiatry 53:247, 1990.

57a. Prescott E, Jacobsen S, Kjoller M, et al: Fibromyalgia in the adult Danish population: II. A study of clinical features. Scand J Rheumatol 22:238, 1993.

58. Ramsay AM: Epidemic neuromyasthenia 1955–1978. Postgrad Med J 54:718, 1978.

59. Ricker K and Moxley RT: Autosomal dominant cramping disease. Arch Neurol 47:810, 1990.

60. Serratrice G, Pellissier JF, Roux H, and Quilichini P: Fasciitis, perimyositis, myositis, polymyositis, and eosinophilia. Muscle Nerve 13:385, 1990.

61. Shafran SD: The chronic fatigue syndrome. Am J Med 90:730, 1991.

62. Shumate JB: Myoadenylate deaminase deficiency. Semin Neurol 3:242, 1983.

62a. Sietsema KE, Cooper DM, Caro X, Leibling MR, and Louie JS: Oxygen uptake during exercise in patients with primary fibromyalgia syndrome. J Rheumatol 20:860, 1993.

63. Simms RW, Goldenberg DL, Felson DT, and Mason JH: Tenderness in 75 anatomic sites: Distinguishing fibromyalgia patients from controls. Arthritis Rheum 31:182, 1988.

64. Sladek GD, Vasey FB, Sieger B, Behnke DA, Germain BF, and Espinoza LR: Relapsing eosinophilic myositis. J Rheumatol 10:467, 1983.

65. Stokes MJ, Cooper RG, and Edwards RHT: Normal muscle strength and fatigability in patients with effort syndromes. Br Med J 297:1014, 1988.

66. Straus SE, Dale JK, Tobi M, et al: Acyclovir treatment of the chronic fatigue syndrome: Lack of efficacy in a placebo-controlled trial. N Engl J Med 319:1692, 1988.

67. Straus SE, Tosato G, Armstrong G, et al: Persisting illness and fatigue in adults with evidence of Epstein-Barr virus infection. Ann Intern Med 102:7, 1985.

68. Stokes MJ, Colter C, Klestov A, and Cooper RG: Normal paraspinal muscle electromyographic fatigue characteristics in patients with primary fibromyalgia. Br J Rheumatol 32:711, 1993.

69. Taylor DJ, Styles P, Matthews PM, et al: Energetics of human muscle: Exercise-induced ATP depletion. Magn Reson Med 3:44, 1986.

70. Telerman-Toppet N, Bacq M, Khoubesserian P, and Coërs C: Type 2 fiber predominance in muscle cramp and exertional myalgia. Muscle Nerve 8:563, 1985.

71. Thompson JM: Subspecialty clinics: physical medicine and rehabilitation: Tension myalgia as a diagnosis at the Mayo Clinic and its relationship to fibrositis, fibromyalgia, and myofascial pain syndrome. Mayo Clin Proc 65:1237, 1990.

72. Waddy H, Wessely S, and Muray NMF: Central motor conduction studies in chronic postviral fatigue syndrome. Electroencephalogr Clin Neurophysiol 75(Suppl):5160, 1990. Abstract.

73. Walters A, Hening W, Côté L, and Fahn

S: Dominantly inherited restless legs with myoclonus and periodic movements of sleep: A syndrome related to the endogenous opiates? Adv Neurol 43:309, 1986.

74. Walters AS, Hening WA, Kavey N, Chokroverty S, and Gidro-Frank S: A double-blind randomized crossover trial of bromocriptine and placebo in restless legs syndrome. Ann Neurol 24:455, 1988.

75. Walters AS, Wagner ML, Hening WA, et al: Successful treatment of the idiopathic restless legs syndrome in a randomized double-blind trial of oxycodone versus placebo. Sleep 16:327, 1993.

76. Weller B, Karpati G, and Carpenter S: Dystrophin-deficient mdx muscle fibers are preferentially vulnerable to necrosis induced by experimental lengthening contractions. J Neurol Sci 100:9, 1990.

77. Wessely S and Powell R: Fatigue syndromes: a comparison of chronic "postviral" fatigue with neuromuscular and affective disorders. J Neurol Neurosurg Psychiatry 52:940, 1989.

78. Wolfe F: The clinical syndrome of fibrositis. Am J Med 81(Suppl 3A):7, 1986.

79. Wolfe F, Smythe HA, Yunus MB, et al: The American College of Rheumatology 1990 criteria for the classification of fibromyalgia: Report of the multicenter criteria committee. Arthritis Rheum 33:160, 1990.

80. Woods JJ, Furbush F, and Bigland-Ritchie B: Evidence for a fatigue-induced reflex inhibition of motoneuron firing rates. J Neurophysiol 58:125, 1987.

81. Yunus M, Masi AT, Calabro JJ, Miller KA, and Feigenbaum SL: Primary fibromyalgia (fibrositis): Clinical study of 50 patients with matched normal controls. Semin Arthritis Rheum 11:151, 1981.

Chapter 12

PREVENTION AND MANAGEMENT OF MEDICAL COMPLICATIONS OF MYOPATHIES

RESPIRATORY MANAGEMENT
CARDIAC MANAGEMENT
PREVENTION OF EDEMA
DIETARY MANAGEMENT:
  PREVENTION OF OBESITY
SWALLOWING ABNORMALITIES
OTHER GASTROINTESTINAL
  COMPLICATIONS

The patient with progressive, disabling weakness, for whom there is no specific treatment, presents a major challenge to the fortitude and creativity of the physician. Those patients who require a wheelchair may even be unable to reach many physicians' offices. This chapter describes supportive measures that may help such patients.

Most myopathies are seldom fatal. As a rule, only respiratory and cardiac complications are life-threatening and these can sometimes be successfully treated. Careful surveillance for coincidental illness such as malignancy and atherosclerosis is necessary but is often neglected because of the difficulties involved with performing appropriate screening studies in severely disabled patients or those confined to a wheelchair.

RESPIRATORY MANAGEMENT

Normal Respiratory Muscle Function

The muscles normally active during respiration include the diaphragm, abdominal muscles, intercostal muscles, and accessory muscles (sternocleidomastoid and scalene muscles). All are active during breathing at rest.[23] During quiet breathing the intercostal and abdominal muscles function to maintain the mechanical advantage of the diaphragm by optimizing its length.[57] During expiration the diaphragm is lengthened by the abdominal muscles. During inspiration, abdominal and rib cage movements operate to lengthen the diaphragm. Because the force developed by skeletal muscle, including the diaphragm, declines as the speed of shortening increases,[21] the ability of other muscles to maintain the diaphragm in a relatively isometric state provides for maximal force generation by the diaphragm.

Abnormalities of Respiratory Function

Evidence of respiratory dysfunction can be found in most patients with my-

408

opathies or other neuromuscular diseases, although only a minority develop related symptoms. Abnormalities include:

- Decreased respiratory muscle strength, either generalized or selective
- Impaired glottic function, leading to an ineffective cough
- Impaired central nervous system ventilatory drive
- Upper airway obstruction during sleep
- Abnormal swallowing function leading to recurrent aspiration

Generalized respiratory muscle weakness produces restrictive lung disease with a reduction in vital capacity, a decrease in total lung volume, and a decrease in lung compliance. The earliest detectable abnormality is a reduction in static pressures. Maximum expiratory pressure (MEP) is reduced to a greater extent than maximum inspiratory pressure (MIP). (MIP is also referred to as negative inspiratory pressure.)[5,29]

Paralysis produced experimentally in normal subjects given curare leads to a similar disproportionate decrease in static pressures.[58] With decreasing lung volumes, the expiratory muscles are placed at a mechanical disadvantage during expiration and at an advantage during inspiration.[8] This accounts for the greater reduction in MEP than in MIP. If the diaphragm is selectively involved prior to other muscles becoming weak, vital capacity is reduced to a much greater extent when the patient is supine (orthopnea).[19] Chest roentgenogram or ultrasound evaluation shows decreased diaphragm excursion (Fig. 12–1). In such patients, diaphragmatic weakness can be suspected on physical examination when the abdominal muscles show paradoxical inward movement during inspiration. On the other

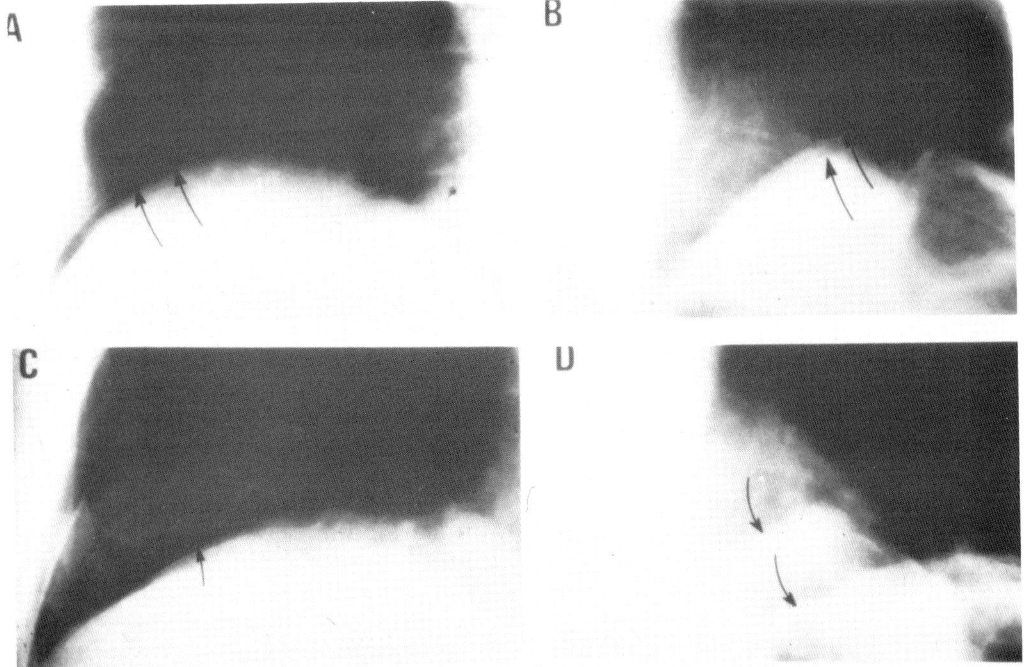

Figure 12–1. Inspiration and expiration chest roentgenograms from patient with selective involvement of the diaphragm. When the patient is supine there is minimal movement (A and B). When seated, there is more than 3 cm expansion from inspiration (C) to expiration (D).

hand, patients with cervical cord transection and selective preservation of diaphragmatic function show paradoxical inward movement of the upper rib cage during inspiration.[49]

DISORDERS CAUSING RESPIRATORY FAILURE

Much can be done to prevent respiratory failure. Early recognition of respiratory muscle weakness is often life-saving. Patients with myopathies in which respiratory failure is frequent (Table 12–1) should have sequential clinical and laboratory studies of lung function beginning at the time of diagnosis. Certain myopathies, most notably acid maltase deficiency, may present with respiratory failure as the first sign of an underlying muscle disease (Table 12–2). These disorders must be considered in patients with unexplained respiratory failure, but amyotrophic lateral sclerosis is a more likely diagnosis in such patients.[62] *Even if laboratory data such as creatine kinase (CK) levels or biopsy suggest myopathy, amyotrophic lateral sclerosis should be considered in the elderly patient with respiratory failure caused by muscle weakness.*

Respiratory muscle weakness leading to respiratory failure seldom affects pa-

Table 12–1 MYOPATHIES CAUSING RESPIRATORY FAILURE

MUSCULAR DYSTROPHIES
  Duchenne
  Becker
  Myotonic
  Limb-girdle
  Congenital
  Emery-Dreifuss

CONGENITAL MYOPATHIES
  Nemaline
  Centronuclear

METABOLIC MYOPATHIES
  Deficiencies of acid maltase and carnitine
  Mitochondrial myopathies

INFLAMMATORY MYOPATHY
  Polymyositis

Table 12–2 MYOPATHIES *PRESENTING* WITH RESPIRATORY FAILURE

Myotonic dystrophy
Centronuclear myopathy
Nemaline myopathy
Acid maltase deficiency

tients with certain myopathies, including facioscapulohumeral dystrophy, oculopharyngeal dystrophy, central core disease, dermatomyositis, inclusion body myositis, and most myopathies of systemic disease. Accordingly, severe pulmonary symptoms in patients with these disorders are usually the result of coincidental illness.

The electrophysiologic methods used to determine if neuromuscular disease is responsible for respiratory failure include phrenic nerve conduction and diaphragmatic EMG.[7a]

RECOGNITION OF IMPENDING RESPIRATORY FAILURE

Symptoms. *Acute* respiratory failure is usually precipitated by a readily recognized event such as pneumonitis, bronchitis, atelectasis, aspiration, pneumothorax, or congestive heart failure. *Chronic* respiratory failure, however, usually presents insidiously with symptoms of nocturnal oxygen desaturation, such as morning headache and lethargy. Generalized fatigue, unexplained weight loss, or cough are also symptoms that should raise the suspicion of respiratory failure in a patient with neuromuscular disease. Chronic hypoxia increases pulmonary vascular resistance, which may in turn lead to symptoms of cor pulmonale: ankle edema, nocturia, and orthopnea. *Dyspnea is uncommon* as a presenting symptom.

Disorders affecting swallowing may predispose to aspiration, with symptoms of coughing or dyspnea during or following meals. As described earlier, patients with selective diaphragmatic weakness often experience severe orthopnea.[48]

Physical Findings. Examination of the chest of patients with respiratory compromise usually shows: (1) diminished breath sounds and atelectatic (paninspiratory) rales at lung bases; (2) diminished diaphragmatic excursion as detected by percussion of the chest, comparing diaphragm descent from *maximum* expiration to maximum inspiration; and (3) decreased effectiveness of the cough. Signs of cor pulmonale, such as cardiomegaly, hepatomegaly, distended neck veins, and papilledema may be present. Many patients, particularly those with Duchenne dystrophy, learn the trick of glossopharyngeal, "frog" breathing, in which rapid cycling of the tongue muscles forces air into the lungs. If the diaphragm is selectively weakened, a seemingly paradoxical breathing pattern occurs during which the patient's abdomen flattens or moves inward during inspiration.

Routine Testing of Pulmonary Function. A spirometer with a low expiratory resistance must be used to obtain an accurate measurement of vital capacity in a patient with muscle weakness.[29] Certain electronic spirometers are suitable.[14,29] Forced vital capacity should be determined routinely and the flow-volume curve inspected carefully (Fig. 12–2). A decrease in expiratory flow rate indicative of obstructive lung disease may be detected on such curves; on the other hand, it might easily be overlooked. In patients with symptoms, signs, or laboratory tests (e.g., elevated hematocrit) suggesting respiratory failure, the vital capacity should be measured with the patient supine as well as seated.

Static pressures (MEP and MIP) are the most sensitive indicators of respiratory muscle weakness.[5,29] They are extremely helpful in evaluating the patient with muscle weakness and unexplained respiratory symptoms. *If static pressures are normal, respiratory symptoms are not the result of muscle weakness.*

Evaluation of pulmonary function also includes (1) chest roentgenogram to assess heart size, diaphragmatic position, and evidence of atelectasis; (2) electrocardiography to search for signs of cor pulmonale (abnormal P waves, right axis deviation, right ventricular hypertrophy); (3) hematocrit, to detect

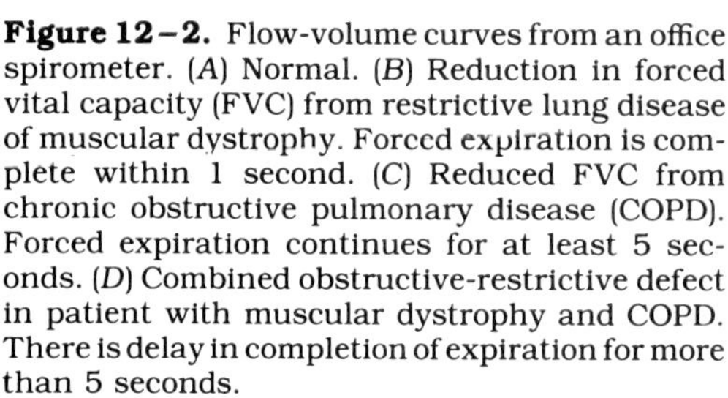

Figure 12–2. Flow-volume curves from an office spirometer. (A) Normal. (B) Reduction in forced vital capacity (FVC) from restrictive lung disease of muscular dystrophy. Forced expiration is complete within 1 second. (C) Reduced FVC from chronic obstructive pulmonary disease (COPD). Forced expiration continues for at least 5 seconds. (D) Combined obstructive-restrictive defect in patient with muscular dystrophy and COPD. There is delay in completion of expiration for more than 5 seconds.

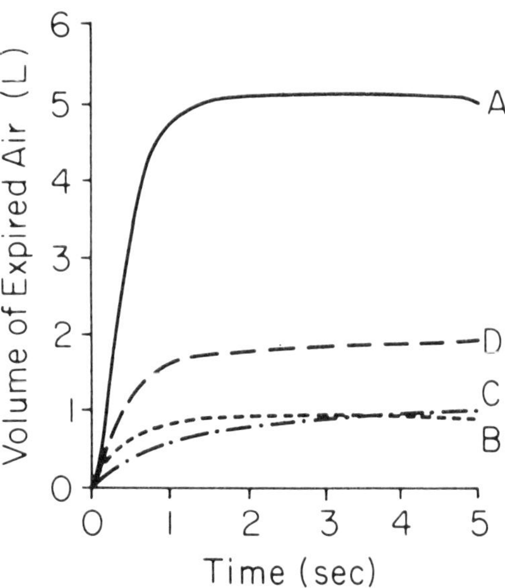

an elevation that may indicate chronic hypoxia; and (4) electrolyte determination, to look for an elevation in bicarbonate, which would indicate metabolic compensation for chronic hypercapnia.

In patients with respiratory symptoms or signs, or in patients with a reduced vital capacity who are not feeling well, additional studies may be indicated, including determination of arterial blood gas levels. Levels of arterial blood gases should also be determined when signs indicate cor pulmonale. *A single normal arterial oxygen value does not exclude intermittent hypoxia.* Noninvasive overnight monitoring of oxygenation with ear lobe or digit oximetry is often necessary.

The following history of a patient with limb-girdle dystrophy illustrates the development of heart failure initially assumed to be the result of severe myocardial disease, but which proved instead to be the result of cor pulmonale.

Case History

A 37-year-old woman with long-standing limb-girdle dystrophy was admitted to hospital because of progressive edema and orthopnea. She had developed proximal weakness before age 10 and had been confined to a wheelchair since age 25. By age 32, early-morning headaches, fatigue, and ankle edema occurred intermittently. For several months she had noted increasing ankle edema and abdominal pain. Nocturnal dyspnea and orthopnea first appeared 2 to 3 weeks before admission. On examination she was lethargic and cyanotic and was tachypneic and tachycardic. The neck veins were distended, with a jugular venous pressure of 200 mm Hg. The liver was enlarged, and hepatojugular reflux was elicited. Bilateral pleural effusions and late-inspiratory rales were present. The heart was enlarged, and a gallop rhythm, along with pulsus alternans, was noted. Marked pitting edema of the legs and thighs was present. Arterial blood gas results were PCO_2 36 mm Hg, PO_2 74 mm Hg, pH 7.31, and blood oxygen saturation 78%. A chest roentgenogram (Fig. 12–3A) showed cardiomegaly, pulmonary edema, and bilateral pleural effusions. An electrocardiogram (ECG) showed evidence of right atrial and right ventricular hypertrophy.

Treatment with diuretics and low-flow oxygen resulted in marked improvement in the patient's signs of heart failure. Increasing

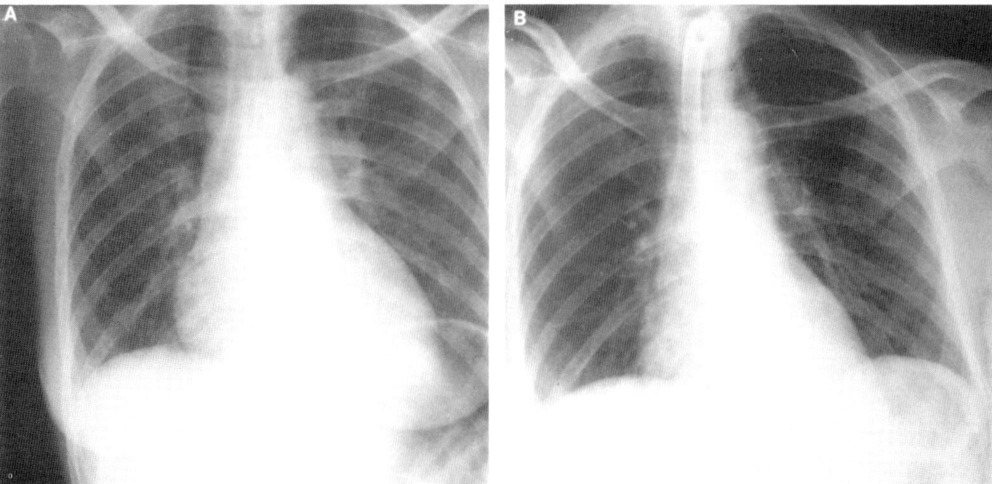

Figure 12–3. Chest roentgenograms from patient with limb-girdle dystrophy (illustrative case) presenting with symptoms of congestive heart failure resulting from cor pulmonale. (*A*) At presentation, cardiomegaly, pleural effusion, and pulmonary edema are present. (*B*) After intubation, correction of hypoxia and resolution of heart failure. Cardiomegaly is resolving.

hypercapnia, however, necessitated respiratory support. Negative pressure devices (pneumobelt and cuirass devices) helped for 6 months, but eventually the patient required tracheostomy and continuous positive pressure ventilation. She has been stable, without signs of heart failure, for the subsequent 6 years (Fig. 12–3B).

Comment: This patient had no previous evidence of cardiac enlargement and no loss of myocardial forces on ECG. Patients with limb-girdle dystrophy can develop a primary myocardiopathy. In this woman, however, signs of heart failure disappeared following the correction of hypoxia, and she has developed no evidence of heart failure in the ensuing 6 years of respiratory support. Cor pulmonale, rather than myocardial fiber disease, was the cause of heart failure.

Prevention of Respiratory Complications

In disorders where respiratory muscle involvement is frequent, forced vital capacity (FVC) should be determined at least annually. A chest roentgenogram and ECG should be obtained if respiratory compromise is detected. All patients should receive a one-time prophylactic immunization for pneumococcal infections,[34] and if the FVC is less than 30% of normal, annual immunization should be given for influenza viral infection.[35]

In patients at risk for respiratory failure because FVC is less than 30% of normal or because of an ineffective cough, respiratory muscle exercises with either incentive spirometry or blow bottles should be considered,[36] although such exercises may not be beneficial if they cause fatigue.[63] Upper respiratory infections should be treated by postural drainage and cupping (vigorous chest percussion with the *cupped* hands) to prevent atelectasis[49] and by administering antibiotics to prevent secondary infection. Such therapy has been shown to be effective against disorders such as chronic bronchitis.[65] Although intermittent positive pressure breathing (IPPB) improved lung compli-

ance in patients with chronic respiratory compromise from scoliosis,[61] it did not achieve this result in patients with muscular dystrophy.[42] Adequate hydration must also be maintained to assure easy mobilization of secretions. Keeping the urine specific gravity between 1.010 and 1.015 usually accomplishes this goal. The patient and family can check specific gravity daily and encourage adequate fluid intake accordingly.

Acute Respiratory Failure

ANTICIPATION OF RESPIRATORY FAILURE

When the FVC falls below 30% of normal in patients with late-stage Duchenne dystrophy and other myopathies where there is severe compromise of respiratory function, both patient and family should be informed of the risk of both acute and chronic ventilatory failure, and the management of acute and chronic respiratory failure should be discussed. The opinions and wishes of patient and family should be considered, and a "plan of action" (or inaction) charted. *If such discussions are not held, decisions concerning respiratory supportive measures are often made by strangers* such as emergency medical technicians or emergency department physicians.

PRECIPITATING FACTORS

The sudden appearance of respiratory symptoms in myopathy usually results from an acute, often-reversible illness and is seldom due to muscle weakness alone.[28,29,52] The events most commonly precipitating respiratory failure are shown on Table 12–3. The recognition of the causative event is often difficult because of preexisting abnormalities of chest examination, pulmonary function tests, chest roentgenogram, and ECG. Diagnosis is facilitated if these have been monitored regularly. *Atelectasis is the precipitating factor in most patients.* Chest roentgenograms in a pa-

Table 12–3 PRECIPITATING FACTORS LEADING TO ACUTE RESPIRATORY FAILURE IN MYOPATHY

FREQUENT
Atelectasis
Aspiration
Pneumonitis
Obstructive lung disease (over age 40)
Congestive heart failure

INFREQUENT
Pulmonary emboli
Pneumothorax
Bronchospasm (e.g., marijuana)

tient who has acute respiratory symptoms from atelectasis often show no interval change, particularly if they are obtained shortly after the onset of symptoms. Roentgenographic findings of atelectasis often appear during subsequent intravenous hydration.

MANAGEMENT

For patients who are obtunded and for dyspneic patients whose arterial blood determinations show hypoxia and hypercapnia, emergency endotracheal intubation is necessary. If hypoxia alone is present and the patient is alert, oxygen at low-flow rates (<1 L/min) may correct hypoxia without causing hypercapnia. Special equipment is often necessary for providing such low flow rates. If oxygen is administered, it is essential to obtain blood gas determinations frequently enough to exclude developing hypercapnia. *Patients with neuromuscular disease are often intermittently or constantly hypercapneic, and the administration of oxygen often depresses ventilatory drive and exacerbates hypoventilation.*[59,66]

If respiratory failure develops over a matter of hours, there is often time to consider tracheostomy directly rather than first performing oral or nasal endotracheal intubation. *Most patients whose baseline FVC is less than 30% of normal and who develop an acute illness requiring intubation will ultimately require tracheostomy.*

In cases where it has been determined that oxygenation is normal, the treatment of acute respiratory failure depends on the cause of respiratory difficulty. All patients require frequent suctioning, postural drainage and cupping, an alternating pressure mattress or waterbed, and noninvasive monitoring of blood gases (earlobe or digit oximetry and end-expiratory CO_2 monitoring). Pathogens are seldom isolated from bronchial secretions at the time of acute presentation, and antibiotics are indicated only when the character of the sputum and clinical or chest roentgenographic findings indicate infection.[28] Aminophyllin and other bronchodilators may be indicated for patients with obstructive lung disease. Because aminophyllin may improve diaphragmatic contractility[2] and ventilatory drive,[18] and because an obstructive component to respiratory failure can be difficult to recognize, a trial course of medication is indicated in most patients over the age of 40.

Chronic Ventilatory Failure

Most patients with acute ventilatory failure can be returned to independent ventilation with appropriate management of the acute, precipitating event[28,52]; many, however, cannot. In Duchenne dystrophy and many other neuromuscular diseases (see Table 12–1), patients eventually become dependent on a respirator.[27] Patients can easily be maintained on a respirator at home if at least two family members or other individuals are available to aid in their care.

THE DECISION TO
HAVE LONG-TERM
RESPIRATORY SUPPORT

As discussed previously, if at all possible, the patient and family should be made aware of the risk of respiratory failure and options for support in advance of an acute deterioration. A gradual deterioration in respiratory function with symptoms or signs of hypoxia should prompt consideration of the elective institution of respiratory support. Negative-pressure respirators, such as the iron lung (Emerson), cuirass,[17a,32] and plastic "rain coat" devices, help some patients particularly early in the course of respiratory failure.[17a] Recently, the use of nasal positive-pressure mechanical ventilation during sleep has supported respirations in patients who require only nighttime assistance.[55] Patients with Duchenne dystrophy who develop chronic respiratory failure can be supported in this way for more than 3 years.[55] Most patients, however, are more easily managed with tracheostomy and positive-pressure ventilation. Tracheostomy permits normal speech, provides an easy means of clearing tracheal secretions, and provides airway access in an emergency setting.

If tracheostomy is elected, it must be performed in hospital and usually requires 1 to 3 days of hospitalization in an intensive care unit. Subsequently, 1 to 3 weeks of training are necessary for the patient and family to acquire the skills necessary for outpatient management. Atelectasis often develops in the posttracheostomy period and may necessitate a longer hospital stay.

Initiation of chronic respiratory support poses major ethical dilemmas.[43] Full discussion is beyond the scope of this chapter. While many patients are happy on long-term support, others are not. The expense and personal toll borne by family members must also be considered. Patients who are deciding about respiratory support are helped by discussing the procedure with others who are receiving such support. Family members and friends who will be involved can discuss home management with care providers at the same time.

SETTING UP HOME VENTILATORY SUPPORT

The goal of outpatient respiratory support is to return the patient to an active lifestyle and permit the patient and family to maintain activities outside the home. The equipment necessary for such a program includes a lightweight, portable, AC/DC rechargeable ventilator; portable suction equipment; and a wheelchair that can accommodate the ventilator. Patients with swallowing difficulties also may require a gastrostomy.

CARDIAC MANAGEMENT

Symptomatic cardiac disease is uncommon in myopathies (Table 12–4); but ECG, histopathologic, and other lab-

Table 12–4 CARDIAC DISEASE IN THE MYOPATHIES

CONGESTIVE CARDIOMYOPATHY
Muscular dystrophy—	limb-girdle, myotonic, Becker, Emery-Dreifuss
Congenital—	nemaline
Metabolic—	acid maltase (infantile), carnitine deficiency
Inflammatory—	polymyositis

COR PULMONALE
Muscular dystrophy—	Duchenne, Becker, myotonic, limb-girdle
Congenital—	nemaline

ARRHYTHMIAS
Muscular dystrophy—	myotonic, limb-girdle, Emery-Dreifuss
Metabolic—	Kearn-Sayre syndrome, hyperkalemic and hypokalemic periodic paralysis
Inflammatory:	polymyositis

MITRAL VALVE PROLAPSE
Muscular dystrophy—	
myotonic, Duchenne	

Table 12–5 MYOPATHIES *PRESENTING* WITH CARDIAC DISEASE

CONGESTIVE HEART FAILURE
Muscular dystrophy—myotonic; limb-girdle; dystrophinopathy	
Metabolic—	acid maltase, carnitine and CPT deficiencies
Inflammatory—	polymyositis

ARRHYTHMIAS
Muscular dystrophy—myotonic dystrophy, limb-girdle, Emery-Dreifuss	
Metabolic—	Kearns-Sayre syndrome; hyperkalemic periodic paralysis
Inflammatory—	polymyositis

oratory studies demonstrate that myocardial involvement is much more frequent than clinical signs indicate. Patients with myopathy occasionally present with cardiac manifestations (Table 12–5).[25,47a,51] As shown by the Case History on p. 412, respiratory failure with resulting hypoxia often leads to signs of heart failure when intrinsic cardiomyopathy is not present.[9] In such patients, the resolution of signs of congestive heart failure following correction of hypoxia implicates disease of respiratory muscle rather than cardiac muscle.[16] Severe cardiomyopathy can, however, occur, as illustrated by the following case.

Case History

A 54-year-old man developed fatigue and dyspnea and was found to have severe leg edema, ascites, and pleural effusions. Cardiomegaly was noted, and severe congestive heart failure was documented by studies showing biventricular dysfunction. A myocardial gated-pool isotopic scan showed an ejection fraction of only 8% (normal > 60%). Treatment with digitalis and diuretics resulted in symptomatic improvement. Three years later, the patient developed proximal leg and arm weakness. He then became unable to sit up from the supine position and was unable to rise from a chair. Muscle biopsy showed features of inflammatory myopathy typical of polymyositis (see discussion, Chapter 5, pp. 168–169). EMG indicated myopathy with marked spontaneous activity, including fibrillations and small polyphasic potentials. The CK level was elevated 40-fold. The chest roentgenogram

continued to show cardiomegaly consistent with a cardiomyopathy. The ECG (Fig. 12–4) showed ventricular ectopy and a loss of R wave voltage. High doses of corticosteroids resulted in clinical improvement in strength, with a recovery of the ability to stand, to walk, and to sit up. The CK levels returned to normal, but cardiac failure did not improve.

The patient's subsequent course was complicated by four episodes of cerebral embolism, two occurring after anticoagulation therapy. Congestive heart failure persisted and resulted in death 7 years after the onset of illness. Autopsy confirmed the presence of dilated, congestive cardiomyopathy without evidence of coronary artery disease.

Comment: Congestive heart failure is an unusual presenting feature of inflammatory myopathy but is occasionally recognized in polymyositis.[25] Skeletal muscle weakness improved with corticosteroid therapy, but congestive heart failure progressed and ultimately proved fatal.

Recognition of Heart Failure

SYMPTOMS

Early features of heart failure include fatigue (which is surprisingly infrequent in patients with muscle weakness), insomnia, cough, abdominal pain, or ankle swelling. Orthopnea and dyspnea seldom occur as an early sign of heart failure in the myopathies.

ROUTINE SURVEILLANCE

Baseline ECG and chest roentgenogram are indicated in all patients with

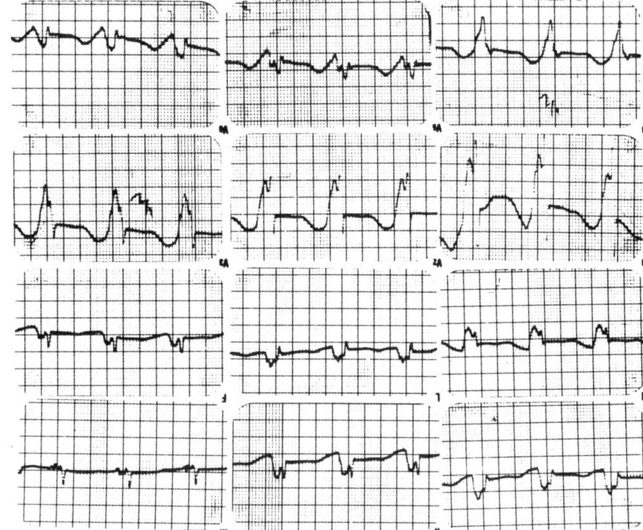

Figure 12–4. ECG of patient with polymyositis with severe congestive cardiomyopathy (illustrative case). A markedly abnormal interventricular conduction of the left bundle type results from myocardial fibrosis. Coronary artery disease was not present.

neuromuscular disease. Serial studies are indicated in those that involve the heart (see Table 12–4). Monitoring of weight, examination for ankle edema, and auscultation of the chest aid in early detection of heart failure.

SIGNS

Congestive heart failure from cardiomyopathy develops insidiously; early signs are pedal edema and pulmonary rales. Noncardiac, dependent edema is frequent in wheelchair-bound patients over age 30, but its presence should still prompt consideration of heart failure, especially in those below that age. Pulmonary rales are frequent in all patients with respiratory muscle weakness but are usually paninspiratory (atelectatic).[15] *Late-inspiratory rales suggest heart failure.*[15] More florid signs of congestive heart failure include tachycardia, right or left ventricular enlargement, gallop rhythm, pulsus alternans, hepatomegaly, and neck vein distention.

LABORATORY EVALUATION

The ECG often provides help with both the diagnosis and management of the neuromuscular disease patient. The ECG shows distinctive and diagnostically helpful changes in Duchenne dystrophy,[31] myotonic dystrophy,[26] infantile acid maltase deficiency,[13] and periodic paralysis[20] (see individual diseases). The presence of first-degree heart block should prompt consideration and careful follow-up for more severe cardiac conduction disorders (see Table 12–4). The occurrence of major myocardial disease can be detected, because replacement fibrosis of myocardium is characterized by a loss of QRS-complex voltage in anterior leads and poor P wave progression.[37] The appearance of Q waves in inferior leads may also accompany fibrosis (see Fig. 12–4).[37]

The chest roentgenogram is usually abnormal if clinically important heart disease is present. It may show a globular heart characteristic of a congestive cardiomyopathy (Fig. 12–5).[37] Echocardiography is also useful, as it can define cardiac chamber enlargement and impaired myocardial contractility.[37] ECG can also identify mitral valve prolapse.[56] Myocardial gated-pool isotope scanning is useful for determining ejection fraction and may be abnormal in patients without other evidence of car-

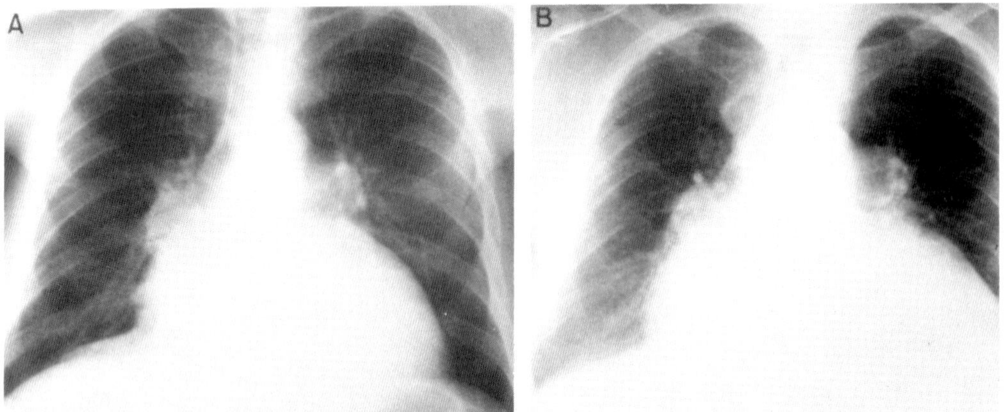

Figure 12–5. Chest roentgenograms from the same patient as Figure 12–4. (*A*) The presence of congestive cardiomyopathy is supported by the enlarged, globular heart. Progressive heart failure occurred (*B*), and pulmonary emboli originating from the heart resulted in sudden death shortly after this film was taken.

diomyopathy.[45] CK testing and determination of CK-MB (see pp. 37–39) is of no value in identifying patients with myocardial disease in the presence of an underlying myopathy.[40,60] Endomyocardial biopsy can identify histologic abnormalities, but because the abnormalities are nonspecific, biopsy is almost never indicated for clinical purposes. Biopsy is helpful only if inflammation is likely.[50]

Treatment

Cor pulmonale is the cause of most heart failure in the myopathies and resolves with correction of hypoxia. Primary myocardial disease is otherwise difficult to treat but fortunately uncommon. Patients in whom cardiomyopathy has resulted in congestive heart failure often develop pulmonary and systemic emboli. In such circumstances, anticoagulation therapy is indicated.[1] We also treat patients with heart failure from cardiomyopathy with measures used in other primary myocardial diseases, including diuretics, afterload reduction, and positive inotropic agents.[37,41] Digitalis is often ineffective and may increase the incidence of arrhythmias, particularly in patients who have cor pulmonale.[22]

The use of kaliuretic diuretics, which cause reduction in total body potassium, poses a special problem in patients with muscle wasting, in whom hypokalemia may exacerbate weakness[6,30]; it must be avoided. At the same time, potassium replacement must be given cautiously because tolerance to potassium decreases because of muscle wasting.[44]

PREVENTION OF EDEMA

Dependent foot, ankle, and leg edema occurs frequently in patients confined to a wheelchair. Such edema should prompt a search for clinical signs of (1) respiratory failure and cor pulmonale, (2) cardiomyopathy, or (3) a coincidental illness, particularly in patients under age 30. In most patients, however, only the lack of muscle-pumping action of the legs can be identified as the cause.

Edema interferes with function because of its mechanical effect and because it increases weight. It also predisposes to skin infection and ulceration. Edema can be diminished by elevating the legs periodically (e.g., with elevating leg rests attached to the wheelchair) and by reducing dietary sodium. Intermittent diuretic therapy often helps, although as usual, the use of potassium-sparing and potassium-depleting diuretics poses risks. Agents such as beta-adrenergic blocking agents, nonsteroidal anti-inflammatory agents, and calcium channel blockers may cause severe edema, precluding their use in many wheelchair-bound patients with myopathies.[47,44]

DIETARY MANAGEMENT: PREVENTION OF OBESITY

There is no evidence that any form of diet improves muscle strength or function in patients with neuromuscular disease. The goal of dietary counseling is to supply nutrition adequate to maintain muscle mass, while preventing obesity. As for any patient with reduced activity, a high-fiber, high-residue diet and adequate hydration are essential to prevent constipation.

Adult patients with progressive myopathies such as the muscular dystrophies have a steadily declining muscle mass.[30] In growing children with myopathy, muscle mass increases at a subnormal rate.[30] The maintenance of the same "normal" weight in an adult patient or a "normal" increase in weight in a growing child with muscle disease thus usually implies an *increase in the proportion of body fat.*[54] Obesity has the obvious disadvantage of decreasing the patient's mobility and ability to exercise; it may also depress ventilatory drive[17] and increase oxygen requirements during exercise.

Caloric Requirements

The basal metabolic rate of patients with myopathies is reduced by about 10% when related to body surface area but increased when related to muscle mass.[38] Estimation of caloric requirements must be reduced because of the inactivity of patients. Patients who are

of normal weight by standard charts may well be obese in terms of total body adipose tissue. Education of the patient and family members to these facts is an essential step in weight control.

The reduced caloric expenditure and high total body adipose tissue (with the high caloric value of fat) of patients with muscle disease means that with dietary treatment, weight loss proceeds very slowly. Nonetheless, successful reduction of weight is often possible. Major weight loss appears to be well tolerated, and at times produces improved muscle function, without loss of muscle mass as assessed by laboratory measurements.[12,24]

SWALLOWING ABNORMALITIES

Abnormalities of swallowing function (deglutition) occur in certain myopathies (Table 12–6) and may be the presenting feature of several disorders. Impaired function of pharyngeal muscles may result in pooling of secretions in the hypopharynx (see Fig. 12–7) and aspiration (see Fig. 12–8). Atelectasis and infection may result but are remarkably infrequent unless weakness of respiratory and glottic muscles impairs cough.

Table 12–6 MYOPATHIES WITH ABNORMALITIES OF DEGLUTITION

MUSCULAR DYSTROPHY
Myotonic*
Oculopharyngeal*
Duchenne (rare)

INFLAMMATORY
Dermatomyositis
Polymyositis
Inclusion body myositis

METABOLIC
Mitochondrial

*Often presenting with dysphagia.

Symptoms and Recognition

Patients with abnormalities of deglutition usually recognize the problem and localize the difficulty themselves. Patients with diseases of the muscles initiating deglutition, such as oculopharyngeal muscular dystrophy, dermatomyositis, and other conditions associated with cricopharyngeal achalasia (see below), indicate that the submental and glottic regions are the site of obstruction. These disorders affect the upper one third of the esophagus, which is striated muscle. Patients localize the problem by indicating a "sticking" of food in the suprasternal region. If the problem is localized to the lower portions of the esophagus and affects smooth muscle (as in scleroderma), the patient will point to the substernal region as the site of obstruction or pain.

Occasionally patients with swallowing abnormalities fail to recognize that their symptoms are caused by weakness of the muscles of deglutition. Occult difficulty with swallowing is frequently seen in oculopharyngeal muscular dystrophy. Patients may present with an unexplained cough or shortness of breath that occurs at or after mealtimes. Unexplained weight loss and the need to mince food into smaller and smaller pieces are occasionally the only signs that patients are having trouble swallowing.

Cricopharyngeal Achalasia

The failure of the cricopharyngeal muscle to contract and permit food to leave the hypopharynx (see Fig. 12–7) is called cricopharyngeal achalasia. The condition is common in oculopharyngeal muscular dystrophy[67] and is seen in other disorders.[39] Cricopharyngeal achalasia is so frequent in oculopharyngeal muscular dystrophy that patients should have studies of swallowing function even if they are asymptomatic. Symptoms can be reversed by cricopharyngeal myotomy.[53]

Management

Severe weight loss or recurrent aspiration may necessitate an invasive procedure to provide adequate nutrition. Long-term enteral feeding is possible with either pharyngostomy or operative or percutaneous gastrostomy. Either form of gastrostomy can be performed without general anesthesia and provide well-tolerated feeding access.

The following case history illustrates the most frequent cause of cricopharyngeal achalasia and emphasizes its successful management.

Case History

A 66-year-old woman developed progressive difficulty swallowing and lost 30 pounds in the 6 months prior to admission. She had a 10-year history of progressive ptosis and ophthalmoparesis and had required surgical correction of bilateral eyelid ptosis 4 years previously. She was of French-Canadian descent and her sister had similar clinical findings. She had never developed chest infections and had no respiratory symptoms. She had slight proximal weakness.

Muscle biopsy had showed changes characteristic of oculopharyngeal dystrophy (Fig. 12–6). Radiographic study of the pa-

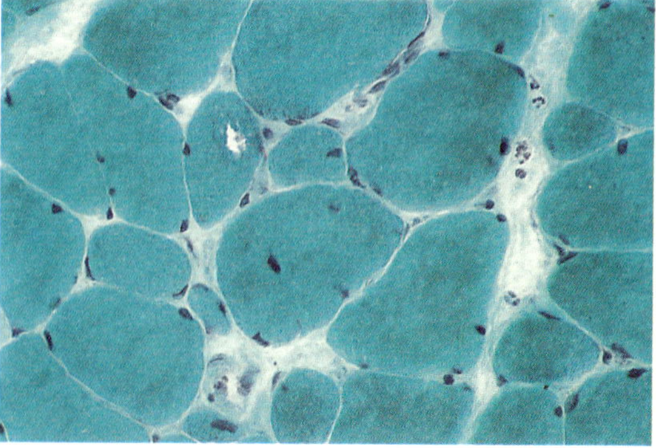

Figure 12–6. Muscle biopsy shows variability in fiber size, internal nuclei, and increased connective tissue surrounding individual muscle fibers. These are nonspecific features found in most muscular dystrophies. In the upper left, there is a fiber with a vacuole characteristic of oculopharyngeal muscular dystrophy (see Chapter 4 for further discussion).

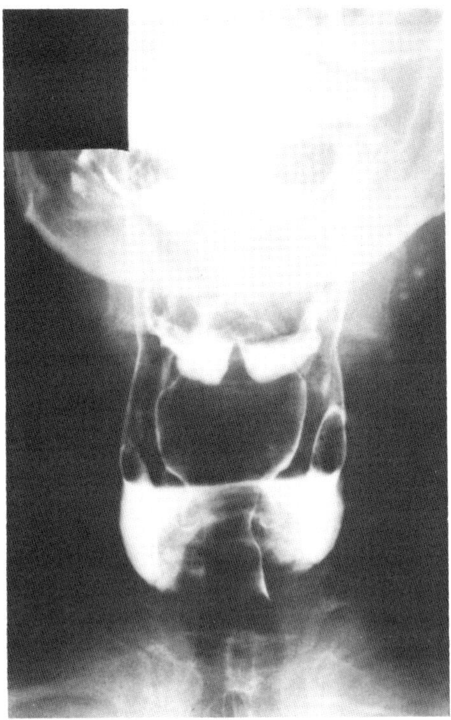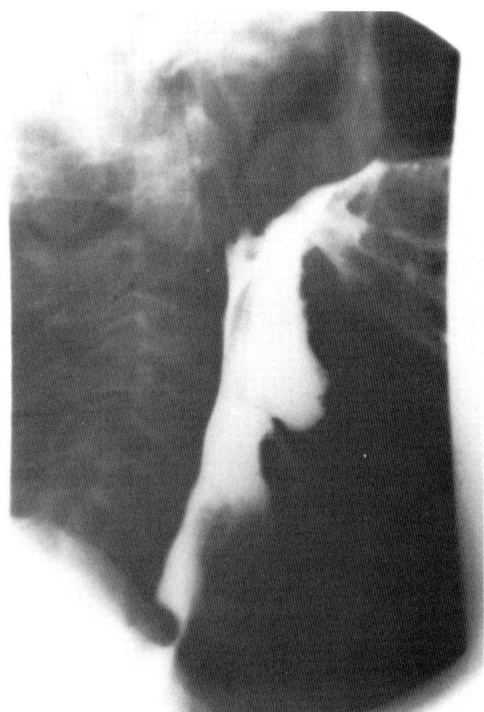

Figure 12–7. Barium roentgenogram of pharynx showing impaired muscle contraction with dilated piriform sinuses and cricopharyngeal achalasia. (*Left*) Posteroanterior view of hypopharyngeal pooling of barium. (*Right*) Lateral view showing the pooling of barium as well as the constriction of the hypopharynx by the cricopharyngeus muscle. Patient with oculopharyngeal dystrophy (illustrative case).

tient's swallowing mechanism showed both marked pooling of barium in the hypopharynx and cricopharyngeal achalasia (Fig. 12–7). There was aspiration of barium with visualization of the bronchial tree (Fig. 12–8). Barium was rapidly cleared from the lung with coughing. She was observed to cough repeatedly during mealtimes, although she had denied cough and other respiratory symptoms. (Her sister had similarly denied cough despite equally severe aspiration.) Following cricopharyngeal myotomy, the patient's swallowing symptoms were completely alleviated. Although she continues to aspirate repeatedly, in the ensuing 11 years she has never developed respiratory infection. Aside from ophthalmoplegia, she remains virtually free of neuromuscular symptoms at age 77.

Comment: This patient's physical findings and swallowing difficulties indicating cricopharyngeal achalasia are characteris-

tic of oculopharyngeal dystrophy. Many patients are of French-Canadian descent. If swallowing difficulty is not alleviated, fatal inanition usually develops.

OTHER GASTROINTESTINAL COMPLICATIONS

Smooth muscle function is abnormal in a relatively small proportion of myopathies: myotonic dystrophy, Duchenne dystrophy, and occasionally mitochondrial myopathy and dermatomyositis.[10] In myotonic dystrophy, gall bladder dysfunction and a variety of esophageal and intestinal disorders are frequent.[10,64,68]

In the MNGIE syndrome (mitochondrial myopathy, peripheral neuropathy, gastrointestinal disease, and encepha-

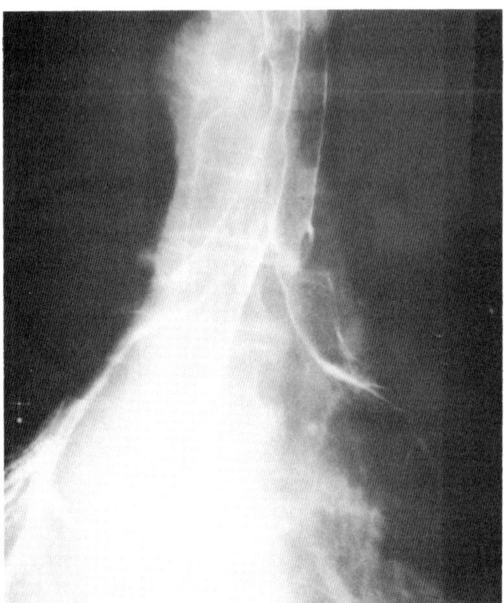

Figure 12–8. Chest roentgenogram during barium swallow study from same patient as Figure 12–7. Aspiration of barium outlines the bronchial tree.

lopathy), intestinal involvement results in severe obstipation and episodes of intestinal pseudo-obstruction caused by severe visceral neuropathy.[11] The syndrome occurs with cytochrome oxidase deficiency,[7] but the specificity of this enzyme abnormality requires confirmation (see pp. 308–311, Chapter 8).

Dermatomyositis is often characterized by severe dysphagia, reflecting involvement of the upper third of the esophagus as well as the pharyngeal muscles.[33] Symptoms include pain on swallowing, weight loss, and aspiration of food. Patients with childhood dermatomyositis can have intestinal perforation resulting from the angiopathy that characterizes the illness.[3] Polymyositis also causes pharyngeal muscular involvement with dysphagia, but other gastrointestinal complications do not develop.

Patients with Duchenne dystrophy have impaired gastric motility resulting from dystrophin deficiency of smooth muscle and may present with severe gastric dilatation and intestinal pseudo-

obstruction.[4] Electrolyte disturbances and aspiration may complicate gastric dilatation. Treatment consists of decompression of the dilated stomach with a nasal gastric tube and the administration of appropriate fluids by a parenteral route.[4] In anecdotal experience, low dose metoclopramide (10–20 mg/d) prevents this complication.

SUMMARY

The medical complications of the myopathies are usually treatable and often preventable. Respiratory muscle weakness leading to ventilatory failure can be the initial sign of some myopathies and is the terminal event in many. Recognition of the physical and laboratory findings of respiratory failure can lead to prevention and treatment of complications, avoidance of which will greatly enhance the quality of living, even in patients with severe diseases. Cardiac muscle involvement can result in congestive heart failure and arrhythmias; cardiac conduction system disease can lead to heart block. Differentiating primary cardiomyopathy from cor pulmonale secondary to hypoxia plays an important role in the management of myopathies. Disordered swallowing can result from disease of the muscles of deglutition and can lead to impaired nutrition and to aspiration of food. Surgical correction of cricopharyngeal achalasia can avert fatal inanition. Smooth-muscle involvement is often underemphasized in the myopathies. Abnormalities of smooth muscle can result in abnormal gastric and intestinal function and be life-threatening in diseases such as Duchenne dystrophy.

In the care of the patient with myopathy, careful attention to respiratory status, cardiac function, and nutrition often detects the development of complications that may be alleviated, and equally importantly, recognizes unrelated or coincidental illness requiring treatment independent of the underlying disease.

REFERENCES

1. Abelmann WH: Treatment of congestive cardiomyopathy. Postgrad Med J 54:477, 1978.
2. Aubier M, DeTroyer A, Sampson M, Macklem PT, and Roussos C: Aminophylline improves diaphragmatic contractility. N Engl J Med 305:249, 1981.
3. Banker BQ and Victor M: Dermatomyositis (systemic angiopathy) of childhood. Medicine 45:261, 1966.
4. Barohn RJ, Levine EJ, Olson JO, and Mendell JR: Gastric hypomotility in Duchenne's muscular dystrophy. N Engl J Med 319:15, 1988.
5. Black LF and Hyatt RE: Maximal static respiratory pressures in generalized neuromuscular disease. Amer Rev Respir Dis 103:641, 1971.
6. Blahd WH, Lederer M, and Cassen B: The significance of decreased body potassium concentrations in patients with muscular dystrophy and nondystrophic relatives. N Engl J Med 276:1349, 1967.
7. Blake D, Lombes A, Minetti C, et al: MNGIE syndrome: Report of 2 new patients. Neurology 40(Suppl 1):294, 1990.
7a. Bolton CF: AAEM Minimonograph #40: Clinical neurophysiology of the respiratory system. Muscle Nerve 16:809, 1993.
8. Braun NMT, Arora NS, and Rochester DF: Force-length relationship of the normal human diaphragm. J Appl Physiol 53:405, 1982.
9. Buchsbaum HW, Martin WA, Turino GM, and Rowland LP: Chronic alveolar hypoventilation due to muscular dystrophy. Neurology 18:319, 1968.
10. Camilleri M: Subject Review: Disorders of gastrointestinal motility in neurologic diseases. Mayo Clin Proc 65:825, 1990.
11. Cervera R, Bruix J, Bayes A, et al: Chronic intestinal pseudoobstruction and ophthalmoplegia in a patient with mitochondrial myopathy. Gut 29:544, 1988.
12. Edwards RHT, Round JM, Jackson MJ, Griffith RD, and Lilburn MF: Weight reduction in boys with muscular dystrophy. Dev Med Child Neurol 26:384, 1984.
13. Ehlers KH, Hagstrom JW, Lukas DS, Redo SF, and Engle MA: Glycogenstorage disease of the myocardium with obstruction to left ventricular outflow. Circulation 25:96, 1962.
14. Florence JM, Brooke MH, and Carroll JE: Evaluation of the child with muscular weakness. Orthop Clin North Am 9:409, 1978.
15. Forgacs P: The functional basis of pulmonary sounds. Chest 73:399, 1978.
16. Frank MJ, Wesse AB, Moschos CB, and Levinson GE: Left ventricular function, metabolism, and blood flow in chronic cor pulmonale. Circulation 47:798, 1973.
17. Fried PI, McClean PA, Phillipson EA, et al: Effect of ketosis on respiratory sensitivity to carbon dioxide in obesity. N Engl J Med 294:1081, 1976.
17a. Fukunaga H, Okubo R, Moritoyo T, Kawashima N, Osame M: Long-term follow-up of patients with Duchenne muscular dystrophy receiving ventilatory support. Muscle Nerve 16:554, 1993.
18. Garay SM, Turino GM, and Goldring RM: Sustained reversal of chronic hypercapnia in patients with alveolar hypoventilation syndrome: Long-term maintenance with noninvasive nocturnal mechanical ventilation. Am J Med 70:269, 1981.
19. Goldman MD, Grassino A, Mead J, and Sears TA: Mechanics of the human diaphragm during voluntary contraction: Dynamics. J Appl Physiol 44:840, 1978.
20. Gould RJ, Steeg CN, Penn AS, and De Vivo DC: Potentially fatal cardiac dysrhythmias and periodic paralysis. Transactions of the American Neurological Association 106:157, 1981.
21. Grassino A, Goldman MD, Mead J, and Sears TA: Mechanics of the human diaphragm during voluntary contraction: Statics. J Appl Physiol 44:829, 1978.
22. Green LH and Smith TW: The use of digitalis in patients with pulmonary disease. Ann Intern Med 87:459, 1977.

23. Green M and Moxham J: The respiratory muscles. Clin Sci 68:1, 1985.

24. Griffiths RD and Edwards RHT: A new chart for weight control in Duchenne muscular dystrophy. Arch Dis Child 63:1256, 1988.

25. Griggs RC: Hypertrophy and cardiomyopathy in the neuromuscular diseases. Circ Res (Suppl 2) 34–35:II-145, 1974.

26. Griggs RC, Davis RJ, Anderson DC, and Dove JT: Cardiac conduction in myotonic dystrophy. Am J Med 59:37, 1975.

27. Griggs RC and Donohoe KM: The recognition and management of respiratory insufficiency in neuromuscular disease. J Chron Dis 35:497, 1982.

28. Griggs RC and Donohoe KM: Emergency management of neuromuscular disease. In Henning RJ and Jackson DL (eds): Handbook of Critical Care Neurology and Neurosurgery. Praeger, New York, 1985, pp 201–225.

29. Griggs RC, Donohoe KM, Utell MJ, Goldblatt D, and Moxley RT III: Evaluation of pulmonary function in neuromuscular disease. Arch Neurol 38:9, 1981.

30. Griggs RC, Forbes G, Moxley RT, and Herr BE: The assessment of muscle mass in progressive neuromuscular disease. Neurology 33:158, 1983.

31. Griggs RC, Reeves W, and Moxley RT III: The heart in Duchenne dystrophy. In Rowland LP (ed): Excerpta Medica International Congress Series No. 404: Pathogenesis of Human Muscular Dystrophies. Excerpta Medica, Amsterdam, 1976, p 661.

32. Holtackers TR, Loosbrock LM, and Gracey DR: The use of the chest cuirass in respiratory failure of neurologic origin. Respiratory Care 27:271, 1982.

33. Horowitz M, McNeil JD, Maddern GJ, Collins PJ, and Shearman DJC: Abnormalities of gastric and esophageal emptying in polymyositis and dermatomyositis. Gastroenterology 90:434, 1986.

34. Immunization Practices Advisory Committee, Centers for Disease Control, Atlanta, Georgia: Pneumococcal polysaccharide vaccine. Ann Intern Med 96:203, 1982.

35. Immunization Practices Advisory Committee, Centers for Disease Control, Atlanta, Georgia: Prevention and control of influenza. Ann Intern Med 103:560, 1985.

36. Iverson LIG, Ecker RR, Fox HE, and May IA: A comparative study of IPPB, the incentive spirometer, and blow bottles: The prevention of atelectasis following cardiac surgery. Ann Thorac Surg 25:197, 1978.

37. Johnson RA and Palacios I: Dilated cardiomyopathies of the adult. N Engl J Med 307:1051–1058; 1119–1126, 1982.

38. Jozefowicz RF, Welle SL, Nair KS, Kingston WJ, and Griggs RC: Basal metabolic rate in myotonic dystrophy: Evidence against hypometabolism. Neurology 37:1021, 1987.

39. Kagen LJ, Hochman RB, and Strong EW: Cricopharyngeal obstruction in inflammatory myopathy (polymyositis/dermatomyositis): Report of three cases and review of the literature. Arthritis Rheum 28:630, 1985.

40. Larca LJ, Coppola JT, and Honig S: Creatine kinase MB isoenzyme in dermatomyositis: A noncardiac source. Ann Intern Med 94:341, 1981.

41. Makabali C, Weil MH, and Henning RJ: Dobutamine and other sympathomimetic drugs for the treatment of low cardiac output failure. Seminars in Anesthesia 1:63, 1982.

42. McCool FD, Mayewski RJ, Shayne DS, Hyde RW, Griggs RC, and Gibson CJ: Short term effects of IPPB on patients with neuromuscular restrictive lung disease. Respiratory Disease 123:188, 1981.

43. Mendell JR and Vaughn AJ: Duchenne muscular dystrophy: Ethical and emotional considerations in long-term management. Semin Neurol 4:98, 1984.

44. Moore-Ede MC, Meguid MM, Fitzpatrick GF, Boyden CM, and Ball MR: Circadian variation in response to potassium infusion. Clin Pharmacol Ther 23:218, 1978.

45. Moorman JR, Coleman RE, Packer DL, et al: Cardiac involvement in myotonic muscular dystrophy. Medicine 64:371, 1985.

46. Mortola JP and Sant'Ambrogio G: Motion of the rib cage and abdomen in tetraplegic patients. Clinical Science and Molecular Medicine 54:25, 1978.

47. Moxley RT: Absence of major side effects of nifedipine following treatment in Duchenne dystrophy [letter]. Pediatrics 75: 1168, 1985.

47a. Muntoni F, Cau M, Ganau A, et al: Brief report: Deletion of the dystrophin muscle-promoter region associated with x-linked dilated cardiomyopathy. N Engl J Med 329:921, 1993.

48. Newsom-Davis J, Goldman M, Loh L, and Casson M: Diaphragm function and alveolar hypoventilation. Q J Med 45:87, 1976.

49. Newton DAG and Stephenson A: Effect of physiotherapy on pulmonary function. A laboratory study. Lancet 2:228, 1978.

50. Nippoldt TB, Edwards WD, Holmes DR Jr, Reeder GS, Hartzler GO, and Smith HC: Right ventricular endomyocardial biopsy: Clinicopathologic correlates in 100 consecutive patients. Mayo Clin Proc 57:407, 1982.

51. Norris FH Jr, Moss AJ, and Yu PN: On the possibility that a type of human muscular dystrophy commences in myocardium. Ann NY Acad Sci 138: 342, 1966.

52. O'Donohue WJ Jr, Baker JP, Bell GM, Muren O, Parker CL, and Patterson JL Jr: Respiratory failure in neuromuscular disease: Management in a respiratory intensive care unit. JAMA 235: 733, 1976.

53. Palmer ED: Disorders of the cricopharyngeus muscle: A review. Gastroenterology 71:510, 1976.

54. Patrick J: Assessment of body potassium stores. Kidney Int 11:476, 1977.

55. Peters SG and Viggiano RW: Subspecialty clinics: Critical care medicine. Home mechanical ventilation. Mayo Clin Proc 63:1208, 1988.

56. Reeves WC, Griggs R, Nanda NC, Thomson K, and Gramiak R: Echocardiographic evaluation of cardiac abnormalities in Duchenne's dystrophy and myotonic muscular dystrophy. Arch Neurol 37:273, 1980.

57. Roussos C and Macklem PT: The respiratory muscles. N Engl J Med 307:786, 1982.

58. Saunders NA, Rigg JRA, Pengelly LD, and Campbell EJM: Effect of curare on maximum static PV relationships of the respiratory system. J Appl Physiol 44:589, 1978.

59. Sieker HO and Hickam JB: Carbon dioxide intoxication: The clinical syndrome, its etiology and management with particular reference to the use of mechanical respirators. Medicine 35:389, 1956.

60. Silverman LM, Mendell JR, Sahenk Z, and Fontana MB: Significance of creatine phosphokinase isoenzymes in Duchenne dystrophy. Neurology 26:561, 1976.

61. Sinha R and Bergofsky EH: Prolonged alteration of lung mechanics in kyphoscoliosis by positive pressure hyperinflation. Am Rev Respir Dis 106:47–57, 1972.

62. Sivak ED and Streib EW: Management of hypoventilation in motor neuron disease presenting with respiratory insufficiency. Ann Neurol 7:188, 1980.

63. Smith PEM, Coakley JH, and Edwards RHT: Respiratory muscle training in Duchenne muscular dystrophy. Muscle Nerve 11:784, 1988.

64. Swick HM, Werlin SL, Dodds WJ, and Hogan WJ: Pharyngoesophageal motor function in patients with myotonic dystrophy. Ann Neurol 10:454, 1981.

65. Tager I and Speizer FE: Role of infection in chronic bronchitis. N Engl J Med 292:563, 1975.

66. Weinberger SE, Schwartzstein RM, and Weiss JW: Hypercapnia. N Engl J Med 321:1223, 1989.

67. Weitzner S: Changes in the pharyngeal and esophageal musculature in oculopharyngeal muscular dystrophy. American Journal of Digestive Diseases 14:805, 1969.

68. Yoshida MM, Krishnamurthy S, Wattchow DA, Furness JB, and Schuffler MD: Megacolon in myotonic dystrophy caused by a degenerative neuropathy of the myenteric plexus. Gastroenterology 95:820, 1988.

INDEX

An "f" following a page number indicates a figure; a "t" indicates a table.